Basic Geriatric Nursing

Contents in Brief

UNIT I Overview of Aging, 1

1 Trends and Issues, 1
2 Theories of Aging, 29
3 Physiologic Changes, 33

UNIT II Basic Skills for Gerontologic Nursing, 78

4 Health Promotion, Health Maintenance, and
   Home Health Considerations, 78
5 Communicating With Older Adults, 95
6 Maintaining Fluid Balance and Meeting
   Nutritional Needs, 111
7 Medications and Older Adults, 140
8 Health Assessment for Older Adults, 158
9 Meeting Safety Needs of Older Adults, 174

UNIT III Psychosocial Care of the Elderly, 191

10 Cognition and Perception, 191
11 Self-Perception and Self-Concept, 214
12 Roles and Relationships, 230

13 Coping and Stress, 241
14 Values and Beliefs, 252
15 End-of-Life Care, 261
16 Sexuality and Aging, 278

UNIT IV Physical Care of the Elderly, 286

17 Care of Aging Skin and Mucous Membranes, 286
18 Elimination, 308
19 Activity and Exercise, 325
20 Sleep and Rest, 353

APPENDIXES

A Laboratory Values for Older Adults, 363
B The Geriatric Depression Scale (GDS), 367
C Daily Nutritional Goals for Older Adults, 368
D Resources for Older Adults, 369

Glossary, 371
Index, 377

Basic Geriatric Nursing

Patricia Williams, RN, MSN, CCRN
Nursing Professor
De Anza College
Cupertino, California

Formerly, Nursing Educator
University of California Medical Center
San Francisco, California

Alumnus, iSAGE Mini Fellowship Program
Successful Aging Project
Stanford University Medical School
Stanford, California

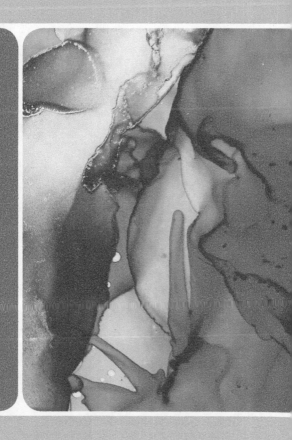

ELSEVIER

Elsevier
3251 Riverport Lane
St. Louis, Missouri 63043

Notice

Practitioners and researchers must always rely on their own experience and knowledge in evaluating and using any information, methods, compounds, or experiments described herein. Because of rapid advances in the medical sciences, in particular, independent verification of diagnoses and drug dosages should be made. To the fullest extent of the law, no responsibility is assumed by Elsevier, authors, editors, or contributors for any injury and/or damage to persons or property as a matter of products liability, negligence or otherwise, or from any use or operation of any methods, products, instructions, or ideas contained in the material herein.

Senior Content Strategist: Brandi Graham
Content Development Specialist: Brooke Kannady
Publishing Services Manager: Shereen Jameel
Project Manager: Vishnu T. Jiji
Design Direction: Renee Duenow

Printed in the United States of America

Last digit is the print number: 9 8 7 6 5 4 3 2 1

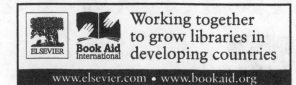

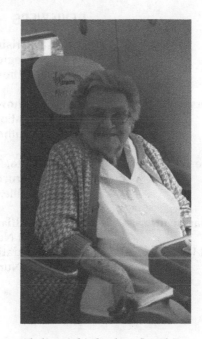

I dedicate this book to Cynthia—
You were deeply loved, are terribly missed,
and your legacy lives on through your grandchildren.

Patricia

Contributors and Reviewers

CONTRIBUTORS

Karen Anderson, MSN, RN
Nursing Faculty and Simulationist,
   San Diego State University,
   San Diego, California
Online Nursing Faculty, West Coast University,
   Irvine, California

Sheri Saretsky, RN, MSN/Ed, DSD
Consultant, Nursing Education, Healthcare Training
   Associates, San Diego, California

Susan M. Schmitz, RN, BSN, PHN
Part-Time Faculty, Health Technology Department,
   De Anza College, Cupertino, California
Flu Nurse and Research Assistant, Flu and Wellness,
   AC Wellness, Cupertino, California

REVIEWERS

Beth Kasparisin, RN, MSN
Associate Degree Director of Nursing, Texas Southmost
   College, Brownsville, Texas

Molly M. Showalter, MSN Ed., RN
Interim Vocational Nursing Program Director,
   Texas Southmost College, Brownsville, Texas

Vaneida Soto, MSN, RN
Faculty Instructor, Texas Southmost College,
   Brownsville, Texas

Brittany Williams, DNP, RN, CMSRN
Doctorate of Nursing Practice, Administration MSN,
   Administration BSN, CMSBN-Certified Medical
   Surgical Nurse, Central Texas College, Killeen, Texas

LPN/LVN Advisory Board

To the Instructor

The changing demographic of today's world presents an immense challenge to health care providers and society as a whole. Nurses must be well prepared to recognize and respond appropriately to the needs of our aging population. The goal of this text is to give the beginning nurse a balanced perspective on the realities of aging and to broaden the beginning nurse's viewpoint regarding aging people so that their needs can be met in a compassionate, caring, and professional manner.

ABOUT THE TEXT

The eighth edition of *Basic Geriatric Nursing* presents the theories and concepts of aging, the physiological and psychosocial changes and problems associated with the process, and the appropriate nursing interventions. The *LPN Threads* design provides consistency among Elsevier's LPN/LVN textbooks. Key features include extensive coverage of cultural issues, clinical situations, delegation, home health care, health promotion, patient teaching, and complementary health approaches. Numerous Critical Thinking exercises provide practice in synthesizing information and applying it to nursing care of the older adult.

LPN THREADS

The eighth edition of *Basic Geriatric Nursing* shares some features and design elements with other Elsevier LPN/LVN textbooks. The purpose of these *LPN Threads* is to make it easier for students and instructors to use the variety of books required by the relatively brief and demanding LPN/LVN curriculum. The following features are included in the *LPN Threads*:

- The **full-color design, cover, photos**, and **illustrations** are visually appealing and pedagogically useful.
- **Objectives** (numbered) begin each chapter and provide a framework for content and are especially important in providing the structure for the TEACH Lesson Plans for the textbook.
- **Key Terms** with phonetic pronunciations and page number references are listed at the beginning of each chapter. They appear in color in the chapter and are defined briefly, with full definitions in the **Glossary**. The goal is to help the student with limited proficiency in English to develop a greater command of the pronunciation of scientific and nonscientific English terminology.

- **Key Points** at the end of each chapter correlate to the objectives and serve as a useful chapter review.
- In addition to consistent content, design, and support resources, these textbooks benefit from the advice and input of the Elsevier **LPN/LVN Advisory Board** (see p. vii).

ORGANIZATION

Unit I presents an overview of aging, examining the trends and issues affecting the older adult. These include demographic factors and economic, social, cultural, and family influences. The unit explores various theories and myths associated with aging and reviews the physiologic changes that occur with aging.

Unit II includes a wide range of information on modifying basic nursing skills for the aging population. There is a strong focus on (1) health promotion and health maintenance for older adults; (2) age-appropriate verbal and nonverbal communication; (3) relevant nutritional and fluid needs, alterations in pharmacodynamics, and concerns related to medication administration for older adults; (4) health assessment of older adults; and (5) meeting safety needs of the older adults.

Unit III addresses the psychosocial needs of the older adult through the nursing process and clinical judgment model. Psychosocial care precedes physiologic care, reflecting the order in which the content is most often taught. Areas of content include (1) cognition problems, (2) self-perception and self-concept, (3) changing roles and relationships, (4) coping and stress management, (5) values and beliefs, and (6) sexuality.

Unit IV addresses the physical needs of the older adult through the nursing process and clinical judgment model. Areas of content include (1) safety, (2) hygiene and skin care, (3) elimination, (4) activity and exercise, and (5) sleep and rest. Units III and IV both offer assessment (data collection), data analysis/problem identification, planning, and implementation of nursing interventions across care settings.

SPECIAL FEATURES

- **Nursing process/Clinical Judgment Model** sections that provide a strong framework for discussing care of older adults in the context of specific disorders
- **Nursing interventions** grouped by health care setting (e.g., acute care, extended care, home care)
- **Special boxes** for critical thinking, clinical situations, health promotion, safety, patient education,

- complementary health approaches, delegation, nurse alerts, and more
- **QSEN** highlighting information related to the six prelicensure competency categories
- Increased **cultural content** on the impact of aging in various cultures
- Focus on **changing demographics** including baby boomers and the impact of their aging on health care
- Additional information on **home health** for both patients and caregivers
- **Review Questions for the Next Generation NCLEX® Examination** at the end of every chapter
- Updated **Laboratory Values for Older Adults** (Appendix A)
- The **Geriatric Depression Scale** (Appendix B)
- **Daily Nutritional Goals for Older Adults** (Appendix C)
- Revised list of **Resources for Older Adults**, including relevant websites (Appendix D)
- **References** grouped by chapter and listed at the end of the book for easy access

TEACHING AND LEARNING PACKAGE

FOR INSTRUCTORS

The comprehensive and free *Evolve Resources with TEACH Instructor Resource* include the following:

- **Test Bank** with approximately 400 multiple-choice and alternate-format questions with topic, step of the nursing process, objective, cognitive level, NCLEX® category of client needs, correct answer, rationale, and textbook page reference
- **6 All New Next Generation NCLEX®Exam–style Case Studies and Review Questions** provide thorough preparation and practice for the Next Generation NCLEX Examination
- **TEACH Instructor Resource** with Lesson Plans, Lecture Outlines, and PowerPoint slides—with Audience Response System questions embedded—that correlate each text and ancillary component

- **Image Collection** that contains all the illustrations and photographs in the textbook

FOR STUDENTS

The *Evolve Student Resources* include the following assets:

- **Answers and Rationales** for Review Questions for the Next Generation NCLEX® Examination
- **Review Questions for the NCLEX® Exam**
- **Study Guide** for additional practice.
- **Audio Glossary** with pronunciations in English and Spanish
- **Calculators** for determining body mass index (BMI), body surface area, fluid deficit, Glasgow Coma Scale score, intravenously administered dosages, and conversion of units
- **Fluids and Electrolytes Tutorial**

ACKNOWLEDGMENTS

I would like to thank Nancy O'Brien, Brandi Graham, Brooke Kannady, Shereen Jameel, Renee Duenow and Vishnu T. Jiji as well as the other staff at Elsevier for their professional expertise, tenacity, insights, infinite patience, and steady encouragement throughout the development of this edition. I would also like to extend thanks to reviewers of this book as well as writers of the ancillary materials—your questions and critique were helpful in making this book even stronger. Thanks also to Dr. V. J. Periyakoil of Stanford University for her mentorship during my mini-fellowship on Successful Aging and for providing valuable resources for this text. Thanks to my colleague Diana Whittiker, RN, MDiv. We had so much fun implementing our Stanford fieldwork with the Hispanic older adults and really brought our projects to life. Last but not least—I thank Karen Anderson, Susan Schmitz, Sheri Saretsky, and Cherie Rebar for their wonderful contributions to and suggestions for the textbook.

A tailored education experience —

Sherpath book-organized collections

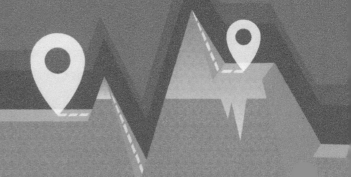

To the Student

Nurses are privileged to share in some of the most intimate aspects of people's lives. We not only help people when they are weak and vulnerable but also help people gain and appreciate new strengths. Although much of our youth and young adulthood focus on achieving independence, our older adult years demonstrate the value in interdependence—being able to rely on others, as well as give back to others in new and different ways. As nurses, we help others compensate for their deficits and build upon their strengths. We rejoice in and point out small successes and help build these to greater successes. It is important to remember that the older person for whom you are caring was once a lot like you. Try to view the older adult under your care not just as the person in need that you see in front of you but rather in the context of their whole life: Was he a three-star general who now needs your help getting dressed? Was she someone who devoted her life to raising children and caring for grandchildren and now needs care of her own? Was he a neurosurgeon who now cannot control his movement because of Parkinson disease? Was she a judge who is now unable to express her preferences because of Alzheimer disease? Care for every older adult the way you would care for your aunt, your grandmother, your grandfather, or the way you wish to be cared for one day. The older adults under your care are fortunate: reaching an advanced age is a privilege not granted to everyone.

READING AND REVIEW TOOLS

- **Objectives** introduce the chapter topics.
- **Key Terms** are listed with page number references, and difficult medical, nursing, or scientific terms are accompanied by simple phonetic pronunciations.
- Each chapter ends with a Get Ready for the Next Generation NCLEX® Examination! **section** that includes (1) **Key Points** that reiterate the chapter objectives and serve as a useful review of concepts, (2) a list of **Additional Resources** including the Study Guide and Evolve Resources, and (3) an extensive set of **Review Questions for the Next Generation NCLEX® Examination** with Answers and Rationales on Evolve.

- **References** at the end of each chapter cite evidence-based information and provide resources for enhancing knowledge.
- A **Glossary** of key terms provides definitions of all the terms that appear at the beginning of chapters.

SPECIAL FEATURES

The following special features are designed to foster effective learning and comprehension and reflect the LPN Threads design:

Clinical Situation boxes relate the text to patient situations and care scenarios.

Complementary Health Approaches boxes address nontraditional and adjunct therapies.

Coordinated Care boxes address leadership and management issues for the LPN/LVN and include topics, such as supervision of ancillary personnel and end-of-life care.

Critical Thinking boxes pose questions designed to stimulate thought and to help students develop and improve their critical thinking skills.

Cultural Considerations boxes provide advice on culturally diverse patient care of older adults.

Health Promotion boxes recommend quality-of-life tips for older adults.

Home Health Consideration boxes give essential information for home care for the older adult.

Medication tables provide quick access to information about medications commonly used in geriatric nursing care.

Nursing Care Plans with Applying Clinical Judgment Questions provide students with real-world examples of nursing care plans and encourage them to think critically about the given scenarios.

Patient Education boxes instruct and inform both older patients and their caregivers about health promotion, disease prevention, and age-specific interventions.

Contents

UNIT I   OVERVIEW OF AGING, 1

1 Trends and Issues, 1

Introduction to Geriatric Nursing, 1
Historical Perspective on the Study of Aging, 1
What's in a Name: Geriatrics, Gerontology, and
    Gerontics, 2
Attitudes Toward Aging, 3
Gerontophobia, 4
    Ageism, 4
    Age Discrimination, 5
Demographics, 6
Scope of the Aging Population, 6
Gender and Ethnic Disparity, 7
The Baby Boomers, 8
Geographic Distribution of the Older Adult
    Population, 8
Marital Status, 8
Educational Status, 8
Economics of Aging, 9
Poverty, 9
Income, 9
Wealth, 13
Housing Arrangements, 13
Health Care Provisions, 16
Medicare and Medicaid, 16
Rising Costs and Legislative Activity, 17
Costs and End-of-Life Care, 18
Advance Directives and Physician Orders for Life-
    Sustaining Treatment, 18
Impact of Aging Members of the Family, 19
Reflection by a Nursing Professor, 20
The Nurse and Family Interactions, 21
Self-Neglect, 22
Abuse or Neglect by the Family, 22
    Physical Abuse, 22
    Neglect, 23
    Emotional Abuse, 23
    Financial Abuse, 23
    Abandonment, 24
    Responses to Abuse, 24
Abuse by Unrelated Caregivers, 25
Support Groups, 26
Respite Care, 26
References, 28

2 Theories of Aging, 29

Biologic Theories, 29
Psychosocial Theories, 31

Implications for Nursing, 32
References, 32

3 Physiologic Changes, 33

The Integumentary System, 34
Expected Age-Related Changes, 34
Common Disorders Seen With Aging, 36
    Melanoma and Nonmelanoma, 36
    Pressure Injuries, 36
    Inflammation and Infection, 36
    Hypothermia, 37
The Musculoskeletal System, 37
Bones, 37
Vertebrae, 38
Joints, Tendons, and Ligaments, 38
Muscles, 38
Expected Age-Related Changes, 39
Common Disorders Seen With Aging, 40
    Osteoporosis, 40
    Degenerative Joint Disease, 41
The Respiratory System, 42
Upper Respiratory Tract, 42
Lower Respiratory Tract, 42
Air Exchange (Respiration), 42
Expected Age-Related Changes, 43
Common Disorders Seen With Aging, 43
    Chronic Obstructive Pulmonary
        Disease, 43
    Influenza, 44
    COVID-19, 44
    Pneumonia, 44
    Tuberculosis, 45
    Lung Cancer, 45
The Cardiovascular System, 45
Heart, 46
Blood Vessels, 46
Conduction System, 46
Expected Age-Related Changes, 47
Common Disorders Seen With Aging, 47
    Coronary Artery Disease, 47
    Coronary Valve Disease, 48
    Cardiac Arrhythmias, 48
    Heart Failure, 48
    Cardiomegaly, 49
    Peripheral Vascular Disease, 49
    Occlusive Peripheral Vascular Problems, 49
    Varicose Veins, 49
    Aneurysm, 49
    Hypertensive Disease, 50

The Hematopoietic and Lymphatic Systems, 50
  Blood, 50
    Erythrocytes, 50
    Leukocytes, 51
    Platelets, 51
  Lymph System, 51
    Lymph Vessels, Fluid, and Nodes, 51
    Spleen and Thymus, 51
    Lymphocytes and Immunity, 51
  Expected Age-Related Changes, 51
  Common Disorders Seen With Aging, 52
    Anemia, 52
    Leukemia, 52
The Gastrointestinal System, 52
  Oral Cavity, 52
  Tongue, 52
  Salivary Glands, 53
  Esophagus, 53
  Stomach, 53
  Small Intestine, 53
  Large Intestine, 53
  Expected Age-Related Changes, 53
  Common Disorders Seen With Aging, 54
    Hiatal Hernia, 54
    Gastritis and Ulcers, 55
    Diverticulosis and Diverticulitis, 55
    Cancer, 55
    Hemorrhoids, 55
    Rectal Prolapse, 56
The Urinary System, 56
  Kidneys, 56
  Ureters and Bladder, 56
  Characteristics of Urine, 56
  Expected Age-Related Changes, 57
  Common Disorders Seen With Aging, 57
    Urinary Incontinence, 57
    Urinary Tract Infection, 57
    Chronic Kidney Disease, 58
The Nervous System, 58
  Central Nervous System, 58
    Medulla, 58
    Pons and Midbrain, 58
    Cerebellum, 58
    Hypothalamus, 59
    Cerebrum, 59
  Peripheral Nervous System, 59
  Expected Age-Related Changes, 59
  Common Disorders Seen With Aging, 60
    Parkinson Disease, 60
    Dementia, 60
    Alzheimer Dementia, 61
    Transient Ischemic Attacks, 63
    Stroke, 63
The Special Senses, 64
  The Eyes, 64
  Refraction, 65
  Expected Age-Related Changes, 65
  Common Disorders Seen With Aging, 66
    Blepharitis, 66

    Diplopia, 67
    Cataracts, 67
    Glaucoma, 67
    Age-Related Macular Degeneration and
      Retinal Detachment, 67
  The Ears, 67
  Expected Age-Related Changes, 68
  Common Disorders Seen With Aging, 68
    Otosclerosis, 68
    Tinnitus, 68
    Deafness, 68
    Ménière Disease, 69
  Taste and Smell, 69
  Expected Age-Related Changes, 69
The Endocrine System, 69
  Pituitary Gland, 70
  Thyroid Gland, 70
  Parathyroid Glands, 70
  Pancreas, 70
  Adrenal Glands, 70
  Ovaries and Testes, 70
  Expected Age-Related Changes, 71
  Common Disorders Seen With Aging, 72
    Diabetes Mellitus, 72
    Hypoglycemia, 73
    Hypothyroidism, 73
The Reproductive and Genitourinary
  Systems, 73
  Female Reproductive Organs, 73
  Male Reproductive Organs, 73
  Expected Age-Related Changes, 74
    Changes in Women, 74
    Changes in Men, 74
  Common Disorders Seen With Aging, 74
    Uterine Prolapse, 74
    Vaginal Infection, 75
    Breast Cancer, 75
    Prostate Cancer, 75
References, 76

UNIT II   BASIC SKILLS FOR
          GERONTOLOGIC NURSING, 78

4 Health Promotion, Health
  Maintenance, and Home Health
  Considerations, 78

Recommended Health Practices for Older
  Adults, 79
  Diet, 79
  Exercise, 79
  Tobacco and Alcohol, 79
  Physical Examinations and Preventive Overall
    Care, 80
  Dental Examinations and Preventive Oral
    Care, 82
  Maintaining Healthy Attitudes, 83
Factors That Affect Health Promotion and
  Maintenance, 83

Religious Beliefs, 84
Cultural Beliefs, 84
Knowledge and Motivation, 84
Mobility, 85
Perceptions of Aging, 85
Impact of Cognitive and Sensory Changes, 85
Impact of Changes Related to Accessibility, 86
Home Health, 86
Unpaid Caregiver, 86
Paid Caregivers, 87
Types of Home Services, 87
Nursing Process/Clinical Judgment Model
for Inadequate Health Maintenance and
Inadequate Health Management, 88
Assessment (Data Collection), 88
Data Analysis/Problem Identification, 89
Planning, 89
Implementation, 89
Nursing Process/Clinical Judgment Model for
Nonadherence With the Treatment Plan, 90
Assessment (Data Collection), 90
Data Analysis/Problem Identification, 90
Planning, 90
Implementation, 90
References, 93

5 Communicating With Older Adults, 95

Information Sharing (Framing the Message), 95
Formal or Therapeutic Communication, 96
Informal or Social Communication, 97
Nonverbal Communication, 97
Symbols, 97
Tone of Voice, 97
Body Language, 98
Space, Distance, and Position, 98
Gestures, 99
Facial Expressions, 99
Eye Contact, 99
Pace or Speed of Communication, 99
Time and Timing, 99
Touch, 100
Silence, 100
Empathy, Acceptance, Dignity, and Respect In
Communication, 101
Active and Empathetic Listening, 101
Barriers to Communication, 101
Hearing Impairment, 102
Aphasia, 102
Dementia, 103
Cultural Differences, 103
Skills and Techniques, 104
Informing, 104
Direct Questioning, 104
Using Open-Ended Techniques, 104
Confrontating, 105
Communicating With Visitors and Families, 105
Delivering Bad News, 105

Having Difficult Conversations, 106
Improving Communication Between the
Older Adult and The Primary Care
Provider, 106
Effective Communication With the Health Care
Team, 106
Telephoning Primary Care Providers, 107
Patient Teaching, 108
References, 110

**6 Maintaining Fluid Balance and Meeting
Nutritional Needs, 111**

Nutrition and Aging, 111
Caloric Intake, 111
Nutrients, 112
Carbohydrates, 113
Proteins, 113
Fats, 115
Vitamins, 115
Minerals, 117
Functional Foods, 118
Water, 119
Malnutrition and the Older Adult, 119
Factors Affecting Nutrition in Older
Adults, 119
Social and Cultural Aspects of
Nutrition, 122
Nursing Process/Clinical Judgment Model for
Risk for Altered Nutrition, 122
Assessment (Data Collection), 125
Appetite Changes, 125
Nutritional Intake, 125
Social and Cultural Factors, 126
Home Care or Discharge Planning, 126
Data Analysis/Problem Identification, 126
Planning, 126
Implementation, 126
Nursing Process/Clinical Judgment Model for
Fluid Volume and Potential for Altered
Intake, 130
Assessment (Data Collection), 130
Fluid Volume Deficit, 131
Fluid Volume Overload, 131
Data Analysis/Problem Identification, 131
Planning, 131
Implementation, 131
Nursing Process/Clinical Judgment Model for
Altered Swallowing Ability, 133
Assessment (Data Collection), 134
Data Analysis/Problem Identification, 134
Planning, 134
Implementation, 134
Nursing Process/Clinical Judgment Model for
Aspiration Risk, 136
Assessment (Data Collection), 136
Data Analysis/Problem Identification, 136
Planning, 136

Implementation, 136
References, 139

7 Medications and Older Adults, 140

Risks Related to Drug Testing Methods, 141
Risks Related to the Physiologic Changes of
Aging, 141
Pharmacokinetics, 141
Drug Absorption, 141
Drug Distribution, 141
Drug Metabolism, 142
Drug Excretion, 142
Pharmacodynamics, 142
Polypharmacy, 142
Potentially Inappropriate Medication Use in Older
Adults, 144
Risks Related to Cognitive or Sensory
Changes, 145
Risks Related to Inadequate Knowledge, 146
Risks Related to Financial Factors, 147
Medication Administration in an Institutional
Setting, 147
Nursing Assessment and Medication, 147
Medication and the Nursing Care Plan, 148
Nursing Interventions Related to Medication
Administration, 148
Right Patient, 148
Right Medication, 150
Right Amount, 150
Right Dosage Form, 151
Right Route, 151
Right Time, 152
Right Documentation, 153
Patient Rights and Medication, 153
Self-Medication and Older Adults, 153
In an Institutional Setting, 153
In the Home, 153
Teaching Older Adults About Medications, 154
Safety and Nonadherence Issues, 155
References, 157

8 Health Assessment for Older Adults, 158

Health Screening, 158
Health Assessments, 159
Interviewing Older Adults, 159
Preparing the Physical Setting, 159
Establishing Rapport, 159
Structuring the Interview, 160
Obtaining the Health History, 160
Physical Assessment of Older Adults, 161
Inspection, 162
Palpation, 165
Auscultation, 165
Percussion, 165
Measuring Vital Signs in Older Adults, 165
Temperature, 165
Pulse, 166

Respiration, 167
Blood Pressure, 167
Sensory Assessment of Older Adults, 168
Psychosocial Assessment of Older
Adults, 168
Special Assessments, 168
The Minimum Data Set 3.0, 168
Assessment of Condition
Change in Older Adults, 170
Fulmer Spices, 170
FANCAPES, 171
References, 173

9 Meeting Safety Needs of Older Adults, 174

Internal Risk Factors, 174
Falls, 175
Fall Prevention, 176
Tools to Assess for Falls, 177
Specific Strategies to Prevent Falls, 177
External Risk Factors, 178
Fire Hazards, 179
Home Security, 179
Internet Safety, 179
Vehicular Accidents, 179
Thermal Hazards, 182
Summary, 183
Nursing Process/Clinical Judgment Model for
Potential for Injury, 183
Assessment (Data Collection), 183
Data Analysis/Problem Identification, 184
Planning, 184
Implementation, 184
Nursing Process/Clinical Judgment Model for
Hypothermia/Hyperthermia, 187
Assessment (Data Collection), 187
Data Analysis/Problem Identification, 187
Planning, 187
Implementation, 187
To Prevent Hyperthermia, 188
To Prevent Hypothermia, 188
References, 189

UNIT III PSYCHOSOCIAL CARE OF THE ELDERLY, 191

10 Cognition and Perception, 191

Normal Cognitive-Perceptual Functioning, 191
Cognitive and Intelligence, 192
Cognition and Language, 192
Nursing Process/Clinical Judgment Model for
Altered Sensory Perception, 194
Assessment (Data Collection), 194
Data Analysis/Problem Identification, 194
Planning, 194
Implementation, 194

Nursing Process/Clinical Judgment Model for
Chronic Confusion, 197
Assessment (Data Collection), 200
Data Analysis/Problem Identification, 201
Planning, 201
Implementation, 201
Nursing Process/Clinical Judgment Model for
Altered Communication Ability, 205
Assessment (Data Collection), 206
Data Analysis/Problem Identification, 206
Planning, 207
Implementation, 207
Nursing Process/Clinical Judgment Model
for Pain, 207
Assessment (Data Collection), 209
Data Analysis/Problem Identification, 210
Planning, 210
Implementation, 210
References, 213

11 Self-Perception and Self-Concept, 214

Normal Self-Perception and Self-Concept, 214
Self-Perception/Self-Concept and
Aging, 216
Depression and Aging, 217
Suicide and Aging, 218
Nursing Process/Clinical Judgment Model for
Altered Self-Perception and Altered Self-
Concept, 218
Assessment (Data Collection), 218
Nursing Process/Clinical Judgment Model for
Altered Body Image, 219
Assessment (Data Collection), 219
Data Analysis/Problem Identification, 219
Planning, 219
Implementation, 219
Nursing Process/Clinical Judgment Model for
Potential for Decreased Self-Esteem, 220
Assessment (Data Collection), 220
Data Analysis/Problem Identification, 220
Planning, 221
Implementation, 221
Nursing Process/Clinical Judgment Model for
Fear, 222
Assessment (Data Collection), 223
Data Analysis/Problem Identification, 223
Planning, 223
Implementation, 223
Nursing Process/Clinical Judgment Model for
Anxiety, 223
Assessment (Data Collection), 224
Data Analysis/Problem Identification, 224
Planning, 224
Implementation, 224
Nursing Process/Clinical Judgment Model for
Decreased Hope, 224
Assessment (Data Collection), 224

Data Analysis/Problem Identification, 225
Planning, 225
Implementation, 225
Nursing Process/Clinical Judgment Model for
Loss of Power, 225
Assessment (Data Collection), 226
Data Analysis/Problem Identification, 226
Planning, 226
Implementation, 226
References, 229

12 Roles and Relationships, 230

Normal Roles and Relationships, 230
Roles, Relationships, and Aging, 231
Nursing Process/Clinical Judgment
Model for Complex Grief, 234
Assessment (Data Collection), 234
Data Analysis/Problem Identification, 235
Planning, 235
Implementation, 235
Nursing Process/Clinical Judgment Model for
Loneliness and Potential for Social Isolation, 236
Assessment (Data Collection), 236
Data Analysis/Problem Identification, 236
Planning, 236
Implementation, 236
Nursing Process/Clinical Judgment Model for
Altered Family Functioning, 237
Assessment (Data Collection), 237
Data Analysis/Problem Identification, 237
Planning, 237
Implementation, 237
References, 240

13 Coping and Stress, 241

Normal Stress and Coping, 241
Physical Signs of Stress, 243
Cognitive Signs of Stress, 243
Emotional Signs, 243
Behavioral Signs, 243
Stress and Illness, 244
Stress and Life Events, 245
Stress Reduction and Coping Strategies, 245
Nursing Process/Clinical Judgment Model for
Limited Coping Ability, 246
Assessment (Data Collection), 246
Data Analysis/Problem Identification, 247
Planning, 247
Implementation, 247
Nursing Process/Clinical Judgment Model for
Disrupted Living Situation and Maladaptive
Response to Disrupted Living Situation, 248
Assessment (Data Collection), 249
Data Analysis/Problem Identification, 249
Planning, 249
Implementation, 249
References, 251

14 Values and Beliefs, 252

Common Values and Beliefs of Older
Adults, 254
Economic Values, 254
Interpersonal Values, 254
Cultural Values, 254
Spiritual or Religious Values, 255
Nursing Process/Clinical Judgment Model for
Spiritual Disconnection, 256
Assessment (Data Collection), 256
Data Analysis/Problem Identification, 257
Planning, 257
Implementation, 257
References, 259

15 End-of-Life Care, 261

Death in Western Cultures, 261
Attitudes Toward Death and End-of-Life
Planning, 262
Advance Directives, 263
*Caregiver Attitudes Toward End-of-Life
Care, 263*
Values Clarification Related to Death and End-of-
Life Care, 263
What Is a "Good" Death?, 263
Where People Die, 264
Palliative Care, 265
Collaborative Assessment and Interventions for
End-of-Life Care, 265
Communication at the End of Life, 265
Psychosocial Perspectives, Assessments, and
Interventions, 267
Cultural Perspectives, 267
Communication About Death, 267
Decision-Making Process, 267
   *Amount and Type of Intervention That Will
   Be Accepted, 268*
   Significance of Pain and Suffering, 268
Depression, Anxiety, and Fear, 268
Physiologic Changes, Assessments, and
Interventions, 269
Pain, 269
Fatigue and Sleepiness, 271
Cardiovascular Changes, 271
Respiratory Changes, 271
Gastrointestinal Changes, 272
Urinary Changes, 273
Integumentary Changes, 273
Sensory Changes, 273
Changes in Cognition, 273
Death, 273
Recognizing Imminent Death, 274
Funeral Arrangements, 275
Bereavement, 275
References, 277

16 Sexuality and Aging, 278

Factors That Affect Sexuality of Older Adults, 278
Age-Related Changes in Women, 279
Age-Related Changes in Men, 279
Impact of Illness on Sexual Health, 280
*Effects of Alcohol and Medications on Sexual Health,
280*
Loss of a Sex Partner, 280
Marriage and Older Adults, 281
Caregivers and the Sexuality of Older
Adults, 281
Sexual Orientation of Older Adults, 281
Sexually Transmitted Infections, 281
Privacy and Personal Rights of Older Adults, 282
Nursing Process/Clinical Judgment Model for
Altered Sexual Function, 282
Assessment (Data Collection), 282
Data Analysis/Problem Identification, 283
Planning, 283
Implementation, 283
References, 285

**UNIT IV   PHYSICAL CARE OF THE
                  ELDERLY, 286**

**17 Care of Aging Skin and Mucous
      Membranes, 286**

Age-Related Changes in Skin, Hair, and Nails, 286
Skin Color, 287
Dry Skin, 287
Rashes and Irritation, 288
Pigmentation, 288
Tissue Integrity, 288
   Pressure Injuries, 289
   *Amount, Distribution, Appearance, and
   Consistency of Hair, 290*
   Tissue of the Feet, 290
   Nails, 290
   Other Common Foot Problems, 293
Nursing Process/Clinical Judgment Model for
Altered Skin Integrity, 293
Assessment (Data Collection), 293
Data Analysis/Problem Identification, 294
Planning, 294
Implementation, 294
Age-Related Changes in Oral Mucous
Membranes, 300
Dental Caries, 301
Periodontal Disease, 301
Pain, 301
Dentures, 302
Dry Mouth, 302
Leukoplakia, 302
Cancer, 302

Alcohol and Tobacco-Related Problems, 303
    Problems Caused by Neurologic Conditions, 303
Nursing Process/Clinical Judgment Model for
    Altered Oral Mucous Membranes, 303
    Assessment (Data Collection), 303
    Data Analysis/Problem Identification, 303
    Planning, 303
    Implementation, 304
References, 307

18 Elimination, 308

Normal Elimination Patterns, 308
Elimination and Aging, 308
Constipation, 309
    Fecal Impaction, 310
Nursing Process/Clinical Judgment Model for
    Constipation, 311
    Assessment (Data Collection), 311
    Data Analysis/Problem Identification, 311
    Planning, 311
    Implementation, 311
        Diarrhea, 313
Nursing Process/Clinical Judgment Model for
    Diarrhea, 313
    Assessment (Data Collection), 313
    Data Analysis/Problem Identification, 313
    Planning, 314
    Implementation, 314
        Fecal Incontinence, 315
Nursing Process/Clinical Judgment Model for
    Fecal Incontinence, 315
    Assessment (Data Collection), 315
    Data Analysis/Problem Identification, 315
    Planning, 315
    Implementation, 316
        Urinary Retention, 316
        Urinary Tract Infection, 316
        Urinary Incontinence, 316
Nursing Process/Clinical Judgment Model For
    Altered Urinary Function, 319
    Assessment (Data Collection, 319
    Data Analysis/Problems Identification, 319
    Planning, 319
    Implementation, 319
References, 324

19 Activity and Exercise, 325

Normal Activity Patterns, 325
Activity and Aging, 326
    Exercise Recommendation for Older Adults, 326
Effects of Disease Processes on Activity, 328
    Nursing Process/Clinical Judgment Model for
        Altered Mobility, 329
        Assessment (Data Collection), 329
        Data Analysis/Problem Identification, 329
        Planning, 329
        Implementation, 330

Nursing Process/Clinical Judgment Model for
    Altered Activity Tolerance, 335
    Assessment (Data Collection), 335
    Data Analysis/Problem Identification, 335
    Planning, 336
    Implementation, 336
Nursing Process/Clinical Judgment Model for
    Problems of Oxygenation, 337
    Assessment (Data Collection), 337
    Data Analysis/Problem Identification, 338
    Planning, 338
    Implementation, 338
Nursing Process/Clinical Judgment Model for
    Altered Self-Care Ability, 341
    Assessment (Data Collection), 341
    Data Analysis/Problem Identification, 342
    Planning, 342
    Implementation, 342
Nursing Process/Clinical Judgment Model for
    Deficient Diversional Activity, 345
    Assessment (Data Collection), 345
    Data Analysis/Problem Identification, 345
    Planning, 345
    Implementation, 345
Rehabilitation, 348
    Negative Attitudes: The Controlling or Custodial
        Focus, 348
    Positive Attitudes: The Rehabilitative Focus, 349
References, 352

20 Sleep and Rest, 353

Sleep-Rest Health Pattern, 353
    Normal Sleep and Rest, 353
    Sleep and Aging, 354
    Sleep Disorders, 355
        Insomnia, 355
        Sleep Apnea, 357
        Circadian Rhythm Sleep Disorders, 358
        Rapid Eye Movement Sleep-Behavior
            Disorder, 358
Nursing Process/Clinical Judgment Model for
    Disrupted Sleep Pattern, 358
    Assessment (Data Collection), 358
    Data Analysis/Problem Identification, 358
    Planning, 358
    Implementation, 358
References, 362

APPENDIXES

A Laboratory Values for Older Adults, 363
B The Geriatric Depression Scale (GDS), 367
C Daily Nutritional Goals for Older Adults, 368
D Resources for Older Adults, 369

Glossary, 371
Index, 377

Trends and Issues

Objectives

1. Describe the subjective and objective ways in which aging is defined.
2. Identify personal and societal attitudes toward aging.
3. Define ageism.
4. Discuss the myths that exist with regard to aging.
5. Identify recent demographic trends and their impact on society.
6. Describe the effects of recent legislation on the economic status of older adults.
7. Identify the political interest groups that work as advocates for older adults.
8. Identify the major economic concerns of older adults.
9. Describe the housing options available to older adults.
10. Discuss the health care implications of a growing population of older adults.
11. Describe the changes in family dynamics that occur as family members become older.
12. Examine the role of nurses in dealing with an aging family.
13. Identify the different forms of elder abuse.
14. Recognize the most common signs of abuse.
15. Describe effective approaches for the prevention of elder abuse.

Key Terms

abuse (p. 22)
ageism (p. 4)
chronologic age (krŏ-nŏ-LŌJ-ĭk, p. 2)
cohort (KŌ-hŏrt, p. 8)
demographics (dĕm-ŏ-GRĂF-ĭks, p. 6)
geriatric (jĕr-ē-ĂT-rĭk, p. 2)

gerontics (p. 2)
gerontology (p. 2)
gerontophobia (p. 4)
mandated reporter (p. 26)
neglect (nĭ-glĕkt, p. 22)
respite (RĔS-pĭt, p. 26)

INTRODUCTION TO GERIATRIC NURSING

HISTORICAL PERSPECTIVE ON THE STUDY OF AGING

Until the middle of the 19th century, only two stages of human growth and development were identified: childhood and adulthood. In many ways, children were treated like small adults. No special attention was given to them or to their needs. Families had to produce many children to ensure that a few would survive and reach adulthood. In turn, children were expected to contribute to the family's survival. Little or no attention was given to those characteristics and behaviors that set one child apart from another.

As time passed, society began to view children differently. People learned that there are significant differences between children of different ages and that children's needs change as they develop. Childhood is now divided into substages (i.e., infant, toddler, preschool, school age, and adolescence). Each stage is associated with unique challenges related to the individual child's stage of growth and development.

Because the substages are related to obvious physical changes or to significant life events, this classification is now accepted as logical and necessary.

Until recently, society also viewed adults of all ages interchangeably. Once you became an adult, you remained an adult. Perhaps society perceived dimly that older adults were different from younger adults, but there was not much concern about those differences because few people lived to old age. In addition, the physical and developmental changes of adulthood are more subtle than those of childhood; therefore these changes received little attention.

Until the 1960s, sociologists, psychologists, and health care providers focused their attention on meeting the needs of the typical or average adult: people between 20 and 65 years of age. This group was the largest and most economically productive segment of the population; they were raising families, working, and contributing to the economy. Only a small percentage of the population lived beyond 65 years of age. Disability, illness, and early death were accepted as natural and unavoidable.

1

In the late 1960s, research began to indicate that adults of all ages are not the same. Then also, the focus of health care shifted from illness to wellness. Disability and disease were no longer considered unavoidable parts of aging. Increased medical knowledge, improved preventive health practices, and technologic advances helped more people live longer, healthier lives.

Older adults now constitute a significant group in society, and interest in the study of aging is growing. The study of aging will be a major area of attention for years to come.

WHAT'S IN A NAME: GERIATRICS, GERONTOLOGY, AND GERONTICS

The term *geriatric* comes from the Greek words *geras*, meaning "old age," and *iatro*, meaning "relating to medical treatment." Thus geriatrics is the medical specialty that deals with the physiology of aging and with the diagnosis and treatment of diseases affecting older adults. Geriatrics, by definition, focuses on abnormal conditions and their medical treatment.

The term *gerontology* comes from the Greek words *gero*, meaning "related to old age," and *ology*, meaning "the study of." Thus gerontology is the study of all aspects of the aging process, including the clinical, psychologic, economic, and sociologic problems of older adults and the consequences of these problems for older adults and society. Gerontology affects nursing, health care, and all areas of our society—including housing, education, business, and politics.

The term *gerontics*, or *gerontic nursing*, was coined by Gunter and Estes in 1979 to define the nursing care and service provided to older adults. Gerontic nursing comprises a holistic view of aging, with the goal of increasing health, providing comfort, and caring for older adults' needs. This textbook focuses on gerontic nursing. It addresses ways in which to promote high-level functioning and methods of giving care and comfort to older adults.

The objectives of this book are to
- Examine trends and issues that affect the older adult's ability to remain healthy
- Explore theories and myths of aging
- Study the normal changes that occur with aging
- Review pathologic conditions that are commonly observed in older adults
- Emphasize the importance of effective communication when working with older adults
- Explore the general methods used to assess the health status of older adults
- Describe the specific methods of assessing functional needs
- Identify the most common patient problems experienced by older adults and discuss nursing interventions aimed at solving these problems
- Explore the effects of medication and medication administration on older adults

The dictionary defines *old* as "having lived or existed for a long time." The meaning of this word is highly subjective; to a great degree, it depends on how old we ourselves are. Few people like to describe themselves as old. A recent study reveals that people younger than age 30 view those older than age 63 as "getting older." People over the age of 65, however, do not think people are "getting older" until they are 75 years old.

Aging is a complex process that can be described chronologically, physiologically, and functionally. Chronologic age, the number of years a person has lived, is most often used when we speak of aging because it is the easiest to identify and measure. Many people who have lived a long time remain functionally and physiologically young. These individuals remain physically fit, stay mentally active, and are productive members of society. Others are chronologically young but physically or functionally old. Thus chronologic age is not the most meaningful measurement of aging.

In using chronologic age as the measure, authorities use various systems to categorize the aging population (Table 1.1). To many people, 65 years is a magic number in terms of aging. The wide acceptance of age 65 as a landmark of aging is interesting. Since the 1930s, the age of 65 has come to be accepted as the age of retirement, when it is expected that a person willingly or unwillingly stops paid employment. However, before the 1930s, most people worked until they decided to stop working, until they became too ill to work, or until they died. When the New Deal established the Social Security program, 65 was set as the age at which benefits could be collected. However, the average life expectancy of the time was 63 years of age. The Social Security program was designed as a fairly low-cost way to win votes because most people would not live long enough to collect the benefits. Although age 65 was considered old then, it certainly is not considered old now. If the same standards were applied today, the retirement age would arrive at age 77. However, society clings to age 65 as the retirement age and resists political proposals designed to move the start of Social Security benefits to a later age. Despite the resistance, the age to qualify for full Social Security benefits is

Table 1.1	Categorizing the Aging Population
AGE (YEARS)	**CATEGORY**
55 to 64	Older
65 to 74	Elderly
75 to 84	Aged
85 and older	Extremely aged
Or	
60 to 74	Young old
75 to 84	Middle old
85 and older	Old old

changing. Individuals born before 1937 still qualify for full benefits at 65 years of age, but there are incremental increases in age for all persons born after that time. Individuals born in 1960 or later must wait until age 67 to qualify for full benefits. Reduced benefits are calculated for individuals who claim Social Security benefits after age 62 but before the full retirement age. To be consistent with other sources, however, this text will refer to individuals of age 65 and above as "older adults."

ATTITUDES TOWARD AGING

Before we look at the attitudes of others, it is important to examine our own attitudes, values, and knowledge about aging. The three following Critical Thinking boxes that follow are designed to help you assess how you feel about aging.

After you have filled out these Critical Thinking boxes, look at the characteristics you described and think about the feelings you experienced as you considered your answers. Do your feelings correspond to your attitudes about aging? In the Critical Thinking Box about Values, were the three people's characteristics similar or different? What do these characteristics say about your values? Our attitudes are the product of our knowledge and values. Our life experiences and our current age strongly influence our views about aging and older adults. Most of us have a rather narrow perspective, and our attitudes may reflect this. We tend to project our personal experiences onto the rest of the world. Because many of us have a somewhat limited exposure to older adults, we may believe quite a bit of inaccurate information. In dealing with older adults, our limited understanding and vision can lead to serious errors and mistaken conclusions. If we view old age as a time of physical decay, mental confusion, and social boredom, we are likely to have negative feelings toward aging. Conversely, if we see old age as a time for sustained physical vigor, renewed mental challenges, and social usefulness, our perspective on aging will be quite different.

? Critical Thinking

Your Current Knowledge About Aging

Respond to the following questions to the best of your knowledge.

You are "old" at age _____

_____.

There are _____

_____ older adults in the United States.

Most older adults live in_____.

Economically, older adults are _____

_____.

With regard to health, older adults are _____

_____.

Mentally, older adults are _____

_____.

? Critical Thinking

Your Views and Attitudes About Aging

- How many older adults do you know personally?
- Do you think they are "old"? Do *they* consider themselves "old"?
- How do you personally define "old"?
- Why is aging an issue today?
- Should Social Security laws be changed to reflect today's longer life expectancy?

Please complete the following statements. Write as many applicable comments as you can. *There are no right or wrong answers.*

A person can be considered "old" when _____

_____.

When I think about getting older, I _____

_____.

Growing older means _____

_____.

When I get older, I will lose my _____

_____.

Seeing an older person makes me feel _____

_____.

Older people always _____

_____.

Older people never _____

_____.

The best thing about aging is _____

_____.

The worst thing about aging is _____

_____.

Looking back at my responses, I feel that aging is _____

_____.

It is important to separate facts from myths as we examine our attitudes toward aging. The single most important factor that influences how poorly or well a person will age is attitude. This statement is true not only for others but also for ourselves.

Throughout time, youth and beauty have been viewed as desirable, and old age and physical infirmity have been loathed and feared. Greek statues portray youths of physical perfection. Artists' works throughout history have shown heroes and heroines as young and beautiful and evildoers as old and ugly. Little has changed to this day. A few cultures cherish their older members and view them as keepers of wisdom. Even in Asia, where tradition demands respect for older adults, societal changes are destroying this venerable mindset.

For the most part, mainstream American society does not value its older adults. The United States tends to be a youth-oriented society in which people are judged by age, appearance, and wealth. Young, attractive, and wealthy people are viewed positively; old, imperfect, and poor people are not. It is difficult for young people to imagine that they will ever be old. Despite some cultural changes, aging continues to have negative connotations. Many people continue to do everything they can to appear young. Wrinkles, gray hair, and other physical changes of aging are actively confronted with makeup, hair dye, and cosmetic surgery. Until recently, advertising seldom portrayed people older than age 50 except to sell eyeglasses, hearing aids, hair dye, laxatives, and other rather unappealing products. The message seemed to be, "Young is good, old is bad; therefore everyone should fight getting old." It is significant that trends in advertising appear to be changing. As the number of healthier, dynamic senior citizens with significant spending power has increased, advertising campaigns have become increasingly likely to portray older adults as the consumers of their products, including exercise equipment, health beverages, and cruises. Despite these societal improvements, many people do not know enough about the realities of aging and, because of ignorance, are afraid to get old. Some media studies have found that people who watch more television are likely to have more negative perceptions of aging.

GERONTOPHOBIA

The fear of aging and refusal to accept older adults into the mainstream of society is known as *gerontophobia*. Senior citizens and younger persons can fall prey to such irrational fears (Box 1.1). Gerontophobia sometimes results in very odd behavior. Teenagers buy antiwrinkle creams. Thirty-year-old women consider facelifts. Forty-year-old women have hair transplants. Long-term marriages dissolve so that one spouse can pursue someone younger. Often these behaviors arise from the fear of growing older.

AGEISM

The extreme forms of gerontophobia are ageism and age discrimination. Ageism involves a negative attitude toward aging and older adults based on the belief that aging makes people unattractive, unintelligent, and unproductive. It is an emotional prejudice or discrimination against people based solely on age. Ageism allows the young to separate themselves physically and emotionally from the old and to view older adults as somehow having less human value. Like sexism or racism, ageism is a negative belief pattern that can result in irrational thoughts and destructive behaviors, such as intergenerational conflict and name calling. Like other forms of prejudice, ageism occurs because of myths and stereotypes about a group of people who are "different."

Box 1.1   Aging: Myth Versus Fact

MYTHS: OLDER ADULTS...
- Are pretty much all alike.
- In general, are lonely and alone.
- Tend to be sick and frail and to live in nursing homes.
- Are often cognitively impaired.
- Have no interest in sex.
- Suffer from depression more than younger adults.
- Become more difficult and rigid in their thinking.
- Have difficulty coping with age-related changes.

FACTS: OLDER ADULTS...
- Are a very diverse age group.
- Typically remain engaged and productive, often working or volunteering or keeping in contact via social networks.
- Usually live independently. Only about 1% of older adults between the ages of 65 and 74 and 2% of those between 74 and 85 live in nursing homes.
- May experience some cognitive decline, but this is usually not severe enough to cause problems in daily living.
- Typically remain sexually active, although frequency may decline.
- In general, have lower rates of depression as compared with younger adults, although the consequences can be more severe.
- Tend to maintain a consistent personality throughout the lifespan.
- Typically adjust well to the challenges of aging.

The combination of societal stereotyping and a lack of positive personal experiences with older adults affects a cross section of society. Studies have shown that health care providers share the views of the general public and are not immune to ageism. Specializing in geriatrics is unpopular by nursing and medical students, even though older adults are frequent users of the health care system (Hebditch et al., 2020); therefore many nurses actually do function as geriatric nurses to a great extent. Some health care providers erroneously believe that they are not fully using their skills when working with the aging population. Working in intensive care, the emergency department, or any other high technology area is viewed as exciting and challenging. Working with older adults is viewed as routine, boring, and depressing. As long as negative attitudes such as these are held by health care providers, this challenging and potentially rewarding area of service will continue to be underrated and the older adult population will suffer for it.

Because ageism can have a negative effect on the way health care providers relate to older patients, such patients can, as a result, have poor health care outcomes. Ageism leads to significantly worse health outcomes worldwide; this can be due to external factors, such as denied access to health services and treatment, or internal factors, as when a recipient of ageism develops a disease-causing inflammation (Chang et al., 2020). Because the older adult population is growing, health care providers need to think carefully about their own attitudes. Furthermore, they must confront signs of ageism whenever and wherever they appear. Activities such as greater positive interactions with older adults and improved professional training designed to address misconceptions regarding aging are two ways of fighting ageism. The Hartford Institute for Geriatric Nursing (HIGN), formed in 1996, has the goal of shaping the health care of older adults by promoting excellent nursing practice. Their website, www.hign.org, is a treasure trove of geriatric nursing resources, including the *Try This* series of assessment tools. Research shows that negative perceptions of aging are predictive of mental and physical decline (Chang et al., 2020); therefore keeping a positive attitude toward aging might just prevent someone from becoming frail in their older years.

AGE DISCRIMINATION

Age discrimination reaches beyond emotions and leads to actions; older adults are often treated differently simply because of their age. Examples of age discrimination include refusing to hire older people, not approving them for home loans, and limiting the type or amount of health care they receive. Age discrimination is illegal. Some older adults respond to age discrimination with passive acceptance, whereas others are banding together to speak up for their rights.

The reality of getting old is that no one knows what it will be like until it happens. But that is the nature of life—growing older is just the continuation of a process that started at birth. Older adults are fundamentally no different from the people they were when they were younger. Physical, financial, social, and political conditions may change, but the person remains essentially the same. Old age has been described as the "more-so" stage of life because some personality characteristics may appear to amplify. Older adults are not a homogeneous group. They differ as widely as any other age group. They are unique individuals with unique values, beliefs, experiences, and life stories. Because of their extended years, their stories are longer and often far more interesting than those of younger persons.

Aging can be a liberating experience. Aging seems to decrease the need to maintain pretenses, and the older adult may finally be comfortable enough to reveal the real person beneath the facade. If a person has been essentially kind and caring throughout life, they will generally reveal more of these positive personal characteristics over time. Likewise, if a person was miserly or unkind, they will often reveal more of these negative personality characteristics with age. The more successful a person has been at meeting the developmental tasks of life, the more likely they will be to face aging successfully. Perhaps the best advice to all who are preparing for old age is to be found in the Serenity Prayer:

O God, give us the serenity to accept what cannot be changed; courage to change what should be changed; and wisdom to distinguish one from the other.

Reinhold Niebuhr

DEMOGRAPHICS

Demographics is the statistical study of human populations. Demographers are concerned with a population's size, distribution, and vital statistics. Vital statistics include birth, death, age at death, marriage(s), race, and many other variables. The collection of demographic information is an ongoing process. The Bureau of the Census conducts the most inclusive demographic research in the United States every 10 years. The most recent census was completed in the year 2020.

Demographic research is important to many groups. Demographic information is used by the government as a basis for granting aid to cities and states, by cities to project their budget needs for schools, by hospitals to determine the number of beds needed, by public health agencies to determine the immunization needs of a community, and by marketers to sell products. The politicians of the 1930s used demographics to formulate plans for the Social Security program. Demographic studies provide information about the present that allows projections into the future.

One important piece of demographic information is life expectancy, or the number of years an average person can expect to live. Projected from the time of birth, life expectancy is based on the ages of all people who have died in a given year. If a large number of infants die at birth or during childhood, the life expectancy of that year's group tends to be low. Life expectancy throughout history has been low because of environmental hazards, wars, accidents, the scarcity of food and water, inadequate sanitation, and contagious diseases.

- During biblical times, the average life expectancy was approximately 20 years. Some people did live significantly longer, but 40 years was considered a good long life.
- By 1776, when the Declaration of Independence was signed, the life expectancy had risen to 35 years. It was very uncommon for anyone to live into their 60s.
- By the 1860s, at the time of the American Civil War, life expectancy had increased to 40 years. The 1860 census revealed that 2.7% of the American population was older than age 65.
- By the beginning of the 20th century, the overall life expectancy had increased to 47 years, and 4% of the American population was 65 years of age or older. In a span of more than 2000 years, life expectancy had increased by only 27 years.
- During the 20th century, the life expectancy of Americans increased by approximately 29 years. A child born in the United States in the year 2004 has an average life expectancy of nearly 77.4 years.
- Projections indicate that a male child born in 2017 will have a life expectancy of 75.97 years and a female child born in the same year will have a life expectancy of 80.96 years (Social Security Administration, 2020a).
- The COVID-19 pandemic has already decreased life expectancy projections by one full year in the United States (Thompson, 2021).

Since the beginning of the 20th century, advances in technology and health care have dramatically changed the world, especially in industrialized nations, where food production exceeds the needs of the population. Diseases such as cholera and typhoid have been eliminated or significantly reduced by improved sanitation and hygiene practices. Dreaded communicable diseases that at one time were often fatal (e.g., smallpox, measles, whooping cough, and diphtheria) are now preventable through immunization. Even pneumonia and influenza are no longer the fatal diseases they once were—or so we thought until the recent COVID-19 pandemic appeared; before effective vaccines were developed, it killed a disproportionate number of older adults. Today, vaccines for many diseases can be given to those who are at higher risk, and treatment can be given to those who become infected.

A longer life is a worldwide phenomenon. Some 9% of the world's population is 65 years of age or older (United Nations, Department of Economic and Social Affairs, Population Division, 2019). Monaco is the top ranked country for longevity; Singapore, Japan, Iceland, and Hong Kong are also in the top 10. The standing of the United States has steadily declined and, according to the Central Intelligence Agency's estimates (Central Intelligence Agency, 2020), it now ranks 43rd of 224 countries. Some possible explanations for the disparity between the United States and other countries include higher levels of accidental and violent deaths, obesity, relatively high infant mortality, and the high cost of health care. Much of the world's net gain in older persons has occurred in the developing countries of Africa, South America, and Asia (Fig. 1.1).

SCOPE OF THE AGING POPULATION

According to the U.S. Census Bureau (2018), by 2034, for the first time in recorded history, the number of people over 65 years of age is projected to exceed the number of children under age 18. In 2018, there were 52.4 million people in the United States, or 16% of the population, who were 65 years of age and older. By 2040, this number is expected to increase to 80.8 million people 65 years of age or older, or roughly 21.6% of the total population. The number of those 85 years of age and older is expected to double from 6.5 million in 2018 to more than 14 million in 2040 (Administration on Aging, 2020). We are becoming an increasingly older society (Fig. 1.2).

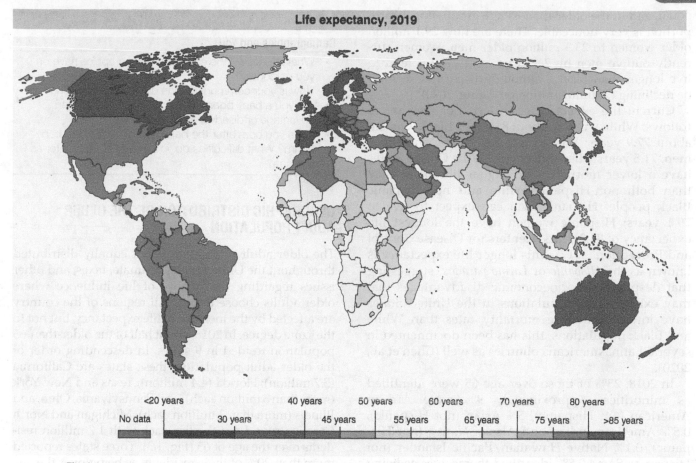

Life expectancy, 2019

| No data | <20 years | 30 years | 40 years | 45 years | 50 years | 55 years | 60 years | 65 years | 70 years | 75 years | 80 years | >85 years |

Fig. 1.1 Life expectancy world map. (From Roser, M., Ortiz-Ospina, E., Ritchie, H. [2013, revised 2019]. "Life Expectancy." Published online at *OurWorldInData.org*. Retrieved from https://ourworldindata.org/life-expectancy [Online Resource].)

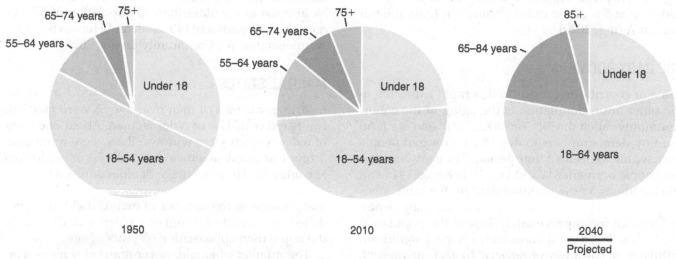

1950   2010   2040
                           Projected

Fig. 1.2 Percentage of the population in five age groups: United States, 1950, 2010, and 2060. (Data from the U.S. Census Bureau.)

GENDER AND ETHNIC DISPARITY

The Administration on Aging (2020) projects that racial and ethnic minority populations will represent 34% of the older population by 2040, an increase from 19% in 2008. It is projected that by 2040, the White non-Hispanic population will increase by 32%. During the same time period, the percentage of racial and ethnic minority persons of the same age cohort is expected to grow by 125% (Hispanics, 175%; African Americans, 88%; American Indian and Alaska Natives, 75%; and Asians, 113%).

Life expectancy within the U.S. population is variable. The populations of men and women are not equal, and in the older-than-65 age group, this dispro-portion is very noticeable. There are now 29.1 million older women to 23.3 million older men. Women cur-rently outlive men by 2.6 years, and Whites tend to live longer than Blacks, although disparities seem to be declining (Administration on Aging, 2020).

Current life expectancies in terms of race are as follows: White women, about 81 years; Black women, about 77.9 years; White men, 76.1 years; and Black men, 71.5 years. Hispanic people in the United States have a lower mortality and higher life expectancy than both non-Hispanic White and non-Hispanic Black people. Hispanic men can expect to live to 79.1 years; Hispanic women have the longest life expectancy of 84.2 years (Centers for Disease Control and Prevention, 2017). This longer life expectancy is known as the *Hispanic* or *Latino paradox*, suggesting that despite any socioeconomic disadvantages that may exist, Latino populations in the United States have lower premature mortality rates than White and Black populations; this has been documented in several Latin American countries as well (Chen et al., 2020).

In 2018, 23% of those over age 65 were identified as minorities. Approximately 9% were African American (not Hispanic), 5% Asian (not Hispanic), 0.5% American Indian and Alaska Native (not His-panic), 0.1% Native Hawaiian/Pacific Islander (not Hispanic). Some 0.8% identified themselves as being descended from two or more races. People identify-ing as "Hispanic origin (who may be of any race)" constituted 8% of the older population (Administra-tion on Aging, 2020).

THE BABY BOOMERS

A major contributing factor to this rapid explosion in the older adult population is the aging of the cohort commonly called the *baby boomers*. *Age cohort* is a term used by demographers to describe a group of people born within a specified time period. The baby boomers are people born after World War II, between 1946 and 1964. Although now outnumbered by the millennials (those born between 1982 and 2000), the baby boom-ers account for approximately 21% of the population (Statistica, 2020b) and continue to have a significant influence in all areas of society. In fact, at present, 10,000 baby boomers reach 65 years of age every day! It remains to be seen whether this group will expe-rience aging in the same way that previous genera-tions have or whether they will reinvent the aging and retirement experience. The oldest baby boomers reached age 65 in 2011; by 2029, all baby boomers will be 65 years of age or older. Based on the sheer size of this group, the older population in 2030 will be twice the size it was in 2000. The implications of this for all areas of society, particularly health care, are unprecedented.

? Critical Thinking

Demographics and You

- What impact will the changing demographics have on you personally?
- How is your community's age distribution changing?
- Are you a baby boomer? Do you find this to be an advantage or disadvantage as you age?
- Were you born after the baby boom? Before the baby boom? What difficulties do you expect to encounter as you age?

GEOGRAPHIC DISTRIBUTION OF THE OLDER ADULT POPULATION

The older adult population is not equally distributed throughout the United States. Climate, taxes, and other issues regarding the quality of life influence where older adults choose to live. All regions of the country are affected by the increase in life expectancy, but not to the same degree. In 2018, about half of the older-than-65 population resided in 9 states. In descending order of the older adult population, these states are California (5.7 million); Florida (4.4 million); Texas and New York (more than 3 million each); and Pennsylvania, Ohio, and Illinois (more than 2 million each). Michigan and North Carolina round out the list, each with 1.7 million resi-dents over the age of 65 (Fig. 1.3). Three states reported more than 20% of their residents as being over the age of 65: Florida, Maine, and West Virginia. Three states—including Alaska, Nevada, and Colorado—have shown an increase in the older-than-65 population of 57% or more (U.S. Department of Health and Human Services, Administration for Community Living, 2020a).

MARITAL STATUS

In 2019, some 69% of men over age 65 were married, compared with 47% of older women. About one-third of older women were widows; there were more than 3 times as many widows (8.9 million) as widowers (2.6 million). The percentage of older adults who were separated or divorced was approximately 15%. A fur-ther increase in the number of divorced elders is pre-dicted as a result of a higher incidence of divorce in the population approaching 65 years of age.

The number of single, never-married seniors rem-ains somewhat consistent at about 5% (women) to 6% (men) of the older-than-65 population (U.S. Depart-ment of Health and Human Services, 2020).

EDUCATIONAL STATUS

The educational level of the older adult population in the United States has increased dramatically over the past 3 decades. In 1970, only 28% of senior citizens had graduated from high school. By 2019, some 88% were high school graduates or more, and 31% had a

Persons Age 65 and Older as a Percentage of Total Population 2018

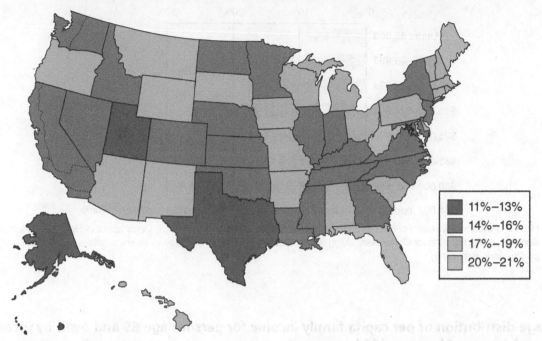

Fig. 1.3 Persons 65 years or older as a percentage of total population, 2018. (From the U.S. Department of Health and Human Services, Administration for Community Living. https://acl.gov/aging-and-disability-in-america/data-and-research/profile-older-americans)

bachelor's degree or higher. Completion of high school varied by race and ethnicity, with Whites (92%) completing high school at higher rates, followed by Asians (80%), African Americans (79%), and Hispanics (59%).

In addition to being better educated, today's older adult population is more technologically sophisticated. The World Economic Forum (2019) reports that 70% of Americans over age 65 use the internet. Also popular among older adults are apps such as Google Maps, with parking spot reminders, and Medisafe, a mobile medication management system. About 81% of adults in their 60s use a smartphone, dropping to 62% after age 70 (AARP, 2020a). Social networking sites, such as Facebook and LinkedIn, are used by a growing number of older adults.

ECONOMICS OF AGING

The stereotypical belief that many older adults are poor is not necessarily true. The economic status of older persons is as varied as that of other age groups. Some of the poorest people in the country are old, but so are some of the richest.

POVERTY

In 2018, over 5.1 million (9.7%) older adults lived at or below the poverty level A second indicator called the Supplemental Poverty Measure—which considers regional variations in housing costs, medical out-of-pocket expenses, and other factors—showed an even greater percentage of older adults (12.8%) living in poverty in 2019. Older women were more likely to be impoverished than older men. The highest rates of poverty were among older Hispanic women who live alone (37.8%).

INCOME

As of 2018, the median income of men over age 65 was $34,267, whereas that for women over age 65 was only $20,431. The median income of households headed by a person 65 years of age or older was approximately $64,023. Median income is the middle of the group, with half earning less and half earning more. It is not an average amount. Median figures can be deceptive because income is not distributed equally among Whites and minority groups (Fig. 1.4).

The major sources of aggregate income for older adults include Social Security benefits, asset income, pensions, and other earnings. Fig. 1.5 shows the sources of income for five different income levels (income quintiles).

Overall, Social Security income accounts for approximately 33% of the income for people age 65 and older. Of older adults who receive Social Security, half of those married and 70% of those unmarried rely on this benefit for 50% of their income. Average monthly Social Security income in 2020 was $1545 for a retired worker (Social Security Administration, 2020b). Low-earning

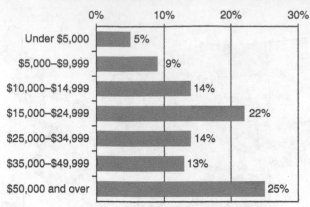

Persons Age 65 and Older Reporting Income, 2018

$25,601 median income for 52.8 million persons 65 and older reporting income.

Fig. 1.4 Percent distribution of the U.S. population by income, 2018. (From the U.S. Department of Health and Human Services, Administration for Community Living. https://acl.gov/aging-and-disability-in-america/data-and-research/profile-older-americans)

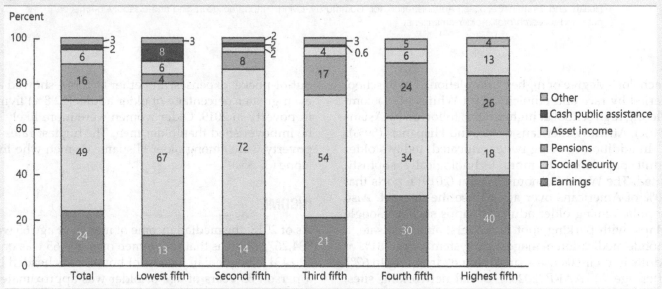

Percentage distribution of per capita family income for persons age 65 and over, by income quintile and source of income, 2014

NOTE: The definition of "other" includes, but is not limited to, unemployment compensation, workers' compensation, veterans' payments, and personal contributions. Quintile limits are $12,492, $19,245, $29,027, and $47,129. Estimates may not sum to the totals because of rounding.
Reference population: These data refer to the civilian noninstitutionalized population.
SOURCE: U.S. Census Bureau, Current Population Survey, Annual Social and Economic Supplement.

Fig. 1.5 Sources of income in the United States. (From the U.S. Census Bureau. https://agingstats.gov/docs/LatestReport/Older-Americans-2016-Key-Indicators-of-WellBeing.pdf)

individuals and couples are more likely to rely on Social Security as their major source of income. High earners are less reliant on Social Security.

Social Security funding may become inadequate as the number of retirees drawing benefits increases, while the pool of workers paying into the system decreases. There are presently 2.8 workers for each Social Security beneficiary; by 2035, this number will decrease to 2.3. People both within and outside the government have proposed plans to ensure the long-term survival of the Social Security program. If no changes are made, it is estimated that Social Security cash reserves will be depleted in 2034 (AARP, 2020b). This does not mean that the program will be bankrupt; rather, it will be able to pay out only what it collects through Social Security taxes.

Asset income—or income derived from investments such as stocks, bonds, and other retirement accounts—has dropped drastically since 2008. The economic downturn has been compared in severity with the Great Depression of the 1930s. Many retirees and those near retirement lost a large percentage of the monies they had saved and invested for retirement. Many of those who invested personally and those who had their money in employer-directed programs were severely affected. These financial losses have forced many individuals nearing retirement to continue working.

Approximately one-fifth of people age 65 and older receive pensions from public or private sources, although this varies by income quintile (see Fig. 1.5). People who retire from a government agency are more likely to receive a pension than those who retire from a private industry. Not only are former government employees more likely to receive pensions, but government pensions also tend to be more generous than those in the private sector because government wages have historically been below those of the private sector. The median federal government pension in 2018 was $30,061, the median state or local government pension was $22,546, and the median private pension or annuity was $9827 (Pension Rights Center, 2020).

Early retirement was popular from the 1970s until about 1985. Since then, the trend has shown more people working for pay after age 65. For those over age 65 who worked, the median weekly wage in the third quarter of 2020 was $1006 ($52,000 annually) (Bureau of Labor Statistics, 2020). This is typically significantly less than what the person earned earlier in life and reflects a decrease in hours worked and in wages. Additionally, these data were gathered during a pandemic that imposed unusual work practices on all people, but they are consistent with data trends of prior years.

Earnings make up a substantial portion of income for many people over age 65. Those who are in higher income brackets, generally professionals, may continue to work well beyond age 65 as long as they are healthy and interested in what they are doing. Socialization, time away from a retired spouse, intellectual challenge, and a sense of self-worth are verbalized as reasons for working, particularly by those in the baby boom generation. Some baby boomers need to continue to work to maintain the standard of living they desire. Some need to work because they neglected to save enough for retirement or need to make up for losses in their investments. Those in lower income brackets may need to continue to work, or to seek work, to pay for necessities of life or a few luxuries.

Legislation and political activism among older people have helped improve the economic outlook for older adults (Table 1.2). Beginning in 1965, key legislation was passed, including Medicare and Medicaid, establishment of the Administration on Aging, and the Older Americans Act, which supports numerous home- and community-based services such as Meals

Table 1.2	Legislation That Has Helped Older Adults
YEAR	**LEGISLATION**
1965	Medicare and Medicaid established Administration on Aging established Older Americans Act (OAA) passed
1967	Age Discrimination Act passed
1972	Supplemental Security Income Program instituted
	Social Security benefits indexed to reflect inflation, cost-of-living adjustment
	Nutrition Act passed, providing nutrition programs for older adults
1973	Council on Aging established
1978	Mandatory retirement age changed to 70 years
1986	Mandatory retirement age eliminated for most employees
1988	Catastrophic health insurance made part of Medicare
1990	Americans With Disabilities Act passed
1992	Vulnerable Elder Rights Protection Program initiated
1997	Balanced Budget Act (Medicare Part C) passed
2000	Amendment to Older Americans Act (nutrition programs) passed
2006	Drug Benefit Program added to Medicare
2010	The Patient Protection and Affordable Care Act passed
2016	Reauthorization of the Older Americans Act
2020	CARES Act passed

on Wheels, in-home services for older adults, elder abuse prevention, and caregiver support. In 2020, the Coronavirus Aid, Relief, and Economic Security (CARES) Act provided nearly $1 billion in grant funding to assist older adults who wished to shelter in place, pay for home-delivered meals, and offer many other resources designed to minimize exposure to COVID-19 (U.S. Department of Health and Human Services, Administration for Community Living, 2020b). Through activist organizations, older adults have united to consolidate their political power and to use the power of the vote to initiate programs that benefit them (Box 1.2). Over the past 25 years, these groups have helped to improve the economic welfare of older adults. The Federal Housing Authority and other lending agencies have proposed the use of reverse mortgages, which are plans that allow older adults to remain in their homes and receive monthly payments based on their home equity. Monthly income realized from these plans could range from hundreds to several thousands of dollars, depending on the property value and the age of the residents. The most common type of reverse mortgage is a Home Equity Conversion Mortgage (HECM). This money could be a much-needed income supplement for many older adults.

Box 1.2 **Politically Active Senior Citizen Groups**

AARP (FORMERLY KNOWN AS THE AMERICAN ASSOCIATION OF RETIRED PERSONS)

- Membership is open to people who are at least 50 years of age and their spouses (regardless of age).
- Currently has 38 million members.
- Uses volunteers and lobbyists to advance the political and economic interests of older adults.
- Provides a wide variety of membership benefits, including insurance programs and discounts.
- Was instrumental in helping to enact Medicare in 1965.

AMERICAN SENIORS ASSOCIATION (ASA)

- Does not report current numbers but claims to be the fastest-growing senior advocacy group in America.
- Describes itself as the "conservative alternative to AARP."

ALLIANCE FOR RETIRED AMERICANS (ARA)

- Reports 4.3 million members.
- Focuses on political and legislative issues.
- Formerly known as the National Council of Senior Citizens.
- Occasionally clashes with AARP on issues such as Medicare drug benefits.

NATIONAL COUNCIL OF GRAY PANTHERS NETWORKS (NCGPN, FORMERLY GRAY PANTHERS)

- As a social justice action network, is involved in the promotion of economic security, civil rights, marriage equality, and other issues.
- Has approximately 500 activists from 32 states.
- In addition, has 16 local Gray Panthers Networks with an estimated 500 additional activists.
- Issues action alerts on important senior issues; maintains an active NCGPN Facebook page.

Box 1.3 **Factors That Influence the Economic Conditions of Older Adults**

- Many older adults bought their homes when housing costs and inflation were low. If they have paid off their mortgages, their housing costs are limited to taxes, maintenance, and utility bills.
- The number of older adults who receive pensions is greater now than it will be in the future. Businesses now offer smaller pensions to fewer employees, and the traditional "defined benefit" pensions have largely been replaced by "defined contribution" pensions, which are affected by stock market fluctuations.
- Older adults qualify for several tax breaks that are unavailable to younger people.
- Most older adults pay no Social Security taxes; younger working adults pay increasingly higher rates.
- Social Security and government pensions are largely exempt from taxation.
- Taxpayers older than 65 years of age can take additional tax deductions.
- If an older adult is a homeowner and sells the home, a one-time capital gains tax exclusion applies.
- Most older adults qualify for government income programs.
- Some 97% of people over age 60 receive Social Security benefits or will in the future (Center on Budget and Policy Priorities, 2020a).
- More than 61 million people were Medicare recipients in 2015 (Kaiser Family Foundation, 2020).
- More than 2 million low-income, blind, or disabled older adults receive Supplemental Security Income (SSI) (Center on Budget and Policy Priorities, 2018).

Reverse mortgages are not right for everyone, however. Extremely high fees, up to $40,000, are associated with them, and such payments can become due in full if the older person moves out of the home for a year or more—which is not outside the realm of possibilities if the person experienced a serious illness and placement in a care facility. In such a case, it is possible that such a person might need to sell the home to repay the HECM (Nolo.com, 2020).

Some older adults may choose not to seek economic help despite the numerous assistance programs designed for them. Many people are suspicious of "getting something for nothing" or are reluctant to disclose personal financial details, which is necessary to qualify for most assistance programs. Many older people feel that asking for help is humiliating. Some fear that they will lose what little they have if they seek assistance. As in all age groups, other older people have no difficulty seeking or, in some cases, demanding financial assistance or concessions. Factors that can affect the financial well-being of older adults are described in Box 1.3.

Be sensitive in dealing with the financial issues of older adults. The Critical Thinking box should help you assess your attitudes, and therefore your sensitivity, toward these kinds of situations. Many older adults who find it easy to talk about their intimate physical and medical problems are reluctant to discuss finances. Nurses may suspect financial need if an older person lacks adequate shelter, clothing, heat, food, or medical attention. When an economic problem causes real or potential dangers, be prepared to respond appropriately.

? Critical Thinking

Your Sensitivity to the Financial Problems of Older Adults

Respond to the following statements:
- Older adults control all of the money in the country.
- Most older adults are poor.
- Older adults have it easy; the younger working people have it rough.
- Older adults have too much political power, and they get too many benefits and entitlements.
- Older adults worked for what they are getting, and they deserve everything they receive from the government.
- A society that does not care for its older people is cruel and uncivilized.
- The properties of older adults should be used to pay for their physical needs and medical care.

Because regulations covering assistance programs often change, it is difficult for older patients and the nurses trying to help them to keep current and up to date. Nurses may be called on to help older adults deal with the paperwork required when they are applying for assistance, to provide emotional support as they work through frustrating bureaucratic processes, or to arrange transportation to the appropriate agencies. Nurses usually are not expected to be experts in this area, but they should know how to locate appropriate resources. Nurses working in community health should be aware of community agencies providing assistance to older adults so that appropriate referrals can be made. Nurses working in hospitals and nursing homes can initiate referrals to social workers or other professionals who are knowledgeable about assistance programs. Most states and counties throughout the United States have services for older adults or departments on aging. These are typically listed in the government section of a telephone directory or on government websites. Many publish directories of resources available in their specific community.

WEALTH

Although many older people receive less cash on a yearly basis from Social Security and pensions than some younger individuals earn, a substantial number have accumulated assets and savings from their working years. Frugal lifestyles and self-reports by older adults of being "poor" should be viewed cautiously. Some individuals are truly impoverished, whereas others have significant assets.

In 2019, approximately 78% of Americans over 65 years of age owned their homes (Statistica, 2020a). A home is usually an older person's largest asset. Many older people choose not to sell their homes because they fear that they will have nowhere to live. Many prefer to remain "house rich and cash poor," making do on a limited income, rather than sell their homes.

Economic well-being is usually measured in terms of income, which is the amount of money a household receives on a weekly, monthly, or yearly basis. However, this measurement is not always a reliable indicator of financial security in older adults. People older than 65 years of age generally have more discretionary income (i.e., money left after paying for necessities, such as housing, food, and medical care) available than do younger people. Younger individuals, particularly those with growing families, may have a higher income, but they also have higher nondiscretionary demands.

HOUSING ARRANGEMENTS

Many people assume that older adults live in senior citizen housing or nursing homes. They are wrong. Most older adults live either with a spouse or alone. Approximately 3% of adults over age 75 live in institutional settings, such as nursing homes, although this figure increases to about 10% for people over age 85 (Federal Interagency Forum on Aging-Related Statistics, 2020).

Older individuals often try to keep their homes, despite the physical or economic difficulties of doing so. A home is more than just a physical shelter; it represents independence and security. The home holds many memories. Being in a familiar neighborhood close to friends and church is important. A sense of community is important to many older adults, who dislike the thought of leaving security for the unknown. The physical exertion and emotional trauma involved in moving can be intimidating, even overwhelming, to older adults. Moving to a different, often smaller residence is a difficult decision, particularly when it involves giving up precious possessions due to lack of space.

For some older people, keeping the family home is not a sensible option for many reasons. Many of the homes owned by older adults are in central cities with high crime rates. Expenses, such as increasingly high property taxes and ongoing maintenance costs, often put excessive strain on older persons with limited financial resources. Home maintenance, including even simple tasks such as housecleaning, becomes increasingly difficult with advancing age or illness. Ownership may require more effort in terms of money and time than some older people possess, yet many struggle to remain independent and keep their homes.

Some older individuals remain in their own homes and refuse to give them up long after it is safe for them to be alone. They may be able to cope as long as family, friends, and neighbors are willing to help. However, if there is a change in their support system, dangerous, life-threatening situations may arise. Some older people try to live in their homes despite broken plumbing, inadequate heat, and insufficient access to food. Families, health care professionals, and social service agencies may have to step in to protect the welfare of these aging individuals.

Some older people recognize the problems associated with living alone and decide to seek housing arrangements that are better matched to their needs and abilities. They may move into an apartment, condominium, senior complex, or other type of housing. As the older adult population grows, new types of housing and living arrangements are evolving (Fig. 1.6). The following Critical Thinking box should help you examine your attitudes toward housing for older adults.

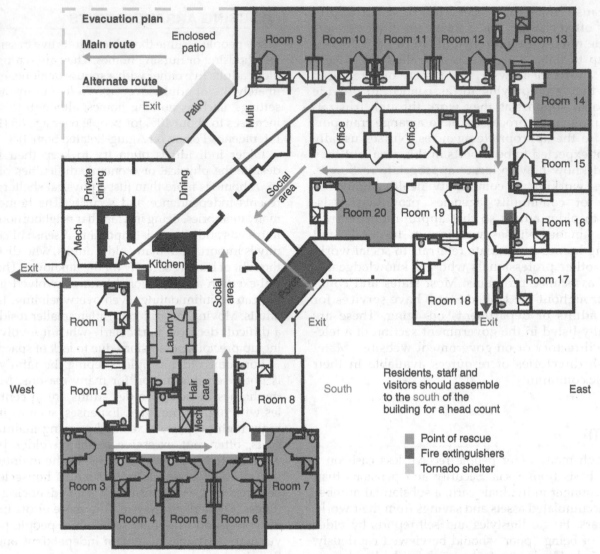

Fig. 1.6 A living plan for a community-based residential facility with evacuation plan. (Courtesy Elness Swenson Graham Architects, Inc., Minneapolis, MN.)

? Critical Thinking

Your Attitudes Toward Housing for Older Adults

- Is it safe for older adults to remain indefinitely in their own homes?
- When should an older person sell their home?
- Once a home is sold, what are the best types of living accommodations for older adults?
- What kinds of alternative housing for older adults are available in your community?
- Should older adults live in housing that is separated from people in other age groups? Why? Why not?

Independent or assisted living centers are becoming common. These centers combine privacy with easily available services. Most consist of private apartments that are either purchased or rented. For additional charges, the residents can be served meals in restaurant-style dining rooms and receive laundry and housekeeping services (Fig. 1.7). Different levels of medical, nursing, and personal care services are

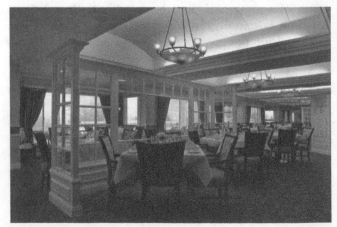

Fig. 1.7 Dining room in an assisted living facility. (Photo courtesy Era Living, Seattle, WA.)

available. Health care services may include assistance with hygiene, routine medication administration, and even preventive health clinics. Many centers have communal activity rooms, arts-and-crafts hobby centers, swimming pools, lounges, beauty salons, mini-grocery stores, greenhouses, and other amenities. Transportation to church, shopping, and other appointments is provided by some of these facilities. Most independent and assisted living facilities are privately operated, and costs are significant—although far cheaper than nursing home care. Some states offer subsidies to older individuals with limited resources because these living arrangements are often more cost-effective than other housing alternatives.

? Did You Know?

Cruise Care

Some older adults are choosing to live on cruise ships instead of assisted living or long-term-care facilities. The ship provides a higher employee-to-resident ratio, more activities, more and better choices of food, better scenery, and more companionship for a lower price than nursing homes and a comparable price to assisted living facilities. Additionally, they have physicians and nurses on board (Bandoim, 2019). Although not appropriate for individuals suffering from dementia or immune compromise or those who require frequent medical appointments, cruise care might be an option (at least temporarily) for some adventurous seniors.

Life-lease or life-contract facilities are another housing option. For a large initial investment and substantial monthly rental and service fees, older persons or couples are guaranteed a residence for life. Independent residents occupy apartment units, but extended-care units are either attached to the apartment complex or located nearby for residents who require skilled nursing services. If one spouse needs skilled care, the other may continue to live in the apartment and can easily visit the hospitalized loved one. When the occupants die, control of the apartment reverts to the owners of the facility. The costs for this type of housing are high and may be out of the range of the average older adult. However, despite the costs, many find this option appealing because it meets their needs for independence, socialization, and services. Many find security in knowing that skilled care is easily available if needed.

Less wealthy older adults have fewer housing options. Some older adults qualify for government-subsidized housing if they meet certain financial standards and limits. Government-subsidized housing units may be simple apartments without any special services, or they may have limited services, such as access to nursing clinics and special transportation arrangements. Most communities are finding that the demand for these facilities exceeds the availability. Waiting lists with up to 2-year delays are common; some communities award the housing via lotteries. Interpretation of government regulations is causing some concern with regard to senior citizen housing. Residences originally intended for older adults may be required to accept a variety of medically disabled people regardless of age. Some of these younger residents suffer from psychiatric or drug-related problems, and the presence of these individuals may leave older adult residents feeling threatened and unsafe.

Some older adults who are not related to each other are forming group housing plans. In this type of arrangement, unrelated people share a household in which they have private bedrooms but share the common recreational and leisure areas as well as home maintenance tasks. Some communities offer services to help match people who are interested in this option. Roommates are selected so that the strengths of one individual compensate for the weaknesses of the other. In some cases, a large house may shelter 10 or more residents. Not all such arrangements are limited to older adults. In some situations, younger adults who need reasonable housing may be included. By providing services for older adult residents, the younger residents can reduce their rental costs. Both younger and older individuals who have chosen this option report benefits from the extended-family atmosphere.

A more formal type of group home, called a community-based residential facility (CBRF), is available in some communities. For a monthly fee, this type of facility provides services such as room and board, help with activities of daily living (ADLs), medication assistance, yearly medical examinations, information and referrals, leisure activities, and recreational or therapeutic programs. Fees for this type of housing may be paid by the individual or may be provided by county or state agencies. Most of these facilities provide private or semiprivate rooms with community areas for dining and socialization.

Older adults who require more extensive assistance may need placement in nursing homes or extended-care facilities. Nursing homes provide room and board, personal care, and medical and nursing services. They are licensed by individual states and regulated by federal and state laws. Three levels of care are provided by nursing homes: skilled care, intermediate care, and custodial care. Skilled care is daily nursing care, including medication administration and skilled treatments or procedures that require the expertise of licensed nurses. It also includes services performed by specially trained professionals, such as speech, physical, occupational, and respiratory therapists. Intermediate care describes professional care that is not required on a daily basis. It is a step down from skilled care. Custodial care is the next step down and refers to care that is considered nonskilled personal care, such as assistance with ADLs.

Subacute care facilities provide comprehensive inpatient care designed for individuals who have an

? Critical Thinking

Nursing Home Insurance

Medicare will pay for a maximum of 100 days in a skilled care facility after a 3-day hospital stay. After that time, the cost of care is usually the responsibility of the older person or their family unless they qualify for Medicaid. In light of this, do you think that people approaching retirement should purchase nursing home insurance? Why or why not?

acute illness, injury, or exacerbation of a disease process. Subacute care falls between the traditional care provided in an acute care hospital and that provided in a skilled nursing home. For example, a ventilator-dependent patient or someone requiring frequent respiratory treatments would find appropriate care in a subacute facility.

Specialty care facilities—such as residences designed to meet the special needs of people with Alzheimer disease or other memory loss and their families—are gaining in popularity around the country. Other specialty care facilities are numerous and include inpatient hospice facilities, long-term care spinal cord injury facilities, and skilled nursing facilities that provide dialysis treatment.

HEALTH CARE PROVISIONS

Health care is a major area of concern in the United States. Everyone wants the best and most comprehensive medical care for themselves and their families. The expense of this level of care is the problem. At one time, individuals were personally responsible for the payment of physician and hospital bills. This gradually changed, and health care insurance, either individually purchased or paid for by an employer, became the norm. Insurance companies paid the bills, and the individual became less aware and involved in the rising cost of health care.

Government played a minimal role until the establishment of Medicare in 1965.

MEDICARE AND MEDICAID

Medicare is the government program that provides health care funding for older adults and disabled persons. Medicare is a popular program, and most Americans believe that it must be preserved. This has become increasingly difficult as the baby boom generation has become older; by 2030, all people in this cohort will be Medicare eligible. In 2020, Medicare provided coverage for approximately 61.2 million citizens (Kaiser Family Foundation, 2020). By 2050, this number is expected to swell to 90.7 million citizens (Kaiser Family Foundation, 2021). Most Americans older than 65 years of age qualify for Medicare.

Medicare has four distinct programs, none of which pays all of the health care costs. Medicare Part A is hospital insurance. It covers inpatient hospital care; skilled nursing care following hospitalization; some home health services, such as visiting nurses and occupational, speech, or physical therapists; and hospice services, but only after the patient pays an initial deductible and any copayments. During the 1980s, Medicare instituted the diagnosis-related group (DRG) system in an attempt to contain hospital costs. Under this system, a hospital is paid a set amount based on the patient's admitting diagnosis. If the patient is discharged in fewer days than predicted, the hospital keeps the excess money. If the patient needs to stay longer than projected, the hospital absorbs the additional costs. Although DRGs have resulted in cost reduction, they have also led to the discharge of people "quicker and sicker" than in the past. Many older people are released from the hospital before they have actually recovered from their illnesses, placing a greater health care burden on families and home health agencies.

Medicare Part B is medical insurance for outpatient care. It is optional, but most people choose this coverage. This plan covers 80% of the "customary and usual" rates charged by providers after deductibles are met. In addition to providers' fees, Medicare Part B covers medically necessary ambulance transport; physical, speech, and occupational therapy; home health services when medically necessary; mental health services; x-rays and lab tests; chiropractic care; medical supplies and equipment; and outpatient surgery or blood transfusions. The patient is responsible for the remaining 20% of the costs plus the difference between the actual fee and the government's "customary and usual" rate. The true costs of medical care often exceed the amount that the government pays. Many older adults pay for private supplemental health care insurance to cover these expenses rather than pay out of pocket.

Medicare Part C, or Medicare Advantage Plans, are optional plans offered by private companies approved by Medicare to individuals who are eligible for Part A and enrolled in Part B. These plans allow beneficiaries to receive their Medicare benefits through private insurance companies. The older adult enrolls in a private plan, such as a health maintenance organization (HMO) or preferred provider organization (PPO). These plans are designed to cover total costs, so that supplemental insurance coverage is not necessary. They usually also include prescription drug benefits. They do, however, limit the pool of available health care providers, and premiums and rules vary depending on the plan selected.

Medicare Part D, or prescription drug coverage, is a voluntary plan available to anyone enrolled in Part A or B of Medicare. It includes both stand-alone prescription plans and Medicare Advantage drug plans.

Under Part D, prescription drugs are distributed through local pharmacies and administered by a wide variety of private insurance plans. In many plans, there is a significant gap between the cost of the drugs and the benefits provided. After meeting a deductible, recipients of Medicare Part D pay 25% of their prescription costs until they reach the out-of-pocket spending limit and qualify for catastrophic coverage; in 2020, this spending limit was $6350 (Medicare Interactive, 2021).

Supplemental Medicaid (Title 19) assistance may be available for those older adults who meet certain financial need requirements. Many of those who have assets do not qualify; they are left with a Medicare gap (or "medigap") that they must fill (pay for) themselves. Many older people buy private medical insurance—often at unreasonable prices—to pay medical bills that are not covered by Medicare. The Affordable Care Act mandated states to expand Medicaid coverage; however, not all states have expanded coverage at this time.

 Critical Thinking

Medicaid and Personal Assets

Do you think that people should qualify for Medicaid if they hold valuable assets—that is, if they own a home or expensive cars? Or do you think they should liquidate their assets (i.e., sell the home and cars) before receiving Medicaid? Why or why not?

RISING COSTS AND LEGISLATIVE ACTIVITY

The costs of health care have increased dramatically in recent years. The United States spends more money on health care than any other country in the world, yet such care is not provided for all U.S. citizens. Many other nations do a better job of meeting their citizens' health care needs.

The Centers for Medicare & Medicaid Services (2020) reported that the United States spent approximately $3.8 trillion on health care in 2019. This accounts for 17.7% of our gross domestic product. A significant proportion of health care spending is spent on the older adult population. These costs are staggering, especially considering the expanding population of older adults. There has been an upsurge in initiatives to contain health care costs, such as managed care and insurance reform. If we expect to continue to provide adequate health care in the future, we can expect to see more changes in the way health care is financed and delivered. This is a major and often divisive political issue.

The cost of Medicare alone has grown dramatically from $3 billion in 1967, the first year of funding, to $55.5 billion in 1983; $297 billion in 2004; $551 billion in 2012; and $799 billion in 2019. The Congressional Budget Office (CBO) (2019) projects that it will surpass $1 trillion in 2023 and hit $1.5 trillion ($1500 billion) in 2029 (Fig. 1.8). The recipients of Medicare, however, pay quite a bit in out-of-pocket expenses: some 50% of typical Medicare recipients pay approximately 16% of their income on health care and premium costs (Noel-Miller, 2020).

The Patient Protection and Affordable Care Act (PPACA) was signed into law in 2010. It includes numerous health-related provisions designed to take effect over several years. This legislative initiative includes major changes in health insurance, health care funding, student loans, and a wide range of spending considerations. The costs of these provisions are to be offset by a variety of taxes, fees, and cost-saving measures.

There is a great deal of controversy regarding the PPACA because its long-term effects are still unknown. Those in favor of the legislation cite expanded coverage, greater competition among insurance companies, coverage of people with preexisting medical conditions, and closure of the donut hole affecting senior citizens (a large funding gap that placed a burden on older adults for medication payment; the donut hole "closed" in 2020) . Those opposed to the legislation cite cuts in Medicare funding, cuts in the Medicare Advantage program, increases in the Medicare tax, and expansion of Medicaid. They fear increased costs of health care, more taxes, and decreased incentives to primary care providers.

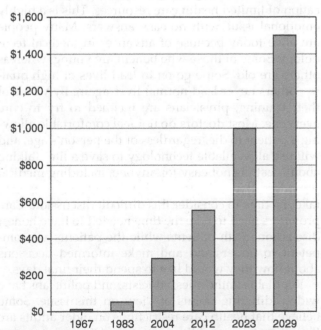

Projected Medicare Spending in Billions of Dollars

Fig. 1.8 Projected Medicare spending in billions of dollars. (Data from Congressional Budget Office, 2019, Medicare—CBO's May 2019 Baseline. https://www.cbo.gov/system/files/2019-05/51302-2019-05-medicare_0.pdf and Congressional Budget Office, 2020, 10-Year Budget Projections and Historical Budget Data. https://www.cbo.gov/about/products/budget-economic-data#2)

Legal challenges regarding the constitutionality of this bill were raised by several states, yet it was ruled constitutional by the U.S. Supreme Court in June of 2012. In writing the majority opinion, however, Justice John Roberts stated that the program is a tax—which may pave the way for different legal challenges. Efforts are now under way to strike down the entire PPACA, which would result in 21 million people becoming uninsured and millions more being denied health insurance due to preexisting conditions (Center on Budget and Policy Priorities, 2020b). Health care providers should pay attention, because this legislation is likely to have an impact on how health care is provided and funded. Other aspects of the law continue to be challenged in court.

COSTS AND END-OF-LIFE CARE

Not all older people use the available health care resources equally. Most health care services are consumed by the very ill or terminally ill minority, many of whom happen to be older adults. It is estimated that between 13% and 25% of all Medicare dollars spent on those 65 years of age or older was spent on beneficiaries in their last year of life (Duncan et al., 2019). Despite this, those patients' personal assets are quite often depleted. Serious questions are being raised about the appropriateness of using intensive, expensive interventions to extend the lives of terminally ill older people.

Financial concerns are forcing health care providers and society to face ethical dilemmas regarding the allocation of limited health care resources. This is a highly emotional issue with no easy answers. Many people are alive today because of advances in medical technology. Some of those who benefit are young, whereas others are old. Some go on to lead lives of high quality; others never lead normal lives again. By virtue of their training, physicians are inclined to try to cure everyone. Most doctors do not feel comfortable allowing a patient to die, regardless of the person's age, and will use all available technology to save a life. Talking about death is not easy for anyone, including medical providers. It is easier to avoid end-of-life issues than to take the time to consider this difficult discussion. Care providers need to take the time needed to have honest discussions with patients while the patients are competent to understand and make informed decisions about how they would like to spend their final days.

Reputable authorities, ethicists, and politicians have widely differing points of view on this issue. Some believe that health care restrictions on older adults are the ultimate in age discrimination. Others argue that the benefits gained, which can usually be measured in months, do not outweigh the costs. Private citizens examining this dilemma are equally confused. Even those who believe that health care costs are excessive frequently want everything possible done to save their lives or those of their loved ones. This moral, ethical, and legal dilemma has no simple solution. Part of the debate regarding health care reform involves differing viewpoints regarding end-of-life care. Perhaps this issue will encourage an honest national discussion among spouses, families, spiritual advisors, physicians, and other health care providers.

The following Critical Thinking box is designed to increase your awareness of and insight into these problems.

? Critical Thinking

Your Understanding of the Health Care Dilemma

- Should an 80-year-old person have coronary bypass surgery at a cost of approximately $123,000? A cardiac transplant at a cost of approximately $1.3 million?
- Should dialysis be provided to individuals older than 65 years of age? Older than 75? Older than 85?
- Should people older than age 65 receive organ transplants?
- Should a ventilator be used on a terminally ill patient?
- Are feeding tubes a part of basic physical care or are they extraordinary means?
- Should the individual, family, or primary care provider decide on the type and amount of medical intervention necessary?
- What should be the role of the government in health care?

ADVANCE DIRECTIVES AND PHYSICIAN ORDERS FOR LIFE-SUSTAINING TREATMENT

All adults who are 18 years of age or older and of sound mind have the right to make decisions regarding the amount and type of health care they desire. Because older adults are more likely to experience significant health problems, the question of what and how much medical care to administer must be addressed. Such important decisions are best made during a stress-free time when the individual is alert and experiencing no acute health problems. A person's wishes can best be communicated using advance directives, which are legally recognized documents that specify the types of care and treatment that individuals desire when they cannot speak for themselves. Typically included in advance directives are: (1) do not resuscitate/do not attempt to resuscitate (DNR/DNAR) and allow natural death (AND) orders, (2) directives related to mechanical ventilation, and (3) directives related to artificial nutrition and hydration.

Two formal types of advance directives are recognized in most states: (1) the durable power of attorney for health care and (2) the living will. Information about both of these is typically provided when someone enters the hospital. Each patient is expected to make a decision about the type and extent of care to be administered if their condition becomes terminal.

These documents are designed to help guide the family and medical professionals in planning care. The family is often relieved to have this information when they are making difficult decisions during a stressful time. Advance directives are generally recognized and respected, but various agencies or health care providers may have beliefs or policies that prohibit them from honoring certain advance directives. Individuals should discuss their wishes with their health care providers when these documents are written. If there are irreconcilable differences between an individual and the care provider, changes in either the document or the care provider must be considered.

A durable power of attorney for health care transfers the authority to make health care decisions to another person, called the *health care agent*. The agent may act only in situations in which the persons involved are unable to make such decisions for themselves. Because the health care agent must be trusted to follow through with the older person's wishes, the agent specified in the document is usually a family member or friend. These wishes are specified in writing and usually witnessed by unrelated individuals so as to reduce the possibility of undue influence. Standardized legal forms are available to initiate a power of attorney for health care.

A living will informs the physician that the individual wishes to die naturally if a terminal illness develops or if the person receives an injury that cannot be cured. Living wills prohibit the use of life-prolonging measures and equipment when the individual is near death or in a persistent vegetative state. Living wills go into effect only when two physicians agree in writing that the necessary criteria have been met.

Usually, either of these documents is adequate to communicate a person's wishes; both are not needed. Those who choose to initiate both documents should ensure that there is no conflict between the directions provided in each document. Either document can be revoked at any time. An advance directive should be stored in a safe place where it can be located easily when needed. A safe deposit box is not recommended for this purpose. Family members and the family lawyer should know the content of the document and its location. An advance directive should be provided to the primary care provider so that it becomes part of the patient's permanent medical record. These documents are often required and kept available for emergency situations when an individual resides in an institutional setting such as an independent or assisted-living apartment, community-based residential facility, or nursing home.

Laws and specifics differ from state to state. Nurses should be aware of the legal standing of such documents in the particular state where they practice and should understand any legal ramifications engendered by these documents. Physician orders for life-sustaining treatment (POLST) is a legal document that has been adopted by almost every state and takes the person's wishes further by creating actual doctor's orders to be carried out by emergency personnel. The POLST contains three or four sections, depending on the state, including specifics about cardiopulmonary resuscitation (CPR) (whether to attempt resuscitation or allow natural death), medical interventions (comfort care, limited interventions, or full treatment including when to transfer to hospital), antibiotics (use freely, use for comfort, or do not use at all), and artificial nutrition (no tube feeding, trial of tube feeding, or long-term tube feeding). The POLST is printed on bright paper, the color of which is determined by the state, and signed by the physician and patient. Sample POLST forms are freely available on the internet.

> ### ? Critical Thinking
>
> **Advance Directives and Physician Orders for Life-Sustaining Treatment (POLST)**
>
> - How would you as a nurse approach a patient regarding the initiation of an advance directive?
> - Can a person who is diagnosed with Alzheimer disease initiate a living will or durable power of attorney?
> - Does your state have POLST?
> - How do hospitals and extended-care facilities identify a patient's advance directive?

IMPACT OF AGING MEMBERS OF THE FAMILY

The family is undergoing significant change in our society. Many factors—including increasing divorce rates, single parenting, coparenting, and a mobile population—are creating a less stable, less predictable family structure. Blended families, extended families, and separated families all present challenges. In addition to these societal changes, the demographic changes discussed previously are having and will continue to have repercussions that we can only begin to appreciate (Box 1.4).

Families today face historically unprecedented situations. Because of the lifespan extension, it is not

> ### Box 1.4   Demographic Changes Affecting the Family
>
> - Because of extended lifespans, the number of family members over age 65 is growing.
> - More people are living with chronic conditions and need some degree of care or assistance.
> - The number of people in the younger generations is decreasing in proportion to the number of older members.
> - There is a growing number of widows who may be unprepared to provide for their own needs and will need assistance.
> - The role of women is changing. As women increasingly must work outside the home, many are attempting to meet the demands of their parents as well as their homes, children, and workplaces.

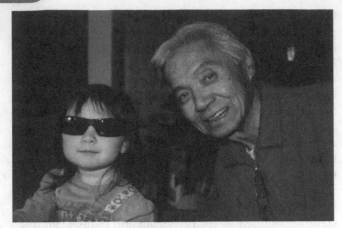

Fig. 1.9 Fun—quality time with granddaughter.

uncommon for 4 or 5 generations of a family to be alive at one time (Fig. 1.9). Until recently, this was unheard of. Using 20 years as a typical generation, a family might resemble the one described in Table 1.3. If the generation time is less than 20 years, even more generations might be alive at the same time.

REFLECTION BY A NURSING PROFESSOR

Some years ago, as death was approaching for a 91-year-old gentleman, his family gathered at the hospital. His wife of 69 years asked that "the children" come into the room. This sounded rather strange because "the children" were all in their 60s, the grandchildren were all mature adults, and the great-grandchildren were fast approaching adulthood. It sounded even stranger to me, because this older man was my grandfather, and my father was "the baby" of the family.

Gloria Wold

Many older adults who need care will receive assistance, both economic and physical, from their families. The problems encountered in such situations can differ widely, depending on the respective ages of the family members. In some families, the "children" who are attempting to provide care for the oldest members are likely to be past age 65 themselves. They may have health problems of their own that make caregiving difficult or impractical. They may also have financial obligations to their own children, such as paying for education.

Table 1.3   The Family

AGE (YEARS)	GENERATION
80+	Parents
60+	Children
40+	Grandchildren
20+	Great-grandchildren
Less than 20	Great-great-grandchildren

Middle-aged family members often become the caregivers. The generation in their 40s and early 50s is sometimes called the *sandwich* generation because its members are caught in the middle—trying to work, to raise their own children, and perhaps provide assistance to one or two generations of aging family members. Sometimes they are also trying to help raise grandchildren by giving financial or physical assistance.

Although the financial, psychologic, and physical demands of assisting aging relatives affect all family members, women are likely to be the most affected. It is estimated that 75% of the caregivers in the United States are female (Box 1.5). Typically, sons contribute financially, but the brunt of the burden of emotional and physical care falls on the daughters. It is estimated that as the population ages, women will spend more time caring for their parents than they did caring for their children.

Families try to help aging family members in many ways. If the older adult is able to live alone, families may assist by visiting frequently and helping with transportation to shopping and medical appointments. Some prepare meals, help with housecleaning, and make major home repairs. Running between two households and trying to maintain both can be mentally and physically exhausting, but many are willing to help their loved ones in any way they can.

A family crisis may occur when the aging person is no longer able to live alone. Important decisions must be made. Most families find that there is no perfect solution. The two most common options are bringing the aging parent into the home of one of the children or placing the parent in an assisted living or long-term care facility. There are problems and concerns with any option that requires a major change in living arrangements. It is essential that the family making this difficult decision consider many factors. The amount of care needed by the parent; the availability of a willing and able family member; the amount of available space in the child's home; the added financial and emotional burden of an additional household member;

Box 1.5   Caregivers in the United States

Data from Family Caregiver Alliance: *Caregiver Statistics: Demographics* https://www.caregiver.org/caregiver-statistics-demographics

- The average caregiver age is 49 years.
- About 49% of caregivers are caring for a parent or parent-in-law.
- Some 75% of caregivers are female, and female caregivers typically spend more time providing care and performing personal care tasks.
- Family caregivers spend an average of 24.4 hours per week in giving care.
- The average duration of caregiving for a family caregiver is 4 years.

the wishes of the parent, the child, and the child's family; and the interpersonal dynamics within the family must all be considered before a decision is made.

Children may take older parents into their homes when the older parents can no longer maintain their own homes. Although this arrangement works well in some families, in others it is problematic for everyone involved. The familiar roles and responsibilities are often reversed when children step in and attempt to take care of their parents. This places the aging person into the role of the child, which they usually resent strongly. "Don't tell your mother what to do!" or "I'm still your father!" is often heard in such parent-child interactions.

Loss of independence is probably the most significant issue that aging parents and their children must face. The aging family members have spent decades making their own decisions. As independent adults, they made their own choices about where to live, what to do, and when to do it. They chose what to eat, obtained their food, and prepared it without interference. They went to bed when and where they chose. They went where they wanted to go without asking permission. They had control of their lives. Most independent adults do not want to ask anyone for help.

As physical changes or diseases affect older adults, some or all of their independent function may be lost. Aging people find it difficult to accept that they can no longer do the things they once did. It is also distressing for the family to watch their loved ones change. While the aging person tries to cope with these changes, the family tries to determine how to respond. If "the right thing to do" is not obvious, family members begin to experience mixed feelings and confusion. Feelings of grief, anger, frustration, and loss are common in all affected individuals.

When an older adult moves in with a child's family, the dynamics within the home are unavoidably changed. The ability of the family to adapt and cope with an additional member of the household varies greatly from situation to situation. If all parties are agreeable to the move and if the older adult can be given enough privacy to maintain independence, the blending of the older person into the child's home may be successful. Some families feel that having a resident grandparent can be rewarding and enriching. However, if the presence of the older person intrudes excessively on the family unit, the situation may be unpleasant for both the family and the older person.

If the older family member requires a substantial amount of physical care, the demands on family members can be intense. Nevertheless, many children feel duty bound to care for their aging parents. This sense of obligation may be based on cultural, religious, or personal beliefs. If the children determine that they are unable to care for their parent and instead opt for nursing home placement, the children often feel that they have failed in their responsibilities. This can lead to intense feelings of guilt even if nursing home placement is the most realistic and reasonable option.

THE NURSE AND FAMILY INTERACTIONS

When we as nurses care for older adults, particularly in hospital or nursing home settings, we see the person only as they are now. We often forget that these people have not always been old. They lived, loved, worked, argued, and wept as we all do. Often, the older adults we care for are very ill or infirm and, as nurses, we tend to focus on their physical needs, cares, and treatments. In our preoccupation with our duties, we can easily lose our perspective of the older patient as both a person and a member of a family.

In hospitals and nursing homes, family members come and go. Some families show a great deal of interest and concern for their aging members, visit regularly, and interact with the patient and staff. This allows us to increase our understanding and appreciation of our patients as people. Other older individuals may never have family members visit them. They seem to be alone in the world, even though the medical record lists children and their telephone numbers for emergencies. Even in home settings, family attention and interaction vary greatly. In some households, a great deal of interest is given to each family member; in others, little or none is shown. Why do we see such a wide variation of family attention?

The answer often lies in family dynamics and processes that began long ago when the older adult was a young spouse and parent. Some families are very stable and cohesive. They are together often and share close, loving bonds. They have developed healthy methods for interacting, responding, and meeting each other's needs. Because of the strong bonds that have developed over many years, these families remain interested in and supportive of their aging members.

Other families never develop the closeness that is ideal in a family. The family unit may have been disrupted by divorce, mental illness, or other serious problems. There may have been problems with abuse, alcohol use disorder, or drugs. Long-term problems that have developed over time do not go away when a person gets old. When the family unit is weak, supportive behavior from family members is unlikely.

Most families we interact with fall somewhere between these extremes. Few families are perfect and few are terrible. Families are made up of human beings who respond to stress in many different ways. Coping with the stresses related to aging is difficult for both the older adult and the family. The behavior we see at any given time is the best that the person is capable of at that moment. That does not mean that it is the best that they will be capable of at some other time. We as nurses need to examine the stresses affecting the family so that we can best respond to the needs of all family members. The following Critical Thinking box should help you determine your stress factors.

You and Your Family

Complete the following:

When my parents are unable to care for themselves, I will
_____.

If both my parents and grandparents were alive and in need of assistance, I would _____
_____.

If both my children and my parents needed help from me, I would _____
_____.

If my parents were in a nursing home, I would want the nurses to _____
_____.

When I grow old, I want my family to _____
_____.

SELF-NEGLECT

Abuse and **neglect** usually involve something done to someone, but, unfortunately, self-neglect is a common problem in the older adult population. Self-neglect is more likely to be seen when an older person has few or no close family or friends, but it can occur despite their presence. Because our society has laws to protect the rights of adults, it may be difficult for concerned parties to intervene until a situation has reached critical or even life-threatening proportions.

Self-neglect is defined as the failure to provide for the self because of a lack of ability or lack of awareness. Indicators of self-neglect include:

1. The inability to maintain ADLs, such as personal care, shopping, meal preparation, or other household tasks
2. The inability to obtain adequate food and fluid, as indicated by malnutrition or dehydration
3. Poor hygiene practices, as indicated by body odor, lesions, rashes, or inadequate or soiled clothing
4. Changes in mental function, such as confusion, inappropriate responses, disorientation, or incoherence
5. The inability to manage personal finances, as indicated by the failure to pay bills or by hoarding, squandering, or giving away money inappropriately
6. Failure to keep important business or medical appointments
7. Life-threatening or suicidal acts, such as wandering, isolation, or substance abuse

Self-neglect in the community is most likely to be recognized by neighbors and reported to the police, public health nurses, or social workers. It may also be suspected by emergency department nurses who see these individuals after they are found injured on the street, after a fire, or in some other state of distress.

Self-neglect is often connected with some form of mental illness or dementia. Once the problem is recognized, legal action through the courts may be needed to place the person in the custody of a family member or adult protective services.

ABUSE OR NEGLECT BY THE FAMILY

Many older adults will need some form of long-term care in the home. Attempts to meet these demands may be accompanied by high levels of stress for the caregivers. The National Council on Aging (2021) estimates as many as 5 million older Americans are the victims of abuse or neglect every year, and that 10% of people over age 65 have experienced some form of abuse. Increased demands on limited resources, physical exhaustion, or mental fatigue can result in deviant behaviors on the part of the caregiver. Inappropriate behavioral responses include abuse and neglect of the older family members. Intentional abuse occurs when any person deliberately plans to mistreat or harm another person. Abusive behavior cannot be justified at any time or in any way. Intentional abuse is most likely to occur in families with preexisting behavioral or social problems. High-risk families include those that have a history of family conflict, those with a history of violence or substance abuse, those with mental impairment of either the dependent person or caregiver, and those with severe financial problems or that are experiencing unemployment.

Not all forms of abuse are intentional, but even unintentional abuse is devastating to older adults. Unintentional abuse or neglect is most likely to occur when the caregiver lacks the knowledge, stamina, or resources needed to care for an older loved one. Often, the caregiver is an older spouse or an aging child who physically cannot meet the high-level demands of care. Situations that trigger abuse are more likely to arise when the older person requiring care is confused or needs continual care.

Continuous demands on caregivers can make them virtual prisoners within their own homes. Stress builds, leaving the caregiver feeling trapped, frustrated, or angry. Unable to cope with the stress of the continual demands, caregivers may strike out at older adults, lock them in a room, restrain them in a chair, or leave them unattended. When the stress is high and the caregivers' coping abilities are low, they may not be able to identify any better options. They may not intend to hurt the older person or may rationalize that they are doing it to only "keep Dad from hurting himself," but the end result is still abuse.

Abuse can be physical, financial, psychological, or emotional. Neglect and abandonment also constitute forms of abuse.

PHYSICAL ABUSE

There are many types of physical abuse. It involves any action that causes physical pain or injury. Abuse may occur in the form of physical attacks on frail older adults who are unable to defend themselves against younger, stronger family members. Older people may be locked in bedrooms, closets, or basements. Older women may be sexually abused or raped by caregivers or family members. Some older people are starved by family members or given food that is unsuitable or unfit for human consumption. Failure to provide adequate food or fluids also constitutes physical abuse. The inappropriate use of drugs, force-feeding, and the use of physical restraints or punishment of any kind are examples of physical abuse. Warning signs of physical abuse include bruising, lacerations, broken teeth, broken glasses, sprains, fractures, burn marks, wounds in various stages of healing, unexplained injuries, torn or bloody underwear, signs of vaginal trauma, delay in seeking medical treatment or a history of "doctor shopping," and refusal by the caregiver to let visitors see the older adult.

NEGLECT

Physical abuse involves one or more actions that cause harm. Neglect is a passive form of abuse in which caregivers fail to provide for the needs of older persons under their care. Neglect, whether intentional on unintentional, accounts for almost half of the verified cases of elder abuse. Neglect includes situations in which caregivers fail to meet the hygiene or safety needs of the older adult. Examples include situations in which a bedridden person is left wet and soiled with body wastes without care or in which an older person suffers from exposure because of lack of adequate clothing. Failure to provide necessary medical care may constitute neglect because, with no means of accessing care, the older person may suffer or die. However, this is not considered neglect if the older person is mentally competent and refuses treatment. Neglect may be deliberate on the part of the caregiver, or it may result from lack of knowledge, inadequate financial resources, or an insufficient support system. Neglect is not uncommon in situations where one older spouse cares for the other. In spite of the best intentions, the caregiving spouse may be unable to provide adequately for the needs of their more dependent partner. It is not uncommon for an older couple to hide these deficits from family members out of fear of losing their independence.

EMOTIONAL ABUSE

Even when physical abuse is absent and adequate physical care is provided, emotional abuse may occur. Emotional abuse is the most subtle and difficult to recognize type of abuse. It often includes behaviors such as isolating, ignoring, or depersonalizing an older adult. Emotional abusers may forbid people from visiting and isolate the older person from more responsible and sympathetic friends or family members. They may prohibit the use of the telephone or interfere with communication by mail or email.

Emotional abusers can use verbal or nonverbal means to inflict their damage. Verbal abuse includes shouting or voicing threats of punishment or confinement. Emotional abusers often threaten older adults with all manners of horrors if they tell anyone about their plight. Displeasure, disgust, frustration, or anger can be communicated nonverbally through sighing, head shaking, door slamming, or other negative body language. Repeatedly ignoring what the older person has to say and avoiding social interaction with the individual are subtle forms of emotional abuse. Signs of emotional abuse may include the lack of eye contact, trembling, agitation, evasiveness, or hypervigilance on the part of the victim.

Negative communications are devastating because they can attack the older person's mind and emotions. These messages can be so subtle and routine that they may not even be recognized as abusive. Emotional abuse is insidious in that it can damage the older adult's sense of self-esteem and can even destroy the victim's will to live without leaving any obvious signs.

FINANCIAL ABUSE

Financial abuse exists when the resources of an older adult are stolen or misused by a person who is trusted by the older adult. Children and grandchildren may take money from the older adult, rationalizing that the money is owed to them for providing care or that it will eventually be theirs anyway. People who expect to benefit from the older person's estate may be afraid that the needs of the older adult will consume all of the money and leave them with nothing; therefore they decide to take it while they can. Regardless of the caregivers' rationalizations in these situations, it is financial abuse if the older person's money is taken and spent by others for their own purposes. On the other hand, it is not abusive to use the older adult's resources to provide for the personal needs of that older adult.

Many older adults are overly trusting of family members, refusing to believe that their children would steal from them. This denial often continues despite clear evidence to the contrary. Often, all of the savings have been spent, the home has been sold, and any objects of value have disappeared before the older person will accept the truth. Even then, some older adults make excuses to try to cope with the harsh reality. Abusive caregivers often abandon older people once all of their assets are gone. In such cases, older adults are left homeless, penniless, and in despair. Signs of financial abuse include unusual banking activity, such as large or frequent withdrawals, missing bank statements, missing personal belongings of value, and signatures on checks or documents that do not match the signature of the older adult.

Some actions that older adults can take to protect their financial assets include (1) arranging for the direct deposit of Social Security, pension, and other benefit checks; (2) taking great care in the selection of anyone appointed to hold the power of attorney or give advice regarding a will; (3) keeping ATM pin numbers and online passwords secure—not writing them in a location where others could see them and not giving the number to anyone; (4) having written agreements regarding expectations and fees for services; (5) keeping valuables in a secure location, such as a safe deposit box; and (6) remembering that home helpers or attendants are employees, not friends: paying a fair and agreed-upon wage and reserving tips and gifts for special occasions.

ABANDONMENT

Abandonment occurs when dependent older persons are deserted by the person or persons responsible for their custody or care under circumstances in which a reasonable person would continue to provide care. Abandonment usually leaves the older person physically, emotionally, and financially defenseless. Older adults who have been abandoned by their families usually become wards of the state.

RESPONSES TO ABUSE

It is natural to think that an older person suffering from one or more forms of abuse would complain, but this is rarely the case. Fear of being treated even worse or fear of being institutionalized or abandoned may prevent the victim from seeking help.

◈ Clinical Situation

Trends and Issues

An 84-year-old woman was admitted to the hospital for dehydration and malnutrition. Six months earlier, she had suffered a mild stroke. Since then, her 86-year-old husband had been caring for her at home. On admission, the woman weighed 91 pounds. Stage 2 pressure injuries were present on both buttocks. Her clothing and undergarments were soiled, and she was in serious need of a bath. She reported episodes of incontinence of bladder and bowel. She said that her only activity consisted of sitting in a lounge chair watching TV. She was wearing a wig, which covered hair that was matted tightly against her scalp. After several days of carefully combing out the snarls, the nurse realized that the woman's shoulder-length hair had not been washed in months. The patient's husband explained, "I tried to do my best, but since she had always looked after this herself, I didn't know what to do." He made sure that she took her prescribed medicines and tried to see to it that she had enough to eat and drink, but he said that she was "picky." He also stated that he was unsure just how to take care of his wife's hygiene needs: "I tried to wash her up, but she said she wanted to be left alone." He explained that he shopped for groceries when she was asleep. He was afraid that if he called anyone for help, they would place his wife in an institution, and he could not cope with this idea. She had not complained to anyone for the same reason. Their children all lived out of state and had not visited since the patient had the stroke. She and her husband had assured their children by phone that everything was all right. It was only when the patient complained of chest pain that they sought medical attention.

Older people who manifest signs of abuse must be assessed carefully (Box 1.6). They may try to protect and defend the abuser, deny that abuse is occurring, or seem resigned to the situation, believing that there is no better alternative.

Nurse Alert

Assessing for Abuse

All questioning about and assessment of abuse must be done with great tact and sensitivity. It is best to question older adults alone, so that they can speak freely and without intimidation from a potential abuser.

When one is questioning or assessing for abuse, the right of older people to determine their own affairs to the full extent of their abilities must be respected. Information obtained must be kept confidential and shared only with agencies that have been authorized by the patient or necessitated by law. All observations, both objective and subjective, must be carefully documented in case legal action is required. Detailed records should be kept regardless of whether legal action is anticipated. Data may become significant only at a later date, when they would be impossible to reconstruct if they were not appropriately recorded. Photographs may be necessary to provide proof of neglect or abuse. These may include pictures of wounds, injuries, or living conditions. It is wise to avoid using the term *abuse* when one is working with older adults because they may become defensive and will probably deny it. Using words such as *problems* or *concerns* is more likely to yield truthful information.

When there is any question of abuse, an experienced professional who is skilled in dealing with elder abuse should oversee the case. Physical abuse and

---

Box 1.6	Signs That an Older Person May Be Experiencing Abuse

- Excessive agreement or compliance with the caregiver
- Signs of poor hygiene, such as body odor, uncleanliness, or soiled clothing or undergarments
- Malnutrition or dehydration
- Burns or pressure injuries
- Bruises, particularly clustered on the trunk or upper arms
- Bruises in various stages of healing, which may indicate repeated injury
- Inadequate clothing or footwear
- Inadequate medical attention
- Lack of food, medication, or care
- Verbalization of being left alone or isolated
- Verbalization of fear of the caregiver
- Verbalization of a lack of control in personal activities or finances

financial abuse are criminal offenses. Nurses have a moral, legal, and ethical responsibility to report any suspected cases of abuse (see Critical Thinking box). Nurses who provide care to at-risk groups, particularly the young and the older adult population, must be aware of their legal obligations with regard to suspected abuse. Nurses must know the state laws pertaining to abuse, the proper authorities to contact, and how to contact them. Once the responsible authorities have been notified, they are obligated by law to investigate and pursue any legal action necessary to ensure the safety of the abused and to protect them from further harm.

? Critical Thinking

Your Knowledge of Elder Abuse

- Is elder abuse increasing today? If so, why?
- What would you do if you thought a close friend or relative was an elder abuser?
- What do you think is the best way to reduce the incidence of elder abuse? Why?
- What would you do if you suspected that a nursing assistant was abusing patients?
- What can you as a student nurse do to prevent elder abuse?
- What resources are available in your community to help prevent elder abuse?

ABUSE BY UNRELATED CAREGIVERS

Understandably, we would like to think that all persons seeking employment as caregivers to older adults were responsible, caring individuals, but, unfortunately, this is not the case. People who are hired to provide for the safety and well-being of older adults can sometimes become their greatest threat. The increasing use of unrelated caregivers exposes older adults to additional risks.

As the older population grows and more frail older adults remain in their homes, the demand for nursing assistants, home health aides, and housekeepers increases. Most people who work as nursing assistants or housekeepers are decent, caring individuals who provide difficult services for little reward. The salaries paid to nursing assistants and housekeepers are low, the hours are long, and the work is emotionally and physically demanding. It can be difficult to find caring, responsible people who are willing to provide this service. When the demand for caregivers exceeds the supply of desirable workers, employers may be forced to hire people who are willing to take these jobs only because they cannot find other employment.

Specific federal and state laws designed to prevent undesirable persons from contact with vulnerable people, such as the young and the older adult population, are in force today; however, sometimes people with

QSEN Considerations: Teamwork and Collaboration

Elder Abuse in Institutions

Abuse in institutional settings is most likely to occur when the nursing assistants are forced to work under stressful conditions and have little ability to deal with that stress. The risk for abuse increases when caregivers perceive that they are not valued, supported, or acknowledged.

The following are ways that may help decrease stress and the likelihood of abuse:

- Create a positive team environment with full staffing levels; convey true respect and appreciation for the work every team member does.
- Encourage staff to take breaks on time and to rest and reenergize with healthy snacks. Provide a staff member responsible for "break relief" so that care may continue during breaks.
- Rotate any "difficult" assignments, to avoid overwhelming any one team member.
- Improve staff training to identify and defuse potential abuse situations.
- Initiate a stress-reduction program, including staff support groups and exercise options.
- Recognize the value of nursing assistants to the team's effort by involving them in care planning and consulting them regarding potential problems and possible solutions.
- Increase the recognition of good, compassionate caregiving through verbal praise, employee-of-the-month recognition, bonuses, and other rewards.
- Institute a "get to know the resident" program, whereby one resident is featured on a monthly basis, noting his or her past accomplishments. Team members may be surprised to learn that the dependent older adult they now care for once served as an elite military Special Forces member, raised 12 children, volunteered as a docent at the local aquarium, or played in a rock band.
- Provide an institutional mechanism for dealing with nursing assistants' complaints and concerns in a proactive rather than punitive manner.

criminal records, inadequate training, or other serious shortcomings manage to gain employment despite safeguards such as state registries, employment histories, and reference checks. Undesirable individuals may unwittingly be hired to provide care for older adults by families, home health agencies, and even health care institutions.

In home settings, unscrupulous caregivers have been known to take money and personal belongings from defenseless older people under their care. They may physically abuse older persons and threaten them with physical harm if the abuse is reported. They may threaten to quit, leaving the older person in fear of being placed in an institution. Using threats enables these individuals to remain undetected until they have caused serious harm. When they are discovered, they often disappear, only to reappear somewhere else and repeat their pattern of abuse.

Even health care institutions are not immune to problems of elder abuse. Most people assume that because hospitals and nursing homes are licensed and regulated, this type of behavior does not occur. Unfortunately, this is wishful thinking. Many institutions have difficulty hiring enough people to meet the required staffing levels. Although most health care institutions and agencies screen applicants in an attempt to find the most qualified individuals and to avoid hiring anyone with a history of abusive or criminal behavior, some unscrupulous people manage to avoid detection and are employed as caregivers to older adults. These unsuitable caregivers may victimize older adults before their behavior can be detected. Nurses who supervise other caregivers must constantly be on the lookout for abusive behaviors (Box 1.7). Nurses are **mandated reporters** of elder abuse, which means that if you suspect elder abuse and do not report it, you are breaking the law. You must know and follow the reporting laws in your state. If you suspect it, report any indication of abuse as soon as possible so that appropriate action can be taken and the abusive person removed.

A wide variety of services to reduce abuse and meet the emotional and physical needs of older adults and their caregivers are available. The availability and type of services vary from area to area. Nurses who work with older adults should become knowledgeable about the services available in their communities. Resources

may include education programs designed to improve the awareness of elder abuse, support groups for caregivers, **respite** care programs, and senior day care centers. Many hospitals and health care agencies provide education in nutrition, medication administration, bedside care, and other aspects of elder care. The need for these programs is growing as the older adult population increases.

SUPPORT GROUPS

Caregivers of older adults are often isolated from other people. The demands of providing care prevent caregivers from getting the rest, encouragement, and support they need. Caregivers who want or need to share their experiences and frustrations have started to form support groups to help one another cope with stress. These groups may be specialized (e.g., for caregivers of people with Alzheimer disease) or more general nature. Support groups allow caregivers to share their feelings and learn new strategies to improve coping skills. Some groups schedule speakers to discuss topics of common interest or offer social activities to promote stress reduction.

RESPITE CARE

Respite care allows the primary caregiver to have time away from the demands of caregiving, thereby decreasing stress and the risk for abuse. Many caregivers are unable to lead normal lives because they cannot leave their responsibilities for very long without fear of some disaster occurring. Respite care gives the primary caregiver the opportunity to attend church, go shopping, conduct personal business, obtain medical care, or simply participate in leisure activities. Respite care may be provided by family members, volunteers, or one of the many service agencies that have proliferated within the past few years. The Veterans Administration (VA) offers respite care for enrolled members of the VA health care system. Caregivers may be reluctant to use respite care out of guilt, fear, or other misguided emotions. Nurses should encourage caregivers to protect their own health and well-being by regularly taking advantage of respite care.

Box 1.7 | Abusive Behaviors in Health Care Settings

- Use of sedative or hypnotic drugs that are not medically necessary
- Use of protective devices when they are not medically indicated
- Use of derogatory language, angry verbal interactions, or ethnic slurs
- Withholding of privileges, such as snacks or cigarettes
- Excessive roughness in handling during care or transfers
- Delay in taking a resident to the bathroom or allowing a resident to lie in body waste
- Consumption of a resident's food
- Theft of a resident's money or personal belongings
- Physical striking or any other assaultive behavior toward a resident
- Violation of a resident's right to make decisions
- Failure to provide privacy

Get Ready for the Next-Generation NCLEX® Examination!

Key Points

- Chronologic age is not always the most reliable way to measure aging because the number of years a person has lived provides little information about his or her physiologic or functional ability.
- Many aging people today live more dynamic, positive lives than ever before.
- Stereotyping and negative perceptions of aging and older adults appear to be on the decline, yet subtle forms of ageism still exist and must be addressed.
- The United States will face significant challenges to meet the costs of providing adequate health care to its aging population.
- Because older adults represent a growing segment of the population, they are having a significant impact on politics, economics, housing, and social family dynamics.
- Providing quality care for an increasingly large aging population places increased demands on both family and professional caregivers.
- Although many positive changes have occurred, the frailest older adults remain vulnerable to physical, emotional, and financial abuse.

Additional Learning Resources

SG Go to your Evolve website at http://evolve.elsevier.com/Williams/geriatric for the additional online resources.

Online Resources
- Official geriatric nursing website of the American Nurses Association (ANA): Geronurse-online.org

Review Questions for the Next-Generation NCLEX® Examination

1. Which statements are true regarding older adults? *Select all that apply.*
   a. Most older adults live independently.
   b. Older adults typically remain sexually active.
   c. Older adults are a very diverse group of people.
   d. Most older adults experience significant personality changes.
   e. Older adults suffer from depression more than younger adults.

2. Which is/are true of the baby boom generation?
   a. Its members were born between 1946 and 1964.
   b. Its members will all be age 65 or older by 2020.
   c. They outnumber the millennials.
   d. It comprises about one-third of the population today.

3. When was Medicare legislation established?
   a. 1940s
   b. 1950s
   c. 1960s
   d. 1970s

4. What is the overall percentage of adults over age 75 who live in an institutional setting?
   a. Approximately 1%
   b. Approximately 3%
   c. Approximately 11%
   d. Approximately 17%

5. What does a durable power of attorney for health care enable the health care agent to do?
   a. Decide whether the older adult should be resuscitated
   b. Act only when the older adult is unable to act for themself
   c. Determine when the older adult should be hospitalized
   d. Change care decisions if that appears to be of benefit to the older adult

6. What is probably the most significant issue to affect the older adult and their family?
   a. Loss of independence
   b. Change in physical appearance
   c. Decreased financial resources
   d. Sensory and cognitive decline

7. A nurse is assessing an older adult who was admitted to the emergency room accompanied by their daughter, with whom they reside. What observation might arouse suspicion of elder abuse? *Select all that apply.*
   a. Bruises are observed on the older adult's arms and upper body.
   b. The daughter answers all questions for her parent.
   c. The older adult has a body odor and soiled clothing.
   d. The older adult's skin is intact, with good turgor.
   e. The daughter states that her parent does not get along with her grandchildren.

8. Which are true statements regarding the economic security of older adults? *Select all that apply.*
   a. Securing a reverse mortgage is the best way to ensure economic security for the older adult.
   b. Fewer older adults will be receiving pensions in the years to come.
   c. Most older adults qualify for government income programs.
   d. The typical older adult lives below the poverty level.
   e. Social Security income accounts for approximately one-third of the income of people aged 65 and older.

9. Which type of document indicates someone's wishes by creating physician orders to be followed at home?
   a. Advance directive
   b. Living will
   c. Durable power of attorney for health care
   d. POLST

REFERENCES

AARP (2020a). Older adults keep pace on tech usage. https://www.aarp.org/research/topics/technology/info-2019/2020-technology-trends-older-americans.html#:~:text=Smartphone%20Savvy&text=Today%2C%20smartphone%20adoption%20is%2086,smartphones%20on%20a%20daily%20basis

AARP (2020b). Social security myths. https://www.aarp.org/retirement/social-security/questions-answers/how-much-longer-will-social-security-be-around.html#:~:text=En%20espa%C3%B1ol%20%7C%20According%20to%20the,will%20be%20depleted%20by%202035

Bandoim, L. (2019). Are luxury cruise ships the new retirement homes? https://theweek.com/articles/837253/are-luxury-cruise-ships-new-retirement-homes

Central Intelligence Agency (2020). The world factbook. https://www.cia.gov/library/publications/the-world-factbook/rankorder/2102rank.html

Centers for Disease Control and Prevention (2017). Life expectancy at birth, at age 65, and at age 75, by sex, race, and Hispanic origin: United States, selected years 1900–2016. https://www.cdc.gov/nchs/data/hus/2017/015.pdf

Centers for Medicare and Medicaid Services (2020). NHE fact sheet. https://www.cms.gov/Research-Statistics-Data-and-Systems/Statistics-Trends-and-Reports/NationalHealthExpendData/NHE-Fact-Sheet

Center on Budget and Policy Priorities (2018). Supplemental Security Income (SSI). https://www.cbpp.org/research/social-security/supplemental-security-income-ssi

Center on Budget and Policy Priorities (2020a). Policy basics: Top ten facts about social security. https://www.cbpp.org/research/social-security/policy-basics-top-ten-facts-about-social-security

Center on Budget and Policy Priorities (2020b). Suit challenging ACA legally suspect but threatens loss of coverage for tens of millions. https://www.cbpp.org/research/health/suit-challenging-aca-legally-suspect-but-threatens-loss-of-coverage-for-tens-of

Chang, E-S, Kannoth, S, Levy, S, Wang, S-Y, Lee, JE, & Levy, BR (2020). Global reach of ageism on older persons' health: A systematic review. *PLoS ONE, 15*(1):e0220857. https://doi.org/10.1371/journal.pone.0220857

Chen, Y., Freedman, N. D., Rodriguez, E. J., et al. (2020). Trends in premature deaths among adults in the United States and Latin America. *JAMA Network Open, 3*(2): e1921085. doi:10.1001/jamanetworkopen.2019.21085. https://jamanetwork.com/journals/jamanetworkopen/fullarticle/2760668

Congressional Budget Office (2019). Medicare—CBO's May 2019 Baseline. https://www.cbo.gov/system/files/2019-05/51302-2019-05-medicare_0.pdf

Duncan, I., Ahmed, T., Dove, H., Maxwell, T. (2019). Medicare cost at end of life. *Am J Hosp Palliat Care, 36*(8), 705–710.

Federal Interagency Forum on Aging-Related Statistics (2020) Older Americans: key indicators of well-being. https://agingstats.gov/data.html

Hebditch, M., Daley, S., Wright, J., Sherlock, G., Scott, J., & Banerjee, S. (2020). Preferences of nursing and medical students for working with older adults and people with dementia: A systematic review. *BMC Med Educ, 20*; 92. doi:10.1186/s12909-020-02000-z. https://www.ncbi.nlm.nih.gov/pmc/articles/PMC7106576/

Kaiser Family Foundation (2020). Total number of Medicare beneficiaries. https://www.kff.org/medicare/state-indicator/total-medicare-beneficiaries/?currentTimeframe=0&sortModel=%7B%22colId%22:%22Location%22,%22sort%22:%22asc%22%7D

Kaiser Family Foundation (2021). Projected change in Medicare enrollment 2000–2050. https://www.kff.org/projected-change-in-enrollment-2000-2050-medicare/

Medicare Interactive (2021). The part D donut hole: Medicare part D costs. https://www.medicareinteractive.org/get-answers/medicare-prescription-drug-coverage-part-d/medicare-part-d-costs/the-part-d-donut-hole

National Council on Aging (2021). Elder abuse facts. https://www.ncoa.org/public-policy-action/elder-justice/elder-abuse-facts/

Noel-Miller, C. (2020). Medicare beneficiaries' out-of-pocket spending for health care. *AARP Public Policy Institute: Insight on the Issues, 151*. June 2020. https://www.aarp.org/content/dam/aarp/ppi/2020/06/medicare-beneficiaries-out-of-pocket-spending.doi.10.26419-2Fppi.00105.001.pdf

Nolo.com (2020). If I get a reverse mortgage, can I leave my home to my heirs? https://www.nolo.com/legal-encyclopedia/if-i-reverse-mortgage-can-i-leave-home-heirs.html

Pension Rights Center (2020). Income from pensions. http://www.pensionrights.org/publications/statistic/income-pensions

Social Security Administration (2020a). Actuarial life table. https://www.ssa.gov/oact/STATS/table4c6.html

Social Security Administration (2020b). Fact sheet: social security. https://www.ssa.gov/news/press/factsheets/basicfact-alt.pdf

Statistica (2020a). Homeownership rate in the U.S., 2019, by age. https://www.statista.com/statistics/1036066/homeownership-rate-by-age-usa/#:~:text=The%20homeownership%20rate%20among%20Americans,are%20occupied%20by%20the%20owners

Statistica (2020b). Population distribution in the United States in 2019, by generation. https://www.statista.com/statistics/296974/us-population-share-by-generation/

Thompson, D. (2021). U.S. life expectancy drops 1 full year due to COVID-19. https://www.webmd.com/lung/news/20210218/us-life-expectancy-drops-1-full-year-due-to-covid19#1

United Nations, Department of Economic and Social Affairs, Population Division (2019). World population ageing 2019: Highlights (ST/ESA/SER.A/430). Available at: https://www.un.org/en/development/desa/population/publications/pdf/ageing/WorldPopulationAgeing2019-Highlights.pdf

U.S. Bureau of Labor Statistics (2020). Usual weekly earnings of wage and salary workers, third quarter, 2020. https://www.bls.gov/news.release/pdf/wkyeng.pdf

U.S. Census Bureau (2018). Older people projected to outnumber children for first time in U.S. history. https://www.census.gov/newsroom/press-releases/2018/cb18-41-population-projections.html

U.S. Department of Health and Human Services, Administration for Community Living (2020a). 2019 profile of older Americans. Available at: https://acl.gov/aging-and-disability-in-america/data-and-research/profile-older-americans

U.S. Department of Health and Human Services, Administration for Community Living (2020b). ACL announces nearly $1 billion in CARES Act grants to support older adults and people with disabilities in the community during the COVID-19 emergency. https://acl.gov/news-and-events/announcements/acl-announces-nearly-1-billion-cares-act-grants-support-older-adults#:~:text=The%20CARES%20Act%20funding%20includes,their%20exposure%20to%20COVID%2D19.&text=%24480%20million%20for%20home%2Ddelivered%20meals%20for%20older%20adults

Objectives

1. Discuss how a theory is different from a fact.
2. Describe the most common biologic theories of aging.
3. Describe the most common psychosocial theories of aging.
4. Discuss the relevance of these theories to nursing practice.

Key Terms

antioxidants (ăn-tē-ŎK-sĭ-dănts, p. 30)
biologic (bī-ō-LŎJ-ĭk, p. 29)
free radical (p. 30)

immunologic (ĭm-ū-nō-LŎJ-ĭk, p. 31)
psychosocial (sī-kō-SŌ-shŭl, p. 29)
theory (p. 29)

There is no single universally accepted definition of aging. It is best looked at as a series of changes that occur over time, contribute to loss of function, and ultimately result in the death of a living organism. Like other living organisms, humans age and then die. The maximal life expectancy for humans today appears to be 122 years. Researchers refer to a "realistic maximum" of 125 years (Smil, 2019), although other researchers state that there may be no limit to how long humans can live (Dolgin, 2018). Why do we age at all? Theories of aging have been considered throughout history as humanity has sought to find ways to avoid aging. The quest to stay young has motivated explorers such as Ponce de Leon, who went to Florida to seek a "fountain of youth." The search for the extension of youth has led some people to seek the potions of conjurers, which have often proved to be more poisonous than beneficial.

No one has identified a single unified rationale for why we age and why different people live lives of different lengths. Theories abound to help explain and give some logical order to our observations. These, including physical and behavioral data, are collected and studied to scientifically prove or disprove their effects on aging.

Studies of families and identical twins show that there is a strong correlation in the life expectancies of genetically related people. If your grandparents and parents lived to be 60, 70, 80, or 90 years of age, you are likely to have a similar lifespan. This is not always the case, however. Some individuals fail to meet genetic expectations, whereas others significantly exceed them. Biologic and environmental factors are being studied to explain these variations.

Although there is no question that aging is a biologic process, sociologic, and psychologic components play a significant role. All of these areas—genetic, biologic, environmental, and psychosocial—have produced theories that attempt to explain the changes seen with aging. Despite extensive interest in this topic, the specific causes and processes involved in aging are not completely understood. Because we do not have definitive reproducible evidence indicating exactly why we age, all of the following remain theories.

BIOLOGIC THEORIES

Biologic theories of aging attempt to explain the physical changes of aging. Researchers try to identify which biologic factors have the greatest influence on longevity. It is known that all members of a species suffer a gradual, progressive loss of function over time because of their biologic structure. Many of the biologic theories of aging overlap because most assume that the changes that cause aging occur at a cellular level. Each theory attempts to describe the processes of aging by examining various changes in cell structure or function.

Some biologic theories look at aging from a genetic perspective. The *programmed theory* proposes that everyone has a certain biologic time line to follow. In this theory, each individual has a genetic "program" specifying an unknown but predetermined number of cell divisions. As the program plays out, the person experiences predictable changes, such as atrophy of the thymus, menopause, skin changes, and graying of the hair. A closely related theory is the *run-out-of-program theory*, which proposes that every person has a limited amount of genetic material that will run out eventually; and the *rate of living theory*, which proposes that individuals have a finite number of breaths or heartbeats, which are used up over time. This was first postulated with the observation that larger animals (e.g., elephants) have a slower metabolism and live longer than do small animals (e.g., mice). The *gene theory* proposes the existence of one or more harmful genes that are activated over time, resulting in the typical changes seen with aging and limiting the lifespan of the individual. Researchers have learned a great deal about our genetic code since 2003, when the Human Genome Project was completed. Scientists can now analyze thousands of genes at a time. This will undoubtedly increase our understanding of biologic aging.

The *molecular theories* propose that aging is controlled by genetic material that is encoded to predetermine growth and decline. The *error theory* proposes that aging is caused by environmental damage that accumulates over time. Errors in ribonucleic acid protein synthesis cause errors to occur in the body's cells, resulting in a progressive decline in biologic function. The *somatic mutation theory* is similar but proposes that aging results from damage to deoxyribonucleic acid (DNA) caused by exposure to chemicals or radiation and that this damage causes chromosomal abnormalities that lead to disease or loss of function later in life.

Cellular theories propose that aging is due to cell damage. When enough cells are damaged, overall functioning of the body is decreased. The free radical theory provides one explanation for cell damage. Free radicals are unstable molecules produced by the body during the normal processes of respiration and metabolism or following exposure to radiation and pollution. These free radicals are suspected to cause damage to the cells, DNA, and the immune system. An excessive accumulation of free radicals in the body is purported to contribute to the physiologic changes of aging and a variety of diseases, such as arthritis, circulatory diseases, diabetes, and atherosclerosis. One free radical, named *lipofuscin*, has been identified to cause a buildup of fatty pigment granules, which cause age spots in older adults. Individuals who support this theory propose that the number of free radicals can be reduced by the use of antioxidants, such as vitamins A, C, and E, carotenoids, zinc, selenium, and phytochemicals.

One variation of this theory is the *crosslink* or *connective tissue theory*, which proposes that cell molecules from DNA and connective tissue interact with free radicals to cause bonds (crosslinks) that decrease the ability of tissue to replace itself, causing cell damage. This results in the skin changes typically attributed to aging, such as dryness, wrinkles, and loss of elasticity. Another variation, the *Clinker theory*, combines the somatic mutation, free radical, and crosslink theories to suggest that chemicals produced by metabolism accumulate in normal cells and cause damage to body organs, such as the muscles, heart, nerves, and brain.

The *wear-and-tear theory* presumes that the body is similar to a machine, which loses function when its parts wear out. As people age, their cells, tissues, and organs are damaged by internal or external stressors. When enough damage to the body's parts has occurred, its overall functioning decreases. This theory also proposes that good health maintenance practices will reduce the rate of wear and tear, resulting in longer and better body function. In a similar vein there is the *reliability theory* of aging and longevity, a complex mathematical model of system failures that was first used to describe the failure of complex electronic equipment. It serves as a model to describe degradation (disease) and failure (death) of human body systems.

The *neuroendocrine theory* focuses on the complicated chemical interactions set off by the hypothalamus of the brain. Stimulation or inhibition of various endocrine glands by the hypothalamus initiates the release of various hormones from the pituitary and other glands, which, in turn, regulate bodily functions, including growth, reproduction, and metabolism. With aging, the hypothalamus appears to become less precise in regulating endocrine function, leading to age-related changes such as decreased muscle mass, increased body fat, and changes in reproductive function. It is proposed that it may be possible to design hormone supplements that could delay or control age-related changes.

Complementary Health Approaches

Complementary Therapies to Slow or Reverse Aging

ANTIOXIDANT THERAPY
- Proposed as a method of neutralizing free radicals, which may contribute to aging and disease processes
- Includes a number of vitamins and minerals—such as vitamins A, B_6, B_{12}, C, and E, beta carotene, folic acid, and selenium
- Generally safe when consumed as fruits and vegetables as part of the overall diet
- High doses of some antioxidants may cause more harm than benefit
- No proof that antioxidants are effective
- Should be discussed with primary care provider before starting use

HORMONE THERAPY
- Proposed to replace a reduction in hormones, which naturally decrease with aging
- Includes hormones such as dehydroepiandrosterone (DHEA), estrogen, testosterone, melatonin, and human growth hormone (HGH)
- Little evidence to support claims made by advocates
- May actually cause more harm than benefit
- Usually requires prescription or supervised medical administration

SUPPLEMENTS

- Proposed to replace or enhance nutritional status; often marketed as "natural" remedies
- Include substances such as ginseng, coral calcium, echinacea, and other herbal preparations
- No proof of effectiveness
- Not regulated by the U.S. Food and Drug Administration, so there is no control regarding the amounts of active ingredients, purity, or quality
- High risk for interaction with prescription medications; primary care provider must be notified if these products are used

CALORIE-RESTRICTED DIET

- Proposes that significant calorie reduction can extend life; based on studies in rats, mice, fish, and worms; not proven in humans
- Severe calorie restriction can result in inadequate consumption of necessary nutrients
- Studies show that severely underweight persons have a higher risk for some diseases and even death
- Dietary changes should be discussed with the primary care provider or nutritionist to ensure that adequate nutrition is maintained

The immunologic *theory* proposes that aging is a function of changes in the immune system. According to this theory, the immune system—an important defense mechanism of the body—weakens over time, making an aging person more susceptible to disease. The immunologic theory also proposes that the increased incidence of autoimmune diseases and allergies seen with aging is caused by changes in the immune system.

A fairly new theory of aging correlates aging with calorie intake. Animal research has shown that a point of metabolic efficiency can be achieved by consuming a high-nutrient, low-calorie diet. It is hypothesized that this diet combined with regular exercise may extend optimal health and the lifespan.

PSYCHOSOCIAL THEORIES

Psychosocial theories of aging do not explain the physical changes of aging; rather, they attempt to explain why older adults have different responses to the aging process. Some of the most prominent psychosocial theories of aging are the disengagement theory, the activity theory, life-course or developmental theories, and a variety of other personality theories.

The highly controversial *disengagement theory* was developed to explain why aging persons separate from the mainstream of society. It proposes that older people are systematically separated, excluded, or disengaged from society because they are not perceived to be of benefit to the society. The theory further proposes that older adults want to withdraw from society as they age—that the disengagement is mutually beneficial.

Critics of this theory believe that it attempts to justify ageism, oversimplifies the psychosocial adjustment to aging, and fails to address the diversity and complexity of older adults.

The *activity theory* proposes that activity is necessary for successful aging. Active participation in physical and mental activities helps maintain function well into old age. Purposeful activities and interactions that promote self-esteem improve overall satisfaction with life, even at an older age. Researchers studying the psychosocial theories of aging recently interviewed a group of centenarians. The research team found that the centenarians stayed active for as long as they could and spent little energy on worrying or trying to change things (Teles & Ribeiro, 2019), lending support to the activity theory of aging.

Life-course theories are perhaps the theories best known to nursing. These theories trace personality and personal adjustment throughout a person's life. Many of them are specific in identifying life-oriented tasks for the aging person. Four of the most common theories—Erikson's, Havighurst's, Newman's, and Jung's—are worth exploring.

Erikson's theory identifies 8 stages of developmental tasks that an individual must confront throughout the lifespan: (1) trust versus mistrust, (2) autonomy versus shame and doubt, (3) initiative versus guilt, (4) industry versus inferiority, (5) identity versus identity confusion, (6) intimacy versus isolation, (7) generativity versus stagnation, and (8) integrity versus despair. The last of these stages is the domain of late adulthood, but failure to achieve success in tasks earlier in life can cause problems later on. Late adulthood is the time when people normally review their lives and determine whether they have been negative or positive overall. The most positive outcomes of this life review are wisdom, understanding, and acceptance; the most negative outcomes are doubt, gloom, and despair.

Havighurst's theory details the process of aging and defines specific tasks for late life, including (1) adjusting to decreased physical strength and health, (2) adjusting to retirement and decreased income, (3) adjusting to the loss of a spouse, (4) establishing a relationship with others in one's age group, (5) adapting to social roles in a flexible way, and (6) establishing satisfactory living arrangements.

Newman's theory identifies the tasks of aging as (1) coping with the physical changes of aging; (2) redirecting energy to new activities and roles, including retirement, grandparenting, and widowhood; (3) accepting one's own life; and (4) developing a point of view about death.

Jung's theory proposes that development continues throughout life by a process of searching, questioning, and setting goals that are consistent with the individual's personality. Thus life becomes an ongoing search for the "true self." As individuals age, they go through a reevaluation stage at midlife, at which point they become aware of the many things they have not done. At this stage, they begin to question whether the decisions and choices they have made were the right choices for them. This is the so-called *midlife crisis*, which can lead to radical career or lifestyle changes or to acceptance of the self as is. As aging continues, Jung proposes that the individual is likely to shift from an outward focus (with concerns about success and social position) to a more inward focus. Successful aging, according to Jung, includes acceptance and valuing of the self without regard to the views of others.

IMPLICATIONS FOR NURSING

Physical theories of aging indicate that, although biology places some limitations on life and life expectancy, other factors are subject to behavior and life choices. Nurses can help individuals to achieve the longest, healthiest lives possible by promoting good health maintenance practices and a healthy environment.

Psychosocial theories help to explain the variety of behaviors seen in the aging population. An understanding of these theories can help nurses to recognize problems and provide nursing interventions that will help aging individuals meet the developmental tasks of aging successfully.

Get Ready for the Next Generation NCLEX® Examination!

Key Points

- Many biologic, environmental, and psychosocial theories have been proposed to explain why we age.
- These theories remain theories because the exact processes that cause the changes seen with aging are not completely understood.
- Further research and study are needed to determine which theory or combination of theories is most accurate.
- Once this has been determined, we will be able to institute measures to slow aging and prolong the human lifespan.
- To date, hormone therapy appears to have more risks than benefits.

Additional Learning Resources

SG Go to your Evolve website at http://evolve.elsevier. com/Williams/geriatric for the additional online resources.

🌐 Online Resources
- American Federation for Aging Research: www.afar.org/

Review Questions for the Next Generation NCLEX® Examination

1. A friend asks the nurse what could be done to improve the chance of a long life. Using current biologic theories of aging, the nurse recommended that her friend discuss this first with her primary care provider but advises that the approach more likely to cause harm than good is which of the following?

   a. Intake of antioxidants, such as vitamins A, B_6, B_{12}, C, and E
   b. Replacement of hormones, such as HGH, DHEA, and estrogen
   c. A calorie-restricted diet
   d. Intake of herbal and nutritional supplements

2. The same friend asks how long humans can live. What is the nurse's best reply?

   a. 100 years
   b. 105 years
   c. 110 years
   d. 122 years

3. According to Erikson, what is the primary developmental task of the older adult population?

   a. Generativity versus stagnation
   b. Trust versus mistrust
   c. Intimacy versus isolation
   d. Integrity versus despair

4. A friend tells you that she thinks her father is experiencing a "midlife crisis" because he purchased a new red sports car, started wearing trendy clothing, and is considering a career change. Whose theory explains this behavior?

   a. Newman's
   b. Jung's
   c. Havighurst's
   d. Erikson's

REFERENCES

Dolgin, E. (2018). There's no limit to longevity, says study reviving human life span debate. *Nature*, July 1, 2018. https://www. scientificamerican.com/article/theres-no-limit-to-longevity-says-study-reviving-human-life-span-debate/#

Smil, V. (2019). Is life expectancy finally topping out? *IEEE Spectrum*, 24 April 2019. https://spectrum.ieee.org/biomedical/ethics/is-life-expectancy-finally-topping-out

Teles, S., & Ribeiro, O. (2019). Activity theory. In D. Gu, & M. Dupre (Eds.), *Encyclopedia of gerontology and population aging*. Springer, Cham. https://doi.org/10.1007/978-3-319-69892-2_748-1

Physiologic Changes

Objectives

1. Describe the most common structural changes observed in the normal aging process.
2. Discuss the impact of normal structural changes on the older adult's self-image and lifestyle.
3. Describe the most commonly observed functional changes that are part of the normal aging process.
4. Discuss the impact of normal functional changes on the older adult's self-image and lifestyle.

5. Identify the most common diseases related to aging in each of the body systems.
6. Differentiate between normal changes of aging and disease processes.
7. Discuss the impact of age-related changes on nursing care.

Key Terms

carcinoma (kăr-sĭ-NŌ-mă, p. 36)
cardiomegaly (kăhr-dē-ō-MĔG-ă-lē, p. 49)
cataracts (KĂT-ă-răkts, p. 67)
dementia (dĕ-MĔN-shē-ă, p. 60)
deterministic gene (p. 62)
diverticulosis (dī-vĕr-tĭk-ū-LŌ-sĭs, p. 55)
gastroesophageal reflux disease (p. 55)
glaucoma (glă-KŌ-mă, p. 67)
hiatal hernia (p. 54)
hypothyroidism (hī-pō-THĪ-royd-ĭzm, p. 62)
intermittent claudication (ĭn-tĕr-MĬT-ĕnt klaw-dĭ-KĀ-shŭn, p. 49)
ischemic (ĭs-KĒ-mĭk, p. 60)

nystagmus (nĭs-TĂG-mŭs, p. 69)
orthostatic hypotension (ŏr-thō-STĂT-ĭk hī-pō-TĔN-shŭn, p. 47)
osteopenia (ŏs-tē-ō-pē- nē-ă, p. 40)
osteoporosis (ŏs-tē-ō-pă-RŌ-sĭs, p. 40)
presbycusis (p. 68)
risk gene (p. 61)
seborrheic dermatitis (sĕb-ō-RĒ-ĭk dĕr-mă-TĪ-tĭs, p. 37)
seborrheic keratosis (sĕb-ō-RĒ-ĭk kĕr-ă-TŌ-sĭs, p. 34)
senile lentigo (SĒ-nĭl lĕn-TĪ-gō, p. 34)
senile purpura (SĒ-nĭl PŬR-pū-ră, p. 36)
xerosis (zĕr-Ō-sĭs, p. 35)

Changes in body function with age are part of a continuum that starts the moment life begins. From the moment of conception, tissues and organs develop in an orderly manner. When fully developed, these organs and tissues perform specific functions and interact in a predictable way. Throughout life, human growth and development occur methodically.

Early in life, the physical changes are dramatic. In only 9 months of gestation, the human organism develops from the union of two almost invisible cells into a unique, functioning individual measuring approximately 20 inches in height and usually weighing between 6 and 9 pounds. For the next 13 to 15 years, rapid physical growth continues. By approximately 18 years of age, the human body reaches full anatomic and physiologic maturity.

The peak years of physiologic function last from the late teens through the 30s—the so-called *prime of life*. Physiologic changes are still occurring during this time, but they are subtle and not easily recognized. Because these changes do not happen as rapidly or

as dramatically as those that occur earlier in life, they may be ignored.

As a person moves into the fifth and sixth decades of life, the physiologic changes become more apparent. In the seventh and eighth decades and beyond, they are significant and no longer deniable.

It is important to recognize that although age-related changes are predictable, the exact time at which they occur is not. Just as no two individuals grow and develop at exactly the same rate, no two individuals show the signs of aging at the same time. There is wide person-to-person variation in when—and to what degree—these changes occur. Heredity, environment, and health maintenance significantly affect the timing and magnitude of age-related changes. Some people are chronologically quite young but appear old. The most severe cases of this occur in a rare condition called *progeria*. When they are only 8 or 9 years of age, children with progeria have the physiology and appearance of 70-year-old adults. At the other extreme, there are persons in their 60s, 70s, and even older who are vigorous and appear much younger than their chronologic age. Most people show the signs of aging at a rate somewhere between these two extremes.

We can observe many normal changes in the body's structure and function during the aging process. There are also changes that indicate the onset of disease or illness. Nurses are expected to be able to distinguish between normal changes and abnormal changes that signify a need for medical or nursing intervention. To identify these differences, nurses must have a good understanding of normal body structures and functions. This knowledge should help them to understand how normal and abnormal changes affect the day-to-day functional abilities of older adults. As nurses, we must be aware of physical changes that are likely to occur, assess each person to determine the extent to which these changes have occurred, and then plan our nursing care in response to that individual's needs.

Some diseases are more common with advanced age. Older adults typically experience one or more chronic conditions. A leading cause of disability for adults in the United States is arthritis and other rheumatic conditions (Centers for Disease Control and Prevention [CDC], 2018). Other common causes are heart disease, stroke, hypertension, diabetes, and cancer. According to the National Vital Statistics Reports (Heron, 2019), the 5 leading causes of death among older adults are (1) heart disease, (2) cancer, (3) chronic lower respiratory disease, (4) stroke, and (5) Alzheimer disease.

Nurses must learn that each aging person is an individual. The types and extent of changes seen with aging are specific and unique to each person. Nurses must avoid falling into the trap of stereotyping older adults. Stereotyping is dangerous because it leads us to accept as inevitable some changes that are not inevitable. Stereotyping can also cause us to mistake early signs of disease for a part of aging.

THE INTEGUMENTARY SYSTEM

The integumentary system—which includes the skin, hair, and nails—undergoes significant changes with aging. Because many of these structures are visible, changes in this system are probably the most obvious and are evident to both the aging individual and others.

The epidermis, the outermost layer of the skin, is an important structure that provides protection for internal structures, keeps out dangerous chemicals and micro-organisms, functions as part of the body's fluid regulation system, and helps regulate body temperature and eliminate waste products. It also contains melanocytes that produce the pigment melanin, which provides protection from ultraviolet radiation.

The dermis contains collagen and elastin fibers, which give strength and elasticity to the tissues. The sebaceous (oil-producing) and eccrine (sweat-producing) glands are located in the subcutaneous tissue, as are the hair and nail follicles and the sensory nerve receptors.

Hair and nails are composed of dead keratinized cells. Hair pigment, or color, is related to the amount of melanin produced by the follicle and, like skin pigmentation, is hereditary. Nails are rigid structures that protect the sensitive, nerve-rich tissue at the tips of the fingers and toes. Nails also aid dexterity in fine finger manipulation.

Subcutaneous tissue consists of areolar connective tissue, which connects the skin to the muscles, and adipose tissue, which provides a cushion over tissue and bone. Subcutaneous tissue provides insulation to regulate body temperature. It is here that white blood cells (WBCs) are available to protect the body from microbial invasion through the skin. Blood vessels in the subcutaneous tissue supply the tissue with nourishment and assist in the process of heat exchange. These superficial blood vessels dilate or constrict as needed to release heat or to conserve heat lost through convection.

EXPECTED AGE-RELATED CHANGES

With aging, the epidermis becomes more fragile, increasing the risk for skin damage, such as maceration and infection. Older skin can be as delicate as rice paper and can easily tear (Fig. 3.1). Rashes caused by contact with chemicals, such as detergents or cosmetics, are increasingly common in older individuals. Skin repairs more slowly in older individuals, increasing the risk for infection.

Melanocyte activity declines with age, and, in light-skinned individuals, the skin may become very pale, making older individuals more susceptible to the effects of the sun. Melanocyte clusters can form areas of deepened pigmentation, a condition called *senile lentigo*; these areas are often referred to as *age spots* or *liver spots* and are most often seen on those body areas that are most exposed to sunlight. In a condition called *seborrheic keratosis*, slightly raised, wart-like macules with distinct edges appear (Fig. 3.2). These lesions, ranging in color from light tan to black, are most often observed on the upper half of the body; they may cause discomfort

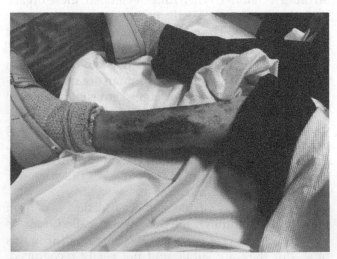

Fig. 3.1 Vertical skin tear from lower leg caught on metal wheelchair footplate during transfer.

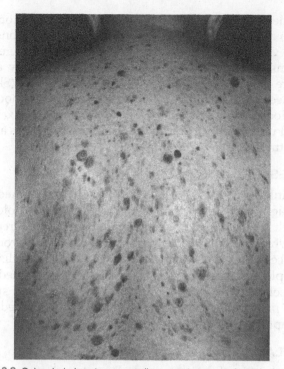

Fig. 3.2 Seborrheic keratoses usually appear at approximately the fifth decade of life and gradually increase in number with age. These superficial, benign growths can enlarge to 20 mm in diameter and have a convoluted surface. (From Dinulos, J. [2021]. *Habif's clinical dermatology*, 7th edition, p. 787. Elsevier.)

and itching. Skin tags, or cutaneous papillomas, are small brown or flesh-colored projections of skin that are most often observed on the necks of older adults.

Aging results in decreased elastin fibers and a thinner dermal layer (Table 3.1). With the loss of elasticity, the skin starts to become less supple. "Crow's feet," or wrinkles, develop. Skin that is very dry or that has had excessive exposure to sunlight or harsh chemicals is more likely to wrinkle at a younger age. Hair color tends to fade or "gray" because of pigment loss, and hair distribution patterns change. Color changes and hair loss patterns tend to be hereditary. The hair on the scalp, pubis, and axillae tends to thin in both men and women. Hairs in the nose and ears often become thicker and more noticeable. Some women experience the growth of facial hair, particularly after menopause. Fingernails grow more slowly, may become thick and more brittle; ridges or lines are commonly observed in them. Toenails may become so thick that they require special equipment for trimming. The function of sweat glands decreases; thus the amount of perspiration also decreases. This results in heat intolerance, because the body's cooling system through evaporation is less efficient.

A decrease in the function of sebaceous and sweat gland secretion increases the likelihood of dry skin, or xerosis (Fig. 3.3). Dry skin is probably the most common

Table 3.1 Integumentary Changes Associated With Aging

PHYSIOLOGIC CHANGE	RESULTS
Decreased vascularity of dermis	Increased pallor in white skin
Decreased amount of melanin	Decreased hair color (graying)
Decreased sebaceous and sweat gland function	Increased dry skin; decreased perspiration
Decreased subcutaneous fat	Increased wrinkling
Decreased thickness of epidermis	Increased susceptibility to trauma
Increased localized pigmentation	Increased incidence of brown spots (senile lentigo)
Increased capillary fragility	Increased purple patches (senile purpura)
Decreased density of hair growth	Decreased amount and thickness of hair on head and body
Decreased rate of nail growth	Increased brittleness of nails
Decreased peripheral circulation	Increased longitudinal ridges of nails; increased thickening and yellowing of nails
Increased androgen/estrogen ratio	Increased facial hair in women

NURSING ASSESSMENTS AND CARE STRATEGIES RELATED TO INTEGUMENTARY CHANGES

NURSING ASSESSMENTS	CARE STRATEGIES
Monitor skin temperature.	Adjust room temperature and provide adequate clothing or covers to prevent chilling.
Assess skin turgor over sternum or forehead, not forearm. Check tongue for furrows.	Provide adequate fluid to prevent dehydration.
Assess for skin breakdown or changes in color or pigmentation.	Institute measures to reduce pressure over bony prominences; possibly facilitate referral to dermatologist.
Assess areas where skin surfaces touch and trap moisture (under breasts, adipose rolls, etc.) for signs of maceration or yeast infection.	Keep skin dry. Pad surfaces to reduce friction. Report abnormal observations for treatment.
Determine adequacy of hygiene and need for toenail trimming.	Modify skin care to reduce drying. Facilitate referral to podiatrist.

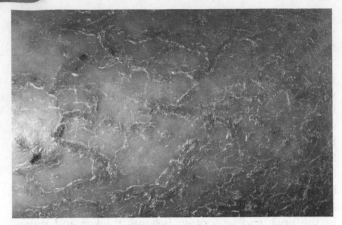

Fig. 3.3 Xerosis. (From Dinulos, J. [2021]. *Habif's clinical dermatology*, 7th edition, p. 109. Elsevier.)

skin-related complaint among older adults, particularly when accompanied by pruritus (itching). This problem is often more severe on the lower extremities because of diminished circulation.

Capillary walls become increasingly fragile with age and may hemorrhage, leading to senile purpura: red, purple, or brown areas commonly seen on the legs and arms. By age 70, the body has approximately 30% fewer cells than at age 40. The remaining cells enlarge, so body mass appears approximately the same. Total body fluid decreases with age. Plasma and extracellular volume remain somewhat constant, but intracellular fluid decreases, increasing the risk for dehydration. Tissue changes include a decrease in subcutaneous tissue, which is visible in the eye orbits and as hollows in the supraclavicular space; sagging of breast and neck tissue also occurs.

COMMON DISORDERS SEEN WITH AGING

MELANOMA AND NONMELANOMA

It is important to distinguish normally occurring changes in the skin from lesions that may be precancerous or cancerous. Skin cancer can be either melanoma or nonmelanoma (usually basal cell carcinoma or squamous cell carcinoma). Cases of skin cancer are commonly observed in older adults who have spent significant amounts of time in the sun. In the United States, more people are diagnosed with skin cancer each year than all other cancers combined. Approximately 20% of Americans will develop skin cancer by age 70. Although melanoma used to cause the majority of skin cancer deaths, squamous cell cancer deaths have increased dramatically in recent years: twice as many people now die from squamous cell cancer than from melanoma. The risk of melanoma doubles if someone has had more than five sunburns at any age (Skin Cancer Foundation, 2021).

Moles of an unusual appearance should be suspected to be melanoma. Irregular shapes, irregular borders, changes in color, changes in size or symptoms, such as itchiness or bleeding, are all considered abnormal. Older men in particular should be taught to screen themselves for changes in the skin because they are more likely than women to die from melanoma (Skin Cancer Foundation, 2021). Suspicious changes should be documented and reported so that they can be examined promptly by a dermatologist. Early diagnosis and treatment are effective at prolonging life.

PRESSURE INJURIES

Shrinkage in the cushion provided by subcutaneous tissue along with vascular changes places the older adult at increased risk for pressure injuries (breakdown of the skin and tissues located over bony prominences). This is a significant problem for immobilized people, such as those who are bedridden or confined to wheelchairs. The staging of pressure injuries and special precautions for their prevention are discussed in Chapter 17.

INFLAMMATION AND INFECTION

Changes in the integumentary system increase the older adult's risk for skin inflammation and infection; these often occur on visible body surfaces such as the face, scalp, and arms, making the conditions distressing to older adults.

Common types of inflammation include rosacea and various forms of dermatitis. Rosacea appears as redness, dilated superficial blood vessels, and small "pimples" on the nose and center of the face (Fig. 3.4); it may spread to cover the cheeks and chin. Left untreated, it can lead to swelling and enlargement of the nose or to conjunctivitis. The exact cause is unknown, but it is most common in postmenopausal women, people who flush easily, and individuals taking vasodilating medications. Treatment of vasodilation includes lifestyle modification, for example avoidance of triggers, such as stressful situations, extreme heat, sun exposure, spicy foods, and alcoholic beverages. Oral and topical

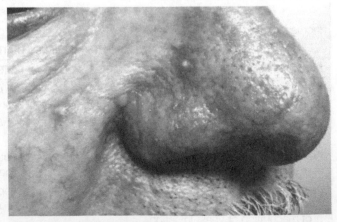

Fig. 3.4 Rosacea pustules and papules. (From Ham, R. J., Sloane, P. D., Washaw, G. A., Potter, J. F., & Flaherty, E. [Eds.] [2014]. *Ham's primary care geriatrics: A case-based approach*, 6th edition. Elsevier.)

medications or light and laser treatments may provide some benefit.

Several forms of dermatitis are common in older adults, including contact, allergic, and **seborrheic dermatitis**. Contact and allergic dermatitis appear as rashes or inflammation that is either localized to certain areas of the body or generalized (Fig. 3.5). Clues to the causative substance are gained from the unique pattern seen on each individual. Identification of the exact irritant may be difficult because of the many chemicals, drugs, and other substances to which an individual is exposed. Treatment consists of avoiding the offending substance.

Seborrheic dermatitis is an unsightly skin condition characterized by yellow, waxy crusts that can be either dry or moist (Fig. 3.6). Caused by excessive sebum production, seborrheic dermatitis can occur on the scalp, eyebrows, eyelids, ears, axillae, breasts, groin, and gluteal folds. There is no known cure, but special shampoos and lotions can help.

Infectious diseases of the skin and nails commonly seen in older adults include herpes zoster (shingles); fungal, yeast, and bacterial infections; and infestation with scabies (mites). Each of these diseases has a unique cause, characteristic appearance, and specific treatment; these, however, are beyond the scope of this text.

HYPOTHERMIA

The decrease in subcutaneous tissue reduces the older adult's ability to regulate body temperature. Very thin older adults lose the insulation provided by subcutaneous and adipose tissue. This loss of insulation is most likely to result in hypothermia if the person is exposed to an environment that is too cold.

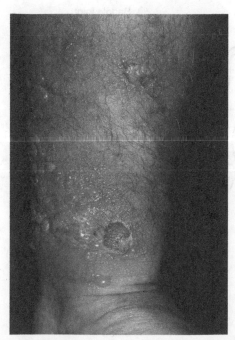

Fig. 3.5 Poison ivy dermatitis with intense blistering. (From Dinulos, J. [2021]. *Habif's clinical dermatology*, 7th edition, p. 1032, Elsevier.)

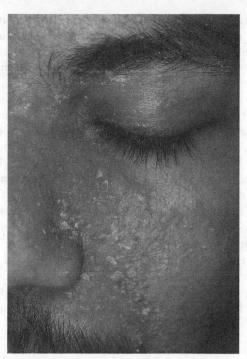

Fig. 3.6 Seborrheic dermatitis is characterized by itching and patches of scales that exfoliate. The most common sites are on the scalp, behind the ears, and on the midface, including the eyebrows and lashes. (From Bolognia, J. L., Schaffer, J. V., Duncan, K. O., & Ko, C. K. [2014]. *Dermatology essentials*. Saunders Elsevier.)

THE MUSCULOSKELETAL SYSTEM

The musculoskeletal system performs many functions. The skeletal bones provide a rigid structure that gives the body its shape. The red bone marrow in the cavities of spongy bones produces red blood cells (RBCs), platelets, and WBCs. Structures such as the ribs and pelvis protect easily damaged internal organs. The muscles provide a power source to move the bones. The combined functions of bones and muscles allow free movement and participation in the activities necessary to maintain an active life.

BONES

Bone consists of protein and the minerals calcium and phosphorus. Calcium is necessary for bone strength, muscle contraction, myocardial contraction, blood clotting, and neuronal activity. This mineral is normally obtained by eating dairy products and dark green leafy vegetables. Vitamin D is needed for the absorption of calcium and phosphate through the small intestine; vitamins A and C are needed for ossification, or bone matrix formation.

For the long bones to remain strong, adequate dietary intake of these nutrients is important. However, the dietary intake of minerals alone does not maintain bone strength. It is also necessary to apply stress to the long bones to keep the minerals in the bones. This needed stress is best provided by weight-bearing activities, such as standing and walking. The calcium that is needed for clotting and nerve and muscle function is constantly being withdrawn from the bone and moved into the bloodstream to maintain consistent blood levels. Calcium is normally redeposited in the bone at an equal rate, replacing the lost calcium. As long as this movement of calcium is in balance, the bone remains strong.

Hormones also play an important role in bone maintenance. Calcitonin, produced by the thyroid gland, slows the movement of calcium from the bones to the blood, lowering the blood calcium level. Parathyroid hormone (PTH) increases the movement of calcium from the bones to the blood, thus raising the blood calcium level. PTH also increases the absorption of calcium from the small intestine and kidneys, thus raising the blood calcium level still further. Insulin and thyroxine aid in the protein synthesis and energy production needed for bone maintenance. Estrogen and testosterone, produced by the ovaries and testes, respectively, help retain calcium in the bone matrix.

VERTEBRAE

The spinal column consists of a series of small bones, called *vertebrae*, which stack up to form a strong, flexible structure. The spinal column supports the head and allows for flexible movement of the back. The segments of the spinal column consist of cervical, thoracic, lumbar, and sacral vertebrae. The muscles that move the back connect at bony processes that protrude from the vertebrae. The spinal cord, the nerve tissue that extends downward from the brain, passes through the vertebral canal, which runs through an opening in each vertebra. The bones of the spinal column protect this nerve tissue from injury.

Fibrous pads, called *intervertebral disks*, are located between the vertebrae and cushion the impact of walking and other activities.

JOINTS, TENDONS, AND LIGAMENTS

Joints are the places where bones meet. The freely moving synovial joints are lined with cartilage, which allows free movement of the joint surfaces. Many of these joints contain a bursa, which is a fluid-filled sac that provides lubrication and thus enhances joint mobility (Fig. 3.7).

Tendons are structures that connect the muscles to the bone, and ligaments are structures that connect bones to other bones.

MUSCLES

There are three types of muscle tissues in the body: cardiac muscle, smooth muscle, and skeletal muscle. Cardiac muscle, located only in the heart, is responsible for the pumping action of the heart that maintains the blood circulation. Smooth muscle is found in the walls

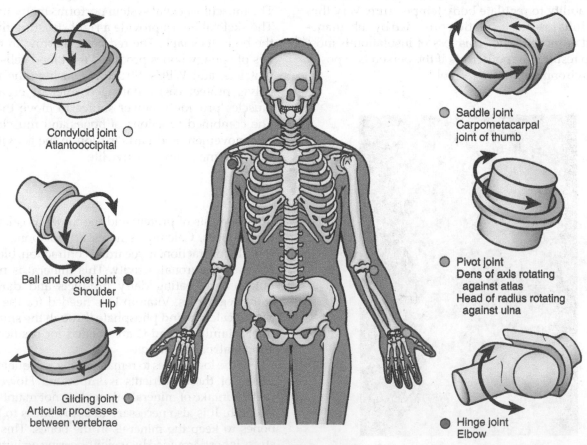

Fig. 3.7 Types of synovial joints: condyloid/ellipsoid joint, ball-and-socket joint, gliding/plane joint, saddle joint, pivot joint, hinge joint. (From Fritz, S. [2013]. *Mosby's fundamentals of therapeutic massage*, 5th edition. Mosby.)

of hollow organs, such as the blood vessels, stomach, intestines, and urinary bladder. Because cardiac and smooth muscle normally cannot be stimulated by conscious effort, they are called *involuntary muscles*.

Skeletal muscle accounts for the largest amount of muscle tissue in the body. The major function of skeletal muscle is to move the bones of the skeleton. Because their actions can be controlled by conscious effort, skeletal muscles are considered *voluntary muscles*. Muscles are connected to bones by tendons. The contraction or relaxation of muscles causes the bones to move. Controlled and coordinated movement of bones and muscles allows us to perform the variety of movements required for activities of daily living (ADLs). Special effort and practice allow us to perform activities such as dancing, participating in sports, and playing a musical instrument.

The amount of muscle mass and type of muscle development differ greatly among individuals. Men normally have larger muscles, or more muscle mass, than women, particularly in the upper body. The male hormone testosterone stimulates muscle development. In both men and women, the largest and strongest skeletal muscles are found in the legs and upper arms; the smallest and weakest are located in the lower back.

Muscle tissue is normally in a state of slight contraction, called tone. Muscle tone is necessary to support the head, keep the spine erect, and perform controlled movement. Muscle mass is built and muscle tone is maintained by exercise. There are two general types of exercise: isometric exercise, which involves muscle contraction without body movement, and isotonic exercise, which involves muscle contraction with body movement. Isometric exercise helps maintain muscle tone and strength but does little to increase muscle size. Isotonic exercise maintains muscle tone and strength and increases muscle mass if it is done repetitively. Aerobic exercise is isotonic exercise that is performed for 30 minutes or longer. Aerobic exercise strengthens the skeletal, cardiac, and respiratory muscles. People who lead inactive or sedentary lifestyles suffer from the lack of isotonic exercise. Regardless of age, unless people undertake exercise programs, they will manifest poor muscle development and strength.

Muscle movement is controlled by impulses from the parietal lobes of the cerebrum and is coordinated by impulses from the cerebellum. The term *muscle sense* describes the brain's ability to recognize the position and action of the muscles without conscious effort. Receptor cells in the muscles, called *proprioceptors*, send information to the brain, which then enables the integration of all body movements. This coordinative function of the brain allows us to walk, bend, or eat without consciously thinking about all of the separate movements and feeling all of the different positions.

Muscles need energy to function. The most abundant source of muscular energy is glycogen. Adenosine triphosphate (ATP), the direct energy source for muscular contraction, is a product of glycogen metabolism.

Glycogen is first broken down into glucose. During cell metabolism, glucose interacts with oxygen transported in the bloodstream by hemoglobin or oxygen stored in the muscle fibers as myoglobin. This reaction involves the production of ATP, heat, water, and carbon dioxide. If muscle fibers do not receive enough oxygen, glucose may not be oxidized completely, and a chemical intermediate, lactic acid, is produced. Elevated levels of lactic acid may result in muscle fatigue and soreness.

EXPECTED AGE-RELATED CHANGES

The major bone-associated change related to aging is the loss of calcium (Table 3.2), which begins between ages 30 and 40. With each successive decade, the skeletal bones become thinner and relatively weaker. Women lose approximately 8% of their bone mass each decade, whereas men lose approximately 3%. Decalcification of various parts of the skeleton—such as the

Table 3.2	Musculoskeletal Changes Associated With Aging
PHYSIOLOGIC CHANGE	**RESULTS**
Decreased bone calcium	Osteopenia (decreased bone density); can lead to osteoporosis; increased curvature of the spine (kyphosis)
Decreased fluid in intervertebral disks	Decreased height
Decreased blood supply to muscles	Decreased muscle strength
Decreased tissue elasticity	Decreased mobility and flexibility of ligaments and tendons
Decreased muscle mass	Decreased strength; increased risk for falls
NURSING ASSESSMENTS AND CARE STRATEGIES RELATED TO MUSCULOSKELETAL CHANGES	
NURSING ASSESSMENTS	**CARE STRATEGIES**
Assess strength and functional mobility.	Provide assistance as needed, modify physical environment, initiate safety precautions to decrease risk of falls, encourage range of motion (ROM) exercise, facilitate referral to physical or occupational therapy.
Assess nutritional intake.	Educate regarding importance of calcium intake, administer supplements as ordered.
Determine activity patterns.	Encourage regular low-impact exercise.

epiphyses, vertebrae, and jaw bones—can increase the risk for fracture, loss of height, and loss of teeth.

The intervertebral disks shrink as the thoracic vertebrae slowly change with aging. The result is a condition called *kyphosis*, which gives the older adult a stooped or hunchback appearance, with the head dropping forward toward the chest. The combination of disk shrinkage and kyphosis results in loss of overall height. A person can lose as much as 2 inches of height by age 70. People who are concerned about their appearance find these changes disturbing because clothing no longer fits properly, and it becomes increasingly difficult to find flattering styles.

Connective tissues tend to lose elasticity, leading to restriction of joint mobility. Loss of flexibility and joint mobility begins as early as the teen years and is common with aging. Regular stretching exercises can help slow or even reverse flexibility problems.

Muscle tone and mass typically decrease with aging, and these decreases are directly related to reductions in physical activity and exercise. People of all ages who exercise regularly have better muscle mass and tone. Hormonal changes, particularly the decrease in testosterone level, tend to reduce muscle mass in aging men. Older men have been shown to lose muscle faster than do older women (Du et al., 2019). Reduced blood supply to the muscles because of aging or disease can lead to changes in muscle function. Less glycogen is stored in aging muscles, thereby decreasing the fuel available for muscle contraction. Any condition that restricts oxygen availability (e.g., anemia or respiratory problems) can lead to an excessive production of waste products such as lactic acid and carbon dioxide. This can increase the incidence of muscle spasms and muscle fatigue with minimal exertion. Decreased endurance and agility may result from a combination of these factors. Neuronal changes in the areas of the brain responsible for muscle control can result in alterations of muscle sense, which may be observed in older adults as an unsteady gait and impairment of other activities that require muscular coordination.

As a person ages, muscle mass decreases, and the proportion of body weight resulting from fatty, or adipose, tissue increases. This has important implications for medication administration. Intramuscular injection sites may not be well muscled, and fatty tissue tends to retain medication differently than does lean tissue. The absorption and metabolism of drugs can be significantly different from those in younger persons.

COMMON DISORDERS SEEN WITH AGING

OSTEOPOROSIS

Excessive loss of calcium from bone combined with insufficient replacement results in osteoporosis. Currently, 54 million Americans have either osteoporosis or osteopenia (decreased bone mass), which places them at risk for osteoporosis (National Osteoporosis Foundation, 2021). This disorder is projected to become even more common as the population ages. Osteoporosis is characterized by porous, brittle, fragile bones that are susceptible to breakage. Spontaneous fracture of the vertebrae or other bones can occur in the absence of obvious trauma. In fact, spontaneous hip fractures may lead to a fall, rather than the fall leading to the hip fracture. Simple falls or other traumas are more likely to result in fractures in people who have osteoporosis. Common fracture sites include the hip (usually the femoral neck), ribs, clavicle, and wrist. Factors that increase the risk for osteoporosis include

- Female gender
- Caucasian or Asian race
- Small body frame
- Family history of osteoporosis
- Gastrointestinal disorders, such as celiac disease, inflammatory bowel disease, or weight-loss surgery
- Menopause (low estrogen levels)
- Lifestyle factors, including lack of exercise/immobility, excess alcohol consumption, cigarette smoking, deficient dietary calcium or vitamin D
- Endocrine or hormonal disorders, including diabetes, hyperthyroidism, hyperparathyroidism
- Long-term use of medications including phenytoin, heparin, aluminum-containing antacids, protein pump inhibitors, oral corticosteroids, and cancer chemotherapy drugs

Bone mineral density (BMD) can be assessed in someone at risk for osteoporosis. Measurement of bone density generally reflects the strength and ability of bones to bear weight. Osteoporosis is best prevented and treated by lifestyle modifications and medications. Lifestyle modifications include a well-balanced diet with adequate amounts of calcium and vitamin D, regular weight-bearing exercise, smoking cessation, and restriction of alcohol intake. Calcium and vitamin D supplements are necessary for individuals who do not consume adequate amounts of these nutrients. Medications for osteoporosis generally fall into two categories: (1) medications that increase bone strength and density (anabolic drugs) and (2) medications that inhibit bone loss (antiresorptive medications). Newer research is suggesting improved effectiveness when these two types of medications are given together. Commonly prescribed antiresorptive medications include alendronate, risedronate, ibandronate, zoledronic acid, and raloxifene. Anabolic medications can also be administered via injection for osteoporosis, including teriparatide and abaloparatide, which are given daily, and romosozumab, which is administered monthly. Menopausal hormone therapy (MHT) has beneficial effects on bone density but also carries an increased risk for heart attack, blood clots, stroke, and breast cancer. Use of MHT is controversial and requires a candid risk/benefit analysis between the patient and primary care provider. Current recommendations are to use the smallest effective dosage for the shortest duration possible. If medications are given for osteoporosis, BMD testing can be done every 2 years to evaluate treatment.

DEGENERATIVE JOINT DISEASE

Osteoarthritis

Osteoarthritis is the most common form of arthritis. It is not considered a normal change of aging; however, the incidence of osteoarthritis increases with age. According to the CDC, osteoarthritis is estimated to affect more than 32.5 million adults in the United States. Women are more likely than men to experience osteoarthritis, especially after age 50 (CDC, 2020f). Some 50% of adults will experience some degree of osteoarthritis during their lifetimes. The exact cause of osteoarthritis is unknown; however, risk factors have been identified, including age, obesity, joint injury or overuse, family history, weak muscles, and female sex (Arthritis Foundation, 2021a). People employed in jobs that place a high amount of physical stress on certain joints are likely to experience changes in those joints later in life. After years of normal joint use, the cartilage on the bones' articulating surfaces thins and begins to wear out. Bony particles or spurs (osteophytes) may form within the joint, causing pain, swelling, and restriction of joint movement. Heberden nodes, which are caused by abnormal cartilage or bony enlargement, may be seen in the distal finger joints. Pain may occur with activity or exercise of the affected joints and may worsen with emotional stress. Synovial membranes of the bursae may become damaged or inflamed. This is particularly true in the weight-bearing joints of the spine, hips, knees, and ankles. Obesity increases the stress on joints and can aggravate symptoms.

Osteoarthritis is treated with a combination of exercise, weight control, joint protection, physical or occupational therapy, and medications. Medication therapy may include acetaminophen, nonsteroidal anti-inflammatory drugs (NSAIDs), or the injection of corticosteroids into the joints. The antidepressant duloxetine has been shown to decrease the pain of osteoarthritis because of its action on serotonin and norepinephrine (mediators of the pain inhibition pathways) and may be recommended for some patients (Kolasinski et al., 2020). Dietary supplements—such as glucosamine, chondroitin sulfate, and various vitamins—have shown benefit for some individuals and are being studied for safety and effectiveness. Like all dietary supplements, however, quality and potency can vary between brands because the products are considered to be food, not drugs, and are not reviewed for safety and effectiveness by the U.S. Food and Drug Administration (FDA, 2019). There are also potential cautions and interactions with prescription medications: chondroitin can potentiate blood thinners, and patients allergic to seafood should avoid glucosamine because it is made from shellfish shells. Intra-articular injection of hyaluronic acid, a joint lubricant, may provide pain relief for some people (Mayo Clinic, 2021b). In severe cases, arthroscopic removal of bone fragments or surgical joint replacements may be necessary.

Rheumatoid Arthritis

Rheumatoid arthritis (RA) is a collagen disease resulting from an autoimmune process; it affects more women than men. RA causes inflammation of the synovium, damage to the cartilage and bone of joints, and instability of ligaments and tendons supporting the joints. Onset is usually between ages 30 and 50, although a significant number of individuals develop the disease after age 60. RA is characterized by periods of exacerbation (sometimes called *flares*), during which the symptoms are severe and cause further damage, alternating with remission, during which the progress of the disease and the damage it causes halt. RA can result in muscle atrophy, soft tissue changes, and bone and cartilage changes. Symptoms of RA include the following:

- Pain and stiffness, particularly after rest
- Warm, tender, painful joints
- Fatigue
- Sense of feeling unwell
- Occasional fevers

The most serious deformities and problems are typically observed when an individual has suffered from this disease for an extended period. Affected individuals are best treated by a rheumatologist, a physician who specializes in rheumatic disorders.

Treatments for RA include lifestyle changes such as stress reduction, balanced rest and exercise, and joint care using splints to support joints. Early and aggressive treatment is often advised—especially if a patient has risk factors (found with antibody testing) indicating the likelihood of persistent disease—to encourage remission and avoid joint damage (Arthritis Foundation, 2021b). Early treatment is defined as within 2 years of symptom onset. Medications from a wide variety of classifications are used to treat RA, including the following:

- NSAIDs—such as aspirin, ibuprofen, and naproxen—to reduce pain and inflammation
- Corticosteroids—such as methylprednisone—to reduce inflammation and pain and to slow joint damage
- Disease-modifying antirheumatic drugs (DMARDs)—such as cyclosporine, azathioprine, sulfasalazine, and methotrexate—to slow disease progression and preserve joint function
- Biologic agents—such as etanercept, infliximab, anakinra, and adalimumab—to interfere with the production of inflammatory chemicals by the body
- When biologic agents are used in conjunction with DMARDs, 85% of patients often demonstrate moderate to good response (Panush, 2019).

 Complementary Health Approaches

Mind-body techniques—such as yoga, biofeedback, and tai chi—can be helpful to patients with rheumatoid arthritis.

Surgical interventions, including synovectomy, tendon reconstruction, and joint replacement—may be performed to reduce pain, improve joint function, and allow the individual to maintain the highest possible level of independent function.

Bursitis

Bursitis, or inflammation of the bursa and the surrounding fibrous tissue, can result from excessive stress on a joint or from a localized infection. Bursitis commonly results in joint stiffness and pain in the shoulder, knee, elbow, and hip, ultimately leading to restricted or reduced mobility. Although bursitis can occur at any age, age-related changes in the musculoskeletal system make it more common in older individuals. Treatment includes resting the joint and administering NSAIDs. Corticosteroid preparations are occasionally injected into the painful areas to reduce inflammation. Mild range-of-motion (ROM) exercise is encouraged to prevent a permanent reduction in ROM or the loss of joint function.

Gouty Arthritis

Gouty arthritis is caused by an inborn error of metabolism that results in elevated levels of uric acid in the body. Crystals of these acids are deposited within the joints and other tissues, causing episodes of severe, painful joint swelling. Some joints, such as those of the great toe, are more commonly affected. Chills and fever may accompany a severe attack. Attacks of gout become more frequent with age. Untreated, this disease can result in joint destruction. It is observed more often in men but is also common in postmenopausal women. Recommendations may include reduction of body weight and decreased intake of alcohol and foods rich in purines, such as liver or dried beans or peas.

THE RESPIRATORY SYSTEM

The respiratory system provides the body with the oxygen needed for life. Without oxygen, cells quickly die. The brain cells are the most sensitive cells in the body; they will die if deprived of oxygen for as little as 4 minutes. Breathing, the process of inhaling to take in oxygen and exhaling to release carbon dioxide, occurs at a rate of 12 to 20 times per minute for our entire lives. The respiratory system is typically divided into two parts: the upper respiratory tract and the lower respiratory tract. The entire respiratory tract is lined with mucous membranes.

UPPER RESPIRATORY TRACT

On its way to the lungs, air passes through the upper respiratory tract, which includes the air passages of the nose, mouth, and throat, all of which are located above the chest cavity. Mucous membranes line the nasal passages and warm and humidify the air that passes through the nose. Cilia and mucus in the nasal passages trap particulate matter (bacteria and debris) and sweep it toward the pharynx, where it is routinely swallowed and destroyed by gastric acid. The cough and sneeze reflexes also help prevent debris and foreign objects from entering the respiratory tract. The pharynx, which is located at the back of the oral cavity, has three segments: the oropharynx, nasopharynx, and laryngopharynx.

The nasopharynx is connected to the middle ear by the eustachian tubes, which help to maintain proper air pressure in the middle ear. The larynx, or voice box, is composed of cartilage rings and folds of tissue, called *vocal folds*. The epiglottis, which is the uppermost cartilage ring, prevents food from entering the airway. During inhalation, the vocal folds move to the sides of the larynx to allow the free passage of air. During exhalation, we can speak and sing by controlling the distance between these folds, which vibrate when air is forced through them and produce sound.

LOWER RESPIRATORY TRACT

The lower respiratory tract includes the lower trachea, bronchial passages, and alveoli, all of which lie within the chest cavity. The trachea is a cartilaginous passageway connecting the larynx to the bronchial passages. The trachea branches into two major bronchi; these further divide like the branches of a tree into smaller and smaller bronchioles. At the ends of the bronchioles are the alveoli, or air sacs, which are the functional units of respiration. A thin layer of fluid lines each tiny air sac, which is surrounded by pulmonary capillaries to allow the efficient exchange of gases by diffusion. It is here that oxygen enters the bloodstream for transport to body tissue and that carbon dioxide from the body leaves the bloodstream. This gaseous exchange is essential for normal cell function and for the maintenance of acid-base balance.

Because the alveoli have a moist lining, their surfaces could adhere if they touched when the alveoli were empty. This is prevented by a special protein substance called *surfactant*.

AIR EXCHANGE (RESPIRATION)

The movement of air into and out of the alveoli is called *ventilation*. Ventilation requires the action of muscles, primarily the diaphragm and the intercostal muscles. During inhalation, the diaphragm contracts and moves downward, although the intercostal muscles pull the ribs upward and outward. These combined activities increase the size of the chest cavity until the air pressure inside the lungs is lower than the atmospheric pressure and air is drawn into the lungs. This process is known as *inhalation* or *inspiration*. When the air pressure inside the lungs equals or exceeds atmospheric pressure, air ceases to enter the lungs. When the diaphragm and intercostal muscles relax, the diaphragm moves upward and the ribs move inward, making the chest cavity smaller. As the chest cavity becomes smaller, the pressure in the lungs becomes greater than the atmospheric pressure. Air is forced out of the lungs until the pressure in the lungs equals the atmospheric pressure. This action is known as *exhalation* or *expiration*. Regulation of respiration is both neurologic and chemical. The respiratory centers in the medulla and pons of the brainstem continuously monitor and control the rate and depth of involuntary respiration. Most breathing is unconscious and involuntary. If we had to think about inhaling and exhaling every breath, we would have little time to do anything else. However, breathing can be conscious and voluntary. When we are swimming, singing, or engaging in other activities that require breath control, we can temporarily alter our breathing patterns.

EXPECTED AGE-RELATED CHANGES

With aging, changes are seen throughout the respiratory tract (Table 3.3; Box 3.1). Years of exposure to air pollution, cigarette smoke, and other hazardous chemicals can damage the air passageways and lung tissue. A decrease in the elastic recoil of the lungs leads to diminished air exchange. Mucous membranes in the nose become drier as the fluid content of body tissue decreases; thus incoming air is not humidified as effectively. The number of cilia decreases, diminishing their ability to trap and remove debris. Decreased vocal cord elasticity leads to changes in voice pitch and quality, and the voice develops a more tremulous character.

Musculoskeletal system changes that occur with aging alter the size and shape of the chest cavity. Kyphosis contributes to a barrel-chested appearance. Costal cartilage at the ends of the ribs calcifies and becomes more rigid, thus reducing the mobility of the rib cage. Intercostal muscles atrophy, and the diaphragm flattens and becomes less elastic. All of these changes reduce lung capacity and interfere with respiratory function, resulting in a decreased ability to inhale and exhale deeply.

Several factors increase the possibility of inadequate oxygenation and the risk for respiratory tract infections in older adults. Ciliary movement inside the lungs decreases. The airways and alveoli become less elastic and there are fewer capillaries surrounding the alveoli, thus interfering with gas exchange. The lung tissue itself has less physical mobility and elasticity, which can lead to the increased pooling of secretions, especially in the lower lobes.

COMMON DISORDERS SEEN WITH AGING

CHRONIC OBSTRUCTIVE PULMONARY DISEASE

Chronic obstructive pulmonary disease (COPD) is an umbrella term for the commonly occurring respiratory disorders of emphysema and chronic bronchitis. Although they may appear independently, these

Table 3.3	Respiratory Changes Associated With Aging
PHYSIOLOGIC CHANGE	**RESULTS**
Decreased body fluids	Decreased ability to humidify air resulting in drier mucous membranes
Decreased number of cilia	Decreased ability to trap debris
Decreased number of macrophages	Increased risk for respiratory infection
Decreased tissue elasticity in the alveoli and lower lung lobes	Decreased gas exchange; increased pooling of secretions
Decreased muscle strength and endurance	Decreased ability to breathe deeply; diminished strength of cough
Decreased number of capillaries	Decreased gas exchange
Increased calcification of cartilage	Increased rigidity of rib cage; decreased lung capacity
NURSING ASSESSMENTS AND CARE STRATEGIES RELATED TO RESPIRATORY CHANGES	
NURSING ASSESSMENTS	**CARE STRATEGIES**
Assess breathing depth and effort.	Position to facilitate ease of respiration. Encourage incentive spirometer or nebulizer as ordered.
Assess cough and sputum production.	Encourage adequate fluid intake. Encourage smoking cessation and avoidance of environmental pollutants.
Assess for signs and symptoms of respiratory infection.	Teach avoidance of individuals with active infection. Teach careful handwashing and disposal of contaminated secretions. Encourage annual influenza vaccination.

Box 3.1	Pulmonary Function Changes Commonly Observed With Aging

- Diminished breath sounds
- Lower maximum expiratory volume
- Increased residual volume
- Reduced vital capacity

disorders often occur together and may coexist with asthma. COPD is common in people who have a history of smoking or who have had a high level of exposure to environmental pollutants. In asthma, the trachea and bronchioles are extremely sensitive to a variety of physical stimuli and emotional stress; these cause constriction of the bronchial passages and increase mucus production within the airways. This narrows the airways and restricts airflow. Asthma used to be considered part of COPD but is now thought of as a related but different disorder. Asthma is typically reversible; COPD is not. Older adults with asthma may be less aware of bronchospasms and be slower to seek emergency care. This can result in poor outcomes. Emphysema is characterized by changes in alveolar structure. The alveoli lose elasticity, become overinflated, and are ineffective in gas exchange. Chronic bronchitis involves inflammation of the trachea and bronchioles. Chronic irritation leads to excessive mucus secretion and a productive cough.

Individuals with COPD manifest symptoms such as productive cough, wheezing, cyanosis, and dyspnea. They are at higher risk for developing respiratory tract infections; in severe cases, respiratory failure can occur. Treatment for COPD includes bronchodilators and anti-inflammatory medications (inhaled corticosteroids). Stem cell therapy is being investigated as a possible future treatment option (University of Houston, 2020).

INFLUENZA

Influenza, often referred to as the *flu*, is a highly contagious respiratory infection caused by a variety of influenza viruses. Many different strains of influenza have been identified, and new forms are continually being found. The various forms of influenza, such as the Hong Kong or Beijing flu, are often named for the area where they were first recognized. Epidemics occur at regular intervals and are seen most often in the winter months. The virus is usually spread by airborne droplets and moves quickly through groups of people who live or work in close contact. The incubation period is brief, often only 1 to 3 days from the time of exposure. The onset of symptoms is sudden; they include chills, fever, cough, sore throat, and general malaise. These may be dramatic and can leave the victim feeling severely ill.

Older adults are at higher risk for serious complications of influenza than younger people. More than 90% of deaths resulting from influenza occur in the population that is above 65 years of age. Influenza presents a special danger for older adults with a history of respiratory disease or other debilitating conditions. Yearly flu shots are recommended for all persons older than 65 years of age to reduce the chance of contracting influenza. Immunizations should be given in the fall, so that the level of immunity is high before the risk for exposure occurs. Immunization should be obtained yearly because the vaccine is different every year. Each year, the vaccine is customized to protect against the particular strain of the virus that is anticipated to be prevalent.

Some people refuse or are hesitant to take the vaccine because of the mild symptoms that may be experienced after inoculation. It is important to explain to older adults that these symptoms are mild and will protect them from more severe problems later. Individuals who are allergic to eggs should not receive the vaccine. Influenza vaccine is cultured in egg protein and can cause a serious allergic reaction in allergic individuals. Given properly, these vaccines are 70% to 80% effective in preventing illness.

COVID-19

COVID-19, another contagious respiratory illness, is cause by a new coronavirus (SARS-CoV-2). It is spread even more easily than influenza and can be more deadly. COVID-19 caused a worldwide pandemic starting in 2020. It has claimed more than three-quarters of a million deaths in the United States as of this writing and has changed much of our daily life. Compared with influenza, when someone is infected with COVID-19, symptoms can occur much later, up to 14 days after infection. The spread of COVID 19 is from person to person, usually in close contact (less than 6 feet apart) through droplets when people talk, sneeze, or cough. COVID-19 may possibly also be spread by physical contact (such as shaking hands) or by touching an infected surface followed by touching the nose, mouth, or eyes (**Centers for Disease Control and Prevention, 2021b**). Symptoms of COVID-19 infection can mimic the flu symptoms described earlier, but they can be more serious, or there may be different symptoms, such as loss of taste or smell. Additionally, the older adult may have very few symptoms yet still be infected with COVID-19. Risk for severe illness with COVID-19 increases with age, leaving older adults over age 85 in the highest risk group. In fact, 80% of people who have died from COVID-19 were over the age of 65 years (**Centers for Disease Control and Prevention, 2021a**). For this reason, in the immunization rollout for COVID-19, older adults were prioritized to receive vaccination first. Whether or not annual vaccination against SARS-CoV-2 will be needed is unclear at this time.

PNEUMONIA

Pneumonia is an acute inflammation of the lungs caused by bacterial, viral, fungal, chemical, or mechanical agents. In response to the agent, the alveoli and bronchioles become clogged with a thick, fibrous substance that decreases the ability of the lung to exchange gases. Pneumonia can progress to a state in which the exudate fills the lung lobes, which then become consolidated or firm. Pneumonia can be detected by radiologic examination. Breath sounds exhibit characteristic changes.

The symptoms of pneumonia differ with the causative organism. Viral pneumonia, sometimes called *walking pneumonia*, is most commonly seen following influenza or another viral disease. Symptoms include headache, fever, aching muscles, and cough with mucopurulent sputum. Treatment for viral pneumonia varies according to the symptoms.

Bacterial pneumonia can be caused by a number of organisms. The most common organisms include

Staphylococcus, Streptococcus, Klebsiella, and *Legionella.* The symptoms of bacterial pneumonia are abrupt and dramatic in onset. Chills, fever up to 105°F, elevated WBC count (leukocytosis), tachycardia, and tachypnea are common, as is pain with respiration, or dyspnea. Because of age-related changes in immunity, the older adult may not have the dramatic fever or leukocytosis that would be expected. The associated cough may be dry and unproductive or purulent and productive. The color of the sputum is significant and should be observed and documented. The type of micro-organism involved can be determined by Gram stain and sputum culture. Bacterial pneumonia is treated with bacteria-specific antibiotics and supportive medical and nursing care.

Aspiration pneumonia is an inflammatory process of the bronchi and lungs caused by inhalation of foreign substances, such as food or acidic gastric contents. The risk for aspiration is highest in older adults with a poor gag reflex, decreased mental status, and in those who must remain supine because these individuals can easily inhale or regurgitate food during oral or tube feeding. Aspiration of highly acidic gastric secretions can lead to cell membrane damage with exudation and ultimately to respiratory distress. Aspiration of large amounts of feeding solution is likely to trigger coughing or choking episodes and dyspnea. If these fluids are not removed immediately by suction, respiratory distress and death may be the result. Aspiration of small amounts of liquid can result in continued and progressive inflammation of the lungs. The person suffering from aspiration pneumonia typically has a rapid pulse and respiratory rate. The sputum is frothy but free of bacteria; however, a superimposed bacterial infection may develop.

TUBERCULOSIS

Tuberculosis (TB) is an infectious disease caused by the bacillus *Mycobacterium tuberculosis,* which spreads by means of airborne droplets. An infected person coughs or sneezes, releasing contaminated droplets into the air. When these droplets are inhaled by other people, the bacillus lodges in their lungs, and the disease spreads. Malnutrition, a weakened immune system, crowded living conditions, poor sanitation, and the presence of systemic diseases such as diabetes and cancer increase the older adult's risk for contracting TB.

The symptoms of TB include cough, night sweats, fever, dyspnea, chest pain, anorexia, and weight loss. The cough may be nonproductive or productive. The sputum may be green or yellow; with hemoptysis, the presence of blood may impart a rusty color.

Because skin tests for TB are not reliable in older adults, diagnosis is based on chest radiography or sputum cultures of acid-fast bacilli. A TB blood test might be needed for someone who was raised outside the United States and received the bacillus Calmette-Guérin vaccine for TB, as such an individual may present with a false-positive skin test (Arumairaj et al.,

2020). Early detection is important to prevent further spread of the disease.

Treatment today consists of drug therapy using a variety of antimicrobial agents, including isoniazid, rifampin, ethambutol, and pyrazinamide. A combination of these drugs is usually administered and continued for 6 to 9 months. With drug-resistant TB, other medications can be added to the drug regimen and treatment can last as long as 30 months. Many of these drugs are associated with numerous adverse effects, particularly in older adults. Nursing care of the older adult with TB focuses on maintaining good nutrition, monitoring adherence with the medication administration schedule, and detecting side effects.

LUNG CANCER

Lung cancer, or bronchogenic cancer, is one of the most deadly forms of cancer in the United States. Most people diagnosed with lung cancer are over age 65, with the average age at diagnosis being age 70. Excluding skin cancer, lung cancer is the second most common type of cancer in both men and women, second to prostate cancer in men and breast cancer in women. Although lung cancer is slightly more common in men, it is by far the leading cause of death in both men and women, with death rates exceeding those of colon, prostate, and breast cancers combined (American Cancer Society, 2021b). The survival rate after the diagnosis of lung cancer is poor, with the 5-year survival ranging from 7% to 63% for non–small cell lung cancer depending on the disease stage upon diagnosis (American Cancer Society, 2021c).

Lung cancer results from exposure to carcinogenic, or cancer-causing, agents, particularly tobacco smoke, air pollution, asbestos, and other hazardous industrial substances. Cough, chest pain, and blood-tinged sputum are typical symptoms, which can easily be missed because they resemble those of pneumonia and other common respiratory conditions of older adults.

The treatment of choice is surgical resection of the lungs—a procedure associated with a high mortality rate in older adults. Other treatments include chemotherapy, radiation therapy, targeted drug therapy, and immunotherapy (American Society of Clinical Oncology, 2020).

THE CARDIOVASCULAR SYSTEM

The cardiovascular system moves blood throughout the body. This continuous closed system is responsible for the transportation of blood with oxygen and nutrients to all body tissues. It also transports waste products to the organs that remove them from the body. Through its action, the cardiovascular system helps the body to maintain homeostasis. The heart pumps the blood, and the blood vessels dilate or constrict to aid in the maintenance of blood pressure and exchange of materials between the blood and body tissues.

HEART

The heart is a muscular organ located centrally in the thoracic cavity between the lungs. The sternum, or breastbone, protects its anterior surface. The heart's tip, or apex, projects toward the left side of the body and extends directly above the diaphragm.

Three pericardial membranes form a sac around the heart. The innermost membrane is on the surface of the heart and is called the *epicardium* or *visceral pericardium*. The middle membrane is the *parietal pericardium*, and the outermost membrane is the *fibrous pericardium*. The space between the epicardium and the parietal pericardium is the pericardial cavity; it contains a small amount of serous fluid that prevents the membrane surfaces from rubbing together during cardiac activity.

The heart, which is composed of cardiac muscle (called *myocardium*), is a hollow organ with four distinct chambers. The right side of the heart consists of the right atrium and right ventricle, which are separated by the tricuspid valve. This side of the heart is a low-pressure pump that moves deoxygenated blood through the pulmonary valve and pulmonary artery and out to the lungs. After the blood has been oxygenated, it returns to the left side of the heart through the pulmonary veins. Because less effort is required to move blood the short distance through the lungs of a healthy individual, the muscle wall of the right side of the heart is relatively thin. The left side of the heart also has two chambers, the left atrium and left ventricle, which are separated by the mitral valve. The pressure within the left side of the heart is higher than that in the right side because the left side is responsible for distributing blood throughout the entire body. To provide the necessary force, the left ventricle has a thicker muscle wall than the right ventricle. When blood leaves the left ventricle, it proceeds through the aortic valve into the aorta and its branches and out to the rest of the body.

The heart's chambers and valves are lined with endocardial tissue. Endothelial tissue continues out from the heart and lines all of the blood vessels. This smooth layer allows the blood to flow freely and reduces the risk for clot formation.

BLOOD VESSELS

The arteries are blood vessels that carry blood away from the heart. With the exception of the pulmonary artery, arteries carry oxygenated blood. The aorta, the largest artery in the body, leaves the heart and branches into a series of progressively smaller arteries and capillaries. These vessels run through the entire body and reach all organs and tissues. Arteries are designed for high-pressure, high-flow situations.

Arterial walls are composed of three layers of tissue. The innermost layer is the endothelium, or tunica intima. This layer is a continuation of the endocardial tissue that lines the inside of the heart. The middle layer, or tunica media, is composed of smooth muscle and connective tissue. This smooth muscle is controlled by the autonomic nervous system and dilates or constricts the artery to maintain the blood pressure. The outermost layer, or tunica externa, is composed of strong fibrous tissue that protects the vessels from bursting or rupturing under high pressure. The relative thickness of the tunica media and externa enables the arteries to perform properly.

The veins are vessels that carry blood toward the heart. With the exception of the four pulmonary veins (two from each lung), veins carry deoxygenated blood. Venules, the smallest veins, are connected to the smallest capillaries. Veins and venules are composed of the same three layers of tissue seen in arteries. The veins use a system of valves, which are created by endothelial tissue folds, to aid in the return of blood to the heart. The valves prevent backflow of blood, which could be a problem when the blood is moving toward the heart against the force of gravity.

The smooth muscle layer of the veins is much thinner than that of the arteries because the veins are not as important in the regulation of blood pressure. The outer fibrous layer is also thinner because blood pressure in the veins is much lower than that in the arteries. Veins are designed for low-pressure, low-flow situations.

A special set of blood vessels, the coronary arteries and veins, supplies the heart with blood enriched with oxygen and nutrients. These arteries are the first branches of the ascending aorta. Because the heart muscle works continuously, it has high oxygen demands. Any condition that obstructs the normal supply of blood to the heart can damage the myocardium. If it is severely deprived of oxygen and nutrients, the heart muscle will die. Too much damaged or destroyed tissue results in cardiovascular system failure and death.

CONDUCTION SYSTEM

To function effectively, the cardiovascular system must work in a controlled, organized, and rhythmic manner. The heart's rhythm is established by specialized cells within the heart muscle; these make up the heart's electrical system. The body's natural pacemaker, the sinoatrial (SA) node, is a group of specialized cells in the right atrium. Impulses generated in the sinoatrial node travel across the atria to the atrioventricular (AV) node in the lower interatrial septum. From there, they are conducted through the bundle of His, through the right and left bundle branches, through the Purkinje fibers, and, finally, to the ventricular myocardium. When the cells of the heart's electrical system depolarize, the myocardium depolarizes and the heart contracts (systole), following which the special cells and the myocardium repolarize as the heart relaxes (diastole). This process alternately empties and fills the chambers, which pump blood through the circulatory system.

EXPECTED AGE-RELATED CHANGES

The heart does not atrophy with aging, as other muscles do. In fact, the heart muscle mass increases slightly with age, and the thickness of the left ventricular wall also increases slightly. This increase in muscle mass may occur to offset some loss of tone. The aging heart may function less effectively even when no pathologic changes are present (Table 3.4). Loss of tone typically leads to the decrease in maximal cardiac output seen in older adults. The normal conduction system, SA node, AV node, bundle of His and its branches all lose cells starting fairly early in life (in the 20s). Cardiac response to autonomic stimulation is decreased because of changes in the receptors. Older persons enhance cardiac output by increasing stroke volume, whereas younger persons increase output by increasing heart rate (cardiac output = stroke volume × heart rate).

The heart valves show some degree of thickening and calcification with aging, resulting in mild degrees of mitral valve regurgitation. The endocardium and endothelium lose elasticity with aging. When these tissues become increasingly fibrous and sclerotic, venous return from the peripheral areas of the body decreases. Orthostatic hypotension occurs because the circulation does not respond quickly to position changes. Less effective pumping by the heart muscle combined with sclerotic changes in the veins can lead to dependent edema and to the appearance of varicosities in the lower extremities. Weakness of the valves in the rectal veins can lead to hemorrhoids.

COMMON DISORDERS SEEN WITH AGING

Cardiovascular disease affects more than 75% of adults over age 60 and 86% of people over age 80, and these individuals frequently have more than one chronic illness (Rodgers et al., 2019). Heart disease is the leading cause of death in the United States, with 80% of cardiac deaths occurring in people older than 65 years of age (CDC, 2020c).

CORONARY ARTERY DISEASE

Some degree of coronary artery disease is present in most persons over age 70. The coronary arteries supply blood to the heart. If these vessels become narrowed or obstructed because of atherosclerosis, the heart may not receive adequate oxygen and nutrients. Many older adults have seriously obstructed coronary arteries, yet they remain essentially asymptomatic. Once circulation to the heart muscle decreases significantly, the amount of oxygen delivered to the heart decreases and ischemia occurs. The pain that may be experienced with ischemia is referred to as *angina pectoris* (literally, chest pain). Although the symptoms of ischemia do include chest pain or pain radiating down the left arm, such pain is not always present or recognized in older adults. Vague gastrointestinal (GI) discomfort or shortness of breath

Table 3.4	Cardiovascular Changes Associated With Aging
PHYSIOLOGIC CHANGE	**RESULTS**
Decreased cardiac muscle tone	Decreased tissue oxygenation related to decreased cardiac output and reserve
Increased heart size, left ventricular enlargement	Compensation for decreased muscle tone
Decreased cardiac output	Increased chance of heart failure; decreased peripheral circulation
Decreased elasticity of heart muscle and blood vessels	Decreased venous return; increased dependent edema; increased incidence of orthostatic hypotension; increased varicosities and hemorrhoids
Decreased pacemaker cells	Heart rate 40 to 100 beats per minute; increased incidence of ectopic or premature beats; increased risk for conduction abnormalities
Decreased baroreceptor sensitivity	Decreased adaptation to changes in blood pressure
Increased incidence of valvular calcification	Increased risk for heart murmurs
Increased incidence of atherosclerosis	Increased blood pressure, weaker peripheral pulses
NURSING ASSESSMENTS AND CARE STRATEGIES RELATED TO CARDIOVASCULAR CHANGES	
NURSING ASSESSMENTS	**CARE STRATEGIES**
Assess apical and peripheral pulses.	Observe closely for abnormal sounds and irregularity of rhythm; determine presence and strength of peripheral pulses comparing both sides of the body. Auscultate heart sounds/palpate pulse for full minute. When assessing lower extremities, start distally and move toward trunk.
Assess blood pressure lying, sitting, and standing.	Hypotension is likely to occur while changing position; encourage patient to change positions slowly and to seek assistance if dizzy.
Assess ability to tolerate activity.	Instruct patient to rest if short of breath or fatigued.

may be reported, or there may be no symptoms at all. People experiencing an anginal attack are advised to decrease their activity and rest until the episode passes. Physicians usually prescribe coronary vasodilators—such as nitroglycerin or β-adrenergic blocking agents—for people with ischemic heart disease.

When one or more coronary arteries become totally obstructed by atherosclerosis or embolus, the person is said to be experiencing a myocardial infarction (MI), or heart attack. The mortality rate from MI is much higher in older adults compared with younger adults. Symptoms of a heart attack in older adults are more variable than in younger people. Some older people who are having heart attacks might think that they are simply suffering from the flu. Older adults are likely to have symptoms such as sudden onset dyspnea or chest discomfort, confusion, and syncope. Diaphoresis is uncommon. Many older adults who have heart attacks die suddenly (Box 3.2).

If severe atherosclerotic occlusion of the coronary arteries is detected before MI, angioplasty, stent placement, or coronary bypass surgery may be performed. The age and overall health of the individual are considered before any of these surgical procedures are attempted. MI caused by an embolus that is detected quickly can be treated using thrombolytic agents, such as streptokinase or tissue plasminogen activator; but the use of these drugs may increase the risk for stroke.

Occlusion of the coronary arteries decreases the nutrient and oxygen flow to the myocardium. Total oxygen deprivation results in myocardial tissue necrosis, which is irreversible. The types of problems experienced after an MI depend on the location and extent of the damage to the heart muscle. Mild damage may not be associated with symptoms and may be detectable only on the electrocardiogram. This type of infarction is often referred to as a *silent* heart attack. Moderate damage may limit a person's physical activity. Extensive damage or damage to a critical area of the heart may result in death.

CORONARY VALVE DISEASE

The heart valves become less pliable over time. In addition, calcium deposits may develop on the valves, preventing them from sealing completely. This can result in mitral valve prolapse, mitral regurgitation, and ultimately heart failure (HF). Symptoms of mitral valve prolapse include chest pain, palpitations, fatigue, and dyspnea. Calcium deposits on the valves roughen the lining and increase the risk for clot formation in the chambers of the heart and in the blood vessels.

CARDIAC ARRHYTHMIAS

Cardiac arrhythmias—including ventricular arrhythmias, atrial fibrillation, and conduction disturbances—are increasingly common with aging. Heart block is a common conduction disturbance caused by disruption of the electrical conduction system of the heart. This disruption can be caused by fibrotic tissue infiltration or MI. Sinus node dysfunction, sometimes called *sick sinus syndrome*, is the primary conduction disorder seen in older adults. This condition causes a disturbance in the rate and rhythm of the cardiac contractions, resulting in symptoms such as light-headedness, fatigue, palpitations, and syncope. When the disturbance is severe, an artificial pacemaker may be implanted to regulate cardiac activity.

HEART FAILURE

HF is primarily a problem of the aging population. According to the American Heart Association, it is estimated that approximately 6.2 million adults suffer from this disorder, a number that has been rising steadily (Virani et al., 2020). The older term *congestive heart failure* described the disease process, in which the patient's lungs are often congested and edema appears because the heart's pumping action is ineffective. HF is not a single disease but rather a syndrome that accompanies and results from many other disorders. A variety of cardiovascular diseases can contribute to the development of HF. Coronary artery disease, MI, hypertension, valve disease, and cardiac infection or inflammation may increase the risk for HF. Diseases of other body systems—including bronchitis, emphysema, asthma, hyperthyroidism, liver disease, kidney disease, and anemia—can also lead to HF. Metabolic changes and fluid and electrolyte imbalances seen with malnutrition can lead to HF. Excessive sodium intake with fluid retention increases the risk for HF. The effects of alcohol, digoxin, hormones, some antineoplastics, corticosteroids, and NSAIDs can directly or indirectly lead to HF.

HF is associated with a wide range of symptoms depending on the type and severity of the underlying disease. Mild chronic HF tends to have a slow, insidious onset. Older adults who experience mild symptoms—such as dyspnea, orthopnea, or paroxysmal nocturnal dyspnea—often decrease their activity spontaneously. They may not recognize these symptoms as serious and may attribute them to "slowing down" with aging. Many older adults do not seek medical attention until they have serious problems and are unable to perform even minimal activities (Box 3.3). Acute HF can result in severe pulmonary congestion or cardiogenic shock and is often fatal in older adults. Chronic HF can become acute HF with increased physical or emotional stress. People with HF are more susceptible to fluid and electrolyte imbalances, infections, and kidney or liver failure.

The medical management of HF includes dietary restriction of sodium to decrease fluid retention, administration of diuretics (e.g., furosemide) to reduce fluid overload, vasodilators (such as nitrates), administration of cardiotonic medications (e.g., digoxin) to

---

Box 3.2 **Signs and Symptoms of Myocardial Infarction in Older Adults**

1. Sudden onset dyspnea
2. Chest tightness or heaviness (usually not crushing pain)
3. Anxiety and confusion
4. Syncope
5. Back pain
6. Jaw (tooth) pain

Box 3.3	Signs and Symptoms of Heart Failure

1. Dyspnea (shortness of breath) with exertion
2. Orthopnea (dyspnea at rest when recumbent)
3. Coughing or wheezing with exertion or at rest
4. Fatigue, weakness, or generalized muscle weakness with minimal exertion
5. Peripheral edema
6. Weight gain without an increase in food intake (as a result of fluid retention)
7. Nausea, vomiting, or anorexia
8. Paroxysmal nocturnal dyspnea (extreme orthopnea during sleep)

increase the heart's pumping efficiency, and planned levels of activity designed to reduce cardiac workload. Invasive therapies including pacemakers and ventricular assist devices may also be used. Heart transplantation may also be considered when all other treatments have failed (Beckerman, 2020).

CARDIOMEGALY

Although aging does not routinely affect the size of the heart, many older adults develop cardiomegaly, or enlargement of the heart, which is often related to chronic HF. As we age, the muscular wall of the left ventricle thickens. Because arteries and veins lose elasticity with age, the heart must pump harder to move blood through the vessels. The muscles of the left ventricle hypertrophy in an attempt to improve the output of blood from the heart to meet the body's tissue demands for oxygenated blood.

The right side of the heart may also hypertrophy. Right-sided enlargement is a result of increased resistance in the pulmonary circulation. When one side of the heart is weakened, the other side is soon affected.

PERIPHERAL VASCULAR DISEASE

Blood vessel changes with aging can lead to problems that may range from mild to severe. In arteriosclerosis, the walls of the arteries become less elastic and plaque forms in the arterial wall, narrowing the lumen and restricting blood flow. Excessive plaque is often related to lifestyle factors or to other disease conditions, most commonly obesity, high cholesterol intake, cigarette smoking, and diabetes mellitus (DM). If the lumen becomes too narrow, blood flow to peripheral sites, particularly the lower extremities, may be restricted. This decreased blood flow deprives the tissues of oxygen and nutrients and causes ischemia. If the lumen is completely obstructed, tissue death may result.

An early symptom of arterial occlusive disease is pain. Intermittent claudication, which manifests as a cramping pain in the legs during or after walking, is common with diminished peripheral circulation. Severe circulatory impairment can result in tissue necrosis and may require amputation.

Acute occlusion may occur if a thrombus or embolus obstructs a blood vessel. Sudden pain, pallor, pulselessness (the "3 Ps"), loss of sensation, or a change in body temperature should be assessed and reported promptly.

OCCLUSIVE PERIPHERAL VASCULAR PROBLEMS

Thrombus formation (clotting) in the lumen of a vein is a common problem, particularly in immobile older adults. These clots can form quickly because of sluggish blood flow within the vessels. Increasing the patient's activity and using antiembolic stockings can help to prevent problems related to venous stasis or pooling.

Thrombi form most often in the veins of the lower extremities, where they irritate and inflame the vessel and cause thrombophlebitis. Signs of thrombophlebitis include edema, swelling, warmth over the affected area, aching, and cyanosis or pallor. Medical management of thrombophlebitis typically includes rest, elevation of the affected leg, application of elastic stockings or wraps, administration of anticoagulant therapy (low-molecular-weight heparin), analgesics, NSAIDs, and sometimes surgical removal of the clot (Nagarsheth, 2021).

If a thrombus breaks loose from the vein and travels in the circulatory system, it is referred to as an *embolus*. Emboli can be life-threatening. They are particularly dangerous if they reach small blood vessels in the lungs or brain, where they can occlude the blood supply to vital tissues.

VARICOSE VEINS

Varicose veins are seen when blood pools in the veins and dilates or stretches them. The decline in vascular muscle tone that occurs with aging increases the risk for this. Varicosities are most often seen as a twisting discoloration in the superficial veins of the lower extremities. Older adults who are obese, are inactive, or spend a great deal of time standing are more likely to have varicosities. The risk for inflamed varicosities increases with age.

Varicosities can result in leg cramps or a dull, aching pain in the legs. Patients can reduce or prevent related problems by avoiding constricting garments such as garters or rolled stockings, refraining from sitting with crossed legs, increasing activity, resting with the legs elevated, and wearing elastic stockings to promote venous return.

ANEURYSM

An aneurysm, or the pouching or ballooning of an artery, is commonly seen in an older adult who suffers from arteriosclerotic blood vessel changes. Older adults with a history of angina, MI, or HF are at increased risk for developing aneurysms. In this process, parts of the muscular walls of the arteries develop plaque and become rigid while other parts of the vessels stretch, dilate, and weaken. The walls of the dilated areas thus become thin and prone to rupture.

The most common aneurysms in older adults are those of the abdominal aorta. Such an aneurysm is sometimes observed as a pulsating mass near the umbilicus, or navel, and the patient may have abdominal pain and GI complaints. Aneurysms in the thoracic aorta are higher up the aorta and can present as back pain, cough, or hoarseness. Thoracic aneurysms are less common than abdominal aortic aneurysms. Aneurysms can also develop in peripheral and cerebral blood vessels. Thrombi can form in aneurysms and block the flow of blood. Rupture of an aneurysm results in massive, life-threatening hemorrhage. Early detection and surgical repair of the damaged area provide the best chance for survival.

HYPERTENSIVE DISEASE

Hypertension is prevalent in the older adult population. More than 70% of persons older than 65 years of age have hypertension, and this figure will continue to rise as our population ages (Agarwala et al., 2020). Hypertension is categorized as essential (primary) or secondary. Essential hypertension, the more common form, has no known cause. Many factors—including heredity, diet, obesity, stress, smoking, increased serum cholesterol levels, and abnormal sodium transport—are known to contribute to essential hypertension. Secondary hypertension occurs as a result of a coexisting disease process or other known cause. Pathologic renal, vascular, and endocrine conditions are among the most common causes of secondary hypertension.

Essential hypertension tends to have a gradual onset and is often asymptomatic until complications arise. Most often, hypertension is discovered during a routine physical examination. It is diagnosed based on two elevated blood pressure measurements taken on three separate days. A reading of less than 120/80 mm Hg is now considered the upper limit of normal in adults (CDC, 2020d).

Essential hypertension cannot be cured, but it can be treated. Treatment includes lifestyle modifications, such as rest, smoking cessation, use of stress reduction techniques, weight loss, and dietary sodium restriction. Pharmacologic approaches typically include administration of a thiazide diuretic, a calcium channel blocker, and either an angiotensin-converting enzyme inhibitor or angiotensin receptor blocker (Sinha & Agarwal, 2019). The person experiencing hypertension must be monitored continuously to determine the effectiveness of therapy. Treatment of secondary hypertension is directed at the underlying pathologic condition.

THE HEMATOPOIETIC AND LYMPHATIC SYSTEMS

Body fluids distribute essential protective factors, nutrients, oxygen, and electrolytes throughout the body. The two major fluids of the body are blood and lymph. These fluids flow through the body within two parallel circulatory systems.

BLOOD

Blood flows within the heart and vessels of the cardiovascular system. The general functions of blood include the transportation of nutrients, waste products, blood gases, and hormones; regulation of fluid-electrolyte balance, acid-base balance, and body temperature; and protection against pathogenic attack by the WBCs and against excessive blood loss through clotting mechanisms.

Blood is 91% to 92% liquid; the remaining 8% to 9% is solid. The liquid of the blood is called *plasma*. As a liquid, plasma is a substance in which many other substances can dissolve and be transported, including nutrients (e.g., glucose, amino acids, and lipids), electrolytes (e.g., sodium, potassium, calcium, and chloride), hormones, vitamins, antibodies, and waste products. Carbon dioxide is carried in the plasma as bicarbonate ion. Plasma contains a variety of proteins. Albumin, the most abundant plasma protein, is important in the maintenance of osmotic pressure needed to regulate blood pressure and volume. In the fibrinogen component are prothrombin, fibrinogen itself, and other clotting factors that circulate until they are required by the body. Globulins function as transport agents for lipids and fat-soluble vitamins; the γ-globulin fraction is composed of antibodies that provide immunity from pathogens. The solid portion of the blood is composed of three types of blood cells: RBCs, WBCs, and platelets.

ERYTHROCYTES

Erythrocytes, or RBCs, live for approximately 120 days; therefore the body produces new RBCs throughout life. They are formed in the red bone marrow by stem cells, which undergo mitosis. For mitosis to occur and thus for RBCs to form, vitamin B_{12} and folic acid are necessary for deoxyribonucleic acid synthesis, a necessary step for RBC production. For maturation, the RBCs need adequate amounts of protein and iron.

When RBCs become old and fragile, they are removed from the circulation by the reticuloendothelial cells of the spleen, liver, and red bone marrow. Their iron is reused in new RBCs formed by the red marrow. Excess iron is stored in the liver for later use. The heme portion of the RBC is converted to bilirubin in the reticuloendothelial system and is then processed by the liver. The liver secretes the bilirubin, or bile pigment, along with the other components of bile, into the duodenum for use in digestion. This bile pigment helps give stool its characteristic brown color. If excessive numbers of RBCs are destroyed or if the liver does not function adequately, excessive amounts of bilirubin remain in the circulation. High bilirubin levels result in jaundice, a yellow discoloration of the sclerae of the eyes and also, in light-skinned individuals, of the skin.

LEUKOCYTES

Leukocytes, or WBCs, have protective functions: they destroy dead or damaged tissue, detoxify foreign proteins, protect from infectious disease, and function in the immune response. WBCs are produced in the lymphatic tissue of the spleen, lymph nodes, thymus, and red bone marrow. The five types of WBCs are neutrophils, eosinophils, basophils, lymphocytes, and monocytes.

PLATELETS

Platelets, more properly called *thrombocytes*, are not whole cells but pieces of cells. They are produced when large cells called *megakaryocytes* fragment and enter the circulation. Platelets, which remain in circulation for approximately 10 days, play an important role in the blood's clotting mechanism.

LYMPH SYSTEM

The lymph and circulatory systems are parallel and interdependent. In fact, the lymph system is sometimes considered part of the circulatory system because it is responsible for returning fluids from the tissues to the circulation. The major components of the immune system—lymphocytes and antibodies—are formed by the lymph system to protect the body from pathogenic micro-organisms, malignant cells, and foreign proteins. The lymph system consists of the lymph vessels, fluid, nodes, and nodules; the spleen; and the thymus gland.

LYMPH VESSELS, FLUID, AND NODES

Lymph vessels are located in most tissue spaces. These permeable vessels absorb fluid and proteins from the tissues. Muscular compression on the vessels moves this fluid through a series of lymph nodes and nodules that trap and phagocytize foreign materials before the fluid enters the circulatory system at the subclavian veins. Lymph nodes and nodules also produce lymphocytes and monocytes, and they phagocytize pathogens. Historically, it was believed the brain contained no lymphatic vessels. However, scientists at the University of Virginia have recently mapped out lymphatic vessels hiding in the meninges; and now it has been discovered that an Italian researcher had mapped this out some 200 years ago! (Sandrone et al., 2019). This finding could have profound implications for the study and treatment of neurologic diseases such as Alzheimer disease.

SPLEEN AND THYMUS

The spleen is responsible for producing lymphocytes and monocytes, which enter the bloodstream. It also contains fixed plasma cells, which produce antibodies to foreign antigens, and fixed macrophages, which phagocytize pathogens and other foreign substances in the blood. Although a person can survive without a spleen, they may be more susceptible to certain bacterial infections, including pneumonia.

The thymus, which is located behind the thyroid gland, is large in fetuses and infants. The embryonic bone marrow and spleen produce the initial T lymphocytes, or T cells, which are responsible for the recognition of foreign antigens and for cell-mediated immunity. The thymus shrinks with age, but once the T cells have become established in the spleen and lymph nodes, they are self-perpetuating.

LYMPHOCYTES AND IMMUNITY

B lymphocytes, or B cells, are also produced in the embryonic bone marrow. These cells are responsible for the recognition of antigens located on a foreign cell and for humoral immunity. In humoral immunity, T cells and B cells often cooperate: sensitized helper T cells detect antigens and induce the B cells to produce antibodies, which are then found in the globulin portion of plasma. When the antigen has been destroyed, suppressor T cells reduce helper T-cell activity and stop the immune process. Conversely, in cell-mediated immunity, antibodies are not produced. Instead, activated T cells divide into memory T cells (which recognize the pathogen) and killer T cells (which destroy bacteria by disrupting their cell membranes).

EXPECTED AGE-RELATED CHANGES

As a person ages, the characteristics of blood change somewhat (Table 3.5). Plasma viscosity increases slightly, a change that is most often related to a general

Table 3.5 Hematopoietic and Lymphatic Changes Associated With Aging

PHYSIOLOGIC CHANGE	RESULTS
Increased plasma viscosity	Increased risk for vascular occlusion
Decreased red blood cell production	Increased incidence of anemia
Decreased mobilization of neutrophils	Less effective phagocytosis
Increased immature T-cells response	Decreased immune response
Lower serum albumin levels	Edema; increased levels of medications that are highly protein bound

NURSING ASSESSMENTS AND CARE STRATEGIES RELATED TO HEMATOPOIETIC AND LYMPHATIC CHANGES	
NURSING ASSESSMENTS	**CARE STRATEGIES**
Monitor laboratory tests, including Hgb, Hct, WBCs, and differential.	Report abnormal findings promptly to primary care provider.
Assess nutritional intake for adequacy of protein, iron, and vitamins; assess for peripheral edema.	Administer nutritional supplements as ordered.

Hct, hematocrit; *Hgb*, hemoglobin; *WBCs*, white blood cells.

decrease in total body fluid. Blood cell production in the bone marrow decreases slightly, resulting in a small decrease in the total number of RBCs and WBCs. Unless extreme physiologic stress or disease is present, blood levels of RBCs, WBCs, and platelets remain within normal limits.

The number of T cells in the body does not appear to decrease with aging, but more of the cells remain immature. The ratio of helper cells to suppressor cells is increased. These T-cell changes lead to a diminished immune response. Consequently, older adults are at greater risk for developing infections, particularly respiratory and urinary tract infections (UTIs). Older adults are also at increased risk for acquiring nosocomial infections. This immune system dysregulation (maladaptive change) in older adults, also known as immunosenescence, can lead to an impaired or altered response to new infections and vaccination. This has significant implications for vaccinations, as for COVID-19, that are important for older adults (Pereira et al., 2020) and may require changes in immunization practices for older adults.

Changes in the immune response may modify the usual signs and symptoms of infection. Such changes may be difficult to recognize in older adults: body temperature may not become significantly elevated until the infection is severe, and pain may not be present to indicate infection. Some examples include (1) absence of fever or chills in older adults with pneumonia, (2) lack of dysuria in older adults with UTIs, (3) absence of pain with peritonitis or appendicitis despite obvious illness, and (4) a delayed or absent physiologic response to TB skin testing as compared with that of a younger individual.

COMMON DISORDERS SEEN WITH AGING

ANEMIA

Anemia is defined as inadequate levels of RBCs or insufficient hemoglobin. The most commonly observed anemias in older adults are iron deficiency anemia, pernicious anemia, and folic acid deficiency anemia.

Iron deficiency anemia results from inadequate nutritional intake, blood loss, malabsorption, or increased physiologic demand. Pernicious anemia is associated with the decreased intake or absorption of vitamin B_{12}. Folic acid deficiency anemia is usually caused by poor nutrition, alcohol use disorder, or malabsorption syndromes, such as Crohn disease. Anemia is common in the older adult population, and these problems are explored further in other chapters.

LEUKEMIA

Leukemia is due to the excessive production of immature WBCs. There are both acute and chronic forms, and leukemia is also classified by the types of abnormal cells present. Other blood disorders (e.g., anemia) and hemorrhage (related to a decrease in the number or function of platelets) are commonly seen with leukemia. Chronic lymphocytic leukemia is the form most often seen in older adults. The average age at diagnosis is 70 (American Cancer Society, 2021a). Depending on the stage of the disease and the patient's overall health, life expectancy may vary from a few to as many as 20 years after diagnosis.

THE GASTROINTESTINAL SYSTEM

Food and fluids containing the nutrients needed for survival normally enter the body through the GI tract. Although it is possible to live without food for several days, the cells require a regular supply of nutrients to support their normal physiologic activities.

As appealing as a crispy salad, turkey dinner, or bowl of strawberries may be to us, these foods are useless to our cells until they are broken down into simple, usable forms by the GI system. The GI tract prepares food for digestion. It then digests, processes, and absorbs the nutrients, which are used by the cells of the body. The GI system also stores and discards wastes and plays a major role in maintaining fluid balance by absorbing water. After we chew and swallow food, we do not need to think about its further processing, because the GI system takes care of removing the nutrients and discarding the waste. However, in unusual situations, the GI tract can be bypassed by administering specially prepared nutrients directly into the bloodstream (parenteral nutrition).

The GI tract begins at the mouth and ends at the anus. Each part of the GI tract performs its own distinct functions.

ORAL CAVITY

Food normally enters the body through the mouth and is prepared for digestion in the oral cavity. The teeth mechanically process food by biting, tearing, grinding, and chewing it, a process called *mastication*. The normal adult has 28 to 32 permanent teeth with shapes and sizes that vary depending on their function. The incisors are used to bite, the canines to tear, and the premolars and molars to chew and grind. Each tooth is composed of a crown, which is the part visible above the gingiva (gum), and a root, which is imbedded in a socket in either the mandible or maxilla of the jaw. The periodontal membrane lines the tooth socket and holds the teeth in place. The crown of the tooth is protected by an extremely hard casing called *enamel*. The pulp cavity of the tooth contains blood vessels and nerve endings.

TONGUE

The tongue is a highly flexible structure controlled by and composed primarily of skeletal muscle. Papillae, which contain the taste buds, are located on the upper surface of the tongue. Cranial nerves control the movement of the tongue and carry the impulses for taste perception. The tongue aids in mechanical digestion by positioning food between the teeth and mixing it with saliva in the oral cavity.

SALIVARY GLANDS

Three pairs of salivary glands excrete saliva into the oral cavity. Saliva is composed primarily of water but also contains the enzyme amylase, which begins the digestion of starch. Saliva production normally increases in response to the sight or smell of food. Inadequate amounts of saliva result in a dry mouth and difficulty swallowing. When adequately mixed with saliva, food reaches a consistency that makes it more suitable for chemical digestion. The tongue lifts against the hard palate, pushing the bolus of food to the pharynx at the back of the oral cavity. From here, the food bolus enters the esophagus.

ESOPHAGUS

Once in the esophagus, food is moved by a process called *peristalsis*, a wavelike motion of the smooth musculature that propels material through the entire GI tract. The esophagus is a hollow muscular tube that passes from the pharynx through the flat layer of diaphragm muscle and to the stomach. The esophagus is located above the diaphragm and the stomach is located immediately below the diaphragm. The lower esophageal sphincter, also called the *cardiac sphincter*, is at approximately the same level as the diaphragm, where the esophagus meets the stomach. It allows food to enter the stomach but prevents the stomach contents from moving backward (refluxing) into the esophagus.

STOMACH

The stomach is a muscular sac in which both mechanical and chemical digestion take place. The stomach is lined with mucous membrane, which helps to prevent damage to the muscle walls. Special stomach glands secrete mucus; others secrete enzymes, intrinsic factor, and hydrochloric acid. This mixture of enzymes and acids is called *gastric juice* or *digestive juice*. The pyloric sphincter at the distal end of the stomach retains the food bolus and the digestive juices within the stomach, where they can be churned, mixed, and further broken down for later digestion and absorption. Once the food has been processed in the stomach, it is referred to as *chyme*. After adequate mixing, small amounts of chyme are released through the pyloric sphincter into the small intestine.

SMALL INTESTINE

The small intestine is more than 20 feet long and is divided into three segments called the duodenum, the jejunum, and the ileum (in order of progression away from the stomach). Additional substances are added to chyme in the small intestine to complete digestion. Intestinal digestive glands secrete intestinal juice, which is alkaline and contains many enzymes. The common bile duct and pancreatic duct converge and enter the duodenum at the sphincter of Oddi. Bile, which is produced in the liver and stored in the gallbladder, breaks down fat by emulsifying it. Pancreatic juice contains enzymes that break down proteins. The pancreas also produces sodium bicarbonate; when released into the duodenum, it neutralizes the hydrochloric acid from the stomach. After all of these chemicals have acted on the material in the GI tract, the process of digestion is completed and the nutrients are in elementary forms (e.g., glucose and amino acids) that can be used by the body's cells.

Absorption of nutrients occurs primarily in the small intestine. Special villi, finger-like projections of the lining of the small intestine that are rich in capillaries and lymphatic vessels, increase the surface area of the lining. As the digested nutrients pass over these villi, they are absorbed into the blood and lymph by the capillary network and lymphatics.

Once the nutrients have been absorbed, undigested material and water are propelled into the large intestine by peristalsis. A structure called the *ileocecal valve* is located between the ileum of the small intestine and the cecum of the large intestine. This structure prevents waste products from moving backward into the small intestine.

LARGE INTESTINE

The large intestine is approximately 5 feet long and is divided into segments called the *ascending, transverse, descending,* and *sigmoid colon* and the rectum. The major functions of the large intestine are the absorption of water, minerals, and vitamins and the storage and elimination of indigestible wastes.

As the effluent, or discharge of waste products, moves through the large intestine, water is absorbed and the mass becomes increasingly solid in consistency. It is stored in the sigmoid and descending colon. When peristalsis causes the effluent to enter the rectum, its presence there triggers the defecation reflex, in which strong peristaltic movements propel the mass from the rectum and through the anus. Another reflex like action, the gastrocolic reflex, occurs when the stomach is distended with food, stimulating vigorous peristalsis of the rectum and a desire to defecate. The internal anal sphincter is an involuntary muscle that relaxes when the rectum is full. The external anal sphincter, which is usually under voluntary control after 2 to 3 years of age, may be contracted to prevent defecation. When the external sphincter relaxes, wastes are eliminated from the large intestine.

EXPECTED AGE-RELATED CHANGES

Over time, changes in the GI tract can interfere with normal digestion and medication absorption (Table 3.6). In the oral cavity, gingival tissue may

Table 3.6   Gastrointestinal Changes Associated With Aging

PHYSIOLOGIC CHANGE	RESULTS
Increased dental caries and tooth loss	Decreased ability to chew normally; decreased nutritional status
Decreased thirst perception	Increased risk for dehydration and constipation
Decreased gag reflex	Increased incidence of choking and aspiration
Decreased muscle tone at sphincters	Increased incidence of heartburn (esophageal reflux)
Decreased saliva and gastric secretions; increased gastric pH	Decreased digestion and absorption of nutrients; altered absorption of some medications that are pH-dependent
Decreased gastric motility and peristalsis	Increased flatulence, constipation, and bowel impaction
Decreased liver size and enzyme production	Decreased ability to metabolize drugs, leading to increased risk for toxicity

NURSING ASSESSMENTS AND CARE STRATEGIES RELATED TO GASTROINTESTINAL CHANGES	
NURSING ASSESSMENTS	**CARE STRATEGIES**
Assess oral cavity for dentition, condition of mucous membranes, and hygiene.	Educate regarding importance of good oral hygiene; stress need for adequate fluid intake. Facilitate dental referral as necessary.
Assess swallow and gag reflexes.	Encourage posture that facilitates swallowing. Consult with speech therapy for swallow studies and safe dietary regimen.
Monitor weight changes.	Measure and record weight at least once per month, more often if fluid balance issues develop.
Assess intake of nutrients and fluid.	Educate regarding recommended dietary intake. Establish calorie count and intake and output if problems are suspected.
Assess bowel sounds and bowel elimination patterns.	Establish bowel routines. Teach importance of adequate fluid, fiber, and activity. Administer laxatives, stool softeners, suppositories, or enemas as needed to prevent constipation and impaction.
Assess effectiveness of medications.	Observe for therapeutic effects (or lack thereof); observe for signs of toxicity.

recede and the periodontal bonds holding the teeth in place may loosen. If the teeth are not structurally sound, the ability to bite and chew can be impaired. Good oral hygiene can slow these changes. It is not considered normal for older adults to lose some or all of their teeth.

Dental caries (cavities) can soften the enamel and expose nerves in the tooth pulp. The resulting pain can decrease the ability and desire to eat.

Esophageal dilation and problems related to swallowing may be observed with aging. Commonly, the gag reflex is depressed in older adults, even in those without neurologic problems. This can lead to episodes of choking and aspiration. Sphincter muscle tone, particularly the lower esophageal sphincter, may decrease, increasing the incidence of esophageal reflux or heartburn.

In the stomach, atrophy of gastric glands may result in a decreased production of intrinsic factor and hydrochloric acid; this, in turn, can interfere with normal digestion and absorption of nutrients. These changes can contribute to anemia and other malabsorptive problems. A decrease in gastric mucus production leads to risk for injury and bacterial penetration into the systemic circulation. Decreases in gut-associated lymphoid tissue can affect the immune response. Peristalsis slows with aging, increasing the likelihood of constipation and the incomplete elimination of feces.

COMMON DISORDERS SEEN WITH AGING

HIATAL HERNIA

A hiatal hernia is the protrusion of the stomach into the thoracic cavity through the esophageal opening in the diaphragm (Fig. 3.8). The primary risk factors for hiatal hernia are obesity and being over age 50. Older adults have the highest incidence of hiatal hernia. Some demonstrate no symptoms; others complain of severe distress that may be intermittent or continuous. Complaints may include heartburn, acid reflux, or generalized epigastric distress. Sometimes the symptoms can resemble an anginal attack. Hiatal reflux episodes are most likely to occur after meals (especially when lying down immediately after eating) or when the person is at rest; in contrast, anginal attacks are

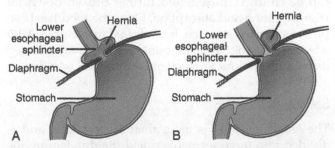

Fig. 3.8 Hiatal hernia. **A,** Sliding hernia. **B,** Rolling or paraesophageal hernia. (From Harding, M., Roberts, D., Reinisch, C., et al. [2020]. *Lewis's medical-surgical nursing,* 11th edition., Elsevier.)

most likely to occur with physical exertion. Vital signs do not normally change in response to problems with hiatal hernias.

Gastroesophageal reflux disease (GERD) is a major problem that can occur with hiatal hernias. With GERD, the gastric contents move backward into the esophagus, where they increase the risk for aspiration. This can present serious concerns in older adults who have diminished gag or cough reflexes. Occasionally, the hernia through the diaphragm is reduced surgically, but typical treatment involves the use of antacids, histamine antagonists, proton pump inhibitors, and dietary modifications. Fatty foods, carbonated beverages, alcohol, and foods that contain caffeine (e.g., coffee, cola, and chocolate) should be avoided to reduce problems with reflux. Smaller, more frequent meals are often beneficial because overeating is likely to enlarge the stomach and cause it to bulge into the diaphragm. It is recommended that food and fluids be restricted after the normal evening meal, and affected persons should avoid lying down too soon after eating. In severe cases, the head of the bed may need to be elevated during sleep to reduce the risk for aspiration.

GASTRITIS AND ULCERS

Chronic atrophic gastritis is an inflammatory change in the mucous membranes of the stomach in which the mucosa becomes thin and abnormally smooth and may develop hemorrhagic patches. All or part of the stomach may be involved.

The term *peptic ulcer* refers to both gastric and duodenal ulcers. Either can occur with aging, but gastric ulcers are more common. A bacterium, *Helicobacter pylori*, or *H. pylori*, has been implicated as the major cause of gastric ulcers because it damages the protective mucous coating that lines the stomach and duodenum. Drug-induced ulcers related to the use of iron supplements, aspirin, and other NSAIDs can also occur in older adults. Diet and nutrition do not appear to play a role in causing or preventing peptic ulcers. However, smoking and alcohol may contribute to the development of ulcers (Yim et al., 2021).

Peptic ulcers in older adults do not cause the classic epigastric pain that is seen in younger people. Older adults suffering from ulcers are more likely to complain of generalized pain and to exhibit a decreased activity level, decreased appetite, and weight loss. Vomiting, melena (dark "tarry" stool containing blood), and generalized signs of anemia may result from gastric bleeding. If a gastric ulcer progresses to the point of perforation, severe hemorrhage can result. If the person has already been weakened by occult (hidden) bleeding, hemorrhage may be serious enough to result in death.

The early recognition and reporting of symptoms by the nurse is important so that treatment can be started before serious problems occur. Medical treatment of ulcers in older adults is generally preferred to surgical correction (Box 3.4).

Box 3.4	**Medical Treatment of Ulcers**

- If caused by *Helicobacter pylori*: antibiotic regimen as prescribed
- If caused by nonsteroidal anti-inflammatory drugs: substitution of a different medication or lowering of the dose if no effective alternative is available
- Administration of proton pump inhibitors (stops acid being pumped into the stomach), such as omeprazole and lansoprazole
- Administration of histamine H_2-blocking agents (blocks histamine, thereby reducing acid secretion), such as famotidine or cimetidine
- Avoidance of tobacco and alcohol, which stimulate acid release
- Administration of antacids to reduce acidity (may not be advised if antibiotics are being prescribed to treat an ulcer caused by *H. pylori* as it may interfere with medication absorption)

DIVERTICULOSIS AND DIVERTICULITIS

Diverticula are small pouches or sacs that develop because of weaknesses in the intestinal mucosa. Half of the population of the United States will have some diverticula by age 60, and by age 80 nearly everyone will have diverticulosis (American Society for Gastrointestinal Endoscopy, 2020). Most people with diverticula experience no symptoms, and there is no specific treatment unless symptoms occur. The patient should continue to eat a normal diet with adequate fluids and fiber. If rectal bleeding occurs, medical intervention is necessary to determine the source.

Diverticulitis involves inflammation of one or more diverticula. This may result in bowel obstruction, perforation, or abscess formation. In cases of severe diverticulitis, the patient may need hospitalization. Oral food intake is restricted, and intravenous fluids are administered to "rest" the diseased area. Surgical correction, including bowel resection or colostomy, may be required if conservative medical treatment is unsuccessful.

CANCER

The risk of colorectal cancer increases with age. Most cases occur after age 50, although the typical age of diagnosis is age 68 for men and 72 for women (American Society of Clinical Oncology, 2019). Carcinoma of the colon is more common in women, whereas rectal carcinoma is more common in men. Any changes in bowel elimination should be viewed with suspicion, especially signs of obstruction or bleeding. Routine screening for colorectal cancer for the person at average risk is recommended to start at age 45 (American Cancer Society, 2020a).

HEMORRHOIDS

Hemorrhoids are common at all ages but may be particularly troublesome to older patients. People with chronic constipation and people with obesity are most likely to have problems with hemorrhoids. Pain and small amounts of bright red blood at the rectum may occur. Most patients with hemorrhoids do not require surgery. Dietary changes, stool softeners, or bulk laxatives are usually effective in reducing problems related to constipation and hemorrhoids.

RECTAL PROLAPSE

Bulging of the rectum through the anus is most likely to occur in women older than age 60, especially those who have given birth to many children. Surgical correction is the typical treatment for this condition, although insertion of a wire loop at the anal sphincter instead of surgery may be attempted in older adults who are too frail for surgery.

THE URINARY SYSTEM

The urinary system consists of two kidneys, two ureters, the urinary bladder, and the urethra. The urinary system supports homeostasis by eliminating wastes and excessive fluid from the body. The kidneys continuously filter the blood and selectively save or eliminate water, electrolytes, and wastes. Those substances not reabsorbed by the kidneys are eliminated from the body as urine.

KIDNEYS

The kidneys are two bean-shaped organs located on each side of the spine behind the peritoneal lining of the abdomen and at the lower edge of the rib cage. The left kidney is usually located slightly higher than the right. Each kidney is surrounded by an adipose tissue pad and is further protected from trauma by the muscles of the back. Within each kidney is a maze of nearly a million nephrons, the functional portion of the kidney. Blood is filtered in the glomerulus of the nephron, and this filtrate is destined to become urine. This highly vascular organ receives blood from the renal artery, which branches off the abdominal aorta. Blood returns to the circulation through the renal vein, which connects to the inferior vena cava. Adequate blood flow to the kidneys is very important; any condition that decreases renal blood flow will interfere with normal kidney function.

The kidneys play an important role in fluid and electrolyte balance and acid-base balance in the body. They remove nitrogenous wastes, excess glucose, and drug metabolites from the bloodstream. They also help to regulate blood pressure. The kidneys typically produce between 1 and 2 L of urine every 24 hours. If excessive fluid is lost elsewhere (e.g., in perspiration or diarrhea), urine output normally decreases. Excessive fluid or alcohol intake tends to increase urine production. A single kidney can meet the needs of the entire body.

URETERS AND BLADDER

The ureters are tubes of smooth muscle that allow urine to drain from each kidney into the bladder. When the body is upright, urine drains by means of gravity. Pressure of the enlarging bladder against the lower portion of the ureter keeps the ureter closed and prevents urine from flowing back toward the kidneys.

The bladder is a hollow muscular sac located below the peritoneum; it normally lies entirely within the pelvic cavity. The bones of the pelvis protect the bladder from trauma. In women, the bladder is located anterior to the uterus; in men, it is superior to the prostate gland.

The muscular wall of the bladder is lined with a mucous membrane and is capable of stretching to hold large volumes of urine (up to 1000 mL or more). Urine is retained in the bladder by means of the sphincter muscles. The internal sphincter is located at the outlet from the bladder into the urethra. Control of the internal sphincter is involuntary. The external urethral sphincter comes under voluntary control at approximately 2 to 3 years of age. Voluntary contraction of the external sphincter prevents urine from leaving the body. Relaxation of the external sphincter allows urine to drain from the body. Voluntary control of urination may be overcome if the bladder becomes overly enlarged with urine. In adults, the urge to urinate typically occurs when urine volume in the bladder reaches approximately 200 to 400 mL.

The urethra is a tubelike passage that leads from the bladder to the outside of the body. At the point of exit, it is referred to as the *urinary meatus*. The female urethra is 1 to 1.5 inches long; the male urethra is 7 to 8 inches long. The urethra is part of the reproductive system in men and serves to transport semen as well as urine; however, ejaculation and urination cannot take place simultaneously. The prostate gland surrounds the urethra. Although this normally causes no problems, an enlarged prostate can interfere with urination.

CHARACTERISTICS OF URINE

Urine is approximately 95% water, with the remainder composed of waste products and salts. The specific gravity (which measures the amount of solids dissolved in water) of urine is normally maintained within close limits. A specific gravity of 1.010 to 1.025 is considered normal. Dilute urine has a low specific gravity; concentrated urine has a high specific gravity. Urine is normally clear, and its color ranges from pale yellow to dark amber. It may be alkaline or acidic, depending on the individual's diet. High protein diets tend to make the urine more acidic; vegetarian diets tend to lead to alkaline urine. Acidic urine is less compatible with bacterial growth than alkaline urine and may help to reduce the risk for a UTI.

EXPECTED AGE-RELATED CHANGES

The kidneys decrease in size from approximately 400 g at age 40 to only 250 g by age 80. By age 70, they lose approximately one-third of their efficiency and they lack functional reserve. Despite this, the kidneys are usually able to remove waste adequately to maintain normal blood levels. As a person ages (Table 3.7), the number of functional units or nephrons decreases. In addition, the kidneys lose mass and decrease in size. Vascular changes, such as those that occur with atherosclerosis or arteriosclerosis, lead to a decreased blood supply to the kidneys. Decreased blood flow results in a diminished glomerular filtration rate. At 90 years of age, the glomerular filtration rate can be as little as half of what it was at age 20. The blood urea nitrogen remaining in the blood increases significantly with age, from a normal of 10 to 15 mg/dL in young adulthood to 21 mg/dL by age 70.

Table **3.7**	Urinary Changes Associated With Aging
PHYSIOLOGIC CHANGE	**RESULTS**
Decreased number of functional nephrons	Decreased filtration rate with decrease in drug clearance
Decreased blood supply	Decreased removal of body wastes; increased concentration of urine
Decreased muscle tone	Increased volume of residual urine
Decreased tissue elasticity	Decreased bladder capacity
Delayed or decreased perception of need to void	Increased incidence of incontinence
Increased nocturnal urine production	Increased need to awaken to void or episodes of nocturnal incontinence
Increased size of prostate (male)	Increased risk for infection; decreased stream of urine; increased hesitancy and frequency of urination
NURSING ASSESSMENTS AND CARE STRATEGIES RELATED TO URINARY CHANGES	
NURSING ASSESSMENTS	**CARE STRATEGIES**
Monitor for signs of drug toxicity.	Promptly notify primary care provider of relevant observations.
Assess for urinary frequency.	Palpate bladder after voiding or use ultrasound bladder scanner to determine whether bladder is emptying completely.
Assess for signs and symptoms of urinary tract infection.	Obtain a urine specimen for analysis.
Assess frequency and timing of episodes of incontinence.	Establish a toileting schedule based on assessment data.

The nephrons and collecting system of the aging body are less sensitive to the effects of antidiuretic hormone. Less sodium and water are reabsorbed and more potassium is lost, resulting in the production of less concentrated urine with aging.

Aging results in reduced urinary bladder size, which leads to decreased bladder capacity (i.e., the volume of urine the bladder can hold before a person experiences the urge to void). Many older people need to void when only 100 mL of urine is present. In addition, overactivity of the detrusor muscle can result in contraction of the bladder before the bladder is full. Either or both of these factors can lead to the urinary urgency and frequency that are common in older adults. To further aggravate the situation, loss of muscle tone can impair voluntary control of the external sphincter muscle. Atonic muscular changes may also occur in the wall of the bladder. Loss of tone may result in a reduced urinary stream, incomplete or unsuccessful voiding, continuous dribbling of urine, or urinary retention with overflow voiding (a condition in which the person voids frequently but never completely empties the bladder). Urinary retention contributes to the risk for UTIs, especially in older adults, because retained urine is a good medium for bacterial growth.

The prostate gland enlarges with age. Most men above 60 years of age experience some degree of prostate gland enlargement due to benign prostatic hyperplasia or prostate cancer. Because it surrounds the urethra, an enlarged prostate gland can compress and narrow the passageway, which, in turn, causes problems with voiding. Hesitancy, frequency, the inability to maintain a steady stream of urine, and urinary retention are common indicators of prostatic hyperplasia.

COMMON DISORDERS SEEN WITH AGING

URINARY INCONTINENCE

Urinary incontinence, the involuntary loss of urine, is not a routine or normal occurrence with aging. Incontinence may occur as a result of physiologic changes, other medical problems such as UTIs, neurologic problems, or changes in the ability to function. Several classifications of medication can contribute to incontinence. Urinary incontinence is discussed in greater detail in Chapter 18.

URINARY TRACT INFECTION

The incidence of UTIs increases significantly with age. Women are more 14 times more likely than men to develop a UTI because of differences in anatomy (Platte, 2019); more than half of all women will experience a UTI at some point in their lives. Men also develop UTIs, but they are less common in men and develop at an older age. Both the normal changes of aging and the increased incidence of health problems contribute to this increased incidence of UTIs (Box 3.5).

- Inadequate or improper hygiene related to difficulty in cleansing after toileting
- Urinary stasis and incomplete emptying of bladder resulting from physiologic changes and decreased mobility
- Coexisting diseases, such as diabetes, hypertension, stroke, and dementia
- Medical interventions, including catheterization and repeated use of antibiotics (leading to resistant strains of bacteria)
- Exposure to micro-organisms in hospitals or extended-care facilities

CHRONIC KIDNEY DISEASE

Chronic kidney disease (formerly called *chronic renal failure*) may be a result of other chronic health conditions, such as hypertension, DM, chronic UTIs, or urinary tract obstruction. It may also result from acute kidney injury caused by hypovolemia, hypotension, or antibiotic toxicity.

The symptoms of chronic kidney disease are extensive and often mimic those of other conditions. These symptoms include changes in urine output, malnutrition, muscle weakness, fatigue, peripheral edema, pulmonary edema, hypertension, nausea and vomiting, itchy and dry skin, and numerous neurologic symptoms. Blood tests reveal significant changes, including elevated levels of blood urea nitrogen and creatinine as well as anemia. The treatment of chronic kidney disease requires the use of medications and dietary changes in an attempt to slow the disease process. Chronic kidney disease may become end-stage kidney disease, which is treated by dialysis or kidney transplantation.

THE NERVOUS SYSTEM

The nervous system processes and controls body functions and links us with the outside world. Through the nervous system, we perceive sensations and detect changes in our environment. We store information about the world within the nervous system and use this information to respond to the world. A functioning nervous system is necessary for survival. Internally, the nervous system and the endocrine system maintain homeostasis.

Many of the functions of the nervous system (e.g., regulation of heartbeat and body temperature) occur at an unconscious level. Other activities—such as writing, working with tools, or singing—can be done only with conscious thought and effort. Some activities, such as breathing, occur unconsciously but can also be controlled consciously. The nervous system functions at an unconscious or reflex level at birth; neurologic control is gained with maturation. With advanced age, the nervous system becomes prone to deterioration and is susceptible to many types of injury and illness.

Because of the serious consequences of age-related neurologic problems, it is important to examine this system in greater detail.

The nervous system is composed of highly specialized cells called *neurons*. Each neuron consists of a cell body, which contains the cell nucleus; multiple dendrites, which are fibers that transmit impulses (messages) to the cell body; and one axon, which carries impulses away from the cell body.

Nerve impulses are electrochemical in nature. An impulse travels through the neuron by fast-moving ion shifts across progressive segments of the cell membrane until it reaches the end of the axon. Axons and dendrites do not touch each other. A small gap called a *synapse* separates these structures. Special chemicals called *neurotransmitters* are released by the axon to stimulate a receptor site on another nerve cell. This allows the nerve impulse to move from one nerve cell to another. When the receptor has been stimulated, the neurotransmitter activity is halted by an inactivating chemical that stops the prolonged transmission of impulses. In the peripheral nervous system, the most common neurotransmitters are acetylcholine and norepinephrine. In the central nervous system, dopamine, serotonin, and norepinephrine are important. Each neurotransmitter has a specific inactivator.

The nervous system consists of two major divisions: the central nervous system and the peripheral nervous system.

CENTRAL NERVOUS SYSTEM

The central nervous system is composed of the brain and spinal cord. The brain is the master integrator of the nervous system. Thought, decision making, behavior, and all life processes are controlled by the various segments of the brain.

MEDULLA

The medulla oblongata extends from the spinal column to the pons of the brain. This area controls many vital functions, including heart rate, constriction of blood vessels (affecting blood pressure), and respiration. Reflex centers for coughing, vomiting, swallowing, and sneezing are also located in this area. Severe trauma to this area of the brain is life-threatening.

PONS AND MIDBRAIN

The pons also exerts control over respiratory patterns and works with the medulla to regulate breathing rhythm. The midbrain integrates visual and auditory reflexes and helps maintain balance and equilibrium.

CEREBELLUM

The cerebellum works to coordinate body movement at an unconscious level. It allows excitation of muscles by neurons higher in the brain and inhibits unnecessary impulses; thus it enables smooth movements without jerkiness. Picking up a cup of coffee and bringing it to your mouth in a coordinated way is an example of cerebellar activity. If you had to think consciously of all the individual movements to accomplish this activity, the coffee would be cold before you could drink it.

HYPOTHALAMUS

The hypothalamus, a small area of the brain above the pituitary gland, is the coordinating center for the autonomic nervous system. It also secretes releasing and inhibiting hormones that affect the secretions of the pituitary gland (such as growth hormone–releasing factor) and thus has various effects on the endocrine system. Other hormones, including antidiuretic hormone and oxytocin, are produced in the hypothalamus, move to the pituitary, and are released by that gland. The hypothalamus regulates body temperature, controls food intake, and is involved with visceral responses, such as the increased heart rate that occurs with anger.

CEREBRUM

The cerebrum is the largest part of the human brain. It is divided into lobes, which are named according to the cranial bones under which they lie. Because of the manner in which nerve impulses are routed in the central nervous system, the left lobes control the right side of the body and the right lobes control the left side; they function contralaterally. The frontal lobes control voluntary motor activity, judgment, planning, organization, problem solving, and behavior. The Broca area, which controls the movements related to speech, is found on the left frontal lobe in right-handed individuals. The parietal lobes interpret impulses and sensations from the skin and muscles. In addition, they are responsible for the recognition of faces, shapes, and colors. Taste sensation overlaps both the parietal and temporal lobes of the brain. The temporal lobes receive auditory (hearing) and olfactory (smelling) impulses and are devoted to new memory, learning, music, and emotions. The occipital lobes deal with vision, depth perception, and three-dimensional perception.

PERIPHERAL NERVOUS SYSTEM

The peripheral nervous system consists of the cranial and the spinal nerves; it includes the somatic and autonomic nervous systems. The peripheral nervous system is a relay system that detects changes in both the internal and external environments and relays this information to the central nervous system. It also transmits impulses from the brain and spinal cord to the appropriate end organs. To prevent messages from short-circuiting each other in the peripheral nervous system and to speed impulse conduction, the axons of many types of nerves are surrounded by Schwann cells, which form a protective myelin sheath. Probably because of the myelin sheath, injured peripheral

nerves can be surgically repaired, or they may even regenerate spontaneously if the damage is not too severe. Neurons in the central nervous system lack this guiding sheath; if damaged, they usually die.

EXPECTED AGE-RELATED CHANGES

Many cellular changes have been observed in the aging brain, including a reduction in its size and weight resulting from a decrease in the volume of the cerebral cortex. There is approximately a 3% reduction in brain tissue in each decade from ages 50 to 90. Brain shrinkage has been linked to a decrease in the number of functional cortical neurons (Table 3.8). Mental function is often changed as these cells are lost or undergo functional changes. Cerebral blood flow decreases with aging because of the gradual accumulation of fatty deposits (i.e., arteriosclerosis). Decreased blood flow also results in a slower rate of cerebral metabolism. A progressive decrease in the number of branches and the connections between dendrites occurs over time. Studies of neurotransmitters show that brain transmission of serotonin becomes impaired with aging (Karrer et al., 2019), which can make the older adult vulnerable to developing depression; and norepinephrine levels decrease. Levels of monoamine oxidase, which metabolizes catecholamines, increase. In the peripheral nervous system, the velocity of nerve conduction is strongly associated with aging (Palve & Palve, 2018).

Table 3.8	Neurologic Changes Associated With Aging
PHYSIOLOGIC CHANGE	**RESULTS**
Decreased number of brain cells	Slowed thought processes, decreased ability to respond to multiple stimuli and tasks
Decreased number of nerve fibers	Decreased reflexes, decreased coordination, decreased proprioception
Decreased amounts of neuroreceptors	Decreased perception of stimuli
Decreased peripheral nerve function	Decreased motor responses, increased risk for ischemic paresthesia in extremities
NURSING ASSESSMENTS AND CARE STRATEGIES RELATED TO NEUROLOGIC CHANGES	
NURSING ASSESSMENTS	**CARE STRATEGIES**
Assess alertness level, cognition, and functional abilities.	Report abnormal findings to primary care provider. Facilitate referral for neurologic evaluation.
Assess balance and reflexes.	Educate regarding safety precautions and use of assistive devices. Structure tasks to reduce confusion; allow adequate time to perform tasks.

Because of these physiologic changes, motor responses take longer to occur in older individuals. Simple actions such as walking and talking often become slower with age. Reflex movements become sluggish, and reactions are slowed. Some loss of coordination is common. Tasks that require quick perception of stimuli and highly coordinated responses (e.g., driving in rush-hour traffic) may pose a risk to those with significant neural loss. Many aging people recognize these changes and modify their lifestyles to avoid potentially dangerous situations.

COMMON DISORDERS SEEN WITH AGING

PARKINSON DISEASE

Parkinson disease, also called *paralysis agitans*, is a progressive, degenerative disorder of the central nervous system. The cause of Parkinson disease is unknown. Specific neurons in the brain that produce the neurotransmitter dopamine are lost. Symptoms usually begin after age 40 and appear gradually. The incidence of Parkinson disease increases in older age groups.

People suffering from Parkinson disease may manifest a variety of symptoms. The initial signs of the disease tend to be unilateral and include slight tremors on one side in addition to a more general weakness and slowing down. As the disease progresses, these tremors become typical and obvious at rest and decrease with conscious movement; they are totally absent during sleep. Emotional stress or fatigue often worsens the tremors. Later in the course of the disease, both sides of the body become affected. Tremor increases, the body becomes more rigid, and movements become slower. The face takes on a flat, open-mouthed, masklike expression, and eye blinking decreases in frequency. Speech slows and may be unclear. Swallowing may be affected. Many have trouble either starting to walk or stopping once they have begun. Gait changes, and the affected individual appears to lean forward and walk with short, shuffling steps that occur faster and faster until the person almost runs in an attempt to avoid falling. It is common for people with Parkinson disease to fall both forward and backward, because with increasing rigidity they lose the ability to compensate for shifts in their center of gravity. In severe cases, the affected person may become extremely rigid and unable to move.

Changes in mental processes may accompany physical changes. It has been reported that as many as 50% of people with Parkinson disease will develop dementia within 10 years; it is called *Parkinson disease dementia* (PDD). Early research suggests that there might be structural changes in the dopaminergic layers of the retina that predict the development of PDD (Leyland et al., 2020). Personality changes, frustration, and depression are common with Parkinson disease.

Medical treatment aimed at decreasing the symptoms of Parkinson disease includes medications such as levodopa (combined with carbidopa); dopamine agonists (which act like dopamine in the brain), such as pramipexole; monoamine oxidase B inhibitors (which block dopamine breakdown), such as selegiline; amantadine; and anticholinergic drugs. These medications may allow less severely affected individuals to function almost normally. Unfortunately, the effects of many of these drugs lessen over time, or the symptoms worsen. Various combinations of medications are often ordered to maximize benefit. Because stress worsens the symptoms, it is particularly important to minimize frustration and emotional upset in these individuals. Deep brain stimulation (DBS) is a surgical procedure that can bring dramatic results to some individuals with Parkinson disease. During this procedure, electrodes are surgically implanted into targeted areas of the brain and are connected to an impulse generator similar to a cardiac pacemaker. Although DBS does not cure or even slow disease progression, it can dramatically reduce symptoms and enhance quality of life for some patients.

DEMENTIA

Dementia is a general term for a permanent or progressive organic mental disorder. It is characterized by personality changes; confusion; disorientation; deterioration of intellectual functioning; and impaired control of memory, judgment, and impulses. Dementia can be a result of drug intoxication, trauma, disease processes, hormonal imbalances, and vitamin deficiencies. Some forms are treatable and reversible, particularly when an early diagnosis is made. Other forms do not respond to any known treatment. The most common type of dementia is Alzheimer dementia. Some of the other dementias more commonly found in older adults include the following:

- Vascular dementia, often referred to as vascular cognitive impairment; this is the second most common form of dementia. It results from hemorrhage or ischemic brain lesions, and the exact symptoms depend on the area of the brain affected. Onset of vascular dementia is usually sudden, unlike the gradual onset of Alzheimer dementia, and usually follows an episode of reduced blood flow to the brain, such as after stroke or multiple transient ischemic attacks (TIAs). Persons with hypertension or other types of cerebrovascular disease are most likely to develop this form of dementia. Risk for vascular dementia can be reduced by identifying and treating factors that contribute to the development of vascular disease, including high lipid (cholesterol) levels, elevated homocysteine levels, high blood pressure, smoking, and obesity.
- Dementia with Lewy bodies (DLB) is caused by microscopic protein clumps (Lewy bodies) in the brain that cause damage to nerve cells. In addition to the classic symptoms of dementia, visual

hallucinations are characteristic of this form of dementia. Many individuals with DLB develop Parkinson-like symptoms, including slowness, limb and facial stiffness, and tremors.

- Parkinson disease dementia usually occurs with the progression of Parkinson disease; it is caused by protein clumps in the brain's substantia nigra and can resemble both DLB and Alzheimer dementia.
- Mixed dementia can occur when more than one form of dementia is present. This will present as primarily one type of dementia (e.g., Alzheimer) with features of other dementias.

ALZHEIMER DEMENTIA

Alzheimer dementia is one stage in the continuum of Alzheimer disease. Research has shown that Alzheimer disease begins with pathologic brain changes several years before the appearance of symptoms such as memory loss. The umbrella term *Alzheimer disease* now includes not only people with dementia but also people with mild cognitive impairment as well as those with no symptoms but verified biomarkers of the disease (Alzheimer's Association, 2021).

Alzheimer dementia is the most common form of dementia and is most often seen in people over age 65. From age 65 onward, the incidence of Alzheimer dementia increases dramatically. By age 85, nearly 35% of the population is affected. More women than men have Alzheimer disease, primarily because they live longer, and age is the greatest risk factor for Alzheimer disease. Researchers estimate that the annual number of cases of Alzheimer and other dementias will more than double by 2060 to 13.8 million individuals (Alzheimer's Association, 2021).

🌐 Cultural Considerations

Alzheimer Dementia

- Older Hispanics are 1.5 times more likely to have Alzheimer or other dementias than are older Whites.
- Older Blacks are about twice as likely to have Alzheimer or other dementias as are older Whites.
- The greater incidence of Alzheimer and other dementias in these groups seems not to be related to genetic factors, but rather to the following:
  - Disparities in health conditions, such as a higher incidence of diabetes and cardiovascular disease.
  - Socioeconomic factors, such as higher poverty rates and lower quality of education.
  - Life experiences, including exposure to adversity, discrimination, and structural racism – a broad term that encompasses many features of life including where people are able to live, the quality of community schools, exposure to environmental toxins and pollutants, and other disadvantages (Alzheimer's Association, 2021).
- Despite these higher incidence rates, researchers believe that Alzheimer dementia is underdiagnosed in the Hispanic and Black populations.

Alzheimer disease is a chronic, progressive, degenerative disease in which large numbers of brain cells and tissues are affected by atrophy, beta-amyloid plaques, and neurofibrillary tangles. The level of the neurotransmitter acetylcholine in the brain decreases, leading to a disturbed ability to reason and retain new information. Levels of norepinephrine and dopamine are also decreased in Alzheimer disease.

The disease progresses from mild forgetfulness to a total loss of function. As mentioned previously, changes in the brain may begin up to 20 years before obvious symptoms are noticed. The diagnostic criteria for Alzheimer disease, revised in 2011, reflect this belief (see Box 10.5). The trajectory for Alzheimer disease is a downward one, beginning even before symptoms become evident (Fig. 3.9). The financial and social costs of Alzheimer disease are staggering, as evidenced by the following:

- The Alzheimer's Association states that the cost of care for individuals who suffer from Alzheimer or other dementias for health care, long-term care, and hospice in 2021 was $355 billion.
- This number is expected to increase to $1.1 trillion by 2050.
- Unpaid caregivers for people with Alzheimer and other dementias (often family members) provide more than 15 billion hours per year in care, representing approximately $257 billion in value to the United States (Alzheimer's Association, 2021).
- The cost of care for the final 5 years of life for an individual with Alzheimer or another dementia is more than $285,000 (Wong, 2020).

The cause of Alzheimer disease is unknown, but it likely involves multiple factors. Extensive research is taking place worldwide to identify a cause so that a cure can be found. Advanced age is the biggest risk factor for Alzheimer disease. Family history of the disease is another, with genetics playing a role. Children of people with Alzheimer disease have an increased risk of developing the disease, in which the apolipoprotein E (APOE) gene plays a major role. This gene's allele (APOE e4) has been implicated as a risk factor; however, everyone has some type of APOE gene (other forms are APOE e2 and APOE e3). If a person receives a copy of APOE e4 from one or both parents, the risk of Alzheimer disease increases, as does the risk for disease at a younger age. APOE e4 may be a factor in one-quarter of Alzheimer disease cases. The fact that a person has the risk gene does not mean that they will develop the disease, but the risk will be greater.

🏃 Health Promotion

Recent studies have suggested that people with the APOE e4 gene have a lower risk of dementia when they had more years of early life education, had mentally challenging work in midlife, and had special interests (a strong social network or participation in leisure activity) in later life (Alzheimer's Association, 2021).

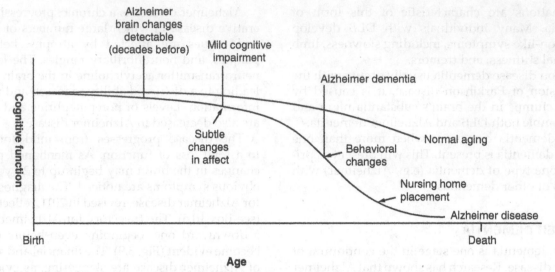

Fig. 3.9 Typical progression of Alzheimer disease.

In addition to risk genes, there are **deterministic genes** that "guarantee" the development of Alzheimer disease in anyone who has these genes. Deterministic genes in the case of Alzheimer disease include those coding three specific proteins. The disease that follows is referred to as *autosomal dominant Alzheimer disease*. These genes, fortunately, are found in only a few hundred extended families worldwide. Members of these families develop the disease at a young age, showing symptoms as early as in their 30s. Less than 1% of Alzheimer cases are true familial cases.

Other factors implicated in Alzheimer disease include head trauma, especially when severe or repeated, and any type of cardiovascular disease. People with more years of formal education have been found to be at lower risk of Alzheimer and other dementias than those without, possibly because of increased neuronal connections or increased "cognitive reserve." Other studies suggest that maintaining social and mental activities while aging can reduce the risk of Alzheimer and other dementias (Alzheimer's Association, 2021).

🌐 Cultural Considerations

Life Stressors and Alzheimer Disease

Life stressors have been associated with the development of Alzheimer disease. A single life stressor, such as losing a child, can increase the risk of developing Alzheimer disease by 4%; the biggest effect is seen in minority populations (Honig & Sano, 2017).

Physical examination and laboratory tests are typically performed to rule out reversible causes of dementia symptoms, such as **hypothyroidism**, vitamin B_{12} deficiency, or medication side effects. Empirical diagnosis is made based on the evaluation of behavioral changes; psychometric testing to measure memory, attention, and problem solving; and brain scans, such as magnetic resonance imaging (MRI), computed tomography (CT), or positron emission tomography (PET).

Until recently, no definitive diagnostic test for Alzheimer disease existed. The only way to confirm the diagnosis was a postmortem examination of the brain tissues. In 2010, researchers in Belgium identified specific proteins that could not only be used diagnostically but also had a high predictive significance for the development of this form of dementia. Spinal fluid levels that are low in beta-amyloid proteins and high in tau and phospho-tau proteins are highly indicative of Alzheimer disease (Jiao et al., 2020). Changes in these protein levels occur slowly and may precede the first classic symptoms of the disease by a decade. These tests are still in the research stage and are not available to the public. More scientific study needs to be done. These studies and others offer promise of earlier detection, better treatment, and hope for a cure for this devastating illness. One area of current research involves blood-based biomarkers of the disease; it is showing promising results in detecting Alzheimer disease with high accuracy (Alzheimer's Association, 2020) and may one day replace spinal fluid analysis, as it is less invasive and better tolerated.

Currently, older adults suffering from Alzheimer disease are treated with several classifications of drugs. Cholinesterase inhibitors are used for patients with mild to moderate disease. These drugs are designed to prevent the breakdown of acetylcholine, the neurotransmitter that plays an important role in memory and thinking skills. Drugs in the class include donepezil, rivastigmine, and galantamine.

Another drug, memantine, has been approved to treat moderate to severe Alzheimer disease. This drug is believed to work by regulating the level of glutamate, a neurotransmitter that helps the brain process, store, and retrieve information. Drugs specific to Alzheimer treatment are often supplemented with antidepressants, anxiolytics, and even antipsychotics, which are prescribed based on the behavioral or psychotic symptoms that frequently coexist with Alzheimer symptoms. The use of antipsychotic medications is controversial, however, as less than one-third demonstrate improvement of behavioral symptoms and the risk of death from these medications is 1.6 to 1.7 times higher than that from treatment with placebo. The FDA has issued a "black box" warning about the risks of these medications when they are used for the treatment of dementia (Rubino et al., 2020). The current practice guidelines for using antipsychotic medications with dementia, issued by the American Psychiatric Association (2016), include numerous recommendations such as using these medications only when symptoms are severe, dangerous, or causing significant patient distress; they also recommend tapering/withdrawing the medications after 4 months to assess the need for continued use.

Alternative Treatments for Alzheimer Disease

Vitamins C and E, coenzyme Q10, selenium, ginkgo biloba, huperzine A, and coral calcium have been recommended as "natural" remedies for the treatment of Alzheimer disease. Dosages vary and have not been evaluated by the FDA for effectiveness or safety. In addition, many older adults, particularly those diagnosed with Alzheimer disease, have lower-than-normal levels of melatonin, a hormone secreted by the pineal gland, that helps to regulate sleep rhythms. There is potential but limited evidence that melatonin, which is available over the counter, or possibly new drugs that have more targeted responses, might provide some benefit by improving sleep patterns and decreasing the incidence of the behavioral changes, called *sundowning*, seen at the end of the day in these patients. Because "natural" remedies can interact with prescription medication, these substances should be used only under the direction of the primary care provider.

Clinical trials are being conducted to determine the potential effectiveness of a vaccine targeting the abnormal beta-amyloid and tau proteins, and positive initial results are being reported, although specific data are lacking (Kuntz, 2021). Many other research projects designed to develop medications or treatments for this devastating disease are currently in the pipeline.

TRANSIENT ISCHEMIC ATTACKS

TIAs are brief episodes of cerebrovascular insufficiency that are usually the result of cerebral blood vessel obstruction. Such obstruction is usually caused by an embolus or atherosclerotic plaque. TIAs occur most commonly in middle-aged and older people.

TIAs occur without warning. Most episodes last only a few minutes, but some may persist as long as 24 hours. A person may have several attacks within a day or may go for months without experiencing another. A variety of symptoms may indicate the occurrence of a TIA. Common symptoms include blurred, tunnel, or double vision; blindness; vertigo; transient numbness and weakness; aphasia or slurred speech; and gait disturbances. The person generally remains conscious throughout the attack. The symptoms of TIAs disappear spontaneously and do not cause permanent neurologic damage.

TIAs may be warnings of an impending stroke, but this is not necessarily the case. Some individuals who suffer from TIAs never have a stroke.

STROKE

Stroke, formerly called *cerebrovascular accident*, is a disturbance of the blood supply to the brain. Most strokes are related to atherosclerosis, hypertension, diabetes, or a combination of these. They can occur at any age, most commonly affecting individuals over age 65. Strokes are often fatal and are the fifth leading cause of death in the United States and a leading cause of disability (American Stroke Association, 2021). The likelihood of stroke fatality increases with advanced age. Stroke occurs slightly more often in men than in women. African Americans are affected more often than other groups, possibly because there is a higher incidence of hypertension in the African American population.

There are two main categories of stroke: (1) *ischemic*, where there is lack of blood and oxygen flow caused by embolus or thrombus, comprising 87% of all strokes, and (2) *hemorrhagic*, in which weakened vessels or aneurysms rupture spontaneously or as a result of hypertension. Although hemorrhagic stroke is less common, it accounts for 40% of all stroke deaths (Han & Higuera, 2019).

> **⚠ Nurse Alert**
>
> If a stroke is suspected, care is directed at supporting essential life functions—maintaining an open airway, providing adequate oxygenation, and preventing trauma. Stroke is a medical emergency requiring a 911 call (or Code Stroke Alert if the patient is hospitalized). Immediate hospitalization is critical to enable the patient to be eligible for the best care possible, which would comprise intravenous recombinant tissue plasminogen activator (IV r-tPA) and possible endovascular therapy (mechanical thrombectomy). If one or both of these procedures are performed in a timely manner, the clot can be dissolved or removed, the damage minimized, and rehabilitation shortened significantly. Intravenous r-tPA must be administered within 4.5 hours of symptom onset; however, with newer imaging studies, the time window for thrombectomy is expanding to 24 hours in some cases (Filho & Samuels, 2021). Because some strokes are hemorrhagic, this must be ruled out first with computed tomography (CT). CT angiography is used to identify the clot for endovascular therapy.

Unfortunately, as many as 25% of stroke patients are discovered in the morning by a family member; if the onset of symptoms is unknown, they are ineligible for tPA and often endovascular therapy as well (MacGrory et al., 2021). The length of hospitalization and rehabilitation or extended care is based on the individual's situation. The onset of a stroke may be sudden, or symptoms may progress gradually. The nature of symptoms varies with the type of stroke, the area of the brain affected, and the extent of the damage (Boxes 3.6 and 3.7). Because the two sides of the brain serve very different functions, the symptoms depend on which side is affected. Effects of strokes are contralateral: damage to the right hemisphere affects the left side of the body; damage to the left hemisphere affects the right side of the body. Some individuals manifest mild symptoms, whereas the symptoms are more severe in others. A few victims of stroke recover completely, but most have some lingering deficits. Most improvement occurs within the first 6 months after a stroke. Any deficit lasting longer than 6 months is likely to be permanent. Recurrence of stroke is common, and each occurrence is likely to cause additional problems.

Box 3.6 Signs and Symptoms of Damage to the Right Hemisphere of the Brain

- Left hemiparesis (weakness of the left arm and/or leg)
- Impaired sense of humor
- Disorientation to time, place, and person
- Difficulty recognizing people
- Visual/spatial problems, including loss of depth perception
- Neglect of the left visual field (patient may not see objects or hazards on the left side of body)
- Loss of impulse control (patient may strike out, cry, or shout if upset)
- Unaware of neurologic function loss (patient may try to stand or walk despite hemiparesis)
- Poor judgment (patient may deny illness or problems or tend to overestimate her or his the ability to perform activities)
- Inappropriate responses (patient may smile continually or demonstrate euphoric behavior even in serious or tragic situations)
- Confabulation (patient may make up detailed but inaccurate explanations to compensate for memory losses, which can be very believable to persons who are not aware of the facts)

Box 3.7 Signs and Symptoms of Damage to the Left Hemisphere of the Brain

- Right hemiparesis (weakness of the right arm and/or leg)
- Language disturbances
- Aphasia—defective or absent language skills that may be expressive (motor), in which words cannot be formed; receptive (sensory), in which language is not understood; or mixed, in which both processes are affected
- Agraphia—loss of the ability to write
- Alexia—inability to comprehend written words; reading problems
- Neglect of the right visual field (patient may not see objects or hazards on the right side of body)
- Behavioral changes (patient may be slow, cautious, and anxious in attempting new activities)
- Mood changes (tendency to worry or feel depressed; patient may verbalize feelings of worthlessness, guilt, anger, and frustration)

THE SPECIAL SENSES

The special senses—including sight, hearing, balance, smell, and taste—are integrally connected to the central nervous system by the cranial nerves. The other senses include touch, pressure, and proprioception, or the awareness of body movement and position in space. These senses are the means by which we gather information from the world around us and about our relationship to this world. The special senses provide our first line of protection against environmental hazards. Unless all of these senses function properly and provide us with accurate information, we are at risk for suffering from these hazards.

It is important to understand the visual and auditory changes that occur with aging, because these changes may have serious safety implications. A great deal of the information that we receive and respond to comes to us through our senses of sight and hearing. We may think that older adults are confused or senile when actually their sensory perceptions are merely impaired because of the changes associated with aging.

THE EYES

The eyes are two globe-shaped structures located in the orbits of the skull, one on each side of the nose. Because the eyes are so important, they have surrounding structures designed to protect them from both physical and biologic hazards.

The eyelids are controlled by skeletal muscle and lined with a smooth mucous membrane called the *conjunctiva*. The eyelids can close; thus they and the eyelashes located on their margins provide protection from dust and flying debris. Tears are produced by the lacrimal glands, located at the upper and outer corners of the eye. These glands lubricate the eye, prevent particles of debris from scraping the surface, and inhibit bacterial growth by means of the enzyme lysozyme. Tears leave the eye at the medial corner through the lacrimal sac and the nasolacrimal duct that drains into the nose.

The eye itself is composed of three layers. The outermost layer, the sclera (commonly called the *white of the eye*), is composed of fibrous connective tissue and supports the inner eye structures. The anterior part of the sclera is the cornea, a transparent structure that refracts or bends light rays. The sclera contains small capillaries that are sometimes visible on its surface. The cornea does not contain any capillaries or nerves.

The middle layer of the eye, the choroid, contains pigments that absorb light and keep the interior of the eye dark. The choroid is highly vascular and supplies nourishment to the surrounding tissue. Located in the anterior portion of the choroid are the iris (the colored portion), the pupil (an opening in the iris through which light enters the eye), the lens (a transparent oval disk), and the ciliary body (muscles that change the shape of the lens to refract light waves). The lens does not contain any capillaries or nerves.

The innermost layer of the eye is the retina. This structure covers the posterior two-thirds of the eye and contains the visual receptors—highly specialized structures called *rods* and *cones*. These receptors use chemical changes in their pigments to detect light. Cones are most abundant near the center of the retina. They detect color and discriminate among different colors based on the wavelength of the incoming light. Rods are more abundant near the periphery of the retina and detect the presence or absence of light. Vitamin A is essential to the formation of the pigment in the rods that enables their response. Rods are important for vision in low-light situations. Nerves in the retina transmit messages from the rods and cones to the optic nerve, which sends the information to the vision centers of the brain. The macula lutea (yellow spot) is an area less than 2 mm in size near the center of the retina that provides sharp central vision.

The greatest part of the eye mass is made up of two fluid-filled cavities. The small anterior cavity is located between the cornea and the lens; it contains *aqueous humor*, a fluid formed by capillaries in the choroid. This fluid passes from the posterior chamber through the pupil to the anterior chamber and supplies nourishment for the lens and cornea, which have no blood supply. Because aqueous humor is produced continuously, some must be absorbed or the amount of fluid would become excessive. Normally, absorption takes place through small veins located at the juncture of the iris and cornea. The presence of excess fluid increases the pressure in the anterior chamber. The posterior cavity of the eye, the vitreous, is much larger and contains a gelatinous substance called the *vitreous humor*. It holds the retina in contact with the choroid of the eye.

REFRACTION

The eye functions much like a camera. Light waves enter it through the cornea and then pass through the aqueous humor, lens, and vitreous humor to the retina. When light waves strike the retina, they stimulate the receptors in the cones and rods. The rods react chemically to the amount of light and regulate nerve impulses to the brain based on this information. Different cones respond to different wavelengths (different colors) of light rays, thus determining the perceived color of objects. Based on information gathered from the rods and cones, the image projected onto the retina is translated into nerve impulses by the retina, which then sends the information through the optic nerves to the visual centers of the cerebral cortex in the occipital region. The optic nerves from both eyes meet at the optic chiasm just under the pituitary gland. At the optic chiasm, the medial fibers (from the image on the part of the retina closest to the nose) cross to the opposite side of the brain, whereas the lateral fibers (from the outside part of the retina) do not cross. This allows visual centers on both sides of the brain to process messages from both eyes and is important for binocular vision. Because of its position, each eye "sees" things somewhat differently from the other and sends slightly different messages to the brain. The brain receives messages from both eyes, correlates the information, and makes sense of it. Binocular vision is also important for depth perception, the sense of how far you are from another person or object.

For information to be received accurately, all of the eye's structures must function together to focus the light rays. The lens's shape is controlled by the ciliary body, whose muscles relax or contract to change the shape of the lens, so that it can bend the light waves correctly and bring an object into clear focus. This change in lens shape is called *accommodation*.

EXPECTED AGE-RELATED CHANGES

Refractive errors, or errors in focusing ability, occur when the cornea is misshapen or the lens cannot appropriately change shape to focus images.

With aging, many structural and functional changes may occur in the eye (Table 3.9). The eyelids become less elastic and sag. Eyelashes tend to be shorter, thinner, and in some cases absent. A grayish haze of the peripheral cornea, referred to as arcus senilis (Fig. 3.10), develops with aging and is more common in dark-skinned persons.

Legal blindness is defined as visual acuity of 20/200 or less in the worse eye even with the best correction, or a visual field extent of less than 20 degrees in diameter. Vision impairment is defined as having vision 20/40 or worse with correction. Most blind people are age 65 or older, with the rate increasing sharply with age. According to the Centers for Disease Control and Prevention (CDC, 2020a), the number of adults with blindness will more than double by 2050 because of aging, diabetes, and other chronic diseases.

Refractive errors are the most common visual problem in the United States. Most people older than 50 years of age experience some degree of farsightedness, also called *hyperopia* or *presbyopia*, which literally means "aging eye." Refractive errors become increasingly common as the ciliary muscles lose their ability to contract

Table 3.9 **Vision Changes Associated With Aging**

PHYSIOLOGIC CHANGE	RESULTS
Decreased number of eyelashes	Increased risk for eye injury
Decreased tear production	Increased risk for eye irritation
Increased discoloration of lens	Decreased color perception
Decreased tissue elasticity	Increased blurring
Decreased muscle tone	Decreased diameter of pupil; increased refractive errors; decreased night vision; increased sensitivity to glare, decreased peripheral vision

NURSING ASSESSMENTS AND CARE STRATEGIES RELATED TO VISUAL CHANGES	
NURSING ASSESSMENTS	CARE STRATEGIES
Assess for signs of irritation, inflammation, and dryness.	Encourage regular use of synthetic tear preparations to help reduce irritation caused by inadequate tear production.
Assess visual acuity.	Encourage or schedule regular professional eye examinations. Educate regarding importance of adequate light with minimum glare. Explain importance of using eyeglasses appropriately for reading or distance, particularly when driving.
Assess ability to detect objects within the environment.	Provide adequate lighting and contrast in colors to highlight important structures, such as the edge of stairs, light fixtures, faucets, etc.

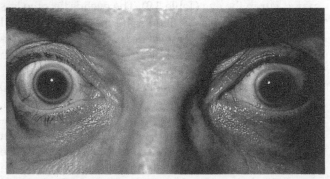

Fig. 3.10 Arcus senilis. (From Yanoff, M., & Finem, B. S. [2020] *Ocular pathology*. Mosby.)

easily, and progressive rigidity of the lens restricts accommodation. A combination of these changes makes it increasingly difficult to focus on close objects, perform detailed close work, or read. Presbyopia is usually corrected by the use of contact lenses or eyeglasses that help the older adult focus on close objects. Laser surgery is an option for some individuals.

Astigmatism, a malformation of the cornea, causes the blurring of images at all distances. People of all ages can have astigmatism, but younger people compensate for it by quickly refocusing the blurred and unblurred images. When this ability decreases with aging, astigmatism appears to worsen. Corrective lenses help with this.

A decrease in tear production is common in older adults because the volume of body fluids and secretions decreases with age. An 80-year-old person produces only 25% of the tears they produced during the teenage years. Environmental factors—such as central heating, dry climate, and wind or air pollution—can worsen the problem. Many older adults complain of dry, burning, or itching eyes caused by friction from the lids or from small particles of debris. The decline in tear production also reduces the antibacterial protection provided by enzymes and can contribute to bacterial eye infections.

Older adults may have poor dark adaption response and may have a decreased ability to adjust from light to darkness and darkness to light. Night blindness, the inability to see well in dim light, grows increasingly common with age.

Color vision and the ability to detect changes in color contrast are affected by aging. The lens of the eye tends to yellow with age, possibly leading to the misperception of color. All dark colors may be perceived as black, and subtle differences in shades may not be detectable. Younger people who find "blue-haired women" amusing should look at them through a lens that is slightly tinted yellow. Amazingly, their hair will look clean and white.

Peripheral vision and depth perception often decrease with aging. It is important to recognize these changes because they significantly increase the risk for accidents and injuries.

Another common occurrence with aging is the development of floaters. Many older adults report seeing flecks, spots, cobwebs, or brilliant crystals in their visual field. These are harmless but can be frustrating because they interfere with many visual activities such as reading, sewing, or doing other detailed work.

COMMON DISORDERS SEEN WITH AGING

BLEPHARITIS

Blepharitis, a chronic inflammation of the eyelids caused by bacteria and oily flakes at the base of the eyelid, is one of the most common disorders of the eye. Symptoms of blepharitis include burning, itching, and sensitivity to light. Discomfort is often worse on awakening. Blepharitis can be caused by *Staphylococcus* bacteria, by sebaceous gland dysfunction, or in conjunction with skin conditions, such as seborrhea or rosacea. There is no definitive cure for this disorder, but treatment can reduce the severity of the problem. Common treatment includes the use of warm compresses, eyelid massage, lid scrubs, and the use of antibiotic ointments. Skin and eyelid hygiene is very important; baby shampoo is recommended.

DIPLOPIA

Diplopia, or double vision, is not normal and indicates some disturbance of the nervous system that requires further investigation by the primary care provider.

CATARACTS

Cataracts, which cause a clouding of the lens of the eye, are increasingly common with aging. Cataracts can occur in persons in their 40s and 50s; by age 80, over half of Americans have a cataract. Factors that increase the risk for cataracts include smoking, alcohol consumption, diabetes, and prolonged sunlight exposure. Cataracts develop over time and result in progressive, painless vision loss. The amount of vision loss depends on the degree of lens opacity and the area of the lens that is affected. The ability to see in bright light or with glare may be particularly compromised with certain types of cataracts. Individuals with cataracts require frequent changes in eyeglass prescriptions while the cataract matures. When vision is severely affected, surgical removal of the cataract or the lens is the treatment of choice. Today, this surgery is common and, in most cases, can be performed on an outpatient basis. Once the cataract has been removed, vision is usually corrected with surgically implanted lenses; in some individuals, contact lenses or cataract glasses may be needed.

GLAUCOMA

Glaucoma is a disease characterized in most cases by increased fluid pressure (intraocular pressure) within the eye, which may damage the retina. Initially, peripheral vision is affected. Tunnel vision and, eventually, permanent blindness may result. The incidence of glaucoma increases with age. Additional risk factors include family history; diabetes; African American, Asian, or Native Alaskan ancestry; hypertension; history of eye injury; heart disease; and prolonged use of corticosteroids. African Americans are at increased risk beginning at age 40 (American Optometric Association, 2021).

Persons with glaucoma seldom experience obvious symptoms, so serious damage usually occurs before the disease is even recognized. However, a test for increased intraocular pressure can be performed easily; it is simple, painless, and takes only minutes. It is normally part of a routine ophthalmic examination, and everyone over age 40 should be tested regularly. Early detection and treatment can delay disease progression. Medications, surgery, and laser therapy can be used to treat glaucoma, but any damage already done cannot be reversed.

AGE-RELATED MACULAR DEGENERATION AND RETINAL DETACHMENT

The macula, the small area in the center of the retina where visual acuity is best, is susceptible to damage and destruction. Age-related macular degeneration (AMD) occurs most often in people over age 50. The incidence of this disorder increases significantly after age 75, and it is more common in Whites, people who smoke, and those with family history of AMD. The exact cause of macular degeneration remains unknown, but two types of the disorder have been identified. The more common atrophic form, also called *dry AMD*, is a result of inadequate nutrient supply or waste removal from the eye due to vascular changes. When its cells atrophy or die, the macula is damaged and central vision is significantly diminished. Vision is restricted but not totally lost because noncentral vision remains. A major clinical trial with 3600 participants, the Age-Related Eye Disease Study (AREDS), demonstrated that a precise formula of antioxidants and zinc, the *AREDS Formulation*, can reduce the risk of developing AMD by 25%. This formulation consists of *specific doses* of vitamins C and E, beta-carotene, zinc, and copper. A second study, AREDS2, replaced beta-carotene with lutein and zeaxanthin (from the same nutrient family but safer to use in smokers) and added omega-3 fatty acids. The second study found that replacing beta-carotene with lutein and zeaxanthin may further reduce the risk for AMD (National Eye Institute, 2020). Of course, these substances should be used at the direction of one's primary care provider.

The neovascular form of macular degeneration, also called *wet AMD*, results from the abnormal growth of tiny blood vessels (neovascularization) under the retina. These vessels ruin vision by leaking fluid and blood, which cause the retina to become swollen and distorted. This form is more likely to cause severe vision loss. Laser surgery or microsurgery may be attempted to seal leaking vessels, slow their growth, and prevent further vision loss.

Circulatory changes in the blood vessels of the eyes are common with DM, resulting in *diabetic retinopathy*. This condition is characterized by the hemorrhaging of small blood vessels into the vitreous humor and has effects similar to those of neovascular macular degeneration (i.e., loss of vision). According to the CDC (2020b), diabetic retinopathy is the leading cause of blindness in American adults. Retinopathy is related not to age but rather to the severity and duration of hyperglycemia. Diabetic retinopathy is increasing at a rapid rate in older adults because of the growing incidence of diabetes in the older adult population.

Normal shrinkage of the eye and changes in the consistency of the vitreous humor are common with aging and may result in retinal detachment, which is the separation of the retina from the choroid. Any or all of these changes can result in the loss of central vision.

THE EARS

The ear is composed of three distinct portions: the outer, middle, and inner ear. The two main functions of the ear are the detection of sound and the maintenance of balance.

The outer ear consists of the visible curved structure called the *pinna*, or *auricle*, and the external ear canal.

The pliable auricle is made of cartilage. The size and shape of the external ear have little influence on hearing.

The middle ear begins at the eardrum, or tympanic membrane. This transparent membrane stretches across the end of the ear canal and separates it from an air-filled chamber called the *middle ear*. Air pressure in the middle ear is controlled through the eustachian tube, which connects the middle ear to the nasopharynx. Attached to the tympanic membrane is a series of three small bones: the malleus (hammer), incus (anvil), and stapes (stirrup). Sound waves enter the ear through the external ear canal and cause the tympanic membrane to vibrate. This, in turn, causes movement of the three small bones, which then transmit the vibrations to the oval window, the opening into the inner ear.

The inner ear is a complex fluid-filled structure that has several functions. A portion called the *cochlea* contains the hearing receptors, which consist of hair cells with fine movable projections that are set in motion when sound waves reach their fluid surroundings. When these hairs move, impulses are carried through the auditory nerve (a cranial nerve) to the midbrain and then to the temporal lobe of the brain, where the sound is heard.

Other specialized hair cells are found elsewhere in the inner ear: the vestibule and the semicircular canals. Hair cells from these structures transmit information in response to gravity, change of position, and motion through the cranial nerves. The central nervous system processes this information and maintains equilibrium.

EXPECTED AGE-RELATED CHANGES

Just as other body tissues become thinner with age, so does the tympanic membrane (Table 3.10). The small muscles that support the membrane show signs of atrophy with advanced age. Arthritic changes affect the joints between the small bones of the middle ear, and hair cells in the inner ear often deteriorate.

Presbycusis, defined as an alteration in hearing capacity related to aging, affects two-thirds of Americans over age 70 (Cheslock & De Jesus, 2021). Men are more affected by this problem than women. The aging person with presbycusis loses the ability to perceive high-frequency tones. Speech sounds, such as *s*, *sh*, *ch*, and soft *t* may not be audible, so the aging person may hear only parts of spoken words. Simple words, such as *cat*, *hat*, *sat*, and *that* may all sound the same. If other noises are present in the environment, sounds become even less distinct. The aging individual may have difficulty sorting out words and making sense of what is being said.

COMMON DISORDERS SEEN WITH AGING

OTOSCLEROSIS

Otosclerosis, a hardening or fixing of the stapes to the oval window, interferes with the transmission of sound waves to the inner ear. This condition occurs slightly more often in women than in men. Surgical correction is possible.

Table 3.10	Auditory Changes Associated With Aging
PHYSIOLOGIC CHANGE	**RESULTS**
Decreased tissue elasticity	Decreased ability to distinguish high-frequency sounds
Decreased joint mobility	Decreased hearing ability
Decreased ceruminous cells in external ear canal	Increased risk for cerumen impaction causing conductive hearing loss
Atrophy of vestibular structures and in the inner ear	Increased problems with balance; decreased number of hair cells
NURSING ASSESSMENTS AND CARE STRATEGIES RELATED TO AUDITORY CHANGES	
NURSING ASSESSMENTS	**CARE STRATEGIES**
Assess hearing and balance.	Facilitate referral for audiometric testing as needed.
Inspect ear canal for cerumen impaction.	Administer prophylactic drops to reduce likelihood of impaction formation. Irrigate if impaction is present.
Assess functioning of hearing aid if used.	Check that batteries are working and that device is not plugged with cerumen. Keep an amplifying device on each patient care unit to use with hard of hearing individuals who do not have a functional hearing aid.
Assess for social isolation or behavioral background noise.	Encourage socialization in areas without excessive changes.

TINNITUS

Tinnitus, or ringing in the ears, is commonly reported by aging people. Tinnitus may be a result of trauma to the ear, pressure from cerumen against the eardrum, otosclerosis, presbycusis, or Ménière disease. Tinnitus can also be caused by certain medications, such as antibiotics and diuretics. If tinnitus is suspected to be medication-related, it must be reported promptly, as it can indicate medication toxicity and risk of (preventable) deafness.

DEAFNESS

Deafness, the inability to hear sounds fully, may be temporary or permanent, depending on the cause. Deafness can be unilateral (affecting one ear only) or bilateral (affecting both ears).

Conductive hearing loss occurs when something interferes with the transmission of sound waves. A plug of cerumen (earwax) in the external canal, eardrum rupture or scarring, the presence of fluid or infection in the middle ear, or any condition that interferes with movement of the middle ear's small bones may result in conductive hearing loss or deafness.

Nerve or sensorineural deafness occurs when either the receptors in the inner ear or the cranial nerves are damaged or destroyed. Some antibiotics and viral infections can cause nerve deafness. Chronic exposure to loud noise can speed up the degeneration of hair cells. Many young people today are experiencing significant hearing loss from excessive exposure to extremely loud music, and this will have serious implications as they age. Work-related noise has also been shown to impair hearing. Many aging individuals who worked in foundries or other noisy places may have suffered employment-related hearing loss. The Occupational Safety and Health Administration now requires employers to protect employees from excessive exposure to loud noise on the job.

Central deafness is caused by trauma or disease in the temporal lobes of the brain. This may be a result of tumors, stroke, or injury. Central deafness is not common.

MÉNIÈRE DISEASE

Ménière disease is a chronic disorder of the inner ear observed in people after age 40. Persons suffering from this disorder experience severe vertigo (not simple dizziness) to the point that they may be unable to stand or walk. They may also report nausea, tinnitus, hearing loss, and a sensation of pressure in the ear. Diaphoresis, vomiting, and nystagmus (rapid, involuntary eye movement) may also occur. Episodes generally appear suddenly and may last for minutes or hours. The frequency of attacks is unpredictable. Ménière disease tends to affect one ear, and it can result in nerve deafness that sometimes persists even if treatment relieves the other symptoms.

TASTE AND SMELL

The receptors for the sense of taste are located in the papillae, or taste buds, on the superior surface of the tongue. The papillae contain chemical receptor cells that are sensitive to salty, sweet, sour, and bitter chemicals. When mixed with moisture, such as saliva or water, food releases chemicals that are detected by these receptors. Foods get their subtle flavors by their unique interaction with various receptors. The detection of odors occurs when the olfactory receptors in the upper nasal cavities respond to airborne chemicals. When vapors escape from food or other volatile substances, they enter the nose and stimulate the receptors.

Information from both taste and smell receptors is then transported to the nervous system through the cranial nerves. When these senses are intact and functioning well, many people salivate and can "taste" a meal while it is being prepared. Without a sense of smell, a person can discern little flavor in food. People who have severe nasal congestion from colds or allergies find that without smell, food has either a strange taste or no taste at all. Some individuals with chronic nasal congestion report ongoing problems with appetite because to them, food has little flavor or appeal. People with permanent damage to the olfactory senses report a permanent change in taste (hypogeusia), which often results in a loss of appetite. Alterations in taste sensation may also be a side effect of brain tumors, gingival disease, periodontitis, systemic disorders such as diabetes or hypothyroidism, and medications. Loss of smell may be present with diseases including Alzheimer disease, Parkinson disease, or multiple sclerosis (Lava, 2019). Loss of taste and smell can occur with COVID-19 (Marshall, 2021).

EXPECTED AGE-RELATED CHANGES

With aging, there is a decrease in the number of functional receptors in both the nasal cavities and the papillae on the tongue (Table 3.11). By age 60, it is estimated that half of all adults will experience some alteration in smell and taste. The changes in taste particularly affect the receptors for sweet and salty tastes. Because salt enhances the flavor of food, older adults often add salt in an attempt to add flavor. Complaints of flavorless food are common even if the food seems well seasoned and tasty to younger individuals. Good oral hygiene, better food preparation, and flavor enhancers are sometimes helpful in improving taste.

The term *burning mouth syndrome* is used to describe an oral sensation of burning or tingling. This may be associated with a vitamin B deficiency, inadequate saliva production, allergies, GERD, trauma, and diabetes.

THE ENDOCRINE SYSTEM

The endocrine system and the nervous system perform the major integrating and regulating functions of the body. The endocrine glands secrete chemical substances, called *hormones*, that regulate body processes. Hormones are secreted directly into the capillaries of the bloodstream, where they circulate until they reach their target organs and cause specific effects. Some endocrine glands produce a single hormone; others produce

Table 3.11	Olfactory Changes Associated With Aging
PHYSIOLOGIC CHANGE	**RESULTS**
Decreased number of papillae on tongue	Decreased ability to taste
Decreased number of nasal sensory	Decreased ability to receptors and to detect smells
NURSING ASSESSMENTS AND CARE STRATEGIES RELATED TO OLFACTORY CHANGES	
NURSING ASSESSMENTS	**CARE STRATEGIES**
Assess ability to smell and taste.	Teach importance of storing food properly and checking expiration dates. Keep drugs and chemicals separated from foods.

several different hormones. Some hormones have only one target organ; others target multiple organs. The production of hormones is regulated by a negative feedback process in which the endocrine glands constantly monitor the effects of hormones circulating in the system. If the effect is adequate, the gland decreases production. If it is inadequate, the gland increases production. The process of regulation is similar to that of a thermostat and furnace in a home. When the temperature reaches that for which the thermostat is set, the thermostat signals the furnace to stop producing heat. If the temperature drops below the preset level, the thermostat signals the furnace to produce more heat. In a highly complex manner, the endocrine glands constantly monitor the effects and levels of the many hormones circulating in the body and increase or decrease production as needed to meet the body's demands.

PITUITARY GLAND

The pituitary gland is often referred to as the body's *master gland* because of the many functions it regulates. It is located within the skull cavity and is connected directly to the hypothalamus. There are two major segments of the pituitary gland: the anterior pituitary and the posterior pituitary. The posterior pituitary is the site of connection between the nervous system and the endocrine system. The posterior pituitary hormones are actually produced in the hypothalamus of the brain and are stored in the posterior pituitary until needed. The major secretion of the posterior pituitary gland is antidiuretic hormone (ADH). This hormone maintains fluid balance in the body by causing the kidneys to reabsorb fluid; in the absence of ADH, the kidneys excrete more fluid. By controlling fluid balance, ADH helps blood to regulate blood pressure. Oxytocin, another posterior pituitary hormone, stimulates uterine contraction during childbirth and milk ejection from the breast during lactation.

The anterior pituitary produces many hormones. Growth hormone increases the rate of protein synthesis and aids in the transport of amino acids to cells. In adults, this hormone also participates in the release of fat from adipose tissue and the use of this fat as energy. Thyroid-stimulating hormone stimulates the normal growth and activity of the thyroid gland. Adrenocorticotropic hormone (corticotropin) stimulates the activity of the adrenal cortex. Gonadotropic hormones include follicle-stimulating hormone and luteinizing hormone, which are responsible for the maturation and function of the gonads, and prolactin, which supports lactation.

THYROID GLAND

The thyroid gland surrounds the trachea and is located just below the larynx. The major hormones produced by the thyroid gland are thyroxin, triiodothyronine, and calcitonin. The thyroid hormones triiodothyronine and thyroxin increase metabolic rate; regulate the metabolism of fat, carbohydrates, and protein in the cells; and increase body temperature. They also affect cardiac, neurologic, and musculoskeletal functions. The function of calcitonin is to keep calcium and phosphate within the bone matrix.

PARATHYROID GLANDS

The parathyroid glands are located on the posterior surface of the lobes of the thyroid gland. PTH, an antagonist of calcitonin, stimulates the movement of calcium and phosphorus from the bones into the blood.

PANCREAS

The pancreas is both an exocrine and endocrine gland. It functions as an exocrine gland during digestion by secreting pancreatic fluid into the duodenum. The endocrine secretions of the pancreas are produced by α cells and β cells in the islets of Langerhans. The α cells produce glucagon, which stimulates the liver to convert glycogen to glucose. The β cells produce insulin, which increases the permeability of cell membranes and enables the cells to use glucose, amino acids, and fatty acids.

ADRENAL GLANDS

The adrenal glands are located on the top of each kidney. The adrenal medulla is the inner portion of the gland; the adrenal cortex is the outer portion. The adrenal medulla secretes epinephrine and norepinephrine, which are the major neurotransmitters of the sympathetic portion of the autonomic nervous system. The adrenal medulla can be viewed as the "crash cart" of the body. Its hormones increase cardiac activity and blood pressure, release of energy reserves, and control other functions needed for survival when a person is faced with danger while also decreasing functions that are less important at that time.

The adrenal cortex releases mineralocorticoids, glucocorticoids, and small amounts of sex hormones. The mineralocorticoid aldosterone is important in the regulation of fluid and electrolyte balance and blood pressure maintenance. The glucocorticoid cortisol is involved in the conversion of glycogen to glucose and in antiinflammatory activities.

The body can convert the hormone dehydroepiandrosterone (DHEA) into estrogen and testosterone. Production of this hormone increases dramatically at puberty and peaks in the mid-20s. Levels then decrease over the years, so that only about 20% remains by age 70.

OVARIES AND TESTES

The testes and ovaries secrete the hormones involved in sexual maturation and function. The primary hormones secreted by the ovaries are estrogen and progesterone. These hormones are responsible for maturation of the ova, stimulation of the uterine endometrium, and the development of the secondary female sexual characteristics. The testes secrete the major male sex hormone, testosterone, which is responsible for sperm maturation and the development of secondary male sexual characteristics.

EXPECTED AGE-RELATED CHANGES

With aging, a variety of changes in endocrine function occur (Table 3.12). The pituitary gland continues to produce adequate levels of critical hormones throughout life. It produces less growth hormone with age, leading to decreased muscle mass.

A decrease in the production of thyroid-stimulating hormone is seen in some older adults. The basal metabolic rate begins to decrease in young adulthood and continues to decrease gradually throughout life. Because lean body mass also decreases, the overall metabolic rate does not change significantly. In response to a decrease in thyroid function, some older people become more sensitive to cooler temperatures.

Studies of the function of the parathyroid gland offer conflicting information. PTH appears to decrease with age except in osteoporosis, where it appears to increase. Elevated levels of PTH may lead to increased blood calcium levels. This is of concern particularly for older women, who may manifest symptoms of confusion, kidney stones, and osteoporosis.

Pancreatic function appears to decrease with aging; however, barring the onset of some form of diabetes, its function remains adequate to meet normal body functioning.

Adrenal function is not altered significantly with advancing age. Adequate hormone levels are produced to meet bodily needs.

The levels of gonadotropic hormones decrease more significantly in women than in men. After menopause, the production of estrogen and progesterone drops significantly. As the production of female sex hormones decreases with aging, some changes in secondary sexual characteristics may be observed, such as the development of facial hair and genital atrophy. Studies indicate that estrogen depletion in postmenopausal women has negative effects on bone density, cardiovascular function, memory, and cognition. Because production of the male hormone testosterone decreases gradually with aging, such changes are gradual and often barely noticeable. Physical exercise, however, may help restore endocrine changes that occur with aging (Copeland, 2020).

Complementary Health Approaches

Attempts to Combat Endocrine Aging

Soy products may improve vaginal dryness and hot flashes. Studies suggest that when such products are used with collagen peptides, they may slow the aging of skin (Zhang et al., 2020.)

Clinical hypnosis may improve hot flashes.

Menopausal hormone therapy (MHT)—long thought to prevent cardiac problems, osteoporosis, vaginal discomfort, and skin changes in women—was frequently prescribed in the past. However, studies have shown significant risks, including the risks of breast cancer and stroke.

Other possibly effective therapies. There are many popular therapies—yoga, hypnosis, relaxation techniques, acupuncture, exercise, stress reduction, relaxation therapy, black cohosh, and ginseng—but they have not been consistently proven to relieve menopausal symptoms any better than placebo (Hutton et al., 2020).

Human growth hormone (HCG) therapy, costing up to $5000 per month, has been marketed as a "cure" for aging; claims include that it increases muscle and bone mass, among other things. Early studies demonstrated a significant increase in muscle mass when HCG was administered to older men. Subsequent studies, however, demonstrated that this benefit was no better than the effect of exercise alone (Endo et al., 2020). Although HCG does have specific medical uses, medical experts recommend against it when used for aging or age-related conditions.

Dehydroepiandrosterone, or *DHEA:* There are unsupported claims that supplementary use of synthetic DHEA can help to fight aging, yet there is little or no conclusive evidence. Some organizations (e.g., the National Collegiate Athletic Association) even ban its use. The Mayo Clinic (2021a) states that there is little evidence supporting the antiaging claims and recommends against using DHEA because of potential serious side effects, interactions with medications, and the increase in risk of certain cancers.

| Table 3.12 | Endocrine Changes Associated With Aging |

PHYSIOLOGIC CHANGE	RESULTS
Decreased pituitary secretions (growth hormone)	Decreased muscle mass
Decreased production of thyroid-stimulating hormone	Decreased metabolic rate
Decreased insulin production or increased insulin resistance	Increased risk for type 2 diabetes mellitus
Decreased production of parathyroid hormone	Increased blood calcium levels (seen with osteoporosis)

NURSING ASSESSMENTS AND CARE STRATEGIES RELATED TO ENDOCRINE CHANGES	
NURSING ASSESSMENTS	CARE STRATEGIES
Monitor laboratory values, paying special attention to minerals, such as calcium and sodium levels, and blood glucose.	Educate patient regarding dietary needs and self-testing of blood glucose.
Assess for body temperature, weight, hair distribution, or behavioral changes, which may indicate endocrine imbalance.	Notify primary care provider of assessment findings.

COMMON DISORDERS SEEN WITH AGING

DIABETES MELLITUS

The incidence of DM increases with age. The likelihood of acquiring diabetes rises sharply with each decade of life. According to the CDC (2020e), 13% of adults in the United States have diabetes; this statistic more than doubles to nearly 27% for those over 65 years of age. DM is a disease with multiple causes that is characterized by the abnormal metabolism of carbohydrates, protein, and fats, resulting in elevated plasma glucose levels. Long-term complications include retinopathy (resulting in a loss of vision), nephropathy (resulting in kidney failure), peripheral neuropathy (resulting in foot ulcers and amputation), autonomic neuropathy (resulting in GI, genitourinary, and cardiovascular symptoms and sexual dysfunction), atherosclerotic vascular problems (resulting in an increased incidence of cardiovascular, cerebrovascular, and peripheral vascular disease), hypertension, cognitive changes, and periodontal disease.

The most current classification system categorizes DM according to its etiology, or cause. The first category, type 1 DM, is defined as being a result of either autoimmune destruction of the β cells of the pancreas or unknown idiopathic causes. The second category, type 2 DM, results from a combination of resistance to the action of insulin and inadequate compensatory insulin secretion. In the third category, other specific types of DM are identified by their unique etiologies, including genetic defects or syndromes, exocrine diseases of the pancreas, diseases of the endocrine system, drugs or chemicals, infections, or other uncommon immune-mediated disorders. A fourth category, gestational DM, exists only during pregnancy. The diagnosis of DM is made on the basis of symptoms and elevated plasma glucose levels. A casual (unrelated to meals) plasma glucose level of 200 mg/dL or higher, particularly with symptoms, warrants further testing. This can be done using the oral glucose tolerance test, the fasting plasma glucose (FPG) level (requiring no calorie intake for at least 8 hours), or the level of hemoglobin A1C (HbA1C). The FPG and HbA1C levels are the more commonly accepted tests because they are less costly and less time-consuming. FPG levels below 99 mg/dL are considered normal. FPG levels between 100 and 125 mg/dL are classified as prediabetes (impaired fasting glucose). FPG levels of 126 mg/dL or higher warrant a provisional diagnosis of diabetes. Abnormal results must be confirmed on a subsequent day to make the diagnosis. The HbA1C test, however, requires only one blood sample because it measures average blood glucose control over the previous 2 to 3 months with no fasting requirement. An HbA1C of 5.7% to 6.4% indicates prediabetes; diabetes is diagnosed by an HbA1C of 6.5% or higher (CDC, 2019).

Type 1 Diabetes Mellitus

Type 1 DM can occur at any age, but it is usually diagnosed before age 25. Approximately 5% of people with diabetes have type 1 DM (Weatherspoon, 2019), which typically has a sudden onset. It may also occur slowly, depending on the rate of destruction of pancreatic β cells. People experiencing type 1 DM produce little or no insulin because of β cell destruction. Absolute lack of insulin production results in excessively high levels of glucose in the blood (hyperglycemia) and leads to the classic symptoms of diabetes: polyuria (excessive and frequent urination), polydipsia (excessive thirst), polyphagia (excessive appetite), and weight loss. The patient with type 1 DM is prone to develop further metabolic problems. When the body is unable to use glucose because of its inadequate production of insulin, starvation will occur at the cellular level. The body may attempt to meet the cells' needs by using fat or muscle as a source of fuel. This results in an accumulation of ketones (by-products of the incomplete metabolism of fatty acids) in the bloodstream. As the level of ketones in the blood rises, the acid-base balance is altered, the blood becomes too acidic, and a condition called *ketoacidosis* occurs. The body attempts to maintain acid-base balance through the compensatory systems of the kidneys and lungs. When a severe imbalance occurs, it may lead to ketonuria, and acetone (or "apple pie") breath may be detected when the patient exhales. Severe acidemia can result in a deep and rapid pattern of breathing called *Kussmaul respirations*. If type 1 DM is not recognized and treated, the patient may die.

Type 1 DM requires continuous careful monitoring and medical supervision. Treatment involves a careful balance of diet, insulin therapy, exercise, and stress management. Each patient requires an individualized program that meets their particular needs.

Changes in diet or activity, infections, and stress can easily cause problems for the patient with type 1 DM. The plasma glucose levels of a patient receiving insulin therapy must be monitored closely. Plasma glucose levels can be determined by the laboratory or by self-testing devices. Any significant changes in an individual's plasma glucose level should be reported promptly to the primary care provider.

Patients with type 1 DM who live independently must be taught the importance of following the prescribed balance of diet, insulin, and exercise. They should be strongly urged to call their primary care provider immediately if they have any signs of infection, particularly any infection that results in vomiting. Special medical identification bracelets or necklaces are advisable. Such devices can help ensure that proper care will be provided in emergencies.

Type 2 Diabetes Mellitus

The form of DM that is most often observed in older adults is type 2 DM, which accounts for 90% to 95% of all persons with diabetes. This form of DM is more commonly observed in individuals who are older than 40 years of age, who have obesity, or whose family history includes type 2 DM. The symptoms of type 2 DM are usually mild and may be unrecognized by an older adult. Diagnosis often occurs during routine medical visits or when the person seeks medical attention for visual disturbances, delayed wound healing, or recurrent vaginal or yeast infections.

With type 2 DM, the individual may have normal or even elevated levels of insulin. Despite this, glucose does not enter the cells normally. It is suspected that a problem with the receptor sites on the cells prevents normal cellular functioning.

Medical providers initially prefer to control type 2 DM by encouraging healthy eating, regular exercise, and weight loss. Weight loss is encouraged because it often results in a spontaneous decrease in plasma glucose levels and reduced insulin resistance. If diet alone is not successful, oral hypoglycemic agents may be prescribed. When under physical stress resulting from infection or surgery, persons with type 2 DM may experience abnormally high plasma glucose levels. In these cases, the classic symptoms of DM may arise and the person may require insulin administration to maintain normal plasma glucose levels. Once these levels are normal and the stressor has been removed, insulin administration is typically discontinued. Plasma glucose levels should be monitored frequently to ensure that they remain within normal limits.

Long-term glycemic control is monitored using the HbA1C test. An HbA1C of 6.5% or less is desirable. Good glucose control has been shown to reduce the risk of vascular complications.

HYPOGLYCEMIA

Hypoglycemia is a potentially serious problem for people receiving insulin or oral hypoglycemic agents. Classic signs of hypoglycemia include headache, nausea, weakness, tremors or trembling sensations, pallor, anxiety, irritability, tachycardia, sweating, and hunger. Many of these symptoms can easily be missed or misinterpreted in the older adult. If hypoglycemia is suspected, the plasma glucose level should be measured promptly. Treatment is based on the specific plasma glucose level. Those with levels of 40 to 60 mg/dL respond best to foods such as milk and crackers, and those with levels of 20 to 40 mg/dL respond best to refined carbohydrates such as honey, juice, or sugar. If unconscious, the patient is treated with an intramuscular injection of glucagon or an intravenous infusion of 50% glucose. Individuals prone to develop hypoglycemia should be taught to carry a carbohydrate source such hard candies or glucose tablets. *One must never administer anything orally to an unconscious patient.*

HYPOTHYROIDISM

Reduced function of the thyroid gland, called *primary hypothyroidism,* is more common in older than in younger persons. Symptoms of hypothyroidism include cold intolerance, dry skin, dry and thin body hair, constipation, depression, and lack of energy. Because many of these changes are commonly observed with aging, they may not be recognized as signs of hypothyroidism. Diagnosis is made by means of blood tests. The treatment of hypothyroidism with very high levels of thyroid hormone has been shown to reduce bone density in older women but not in older men.

THE REPRODUCTIVE AND GENITOURINARY SYSTEMS

In both men and women, the genital and urinary systems are located close to each other. As mentioned previously, many structures in men are used for both the sexual function and elimination. In women, the structures of elimination are completely separate from those of reproduction.

FEMALE REPRODUCTIVE ORGANS

The primary female sexual organs include the ovaries, fallopian tubes, uterus, and vagina. These structures, which are necessary for normal human reproduction, are located in the pelvic cavity between the bladder and bowels. It is important to visualize their location to understand the symptoms that may occur if the size, shape, or position of these organs changes. During the reproductive years, the ovaries produce the hormones estrogen and progesterone. Under the influence of these hormones, the ova mature in the ovaries, and the endometrium of the uterus changes in vascularity to support a possible pregnancy. Upon reaching menopause (sometime between the ages of 45 and 60), ovarian hormone function decreases and then ceases in the female. Recent technology and extensive medical intervention can allow pregnancies to occur after menopause, but the number of women who choose to become pregnant this late in life is likely small. Most women who reach menopause are either resigned or delighted to reach the end of the reproductive stage.

MALE REPRODUCTIVE ORGANS

The male organs of reproduction consist of the testes, which contain a series of ducts and glands, and the penis, which contains the passageway by which sperm, the male sex cells, leave the body in the ejaculate. The testes are suspended in a tissue sac called the *scrotum,* which hangs between the thighs. The testes produce the hormone testosterone, which is responsible for sperm production and maturation. Testosterone is also responsible for the secondary sex changes in men, including body hair patterns, voice changes, and muscle development. A series of ducts and glands provide additional fluid volume to the ejaculate and add nutrients needed for the maturation and development of sperm. The prostate gland is located just below the urinary bladder. It produces an alkaline secretion that increases sperm motility, and it contracts to aid in ejaculation.

EXPECTED AGE-RELATED CHANGES

CHANGES IN WOMEN

Several significant changes occur with menopause (Table 3.13). The production of progesterone and estrogen diminishes. There is no longer a need to produce ova to be fertilized, and there is no need to prepare a site to support a pregnancy. Other changes related to the decline in hormones are not as desirable. Along with other body tissue, the tissues of the external female reproductive organs atrophy because of vascular changes. The tissues of the reproductive organs become less elastic, and the

Table 3.13	Reproductive Changes Associated With Aging	
PHYSIOLOGIC CHANGE	**RESULTS**	
Female		
Decreased estrogen levels	Decreased vaginal secretions	
Decreased tissue elasticity	Decreased pubic hair; increased vaginal tissue fragility; increased tissue irritation; decreased size of uterus; decreased vaginal length and width; decreased size of vaginal opening; increased pain with intercourse (dyspareunia); decreased breast tissue mass	
Increased vaginal alkalinity	Increased risk for infection	
Male		
Decreased testosterone levels	Decreased amount of facial and pubic hair	
Decreased circulation	Decreased rate and force of ejaculation; decreased speed gaining an erection	
NURSING ASSESSMENTS AND CARE STRATEGIES RELATED TO REPRODUCTIVE CHANGES		
NURSING ASSESSMENTS	**CARE STRATEGIES**	
Assess for signs and symptoms of infection or inflammation.	Report unusual vaginal discharge to primary care provider. Administer treatment as prescribed.	
Assess factors that may interfere with sexual activity.	Discuss normal physiologic changes and the possible effects of medications on sexual function. Educate females regarding use of artificial lubrication. Facilitate referral of males to primary care provider for pharmacologic treatment of erectile dysfunction if needed.	

amount of subcutaneous tissue decreases. This results in a flattening of the tissue of the external genitalia, or labia, and a decreased amount and distribution of pubic hair. Vaginal epithelial tissue becomes thinner and less vascular. The tissue of the vagina is drier and more alkaline, and fewer rugae (folds) are present within the vagina. The uterus, cervix, ovaries, and fallopian tubes decrease in size and may be difficult to palpate on examination. The decrease in hormone production and resulting tissue changes may lead to more fragile, more easily irritated vaginal tissue. Decreased vaginal secretions may lead to vaginitis, which can cause vulvar soreness and pruritus or dyspareunia (painful intercourse). Once menopause has occurred, vaginal bleeding is considered abnormal.

The breasts are part of the secondary female sexual organs. Because of the decrease in hormones with aging, breast tissue atrophies. As supporting muscle tissue atrophies, the breasts tend to sag and decrease in size.

CHANGES IN MEN

Male age-related changes in the reproductive system are less noticeable because testosterone continues to be produced into old age, although the amount decreases. Men, even in their late 80s, have successfully fathered children.

With aging, there is some change in the size and firmness of the testes. The penis retains the ability to become erect, although it may take longer to do so and may require more stimulation. Once achieved, erection may last longer than at a younger age. Ejaculation tends to be slower and less forceful in aging men and may not occur during each sexual encounter, particularly if intercourse is frequent.

Enlargement of the scrotum may indicate problems with the testes or part of the duct system. The penis should remain free from any tissue changes, and the presence of ulcers, nodules, or other changes is abnormal. Most aging men experience some degree of prostate gland enlargement. The signs and symptoms most often experienced include urinary frequency, hesitancy, dysuria, decreased force when voiding, dribbling, nocturia, increased incidence of UTIs, and decreased force during ejaculation. In cases of benign prostatic hyperplasia, surgical intervention, such as a transurethral prostatectomy, may help to reduce the symptoms.

COMMON DISORDERS SEEN WITH AGING

UTERINE PROLAPSE

Prolapse of the uterus (into the vagina) is commonly observed in older women. This is particularly a problem for those who have had many pregnancies or for those who delivered children with little medical assistance. Most often, the first signs of uterine prolapse involve changes in either urine or bowel elimination. Urinary frequency, urinary retention, recurrent urinary tract infections (UTIs), back pain, and constipation may be symptoms. In some cases, the cervix and uterus may prolapse through the vagina and be observed protruding outside of the vulva. Surgical correction may be required.

VAGINAL INFECTION

Change in vaginal pH may lead to increased incidence of vaginal infections, particularly yeast infections. This is most often manifested by increased vaginal discharge, irritation, odor, and itching.

BREAST CANCER

Breast cancer continues to be a major cause of cancer deaths in women, and the incidence of this form of cancer continues to increase with age. The current recommendations by the American Cancer Society (2020b) include mammography every other year for women after age 55 and continuing as long as the woman is in good health and expected to live at least 10 more years. Any sign of dimpling; masses; nipple retraction; or breast drainage, discharge, or bleeding is suspicious and requires further medical attention.

PROSTATE CANCER

There are no obvious changes in function to indicate the presence of prostate cancer. Therefore it is important for aging men to have regular medical examinations. A skilled clinician who palpates the prostate may detect changes that indicate malignancy. Prostatic cancer is a major cause of death in aging men.

Get Ready for the Next Generation NCLEX® Examination!

Key Points

- Nurses must possess knowledge about the normal structures and functions of all body systems so that deviations from the norm can be detected.
- All body systems are affected to a greater or lesser degree by aging. Although these changes are normal and expected, they can have a significant impact on the older person's functional ability, self-image, and lifestyle.
- In addition to age-related changes, a variety of diseases are increasingly common in the aging population.
- Nurses must be careful to distinguish between normal physiologic changes and abnormal alterations that indicate the need for prompt medical attention.

Additional Learning Resources

 SG Go to your Evolve website at http://evolve.elsevier. com/Williams/geriatric for the additional online resources.

Review Questions for the Next Generation NCLEX® Examination

1. Your older female patient is complaining because she is having frequent UTIs. Which normal age-related change is most likely to be a contributing factor?

    a. Increased nocturnal urine production
    b. Decreased perception of the need to void
    c. Decreased bladder muscle tone
    d. Urinary incontinence

2. Stan is a 78-year-old widower who has come to your clinic for his annual physical examination. He has numerous physical complaints and says, "This getting old is for the birds!" Although some of the findings will require follow-up by his primary care provider, others are within the realm of normal aging. Which of these findings are normal age-related changes? (Select all that apply.)

    a. Decreased visual acuity
    b. Blood pressure reading of 134/84 mm Hg
    c. Decreased long-term memory
    d. Increased gastric pH
    e. Increased muscle mass

    f. Decreased depth of respiration
    g. Increased calorie requirements
    h. Decreased serum albumin
    i. Increased subcutaneous tissue
    j. Decreased rate of peristalsis

3. What are patients who have had Parkinson disease for 10 years likely to exhibit? (Select all that apply.)

    a. Rigidity and tremors when at rest
    b. Hemiparesis and aphasia
    c. Dementia
    d. Unilateral tremors with movement
    e. Tremors present during sleep

4. An older adult is coming to your clinic for treatment for a gastric ulcer. Which treatment would you expect to be ordered?

    a. Antibiotics
    b. Stress-reduction classes
    c. NSAIDs
    d. Iron supplements before breakfast and dinner

5. What should the nurse explain in discussing expected changes in the female reproductive system in an older adult?

    a. Increased pubic hair is expected
    b. Uterine enlargement is normal
    c. Vaginal tissues become more vascular
    d. Production of vaginal secretions decreases

6. The nurse performs a skin assessment of an older adult. Which finding is abnormal and needs to be reported?

    a. Increased patches of dark pigmentation on exposed skin
    b. A dark, elevated patch that bleeds when touched
    c. Deep wrinkles and frown lines around the mouth and eyes
    d. Numerous brown or flesh-colored skin tags around the neck

7. The nurse encourages the patient to maintain a steady weight in the recommended range to decrease risk of which common endocrine disease observed in older adults?

    a. Hypothyroidism
    b. Hyperthyroidism
    c. Diabetes mellitus
    d. Diabetes insipidus

REFERENCES

Agarwala, A., Mehta, A., Yang, E., & Parapid, B. (2020). Older adults and hypertension: Beyond the 2017 guideline for prevention, detection, evaluation, and management of high blood pressure in adults. American College of Cardiology. https://www.acc.org/latest-in-cardiology/articles/2020/02/26/06/24/older-adults-and-hypertension

Alzheimer's Association (2020). A blood test for Alzheimer's? Markers for tau take us a step closer. https://www.alz.org/aaic/releases_2020/blood-biomarkers-tau.asp#:~:text=As%20reported%20at%20AAIC%202020,finding%20in%20multiple%2C%20diverse%20populations

Alzheimer's Association (2021). 2021 Alzheimer's disease facts and figures. https://www.alz.org/media/Documents/alzheimers-facts-and-figures.pdf

American Cancer Society (2020a). American Cancer Society guideline for colorectal cancer screening. https://www.cancer.org/cancer/colon-rectal-cancer/detection-diagnosis-staging/acs-recommendations.html

American Cancer Society (2020b). American Cancer Society recommendations for the early detection of breast cancer. https://www.cancer.org/cancer/breast-cancer/screening-tests-and-early-detection/american-cancer-society-recommendations-for-the-early-detection-of-breast-cancer.html

American Cancer Society (2021a) Key statistics for chronic lymphocytic leukemia (2021a). https://www.cancer.org/cancer/chronic-lymphocytic-leukemia/about/key-statistics.html

American Cancer Society (2021b) Key statistics for lung cancer. https://www.cancer.org/cancer/lung-cancer/about/key-statistics.html

American Cancer Society (2021c). Lung cancer survival rates. https://www.cancer.org/cancer/lung-cancer/detection-diagnosis-staging/survival-rates.html

American Optometric Association (2021). Glaucoma. https://www.aoa.org/healthy-eyes/eye-and-vision-conditions/glaucoma?sso=y

American Society of Clinical Oncology (2019). Colorectal cancer: Risk factors and prevention. https://www.cancer.net/cancer-types/colorectal-cancer/risk-factors-and-prevention#:~:text=For%20colon%20cancer%2C%20the%20average,with%20regard%20to%20cancer%20treatment

American Society of Clinical Oncology (2020). ASCO answers: Lung cancer. https://www.cancer.net/sites/cancer.net/files/asco_answers_lung.pdf

American Society for Gastrointestinal Endoscopy (2020). Understanding diverticulosis. https://www.asge.org/home/for-patients/patient-information/understanding-diverticulosis

American Stroke Association (2021). About stroke. https://www.stroke.org/en/about-stroke

Arthritis Foundation (2021a). Osteoarthritis. https://www.arthritis.org/diseases/osteoarthritis

Arthritis Foundation (2021b). Rheumatoid arthritis. https://www.arthritis.org/diseases/rheumatoid-arthritis

Arumairaj, A., Park, H., Quesada, F., et al. (2020). Determining the need for additional testing with Quantiferon TB Gold in patients with positive tuberculin skin test and history of BGC vaccination. Chest, 158(4). Suppl. A327)October 01, 2020. https://doi.org/10.1016/j.chest.2020.08.324

Beckerman, J. (2020). Heart failure and heart transplants. https://www.webmd.com/heart-disease/heart-failure/heart-failure-heart-transplant#1

Centers for Disease Control and Prevention [CDC]. (2018). Arthritis-related statistics https://www.cdc.gov/arthritis/data_statistics/arthritis-related-stats.htm

Centers for Disease Control and Prevention [CDC] (2019). Diabetes: diabetes tests. https://www.cdc.gov/diabetes/basics/getting-tested.html

Centers for Disease Control and Prevention [CDC] (2020a). Burden of vision loss. https://www.cdc.gov/visionhealth/risk/burden.htm

Centers for Disease Control and Prevention [CDC] (2020b). Common eye disorders and diseases. https://www.cdc.gov/visionhealth/basics/ced/index.html#:~:text=The%20leading%20causes%20of%20blindness,%2C%20diabetic%20retinopathy%2C%20and%20glaucoma

Centers for Disease Control and Prevention [CDC] (2020c). Heart disease facts. https://www.cdc.gov/heartdisease/facts.htm

Centers for Disease Control and Prevention [CDC] (2020d). High blood pressure: Facts about hypertension. https://www.cdc.gov/bloodpressure/facts.htm

Centers for Disease Control and Prevention [CDC] (2020e). National diabetes statistics report 2020. Atlanta, GA: Centers for Disease Control and Prevention, U.S. Department of Health and Human Services; 2020.

Centers for Disease Control and Prevention [CDC] (2020f). Osteoarthritis. https://www.cdc.gov/arthritis/basics/osteoarthritis.htm

Centers for Disease Control and Prevention (2021a). COVID-19: Older adults. https://www.cdc.gov/coronavirus/2019-ncov/need-extra-precautions/older-adults.html

Centers for Disease Control and Prevention (2021b). The difference between flu and COVID-19. https://www.cdc.gov/flu/symptoms/flu-vs-covid19.htm#:%E2%88%BC:text=COVID%2D19%20is%20caused%20by,can%20be%20contagious%20for%20longer

Cheslock, M., & De Jesus, O. (2021). Presbycusis. [Updated 2021 Feb 18]StatPearls [Internet]. Treasure Island (FL): StatPearls Publishing. 2021 Jan-. Available at. https://www.ncbi.nlm.nih.gov/books/NBK559220/

Copeland, J. L. (2020). Exercise in older adults: The effect of age on exercise endocrinology. In A. Hackney, & N. Constantini (Eds.), Endocrinology of physical activity and sport. Contemporary Endocrinology: Humana, Cham https://doi.org/10.1007/978-3-030-33376-8_23

Du, Y., Wang, X., Xie, H., et al. (2019). Sex differences in the prevalence and adverse outcomes of sarcopenia and sarcopenic obesity in community dwelling elderly in East China using the AWGS criteria. BMC Endocr Disord, 19. 1092019. https://doi.org/10.1186/s12902-019-0432-x

Endo, Y., Nourmahnad, A., & Sinha, I. (2020). Optimizing skeletal muscle anabolic response to resistance training in aging. Frontiers in Physiology, 11, 874. https://doi.org/10.3389/fphys.2020.00874

FDA (2019). Information for consumers on using dietary supplements. https://www.fda.gov/food/dietary-supplements/information-consumers-using-dietary-supplements

Filho, J. O., & Samuels, O. B. (2021). Mechanical thrombectomy for acute ischemic stroke. In J. Biller (Ed.), UpToDate. Retrieved March 20, 2021 from https://www.uptodate.com/contents/mechanical-thrombectomy-for-acute-ischemic-stroke#:~:text=Mechanical%20thrombectomy%20is%20indicated%20for,alteplase%20for%20the%20same%20ischemic

Han, S., Higuera, V. (2019). Stroke severity and mortality: Types, treatments, and symptoms. https://www.healthline.com/health/can-you-die-from-a-stroke#types-of-stroke

Heron, M. (2019). Deaths: Leading causes for 2017National Vital Statistics Reports68. Hyattsville, MD: National Center for Health Statistics.

Honig, L., & Sano, M. (2017). An update on scientific advances and clinical strategies in Alzheimer's disease: Report on the Alzheimer's Association International Conference, https://courses.elseviercme.com/aaic17/7392017

Hutton, B., Hersi, M., Cheng, W., Pratt, M., et al. (2020). Comparing interventions for management of hot flashes in patients with breast and prostate cancer: A systematic review with meta-analyses. Oncology Nursing Forum, 47(7). doi:10.1188/20.onf.e86-e106 #86-E106

Jiao, F., Yi, F., Wang, Y., Zhang, S., et al. (2020). The validation of multifactor model of plasma Aβ42 and total-tau in combination with MoCA for diagnosing probable Alzheimer disease. Front Aging Neurosci, 12. doi:10.3389/fnagi.2020.00212.

Karrer, T. M., McLaughlin, C. L., Guaglianone, C. P., & Samanez-Larkin, G. R. (2019). Reduced serotonin receptors and transporters in normal aging adults: a meta-analysis of PET and SPECT imaging studies. Neurobiology of Aging. doi:10.1016/j.neurobiolaging.2019.03.021.

Kolasinski, S. L., Neogi, T., Hochberg, M. C., et al. (2020). 2019 American College of Rheumatology/Arthritis Foundation guideline for the management of osteoarthritis of the hand, hip, and knee. Arthritis & Rheumatology, 72(2), 220–233. https://doi.org/10.1002/art.41142.

Kuntz, L. (2021). Alzheimer's disease vaccine: Less talk, more numbers. Psychiatric Times. https://www.psychiatrictimes.com/view/alzheimer-disease-vaccine-less-talk-more-numbers. Lava, N. (2019). What is anosmia? https://www.webmd.com/brain/anosmia-loss-of-smell

Leyland, L., Bremner, F. D., Mahmood, R., Hewitt, S., et al. (2020). Visual tests predict dementia risk in Parkinson disease. Neurol Clin Pract, 10(1), 29–39. doi: 10.1212/CPJ.0000000000000719.

MacGrory, B. C., Saldanha, I. J., Mistry, E., et al. (2021). Abstract 1: Thrombolytic therapy for 'wake-up stroke' - A systematic review and meta-analysis. Stroke. Retrieved March 20, 2021 from https://www.ahajournals.org/doi/abs/10.1161/str.52.suppl_1.1.

Marshall, M. (2021). COVID's toll on smell and taste: What scientists do and don't know. Nature Briefing. https://www.nature.com/articles/d41586-021-00055-6

Mayo Clinic Staff (2021a). DHEA. https://www.mayoclinic.org/drugs-supplements-dhea/art-20364199

Mayo Clinic Staff (2021b). Hyaluronic acid (injection route). https://www.mayoclinic.org/drugs-supplements/hyaluronic-acid-injection-route/description/drg-20074557

Nagarsheth, K. H. (2021). Superficial thrombophlebitis treatment & management. https://emedicine.medscape.com/article/463256-treatment

National Eye Institute (2020). Age-related eye disease studies (AREDS/AREDS2). https://www.nei.nih.gov/research/clinical-trials/age-related-eye-disease-studies-aredsareds2

National Osteoporosis Foundation (2021). Preventing fractures: General facts. https://www.nof.org/preventing-fractures/general-facts/

Palve, S. S., & Palve, S. B. (2018). Impact of aging on nerve conduction velocities and late responses in healthy individuals. J Neurosci Rural Pract, 9(1), 112–116. doi:10.4103/jnrp.jnrp_323_17.

Panush, R. S. (2019). Patient education: Complementary and alternative therapies for rheumatoid arthritis (beyond the basics). https://www.uptodate.com/contents/complementary-and-alternative-therapies-for-rheumatoid-arthritis-beyond-the-basics

Pereira, B., Xu, X., & Akbar, A. N. (2020). Targeting inflammation and immunosenescence to improve vaccine responses in the elderly. Frontiers of Immunology, 11, Article 583019. doi:10.3389/fimmu.2020.583019

Platte, R. O. (2019). Urinary tract infections in pregnancy. https://emedicine.medscape.com/article/452604-overview#a6

Rodgers, J. L., Jones, J., Bolleddu, S. I., Vanthenapalli, S., et al. (2019). Cardiovascular risks associated with gender and aging. Journal of Cardiovascular Developmental Disease, 6(2), 19. doi:10.3390/jcdd6020019

Rubino, A., Sanon, M., Ganz, M. L., et al. (2020). Association of the US Food and Drug Administration antipsychotic drug boxed warning with medication use and health outcomes in elderly patients with dementia. JAMA Netw Open, 3(4), Article e203630. doi:10.1001/jamanetworkopen.2020.3630

Sandrone, S., Moreno-Zambrano, D., Kipnis, J., et al. (2019). A (delayed) history of the brain lymphatic system. Nature Medicine, 25, 538–540. https://doi.org/10.1038/s41591-019-0417-3

Sinha, A. D., & Agarwal, R. (2019). Clinical pharmacology of antihypertensive therapy for the treatment of hypertension in CKD. Clinical Journal of the American Society of Nephrology, 14(5), 757–764. https://doi.org/10.2215/CJN.04330418

Skin Cancer Foundation (2021). Skin cancer facts & statistics. http://www.skincancer.org/skin-cancer-information/skin-cancer-facts

University of Houston. (2020). COPD as a lung stem cell disease: Single cell cloning tells the story of abnormal cells. ScienceDaily. Retrieved January 6, 2022 from https://www.sciencedaily.com/releases/2020/04/200415133646.htm

Virani, S. S., Alonso, A., Benjamin, E. J., Bittencourt, M. S., et al. (2020). Heart disease and stroke statistics—2020 update: A report from the American Heart Association. Circulation, 141(9), e139–e596. https://www.ahajournals.org/doi/10.1161/CIR.0000000000000757

Weatherspoon, D. (2019). Statistics and facts about type 2 diabetes. https://www.medicalnewstoday.com/articles/318472

Wong, W. (2020). Economic burden of Alzheimer disease and managed care considerations. American Journal of Managed Care, 26, S177–S183. https://doi.org/10.37765/ajmc.2020.88482

Yim, M. H., Kim, K. H., & Lee, B. J. (2021). The number of household members as a risk factor for peptic ulcer disease. Sci Rep, 11(5274). 2021. https://doi.org/10.1038/s41598-021-84892-5

Zhang, S. Y., Hood, M., Zhang, I. X., Chen, C. L., et al. (2020). Collagen and soy peptides attenuate contractile loss from UVA damage and enhance the antioxidant capacity of dermal fibroblasts. Journal of Cosmetic Dermatology. 23 October 2020. https://onlinelibrary.wiley.com/doi/abs/10.1111/jocd.13805; https://doi.org/10.1111/jocd.13805

4

Health Promotion, Health Maintenance, and Home Health Considerations

http://evolve.elsevier.com/Williams/geriatric

Objectives

1. Describe recommended health maintenance practices and explain how they change with aging.
2. Discuss the relationship of culture and religion to health practices.
3. Identify how perceptions of aging affect health practices.
4. Describe how health maintenance is affected by cognitive and sensory changes.
5. Discuss the impact of decreased accessibility on health maintenance practices.
6. Describe methods of assessing health maintenance practices.
7. Identify older adults who are most at risk for experiencing health maintenance problems.
8. Identify selected problem statements related to health maintenance.
9. Describe nursing interventions that are appropriate for older adults experiencing alterations in health maintenance.
10. Discuss the role of home health as it relates to health promotion and health maintenance in the older adult.
11. Differentiate between unpaid and paid home health care providers.
12. Identify the factors to consider when seeking home health care assistance.

Key Terms

health maintenance (p. 79)
health promotion (p. 79)

nonadherence (p. 90)
prophylactic (prō-fĭ-LĂK-tĭk, p. 81)

As people live longer and the percentage of older adults in the population increases, society faces several major challenges. One of the most significant of these involves meeting the health care needs of an aging population.

Today's older adults are generally healthier than the older adults of previous generations. Improvements in sanitation, public health, and occupational safety implemented during the 20th century have helped raise the age at which a person can expect to experience a life-threatening disease.

Older adults can and do experience acute, life-threatening medical conditions just as younger people do, but acute episodes in older adults are more likely to be associated with chronic conditions. Either an acute condition is caused by a chronic problem, or a chronic problem persists after an acute episode. According to the National Council on Aging (2021), 80% of older adults have at least one chronic illness, whereas almost 70% of Medicare recipients have multiple chronic conditions. Common chronic problems include arthritis, hypertension, diabetes, heart disease, and vision or hearing disorders. Most people with chronic illness are able to manage quite well; however, some require care to meet their needs.

Older adults make up approximately 56% of today's population and account for 58% of all health care expenditures. Female older adults account for more health care spending than their male counterparts, especially in terms of home health care (Centers for Medicare & Medicaid Services, 2019b). The older adult population has primarily benefited from improvements in medical care. Advances in surgery, technology, and pharmacology have enabled us to prolong life in situations that even a few years ago would have been impossible.

This level of care is not without substantial cost. Because a significant portion of older adults' health care expenses is covered by Medicare and Medicaid, the burden on the younger members of society is becoming overwhelming. Despite steady increases in payroll taxes on the working population, Medicare has operated at a deficit since the start of the 21st century. Because there is a fixed amount of taxpayer money, society must identify appropriate and acceptable ways to control health care costs.

One way of dealing with the steady increase in demand for health care services involves rationing the type and amount of care provided to older adults. This approach would prohibit or severely limit the type of care provided, particularly in cases in which the potential for significant improvement in health status is limited. For example, some of the costlier treatments and procedures (e.g., kidney dialysis and cardiac bypass surgery) could be refused if the person were older than a predetermined age. This method has been adopted in some countries but is unpopular in the United States. To avoid rationing health care in this manner, we must find ways to maximize the effectiveness of our health care expenditures. The Patient Protection and Affordable Care Act (see Chapter 1) of 2010 was enacted to reduce spiraling health care costs.

Most studies reveal that it is more cost-effective to prevent problems than to cure or treat them. Therefore more health care providers and the public (including older adults) are beginning to recognize the need to devote more attention to health promotion and health maintenance.

Health promotion is not a new concept. For decades, health care providers have stressed the importance of good nutrition, exercise, and regular medical care. Although most of this information was directed toward younger people, many older people who desired to live longer, healthier lives also paid attention. As the benefits of healthy lifestyle choices became obvious, television, radio, and other media joined health care providers in promoting health awareness. Awareness of the importance of good health maintenance practices increased.

> 🏃 Health Promotion
>
> Nearly one-third of adults 50 years of age or older do not engage in regular physical activity (CDC, 2019a). Encourage physical activity in the older adult in order to decrease the risk of heart disease, diabetes, cancer, and other chronic illnesses.

Many individuals have modified their lifestyles and health care practices to improve their overall health and quality of life (Box 4.1). Those who are unaware or unwilling to heed this advice persist in risky, health-threatening behavior. Nurses need to be aware of the health promotion and maintenance practices that will most benefit

Box 4.1	Advice for the Young and Not-So-Young Adult

- Accept that you are getting older—adjust to the changes and plan for possibilities.
- Explore options for the future—look for things you want to accomplish in your life.
- Find work or creative outlets that make you happy—look for ways to grow throughout your life.
- Modify your lifestyle to promote health—exercise, eat healthy foods, and manage stress.
- Develop and maintain relationships—bonds formed with friends and loved ones provide support; we can never have too many.

older adults and positively reinforce those behaviors. Nurses also need to understand why some older adults choose to adopt positive health behaviors whereas others persist in seemingly self-destructive behavior.

RECOMMENDED HEALTH PRACTICES FOR OLDER ADULTS

DIET

Older adults should consume a well-balanced, plant-based diet with the recommended daily allowances of nutrients. Helpful nutrition guides for healthy eating include "MyPlate for Older Adults" and "Fruits and Veggies: More Matters," promoting the consumption of fruits and/or vegetables (see Additional Learning Resources at end of chapter). Some changes in caloric intake and protein and vitamin needs appear to be desirable with aging (see Chapter 6).

When special diets are indicated, older adults need to learn how to read and interpret the information provided on packaging labels. This is particularly important with sodium-restricted diets, because sodium is commonly found in foods that do not necessarily taste salty, such as bread. It can also be hidden in ingredients such as monosodium glutamate. Because food labels are often printed in very small type, older adults should bring along their eyeglasses or a magnifying glass when they shop. If someone else shops for them, that individual needs to understand the dietary restrictions of the older adult and how to shop wisely.

EXERCISE

Daily exercise should be part of the plan for older adults (Fig. 4.1). Exercise can help keep joints flexible, maintain muscle mass, control blood glucose levels and weight, and promote a sense of well-being. Exercise does not need to be aerobic to benefit older adults. Walking, swimming, golfing, housekeeping, and active lawn work or gardening are all considered exercise. To be most beneficial, exercise should consist of at least 30 minutes of continuous activity. The type, level, and amount of exercise that is best differ for each person and should be based on the recommendations of the primary care provider.

TOBACCO AND ALCOHOL

It is never too late to stop smoking. Even the body of an older person can repair damage once smoking is discontinued. Cessation may be difficult when smoking has been a long-standing habit, but various aids are available to help smokers quit. Before using any of these aids, the older adult should seek guidance from their primary care provider because they may need to follow some special precautions related to existing health problems.

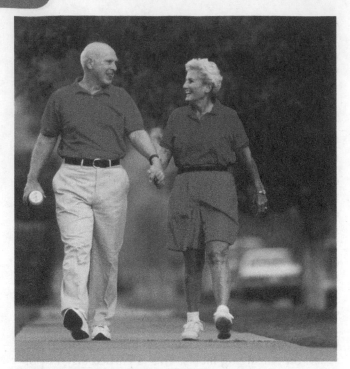

Fig. 4.1 Exercise is important for health promotion and maintenance in older adults. (From Potter, P. A., Perry, A. G., et al. [2014]. *Canadian fundamentals of nursing*, 5th edition. Elsevier.)

Excessive consumption of alcoholic beverages is never recommended. Alcohol use disorder is a common problem in the older adult population for both men and women because alcohol may be used as a means of coping with a variety of problems. Occasional or moderate alcohol consumption by older adults usually is not prohibited unless some medical condition or medication precludes its use. Some primary care providers even recommend a glass of wine or beer as an appetite enhancer in certain situations.

PHYSICAL EXAMINATIONS AND PREVENTIVE OVERALL CARE

Older adults should be examined annually by their primary care providers and more frequently if known health problems exist. Some older adults resist this because of the cost or fear about what the primary care provider may find. Cost is a real concern to many older adults, but inadequate health maintenance should be a greater concern. A delay in the recognition of problems may make them more difficult and expensive to treat. Physical examinations provide an opportunity to detect problems before they become more serious, to monitor and treat chronic conditions, and to prevent some health problems.

Physical examinations in older adults should include evaluations of height and weight, blood pressure, and a rectal examination. Common screening tests for men and women are listed in Table 4.1. Guidelines for various cancer screenings have been issued by multiple organizations, all offering different advice depending on age and risk factors. They all agree, however, that screening decisions should be shared between older adults and their health care providers.

Evaluation of joints, feet, and gait should be part of the physical examination. Problems with the knees and shoulder joints can cause pain, activity limitations, poor sleep, and decreased overall function. Some problems require surgical correction, whereas others can be treated using analgesics, anti-inflammatory medications, or physical therapy. Inspection of the feet often reveals problems. Many older adults have difficulty caring for their toenails because of poor vision, inability to reach their feet, or hypertrophic nail changes. Bunions, calluses, and corns also cause problems for older adults. Neglect of the feet can lead to discomfort, restricted mobility, and a poorer quality of life. If the feet are not properly cared for, the risks for infection and even amputation increase, particularly in those with compromised circulation. Nurses should encourage the older adult to wear properly fitted shoes with good support. Regular visits to a podiatrist can significantly reduce foot problems. Joint or foot problems, illness, pain, and other conditions commonly seen with aging can contribute to gait changes, which can result in imbalance or falls. When gait problems are identified, physical therapy for gait retraining and strengthening exercises, use of assistive devices, and environmental modification may be appropriate.

Vision should be checked yearly to monitor for glaucoma or other eye problems. Refractive examinations can detect the need for a change in eyeglass prescription. Hearing examinations need not be done annually unless a problem is suspected. When signs of diminished hearing are present, audiometric testing is appropriate.

Blood tests for hypothyroidism or diabetes, electrocardiograms, and other diagnostic tests are not routinely part of the physical examination. In the absence of heart disease, blood cholesterol screening should be done every 4 to 6 years (CDC, 2021). Older adults should be aware of the need to communicate any symptoms they experience so that their primary care providers can determine the need for additional testing.

In addition to regular physical examinations, older adults should be sure to obtain immunization against diseases such as pneumonia and influenza, which are more common in older adults. People at greatest risk for developing serious complications from the flu are older adults with one or more chronic health conditions such as diabetes or chronic lung disease. In the COVID-19 pandemic, older adults were among the first groups to be immunized; obtaining booster immunizations, are also important for the older adult community. Because the immune system is less responsive in older adults, it is important that they receive vaccinations in a timely manner.

Table 4.1	Screening Tests for Older Adults		
TEST	**MEN**	**WOMEN**	**BOTH**
Bone density screening	Initial screening at 70 years of age; younger if risk factors are present or if patient experiences bone fracture after age 50	Initial screening at 65 years of age; younger if risk factors are present or if patient experiences bone fracture after age 50	
Cervical cancer screening	N/A	No screening if prior tests were normal and patient not at high risk for cervical cancer	
Colorectal screening			Choices include stool-based tests: Highly sensitive fecal immunochemical test annually Highly sensitive fecal occult blood test annually Multitargeted stool DNA test every 3 years Visual exams: Colonoscopy every 10 years CT (virtual) colonoscopy every 5 years Flexible sigmoidoscopy every 5 years
Mammography	Consider annual if patient has gynecomastia and BRCA1/2 gene mutation exists, starting 10 years before earliest known breast cancer in male family member or at age 50 (whichever comes first)	Every other year (or may choose yearly); continue as long as woman is in good health and expected to live at least 10 more years	

DNA, deoxyribonucleic acid.

Sources: American Cancer Society (2020). American Cancer Society guideline for colorectal cancer screening. https://www.cancer.org/cancer/colon-rectal-cancer/detection-diagnosis-staging/acs-recommendations.html

American Cancer Society (2020). American Cancer Society Recommendations for the Early Detection of Breast Cancer. https://www.cancer.org/cancer/breast-cancer/screening-tests-and-early-detection/american-cancer-society-recommendations-for-the-early-detection-of-breast-cancer.html

National Institutes of Health, National Cancer Institute (2020). ACS's updated cervical cancer screening guidelines explained. https://www.cancer.gov/news-events/cancer-currents-blog/2020/cervical-cancer-screening-hpv-test-guideline

National Osteoporosis Foundation (2021). Bone density exam/testing. https://www.nof.org/patients/diagnosis-information/bone-density-examtesting/

Susan G. Komen Breast Cancer Foundation, Inc. (2020). Breast cancer screening for men at higher risk. https://www.komen.org/breast-cancer/screening/when-to-screen/high-risk-men/

- Pneumococcal vaccine: There are two pneumococcal vaccines. An older adult may be advised by their primary care provider to receive one or both depending on medical history (CDC, 2020b).
- Influenza (flu) vaccine: The influenza vaccine must be obtained on a yearly basis, usually in the fall, because the strain of the virus changes frequently. Flu shots can be obtained from primary care providers, clinics, and most pharmacies. Even with immunization, a larger percentage of older adults contract influenza. It is likely that the COVID-19 vaccine may become part of the annual flu immunization.
- Tetanus, diphtheria, pertussis vaccines: The Tdap vaccine protects against the contagious and deadly diseases *tetanus*, *diphtheria*, and *pertussis*. Tdap is recommended for anyone who has never had the vaccine, including adults over 65 years of age and healthcare personnel (CDC, 2020a). A Td or Tdap booster should also be given every 10 years (or after an exposure to tetanus (e.g., a deep puncture wound) to protect against *tetanus* and *diphtheria*. Although

tetanus is rare in the United States, approximately half of such cases affect the older adult population.
- Shingles (zoster) vaccine: The risk of developing shingles, a herpes zoster infection that causes a classic rash and painful neuralgia, increases with age. A shingles vaccine has been available since 2006; however, the vaccine was expensive and effective only about 50% of the time. A newer, more effective vaccine was approved in 2018 for healthy adults over age 50. This vaccine is still expensive (and may or may not be covered by insurance or Medicare) but is also more effective. It is administered in two doses between 2 and 6 months apart (Amin, 2020). Benefits of this vaccine should be determined based on individual risks, preferences, and the primary care provider's recommendations.
- The need for hepatitis B immunization is based on individual risk factors and should be discussed with a primary care provider.

The **prophylactic** use of medications such as low-dose aspirin (to prevent heart attack or stroke) and vitamin supplements is popular among older adults. If a specific vitamin deficiency exists, vitamins have been proven to be very helpful. Older adults should discuss the possible benefits of this therapy with their primary care providers and follow the recommendations.

Use of prescription and over-the-counter medications is common in the older population. Older adults with medical conditions must understand the reasons for and the importance of their treatment plans. They should keep a card listing all of their medications and the providers who prescribed them. This card should be shown to all licensed professionals they see to prevent serious drug interactions.

Additional precautions regarding the use of medications are discussed in Chapter 7.

 Safety

Older adults must know how and when to take prescribed medications, how to use over-the-counter medications safely, how to store their medications, and when to report side effects. Sharing prescription medications with friends or neighbors is dangerous and must be avoided. Instructions regarding the proper use of medications can be confusing and even overwhelming to many people.

To keep track of medical appointments, older adults should have a calendar or datebook to record appointments and reminders for things such as immunizations. They also should be aware of signs and symptoms that indicate a need to seek medical attention between routine yearly examinations. Signs and symptoms indicating the need for prompt medical attention are listed in Box 4.2.

Older adults with health problems or allergies, those taking medications such as heparin, and those with implanted medical devices such as pacemakers should wear a MedicAlert bracelet or necklace. If they do not wish to wear such a warning device, these individuals should, at minimum, carry cards in their wallets or purses to provide the necessary health information.

 Health Promotion

Medications

- Take prescription medications only as ordered.
- Store medication as directed.
- Report any suspected side effects to your primary care provider.
- Keep a card with names of all medications, dose, and name of primary care provider with you at all times.
- Keep the card up to date.
- Show the card to all health care providers.
- Wear a MedicAlert bracelet or necklace listing serious diseases and allergies.
- Do not use over-the-counter medication or supplements without consulting your primary care provider or pharmacist.
- Do not take anyone else's medication or share your medication with anyone.

Box 4.2	Signs and Symptoms Indicating a Need for Prompt Medical Attention

- Severe pain; radiating or crushing chest, neck, or jaw pain; severe unremitting headache
- Difficulty breathing
- Loss of consciousness
- Loss of movement or sensation in any body part or parts
- Sudden vision changes
- Unusual drainage or discharge from any body cavity
- Wounds that do not heal
- Nausea or vomiting for 24 hours or longer
- Elevated body temperature
- Inability to urinate
- Swelling of the lower extremities
- Excessive (greater than 10%) weight gain or loss
- Sudden or dramatic behavioral changes
- Sudden changes in speech or ability to follow directions

DENTAL EXAMINATIONS AND PREVENTIVE ORAL CARE

Dental examinations should be obtained and an inspection of the oral cavity performed at least annually. Today's older adults are keeping their natural teeth longer than previous generations were able to because of better nutrition and improved dental care. Gum disease and tooth decay are major causes of tooth loss. To prevent or slow the progress of these dental problems, older adults should brush their natural teeth twice daily using fluoride toothpaste and should floss carefully between the teeth. Mouthwash cannot replace regular brushing.

It is recommended that older adults use a soft-bristle brush to clean all tooth surfaces, particularly those suffering from arthritis, because they may have difficulty holding and brushing with a standard toothbrush. Enlarging the brush handle using tape, wide rubber bands, sponges, or polystyrene or lengthening the brush by attaching a wood or plastic strip may make it easier to hold. Some older adults prefer an electric toothbrush that provides the proper movement.

Circular or short back-and-forth brushing works best to clean the teeth. Close attention should be paid to remove all plaque from along the gum line. Red, swollen, or bleeding gums indicate the need to see a dentist. People should have their teeth professionally cleaned twice a year to remove stains and other debris missed by routine brushing.

Older adults who wear dentures still need regular oral examinations because oral cancer occurs more frequently in the older adult population, with the average age at diagnosis of 60 years (NYU Oral Cancer Center, 2021). Good oral hygiene is also necessary. Dentures must be brushed or cleaned at least once a day to remove food debris, bacteria, and stains and to prevent gum irritation or bad breath. Some denture wearers prefer to brush the dentures using a special dentifrice, whereas others prefer to use a soaking solution that works overnight. Either cleansing method is appropriate, but the chemicals should be rinsed off thoroughly before dentures are put back into the mouth.

An older person wearing dentures for the first time needs to become adept at inserting and removing them. Eating with dentures is often awkward, necessitating some relearning so that the wearer will be able to chew effectively. Taking smaller pieces of soft, nonsticky foods and chewing more slowly are recommended. Because dentures make the mouth less sensitive to heat, cold, and foreign objects, such as bone fragments, special care is required when eating.

Poor fit is a major reason why some older adults fail to wear their dentures regularly. This contributes to problems with nutrition and digestion. A few extra appointments with the dentist are often necessary to help achieve a good fit. These adjustments are important because poorly fitting dentures can cause irritation to the gums or mucous membranes of the mouth. Additional adjustments may be needed if the denture wearer gains or loses weight.

Other changes in the oral cavity (e.g., dryness) are also common with aging. Although saliva production does not decrease in all older adults, a variety of medical conditions, medications, and treatments can cause or contribute to dry mouth. This condition can best be relieved by drinking more water. Excessive use of hard candy, caffeinated beverages, alcohol, or tobacco will increase dry mouth.

MAINTAINING HEALTHY ATTITUDES

Strong connections exist between the mind and body. Older adults who maintain a positive outlook on life tend to follow good health practices and remain healthier longer.

Regular interaction with other people of all age groups helps the older adult maintain a positive attitude toward life. It is recommended that older adults get out of the house as often as possible, even if only for shopping or dinner. Keeping in touch with family and friends is important. When spouses or friends are lost through death or relocation, older adults benefit from attempting to establish new relationships by joining church or community social groups. Volunteering in hospitals, schools, literacy centers, or other community agencies is a popular and desirable activity because it helps to promote a sense of value and self-worth (Fig. 4.2). Many older adults continue to remain active in the workforce. They may do so out of financial necessity or as a way of remaining a productive, contributing member of society. A decrease in social interaction can contribute to the deterioration of cognitive and adaptive skills. Nurses cannot force an individual to participate beyond their wishes, but encouragement and information about options can help to stimulate the older person's interests.

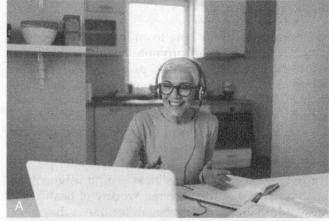

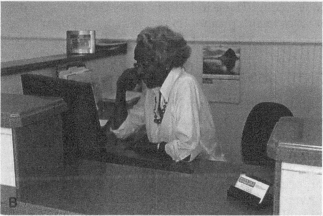

Fig. 4.2   Many older people continue to work and learn after the traditional retirement age. (A, iStock photo [Copyright © istock.com/ PixelsEffect]. B, From Cooper, K., & Gosnell, K. [2015]. *Foundations of nursing*, 7th edition. Mosby.)

FACTORS THAT AFFECT HEALTH PROMOTION AND MAINTENANCE

The actions taken to promote, maintain, or improve health are based on the individual's perception of their health. Health perceptions influence day-to-day choices regarding hygiene practices; nutrition; exercise; use of alcohol, drugs, and tobacco; accessing health care; and many other activities. Health maintenance practices include safety precautions taken to prevent injury from automobile accidents, falls, poisoning, and other hazards. Health perceptions and health maintenance practices in older adults are influenced by personal beliefs, religious and cultural beliefs, socioeconomic status, education, and life experiences.

As people mature, they establish a set of beliefs, perceptions, and values related to health. These perceptions include basic ideas regarding what health is and how to best maintain it. These beliefs form the foundation for each person's health practices. Based on their unique beliefs, most people perform activities they perceive to be helpful in maintaining their health and avoid activities they perceive as harmful. It is difficult to change a person's lifetime health practices. Only those who are highly motivated to change are likely to be successful.

RELIGIOUS BELIEFS

Religious beliefs contribute to an individual's perceptions. These beliefs can promote health maintenance or interfere with good health practices and result in increased health risks. For example, some religions teach that the body is a temple, stressing the importance of avoiding alcohol, tobacco, and other behaviors that are harmful to health. Individuals with these religious beliefs tend to live longer, healthier lives than people who do not share these values. Other people, whose religions teach that illness is a punishment for sins, may feel that they are not worthy of health and must endure illness as atonement for things they have done wrong. These individuals may be less inclined to practice health promotion and may have a more fatalistic approach to health and illness.

CULTURAL BELIEFS

Cultural beliefs and practices also play a significant role in health perception and health maintenance. For example, reliance on home remedies is common in many cultures. Some home remedies are harmless, whereas others are quite dangerous. Problems can occur when home remedies are used in place of conventional medical care, when the remedies interact with prescription medications, or when their use results in delayed care, which can be serious or even fatal if the illness is a serious one. Culture also plays a significant role in the selection of food and the methods used for food preparation. These preferences and practices play an important role in health promotion and maintenance. Plant-based diets consisting mainly of fruit, vegetables, and grains are common in some cultures, whereas diets high in fat and sodium are prevalent in others. These variations can contribute to the good health of some ethnic populations or to the health problems seen in others.

As our society becomes increasingly diverse, nurses need to become more aware of the religious and cultural factors that affect the health maintenance practices of all people (Fig. 4.3). Information about the beliefs and practices of organized religions and major cultural groups is available through sources such as textbooks on transcultural nursing. Although nurses can gain valuable insight from such sources, it is important not to generalize. It is common for two individuals from similar religious and cultural backgrounds to have widely disparate perceptions and practices. A general understanding of cultural factors is important; however, the best source of accurate information about a person's beliefs and practices is that individual. An overview of common health practices helps nurses understand the underlying values and beliefs that motivate each person.

KNOWLEDGE AND MOTIVATION

Factors other than religious and cultural beliefs also play a part in health perceptions and health maintenance practices. Knowledge plays a key role in maintaining health and promoting safety; knowledge of recommended health practices is essential to make good choices. Health and safety teaching must start early and be reinforced throughout life. Whenever there is a significant change in a person's health status, additional teaching is necessary to ensure the safety and highest possible level of wellness for that individual. People cannot make informed decisions regarding their health and safety unless they know the ramifications of various behaviors. Individuals experiencing cognitive changes resulting from disease processes or chemical

---

🌐 Cultural Considerations

Biocultural Differences

Considerable evidence still exists that race and ethnicity contribute to disparities in health throughout the United States. The following groups have higher rates of the following disorders:

- Hypertension: Non-Hispanic Black population
- Diabetes: American Indians/Alaska Native, non-Hispanic Black, and Hispanic populations
- Stomach cancer: Non-Hispanic Black, Hispanic, and Asian American populations
- Cervical cancer: Hispanic and non-Hispanic Black women
- Breast cancer: White women (higher incidence), Black women (higher mortality rate)
- Obesity: Non-Hispanic Black, Hispanic, and non-Hispanic White populations

Sources: American Diabetes Association (2021). Statistics about diabetes. https://www.diabetes.org/resources/statistics/statistics-about-diabetes; Saeed, A., Dixon, D. L., Yang, E. (2020). Racial disparities in hypertension prevalence and management: A crisis control? *American College of Cardiology.* https://www.acc.org/latest-in-cardiology/articles/2020/04/06/08/53/racial-disparities-in-hypertension-prevalence-and-management; Shah, S. C. (2021). Gastric cancer: A neglected threat to racial and ethnic minorities in the USA. *The Lancet, 6*(4): 266–267; Centers for Disease Control and Prevention (2020). HPV-associated cervical cancer. https://www.cdc.gov/cancer/hpv/statistics/cervical.htm; Breastcancer.org (2020). Breast cancer risk factors: Race/ethnicity. https://www.breastcancer.org/risk/factors/race_ethnicity; Centers for Disease Control and Prevention (2021). Adult obesity facts. https://www.cdc.gov/obesity/data/adult.html

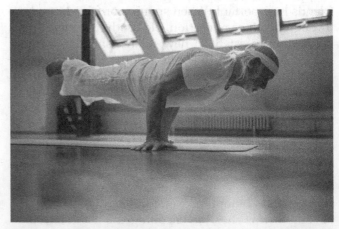

Fig. 4.3 Older adult doing peacock yoga pose. (Copyright © istock. com/BrauwnS.)

dependence may not be able to understand the need for safety or health maintenance practices despite repeated teaching. People with severe cognitive or perceptual problems are likely to experience injuries and alterations in health maintenance practices.

Health maintenance requires motivation in addition to knowledge. People experiencing grief, depression, hopelessness, or low self-esteem may not be motivated to maintain good health practices. Motivating individuals to maintain health is often difficult. All of the teaching in the world will not replace the desire to live a healthy life.

MOBILITY

Even people who are knowledgeable and motivated to maintain their health may have trouble if they cannot obtain the goods or services they need. People with limited physical mobility, lack of access to transportation, or little money are likely to experience difficulty. A person who knows the importance of nutritious food but cannot get to a store or afford to buy the food will have difficulty maintaining good health. A person who knows that it is important to see their primary care provider but cannot get to the office or pay for the care is similarly at risk.

Assessment of the values, perceptions, knowledge level, motivations, and lifelong health practices of individuals provides an understanding of the likelihood of problems with health maintenance. Previous behavior is a good indicator of future practice and motivation.

Many adaptive and assistive devices have been developed to promote safe mobility for people experiencing difficulty moving about or performing many of the activities of daily living (ADLs). The Department of Health and Human Services' website has information on thousands of products designed to assist people with physical limitations to help themselves (see Additional Learning Resources at end of chapter).

PERCEPTIONS OF AGING

Many beliefs about health and health maintenance are formed early in life. The longer a belief is held, the harder it is to change that belief. Therefore it can be difficult to change the health behaviors of older adults.

Perceptions of good health and good health practices vary widely among the aging population. Older adults have their own beliefs about what is normal and expected with aging. Some see and accept declining health as a normal part of aging, whereas others do not. Those who perceive a decline in health as normal and expected with aging may do little to prevent loss of function, simply accepting the changes. It is common to hear these older adults say, "Why should I bother to see the doctor? It's just old age." Some older adults often ignore early signs of illness or attribute them to aging. This often results in a delay before seeking medical care. Others, particularly those who have followed good health practices throughout their lives, believe that old age is not synonymous with disease or loss of function. They continue to follow high-level health maintenance practices in all aspects of their lives, including diet, exercise, rest, and medical attention.

Perceptions regarding aging greatly affect a person's motivation and willingness to participate in health maintenance activities. Someone who feels capable and in control of life is more likely to change behaviors and to work at maintaining health. Older adults who feel useless, helpless, or without purpose, particularly the newly widowed or those who are estranged from their families, are less likely to be motivated to maintain their health.

IMPACT OF COGNITIVE AND SENSORY CHANGES

Cognitive and sensory changes related to aging or disease can lead to problems with health maintenance. Even the normal sensory changes of aging can increase the risks for personal neglect or injury. When significant cognitive or perceptual problems occur, the risks are even greater.

An older person with changes in vision and smell may have body odor or wear soiled clothing because they cannot see or smell soiling. Changes in vision, hearing, smell, sensation, taste, and memory can also lead to decreased awareness of normal environmental hazards. Sensory changes increase the risk for injuries from falls, poisoning, fire, and other traumatic events. Vision changes can cause the older person to miss the edge of a step or a curb, resulting in a fall. Changes in smell and taste can result in consumption of spoiled, unsafe food. Changes in sensation can lead to the use of overly hot bathwater, resulting in burns. Changes in the sense of smell can cause the older adult to not perceive a burning odor, leading to the increased likelihood of injury from fire.

Older adults who are seriously impaired either perceptually or cognitively commonly lack awareness of their own needs. They may ignore parts of their hygiene or completely forget to perform routine health maintenance activities such as bathing, eating, or taking medication. Common health practices may be neglected even though the person is physically capable of performing the activities.

Cognitively impaired older adults are at serious risk for injury because they are unable to recognize the danger of their actions or inactions. They may forget to turn off the burner on the stove, forget to put on a coat when going outside in winter, turn up the furnace instead of turning it off, or walk into a busy street without looking for traffic. Severely impaired persons are at great risk for experiencing problems related to safety and health maintenance, often requiring some form of supervised living or institutional care for safety.

IMPACT OF CHANGES RELATED TO ACCESSIBILITY

Older adults are likely to experience more problems accessing goods and services than are younger people. Access may be limited by decreased physical mobility, lack of transportation, or limited finances. If more than one of these factors is present, the risk for ineffective health maintenance increases dramatically.

Physical limitations, including loss of motor skills, decreased strength and endurance, and the presence of disease, make health maintenance activities more difficult. Decreased physical strength and agility can interfere with normal health maintenance practices. Simple acts such as bathing, cooking, and cleaning can be too physically demanding for some older adults, who may be too fatigued to even attempt normal self-care activities. This lack of strength or energy often results in poor health maintenance practices.

Transportation difficulties present many problems for older adults. Simply getting to the grocery store, pharmacy, or care provider's office when necessary can be a major impediment to health maintenance. Even if older adults desire to practice good health maintenance, they may be hindered by a lack of transportation.

Finances cannot be ignored when discussing health maintenance. Although Social Security, Medicare, and Medicaid offset some financial concerns, they do not cover the entire cost of health care prescriptions or meals. The lack of these resources may cause older adults to limit medical care. Many older adults persist in trying to treat themselves before seeking medical attention. They may try to stretch the time between medical visits or take less than the prescribed amount of medications to save money. Financial constraints can also affect the ability of the older person to purchase special foods and equipment necessary to promote or maintain health.

Finances can also affect safety. Many older adults live in older housing, which is more likely to contain safety hazards, such as poor electric wiring, steep stairwells, and inadequate lighting. High crime rates in poorer areas make older adults who live there particularly vulnerable to rape, mugging, and theft. Even if these factors are not a problem, simple home maintenance can increase the risk for injury. Because it is costly to hire people to do even routine home maintenance chores, many older adults attempt these tasks alone. Some fall from chairs or ladders while trying to paint walls, clean windows, or hang pictures. Many injure themselves trying to shovel snow or mow the lawn.

HOME HEALTH

The typical older adult wishes to remain at home for as long as possible. To accomplish this, additional assistance will likely be needed. Some of this assistance can be provided by family members. More complex interventions require the expertise of specialized caregivers. As the number of older adults has increased, the demand for home care services has also increased and promises to continue to grow for the foreseeable future. Home health interventions can both promote health and help the older person maintain the highest level of function possible for as long as possible. Assistance in the home can help overcome problems related to nonadherence by providing motivation, verifying that care is completed, and providing better access to health care services.

According to the Medicare Payment Advisory Commission, more than 3 million people in the United States receive the Medicare home health benefit (Donlan, 2020), and approximately 1.5 million more receive hospice care (National Hospice and Palliative Care Organization, 2019). Medicare and Medicaid spending for home health care reached more than $113 billion in 2019 (Holly, 2020), and it is expected to keep increasing. This massive number does not include unpaid care provided by family members, friends, or volunteers, which makes the true cost even greater. Without the dedicated help of all these individuals, the health care delivery system would be overwhelmed, and many older adults would experience a poorer quality of life.

UNPAID CAREGIVER

Most unpaid caregivers are family or friends of the older adult, although they may be volunteers from a church or other charitable organization. Caregivers can be divided into primary and secondary classifications. Primary caregivers provide for most of the day-to-day needs of older adults. These are usually close family members, such as spouses or children, but they may be paid employees. Secondary caregivers help intermittently with things like shopping, transportation, and home maintenance. Usually, those family members who reside closest to the older person provide the most direct assistance, whereas those who live farther away are less involved. This can be a source of interfamily strife. One family member may be resentful of doing everything while others do little or nothing. Of course, this is not always the case; some families develop a good balance and distribution of effort. Even family members who live at great distances from older relatives can provide high level long-distance support, usually through an intermediary agency.

Most caregivers are women. They are of all ages, with the average being in the mid to late 40s. They come from all ethnic, racial, and religious backgrounds. Most are providing care to older adults in spite of multiple other responsibilities, including their children, homes, and jobs. Many caregivers experience exhaustion, anxiety, depressive symptoms, and burnout as a result of multiple demands, particularly when they feel that their assistance is not appreciated. Often, they will require teaching, guidance, and assistance while learning how to perform new skills and effective ways to respond to the needs of the older adult. This teaching needs to be done in a kind and courteous manner. Nurses should be careful not to denigrate the services or capabilities of these caregivers. Unpaid caregivers should not be criticized or made to feel guilty that they are not doing enough. Instead, the nurse should work to develop a partnership with family caregivers, performing ongoing assessment, teaching, coaching, and offering psychological support and guidance. Nurses and other professionals need to be kind to unpaid caregivers, recognizing the value of their service and providing positive feedback. Box 4.3 lists agencies that provide assistance and information to older caregivers.

PAID CAREGIVERS

Almost any kind of home help can be arranged, from the simplest to the most complex. Agencies that provide home health services have proliferated in recent years. Many of these are highly ethical organizations that provide valuable service to older adults. Others are less scrupulous and may even increase the risks for a vulnerable older person. Informal referrals from friends, senior citizen centers, churches, or volunteer organizations may be helpful in locating a reliable caregiver. Additional help with identifying qualified assistance can be obtained from the local area's Agency on Aging, state or local social service agencies, or tribal councils. Although some assistance may be provided free of charge by volunteer organizations and some may be covered by insurance or Medicare, the services of most independent contractors or private agencies involve considerable out-of-pocket expense. It is wise to verify the cost of services before making any commitments. Home care is usually less expensive than care in an institutional setting, but not always. Much will depend on the extent and complexity of the care needed. Cost is always an issue, whether providers admit it or not.

Even wealthy people need to be cautious that they spend their money wisely; those with average incomes need to pay even more attention to costs.

It is always wise to check references before hiring anyone to work with older adults. Because the caregiver is often alone and unsupervised with the older adult, any signs of unscrupulous or abusive behavior must be investigated. Ideally, paid caregivers will have a history of punctuality and reliability, because an older adult often becomes anxious if the caregiver is unreliable. These caregivers should provide certification that they are free of communicable diseases, including tuberculosis and COVID-19. A background check should be conducted to ensure that they have committed no serious criminal acts. Reputable home care agencies often provide these checks as part of their service and may also bond their employees to protect patients against loss due to theft or property damage. It is also advisable to plan an introductory visit and trial session to determine the compatibility of the caregiver and older adult. Box 4.4 provides a list of important questions to ask in selecting a home health agency.

TYPES OF HOME SERVICES

Older adults require different levels of home assistance. The level of care needed is likely to change as the person's health status changes over time. An older adult who is generally healthy may require only transportation to appointments and assistance with household chores such as mopping, vacuuming, laundry, grocery

---

Box 4.3   Older Adult Information and Services

- Administration for Community Living (www.acl.gov)
- Eldercare Locator (www.eldercare.acl.gov)
- Medicare benefits (www.medicare.gov)
- National Institute of Medicine (www.medlineplus.gov)
- National Institute on Aging Information Center (www.nia.nih.gov)
- National Council on Aging (www.benefitscheckup.org)
- Federal, state, or local government benefits (www.benefits.gov)
- Department of Veterans Affairs (www.va.gov)
- Department of Housing and Urban Development (www.hud.gov)
- Campaign for Home Energy Assistance (www.liheap.org)
- National Resource Center on Supportive Housing and Home Modification (www.homemods.org)
- LeadingAge (www.leadingage.org)

Box 4.4   Questions to Ask When Selecting a Home Health Agency

- How long has the agency been in business in this community?
- What services does the agency provide?
- How much do these services cost? Is financial aid available? How are charges billed?
- Is the agency certified by Medicare? Is it accredited by any organization, such as the Joint Commission Nursing Care Center Accreditation program?
- Does the agency have a bill of rights for older adults?
- Does the agency have a specific written plan of care for the older adult that is developed with patient and family input?
- What kind of screening is done when hiring employees? Are references available to the family?
- How are caregivers trained and supervised?
- What level of professional supervision is provided?
- Is there a registered nurse on call 24 hours a day?
- How and when is information communicated between the agency and the family?
- What is done to protect confidentiality?
- How are conflicts or complaints resolved?

Modified from the U.S. Department of Health and Human Services Administration for Community Living Fact Sheet, "Home Health Care." https://www.acl.gov/sites/default/files/news%202017-03/Home_Health_Care.pdf.

shopping, and meal preparation, all of which are considered unskilled interventions.

An infirm older adult may need additional help with hygiene and dressing. Older adults with altered cognition may also need ongoing supervision for safety and help with medication preparation and administration. More compromised older adults may require assistance with dressing changes, management of wounds, pain management, or other skilled interventions. Even hospice or palliative care may be provided in the home.

A thorough assessment by a trained professional, usually a registered nurse (RN) or social worker, can best determine how much and what kind of help will most benefit each older adult. Working in conjunction with the patient's primary care provider, the case manager (typically an RN) will assess, plan, supervise, and coordinate services.

QSEN Considerations: Teamwork and Collaboration

Home services are best delivered by a team that includes RNs, licensed practical nurses (LPNs)/licensed vocational nurses (LVNs), health aides, housekeepers, dietitians, and social workers as well as occupational, physical, and speech therapists. Nursing supervision of unlicensed personnel is critical for safe home care. Aides must have adequate training to perform safely in the care setting, and they need to know the limits within which they must work. For example, aides are generally not permitted to measure and dispense medications, although they may be permitted to give medications to the older adult if the nurse or a family member first sets these up in prelabeled and timed packaging. Social workers help manage the financial aspects of care as well as to facilitate communication with other agencies or facilities, particularly if the patient needs to be admitted to a hospital or health care facility. Social workers are also responsible for the assessment of family dynamics and possible intervention in suspected cases of neglect or abuse. A chaplain may be part of the team; home hospice is likely to have chaplains available for end-of-life issues. In addition, the case manager may have responsibility for arranging that all necessary equipment and supplies (such as oxygen, wheelchairs, and hospital beds) are available and remain in good operating condition.

❖ NURSING PROCESS/CLINICAL JUDGMENT MODEL FOR INADEQUATE HEALTH MAINTENANCE AND INADEQUATE HEALTH MANAGEMENT

The nursing process is a step-by-step way of identifying and meeting patient needs based on the scientific method. The Clinical Judgment Model adds the layer of context to care planning, as patient situations are dynamic. When nursing care planning is being discussed, steps from the Clinical Judgment Model are also presented. Figure 4.4 provides a visual representation of how the nursing process and Clinical Judgment Model overlap. For further reading, please consult your *Fundamental Concepts* textbook (Fig. 4.4).

Older adults who are unable to identify or seek out help and those who are unable to follow through with

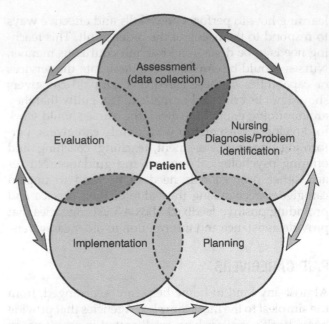

Fig. 4.4 Nursing Process and Clinical Judgment Model: A dynamic, overlapping, continuous process encompassing patient-centered care. (From Williams, P. A. [2021]. *Fundamental concepts and skills for nursing,* 6th edition. Elsevier.)

a therapeutic regimen are at risk for serious health-related problems (see Nursing Care Plan 4.1). An assessment of health perceptions and health maintenance practices is necessary in order to consider the unique problems, beliefs, and perceptions of each older adult. It is important to assess both past and current health management practices because these are good predictors of future health practices.

◆ ASSESSMENT (DATA COLLECTION)

Recognize Cues
- How does the person rate their current health?
- Does the person feel in control of conditions that affect their health?
- What does the person routinely do to maintain their health?
- How does the person manage illnesses?
- What are the person's religious or cultural beliefs regarding health and health practices?
- How do the person's health practices compare with recommended health practices?
- How often does the person see a physician, dentist, or other health professional?
- Does the person engage in high-risk behaviors, such as smoking, excessive alcohol intake, or drug consumption?
- Are there adequate financial resources to maintain their health?
- Does the person have access to the goods and services necessary to maintain health?
- Is the person's knowledge adequate to make informed decisions regarding their health?

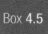

> **Box 4.5** **Characteristics of Older Adults Who Are Likely to Experience Inadequate Health Maintenance**
>
> - Lack of adequate knowledge about recommended health practices
> - Physical limitations
> - Lack of adaptive behaviors to environmental changes
> - Limited financial resources
> - Altered cognitive or perceptual function
> - Difficulty accessing health-related goods or services
> - Loss of motivation because of grief, hopelessness, or powerlessness

See Box 4.5 for a list of the characteristics of older adults who are at risk for inadequate health maintenance.

◆ DATA ANALYSIS/PROBLEM IDENTIFICATION

Analyze Cues and Prioritize Hypotheses: Common problem statements for older adults who are unable to identify or seek out help include

Inadequate Health Management

Inadequate Health Maintenance

◆ PLANNING

Generate Solutions: The nursing goals for an older adult demonstrating inadequate health maintenance are to verbalize appropriate health maintenance practices, demonstrate adequate health maintenance practices, and identify community resources that can assist in health maintenance.

◆ IMPLEMENTATION

Take Action: The following nursing interventions for inadequate health maintenance should take place in hospitals or extended-care facilities:

1. **Assess the older adult's ability to resume adequate health maintenance practices.** After hospitalization or rehabilitation in an extended-care facility, older adults must be assessed carefully to determine whether they are capable of returning home and resuming adequate health maintenance practices. Ideally, discharge from the facility should be delayed until the nurse can be reasonably sure that the patient is ready to take responsibility for their health care needs. If possible, an assessment of the home environment should also be made before discharge and, if necessary, should be modified to promote health maintenance and safety. A referral for a follow-up visit after discharge will help to ensure that the older adult is safe and able to meet the basic requirements of health maintenance.
2. **Teach the skills required to monitor health status when the patient returns home.** Before discharge from a health care institution, older adults should be given a thorough explanation and printed handouts to reinforce the following topics: what they

need to do to maintain health, including when to call or see the primary care provider; what medications are required and when they should be taken; how to perform home screening procedures (e.g., blood glucose monitoring, blood pressure monitoring, and daily weights); and how to keep records and monitor their health.
3. **Consult with the social worker or with agencies that can assist with health maintenance practices.** The community social worker or social agencies may be able to help older adults meet their health maintenance needs by providing transportation, delivering food or groceries, assisting with home maintenance, or offering other services.

The following interventions should take place in the home:

1. **Assess the current health maintenance practices.** The nurse should assess the older person's knowledge of the factors that promote health. Any problem areas should be examined in greater detail. The nurse should also determine what motivates the person to be attentive to these practices, because these motivators may be valuable if modifications in health care practices become necessary.
2. **Explain and reinforce positive health maintenance behaviors.** The nurse should review health practices regarding diet, safety, stress management, exercise, elimination, and sleep. It is important to review when and how to contact their primary care provider, particularly in cases of a serious illness or emergency. If older adults are receiving treatment for any health problems, they should know what health care behaviors are recommended to maintain the highest level of wellness (Box 4.6). They should know what medications to take and when to take them as well as how to perform any special care or treatment.
3. **Assist in identifying family or community resources that promote health maintenance.** Individuals living in their homes may be unaware of services that are available to provide help. Often, a little assistance is all that is needed to enable an older person to live a healthy, independent life. If assistance is delayed, health maintenance may deteriorate to a point at which hospitalization or

> **Box 4.6** **Recommended Health Practices to Maintain Wellness**
>
> - Adopt a well-balanced, plant-based meal plan
> - Establish a regular exercise program
> - Quit smoking
> - Consume alcohol in moderation
> - Get routine immunizations as recommended
> - Stay involved in activities and with others
> - Maintain a healthy attitude
> - See the dentist and primary care provider regularly

institutional placement would be required. These services should be identified before they are required to avoid delays or waiting lists for the services.

4. **Use any appropriate interventions that are used in the institutional setting.**

❖ NURSING PROCESS/CLINICAL JUDGMENT MODEL FOR NONADHERENCE WITH THE TREATMENT PLAN

Several institutions are moving away from the older terminology of noncompliance and toward the term nonadherence because there is less of a negative connotation attached to that term. Truthfully, it is very difficult to adhere 100% to every aspect of a treatment regimen—exercise, diet, medications, annual screening procedures—and it is not uncommon to label a patient as "noncompliant" who has made great strides on many aspects of their health care but has slipped up on one particular part of it. Therefore what might be labeled noncompliance on various nursing diagnoses or patient problem lists will be referred to as nonadherence in this text and on the Priority Problem List shared with our partner texts, *Medical-Surgical Nursing* and *Fundamental Concepts* and *Skills for Nursing*.

A person should be considered nonadherent only when they fail to follow through with recommended health practices despite adequate teaching and resources. Not taking prescribed medications, not attending scheduled medical appointments, and inconsistent following of prescribed meal plans are examples of nonadherent behaviors. Many factors may be related to nonadherence: cognitive impairment, inadequate knowledge, inadequate resources, lack of transportation, fear, anger, decreased self-esteem, substance abuse, and conflict of beliefs or values. Nonadherence should be suspected when a person does not show the expected amount of progress toward wellness, when a person gets worse instead of better, or when a person develops repeated or unexpected complications.

◆ ASSESSMENT (DATA COLLECTION)

Recognize Cues

- Does the person verbalize unwillingness or inability to follow through with the necessary health maintenance or medical care recommendations?
- Does the person verbalize a conflict between personal beliefs or values and the treatment plan?
- Are there unexpected relapses, or do the health problems appear to be getting worse instead of better?
- Does the person often miss medical appointments? What reasons are given?
- Is there more medication left in the bottle than would be expected if it were taken according to directions?

| Box 4.7 | **Characteristics of Older Adults Who Are Likely to Be at Risk for Nonadherence** |

- Cognitive, perceptual, or developmental problems
- Lack of knowledge of the treatment plan
- Lack of adequate financial resources
- Poor self-esteem or altered body image
- Lack of a support system of friends and family
- Lack of motivation
- Substance use or alcohol use disorders
- Negative past experiences with the health care system
- Differing cultural, religious, or health beliefs

- Are there signs of the presence of prohibited foods (e.g., candy for persons with diabetes and a salt shaker for persons with sodium restriction)?

Box 4.7 lists the characteristics of older persons who are at risk for nonadherence.

◆ DATA ANALYSIS/PROBLEM IDENTIFICATION

Analyze Cues and Prioritize Hypotheses: Problem statement for older adults who are adults who are unable to follow through with a therapeutic regimen include the following:

Nonadherence With the Treatment Plan

◆ PLANNING

Generate Solutions: The goals for an older person demonstrating nonadherence are to identify factors that contribute to nonadherent behavior and demonstrate the acceptance of treatment.

◆ IMPLEMENTATION

Take Action: The following nursing interventions for nonadherence should take place in hospitals or extended-care facilities:

1. **Identify the reasons for behavior that is nonadherent with the treatment plan.** A person might not adhere to recommended health maintenance practices for many reasons. Unless the nurse can determine the specific reasons why the person is not following the recommended practices, interventions are likely to be inappropriate and unsuccessful. If the person does not take medication because of forgetfulness, further teaching will not help. If the person refuses medication because they feel unworthy of living, no reminders will help. Interventions must address the root problem. Forgetful people need a system of reminders; people with poor self-esteem need to feel valued before they can accept care. Individuals who exhibit self-neglect may require treatments for depression, dementia, or physical problems that may be hampering their ability for self-care. The individual may need to be monitored so that the nurse can observe and intervene in the event of any excessive deterioration in their health

or level of self-care. Treatment should include home health care provided in a way that does not reduce the person's autonomy any more than necessary. Self-neglect may be an indicator that a person would benefit from assisted living or some other form of residential care. These individuals might improve if they had more opportunities for social interaction. If people are legally determined to be incompetent of making decisions about their own care, they may have a legal guardian appointed and be compelled to accept help. If such individuals are in possession of their mental faculties, they do have the right to refuse treatment.

2. **Provide care in a nonjudgmental manner.** The values and beliefs of older adults are often different from those of their caregivers. If the nurse indicates verbally or nonverbally that the older person's beliefs and practices are in some way inferior, the nurse is not likely to be able to convince the person to adhere to the desired health practices.

3. **Actively include the patient in planning care and adapt or modify the care plan so that it will be more acceptable to the patient.** It is important to develop all plans *with*, not *for*, the older person. Each individual can then incorporate their unique culture, beliefs, and values into the plan being developed. This enables older adults to retain control and responsibility for their own health care. When they "own" the plan and determine the goals, they are more likely to adhere to it.

4. **Emphasize the benefits of adhering to the treatment plan.** Many aging people do not adhere to recommended health care practices because they do not really believe that adherence will help. If people can actually become aware of the benefits that ensue when they do adhere, they are more likely to become actively involved in the process. For example, if a person with diabetes continually sneaks extra food and therefore frequently has high blood glucose levels, the nurse can demonstrate how much lower the blood glucose level is when the person follows the prescribed diet. If less insulin or fewer injections would be required when the blood glucose level is controlled, these benefits should be stressed. Unfortunately, it is not always possible to see any obvious immediate benefits from adherence to the treatment plan.

5. **Acknowledge the aging person's right not to adhere to the treatment plan.** If an alert older person chooses not to adhere to the plan of care despite explanations, teaching, and reminders, the nurse must recognize that this is, in fact, the individual's right.

The following interventions should take place in the home:

1. **Assess the support system.** In the home setting, it is particularly important to identify the strengths of older adults and the amount of support they receive from friends and family. The likelihood of achieving adherence is far greater when patients are willing to learn and to modify their behavior and when they have others who are willing to help. Individuals who resist intervention and receive little support are likely to continue to have problems with adherence.

2. **Help structure the environment to promote adherence to the treatment plan.** Many individuals are nonadherent simply because they are confused or forgetful. Memory devices can catch their attention and verify that critical actions take place. For example, if the person forgets to eat meals, a checklist for the days of the week and the three basic meals can be posted on the refrigerator door. Each time the person fixes a meal, the box is checked. Medications that need to be taken twice a day can be "tagged" to an activity that occurs twice a day, such as toothbrushing. The medication container can be placed next to the toothpaste tube to serve as a reminder. Special divided containers are also available for people who have trouble remembering to take their medication. Medication for an entire week can be prepared by a responsible assistant or nurse. A simple glance in the box lets the person know whether they have taken the right medication at the right time. Bold markings on a calendar, preferably one with large print, can be used to mark special events. Signs in bold letters can be posted in appropriate places. For example, "take a drink" can be posted over the sink of a person whose fluid intake is inadequate.

3. **Enlist the help of family, friends, and neighbors to provide reminders.** Reminder phone calls or texts from friends or family are useful for less frequent occasions, such as doctor visits. It is wise for the friend or family member to call the person the day before the appointment and then again on the day of the appointment to ensure that it is not forgotten. It is even better for a responsible friend or family member to transport the person to the medical appointment. Responsible friends and family members can also provide help in setting up the weekly pillbox and preparing other reminders around the home.

4. **Involve social service agencies in promoting adherence to the treatment plan.** If the person is nonadherent because of financial or transportation problems, a social worker or social service agency may be able to provide assistance that enables the person to adhere to the plan.

5. **Use any appropriate interventions that are used in the institutional setting** (see Nursing Care Plan 4.1).

Nursing Care Plan 4.1

HEALTH MAINTENANCE

Mrs. Fisher is an alert and well-groomed 82 year old female who lives alone. She has a history of type 2 diabetes mellitus. Her blood glucose levels, which you test weekly, are consistently 200 mg/dL or higher. Her primary care provider has prescribed a 1200-calorie diabetic meal plan and an oral hypoglycemic medication.

When you arrive at Mrs. Fisher's apartment early for a home visit, you find an open box of gingersnaps next to the chair where she was sitting. She says, "I like to sit around most of the day and read or watch TV." You ask about the cookies, and she replies, "They're not very sweet; I need to have some food that I enjoy. I won't live forever, you know." You check the bottle of oral hypoglycemic medication and find that she has taken only two tablets in the past week. She states, "I forget to take them. They don't help anyway, and they cost too much."

PROBLEM STATEMENT

Nonadherence With the Treatment Plan

Supporting Assessment Data

- Consistently elevated blood glucose levels
- Inconsistent intake of prescribed medications
- Inconsistent following of prescribed diet
- Statement of lifestyle changes in conflict with personal values and resources

Patient Goals/Outcomes Identification

Mrs. Fisher will do the following:
- Follow prescribed diet
- Increase activity level
- Take medications according to prescribed schedule
- Achieve blood glucose levels of less than 120 mg/dL

NURSING INTERVENTIONS/IMPLEMENTATION

1. Explore reasons for difficulty in adhering to the treatment plan (economic, motivational, etc.).
2. Allow patient to verbalize feelings and problems experienced with activity, diet, and medications.
3. Review daily food intake.
4. Explain long-term benefits of following prescribed diet.
5. Set up reminder system for daily medications.
6. Explore ways of increasing physical activity.
7. Encourage adherence to the plan of care.
8. Praise positive health care behaviors.
9. Continue to monitor blood glucose level, and notify primary care provider if it remains elevated.
10. Arrange a consultation with dietitian at next primary care provider's office visit.

EVALUATION

At the next home visit a week later, you find that Mrs. Fisher's blood glucose level is 174 mg/dL. She states proudly that with the new medication system, she has remembered to take 6 of her oral hypoglycemic tablets and forgot on only a single day. She further states that she has taken 4 short walks with her neighbor. After providing positive feedback on these signs of improved adherence to the treatment plan, you discuss the meal plan with her. Mrs. Fisher states that she has tried to be more careful, but because she still likes an occasional cookie, she will limit herself to 1 or 2 per day. Improvement is demonstrated, and goals are partially met. You will continue with the plan of care and reassess in 1 week.

APPLYING CLINICAL JUDGMENT

1. What additional approaches could be implemented to improve Mrs. Fisher's adherence to her medication regimen?
2. How could you help Mrs. Fisher decrease her snack intake? Can you suggest ways to motivate her to increase her activity?

Get Ready for the Next Generation NCLEX® Examination!

Key Points

- Many of today's older people continue to live independently despite a variety of chronic health problems.
- Health maintenance is an ongoing challenge for older adults, their families, and their health care providers.
- Careful assessment of the older adult's perception of health, health practices, and knowledge of

safety factors is an important part of nursing care in all settings.
- Early detection of problems and early intervention can prevent more serious complications and enable older adults to maintain the highest possible level of wellness and function.
- Home health assistance, both unpaid and paid, can help older adults remain independent for a longer period of time.

Get Ready for the Next Generation NCLEX® Examination!—cont'd

- Nurses play an important role in case management and in providing services to older adults in their homes.
- Caution should be exercised in selecting home care providers for older adults.

Additional Learning Resources

SG Go to your Evolve website at http://evolve.elsevier. com/Williams/geriatric for the additional online resources.

 Online Resources

- Fruits and Veggies: More Matters: https://healthysd.gov/fruits-veggies-more-matters/
My Plate for Older Adults: http://hnrca.tufts.edu/myplate
- National Institute on Disability, Independent Living, and Rehabilitation Research (NIDILRR). https://acl.gov/about-acl/about-national-institute-disability-independent-living-and-rehabilitation-research

Review Questions for the Next Generation NCLEX® Examination

1. What activity best promotes health maintenance for the typical older adult?

   a. One hour of low-impact tai chi per week
   b. One 30-minute walk 3 to 5 times a week
   c. Step aerobics for 20 minutes twice a week
   d. Riding for 5 to 10 minutes on a stationary bike every day

2. The nurse recognizes that regular dental visits are

   a. Necessary only for those older adults who still have their natural teeth.
   b. Recommended on a yearly basis for all older adults, even those with dentures.
   c. Not necessary if the person brushes and flosses properly 3 times a day.
   d. Desirable but not necessary unless pain or another problem occurs.

3. An older adult does not follow through with health recommendations from the primary health care provider. The older adult does not take prescribed medications or keep medical appointments. Which problem statement should the LPN/LVN anticipate seeing on the care plan?

   a. Nonadherence with the treatment plan
   b. Insufficient knowledge
   c. Chronic confusion
   d. Altered family coping

4. Which immunizations should older adults receive on a yearly basis? *(Select all that apply.)*

   a. Pneumonia vaccine
   b. Influenza vaccine
   c. Tetanus vaccine
   d. Polio vaccine
   e. Hepatitis B vaccine

5. In attempting to help an older adult improve his or her health maintenance practices, the nurse will need to assess which factors? *(Select all that apply.)*

   a. Physical strength and endurance
   b. Availability of transportation
   c. Cultural beliefs
   d. Cognitive and sensory changes
   e. Socioeconomic status
   f. Religious beliefs
   g. Social support system
   h. Educational level

6. Your patient, Luz Valencia, a 76-year old widow of Hispanic origin, was recently diagnosed with type 2 diabetes. She takes an oral hypoglycemic medication for blood glucose control. Luz presents to your urgent care clinic with gastrointestinal pain and bloating. Her vital signs are T 98.2 (o), P 96, R 22, and BP 140/86. Her fingerstick blood glucose is 99. She ranks her pain level at 7/10 and states, "My stomach pain is so terrible. I hope it's just gas but I'm scared it might be something more." She has recently tried a new meal plan to help with her diabetes management. From your education, you know that based on Luz's ethnicity, she is at risk for some disorders more than others. From the following list, select those that Luz is at highest risk for based on her Hispanic ethnicity. *(Select all that apply.)*

   a. Obesity
   b. Stomach cancer
   c. Diabetes mellitus
   d. Hypertension
   e. Cervical cancer
   f. Breast cancer

REFERENCES

Amin, S. (2020). Does Medicare pay for shingles vaccine? https://www.medicalnewstoday.com/articles/does-medicare-cover-shingles-vaccine

Centers for Disease Control and Prevention [CDC] (2020a). Vaccines and preventable diseases: diphtheria, tetanus, and pertussis vaccine recommendations. https://www.cdc.gov/vaccines/vpd/dtap-tdap-td/hcp/recommendations.html

Centers for Disease Control and Prevention [CDC] (2020b). Vaccines and preventable diseases: What everyone should know. https://www.cdc.gov/vaccines/vpd/pneumo/public/index.html

Centers for Disease Control and Prevention [CDC] (2021). How and when to have your cholesterol checked. https://www.cdc.gov/cholesterol/checked.htm

Centers for Medicare & Medicaid Services (2019a). Adults need more physical activity. https://www.cdc.gov/physicalactivity/inactivity-among-adults-50plus/index.html

Centers for Medicare & Medicaid Services (2019b). Health expenditures by age and gender. https://www.cms.gov/Research-Statistics-Data-and-Systems/Statistics-Trends-and-Reports/NationalHealthExpendData/Age-and-Gender

Donlan, A. (2020). As older adults are increasingly isolated, advocates call for Medicare home care benefit. https://homehealthcarenews.com/2020/06/as-older-adults-are-increasingly-isolated-advocates-call-for-medicare-home-care-benefit/#:~:text=More%20than%203%20million%20people,into%20Medicare%20is%20not%20new

Holly, R. (2020). National home health spending reaches all-time high of $113.5 billion. https://homehealthcarenews.com/2020/12/national-home-health-spending-reaches-all-time-high-of-113-5-billion/

National Council on Aging (2021). Get the facts on healthy aging. https://www.ncoa.org/article/get-the-facts-on-healthy-aging

National Hospice and Palliative Care Organization. (2019). NHPCO facts and figures (2018 edition). revision 7–2–2019. https://39k5cm1a9u1968hg74aj3x51-wpengine.netdna-ssl.com/wp-content/uploads/2019/07/2018_NHPCO_Facts_Figures.pdf

NYU Oral Cancer Center (2021). Oral cancer: Facts. https://www.nyuoralcancer.org/oral_cancer/oral_cancer_facts.html

Communicating With Older Adults

Objectives

1. Identify communication techniques that are effective with older adults.
2. Define empathetic listening.
3. Identify the significance of nonverbal communication with older adults.
4. Discuss the verbal communication techniques used when sending and receiving messages.
5. Differentiate between social and therapeutic communication.
6. Discuss the ways in which communication is affected by culture.

Key Terms

confrontation (KŎN-frăn-tā-shŭn, p. 105)
empathy (ĔM-pă-thē, p. 101)
proxemics (prŏk-SĒ-mĭks, p. 98)

rapport (ră-PŎR, p. 95)
symbols (SĬM-băls, p. 97)

Communication is the process of exchanging information: sending messages back and forth between individuals or groups of people. Each individual who participates in communication is a unique person with their own values, beliefs, culture, and perceptions. This is particularly important to remember when working with older adults. The older adults of today formed their opinions, values, and beliefs in a very different society from that in which we live today. Today's oldest adults grew up during the Great Depression, when men sold apples on street corners and searched for pieces of coal in railroad yards in order to survive. They lived through a major world war and witnessed the beginning of the nuclear age, when the first atomic bomb was dropped. They grew up in a world without many of today's conveniences, including television and private telephone lines. The upcoming generation of older adults, however, is very different. The baby boomers, who came of age during the Vietnam War, grew up in a world characterized by drugs, protests, and "free love." They grew up with stereos, television, and astronauts walking on the moon. Most baby boomers have adapted to the use of cell phones and computers. Technology was and will continue to be a part of their lives.

Whatever their background, older adults have had time to encounter many situations both good and bad. It may be difficult for a younger person to understand the experiences that have made older adults who they are today. The most effective way to bridge the gulf between the generations is good communication (Table 5.1).

Effective communication is not easy, even among people of the same age group and background. Communication among people from different age groups and backgrounds can be even more challenging. This is particularly true when one of the parties is older; however, effective communication can occur even when people hold significantly different values, beliefs, and perspectives. Effective communication does not mean that we will like or agree with everything another person says but rather that we respect the person's right to think and say it. This atmosphere of mutual respect and understanding helps build trust and rapport. Conscious, ongoing effort is required to become an effective communicator.

Effective communication requires the following:
1. The need or desire to share information
2. Acceptance that there is value and merit in what the other person has to say, demonstrated by a willingness to treat the other person with genuine dignity and respect
3. Understanding of factors that may interfere with or become barriers to communication
4. Development of the skills and techniques that facilitate the effective interchange of information

INFORMATION SHARING (FRAMING THE MESSAGE)

Verbal communication involves sending and receiving messages using words. Some verbal communication is formal, structured, and precise; some is informal, unstructured, and flexible. Formal or therapeutic communications have a specific intent and purpose. Informal

Table 5.1	Communication Dos and Don'ts in Working With Older Adults	
DO	**DON'T**	
Identify yourself.	Assume that the person knows who you are.	
Address the person using their preferred name (e.g., Mrs. Tao and Rahul).	Use "baby talk" or patronizing names, such as "sweetie" or "honey."	
Speak clearly and slowly in a low tone of voice.	Shout.	
Get to know the person.	Make generalizations about older people.	
Listen empathetically.	Pay too much attention to tasks and forget the person.	
Pay attention to body language, yours and theirs.	Consider nonverbal messages as insignificant.	
Use touch appropriately and frequently.	Be afraid to use touch as a method of communication.	

or social conversations are less specific and are used for socialization. Both have a place in nursing. Nurses must be effective in both formal and informal communication and must know how and when to use each type.

Professor Albert Mehrabian (1981), professor emeritus of psychology at the University of California Los Angeles, pioneered the 7%, 38%, 55% rule for communication. Only 7% comes from the actual words we use, 38% depends on paralinguistic cues (i.e., tone, pitch, rate, speed, and volume of voice), and 55% is transmitted by body cues. It is not essential to memorize these percentages; rather, the "take away" message is that more than half of the message we send is transmitted by body language."

FORMAL OR THERAPEUTIC COMMUNICATION

Therapeutic communication is a conscious and deliberate process used to gather information related to a patient's overall health status (physical, psychosocial, spiritual, etc.) and to respond with verbal and nonverbal approaches that promote the patient's well-being or improve the patient's understanding of ongoing care. This type of communication looks easy and natural when performed by an experienced health professional, but it is a skill that requires time, effort, and practice to develop. Careful use of words and language is an art. Knowledge of the other person's health status provides a starting point for conversation. Social discussions often center on past employment, family, or other interests. Greater knowledge of the individual, including educational background enhances one's ability to respond empathetically. Effective verbal communication requires the ability to use a variety of techniques when sending and receiving messages.

When communicating verbally, whether in a formal or informal situation, nurses should know as much as possible about the other person involved. A person's age, marital status, cultural or ethnic orientation, educational background, interests, and the ability to hear and see influence the communication techniques used and the words chosen. We need to be careful to choose words that the patient can understand—not so simple that we are "talking down" to the patient, but also not so technical or "medical" that the meaning is unclear. Avoid acronyms, such as *TURP* (transurethral resection of the prostate) or *CBC* (complete blood count), unless you are sure that the person understands them. Careful listening to the patient's speech can yield clues about the appropriate level of language to be used.

 QSEN Considerations: Patient-Centered Care

Improving Communication

According to QSEN, it is important to understand the principles of effective communication. You should assess your own level of skill in communicating with patients and families, and you should strive for continuous improvement of these skills.

Cultural Considerations

Communication Styles

- Some people tend to be bold and to ask direct questions, particularly in a crisis. We expect the answers to be similarly clear and direct.
- You may find that some people prefer to proceed less directly and need to establish a relationship through "small talk" before addressing more serious concerns. Although this may seem less productive, your awareness that the patient and their family may be more comfortable with this type of communication can contribute to greater success in the long-term relationship.
- You will likely find these differences in communication styles to be true not only in patient care situations but also in communicating with other members of the health care team.

Communication

Misunderstanding of Medical Jargon

A nurse was finishing up her early morning care for a postoperative cardiac surgery patient. The patient was on the ventilator and could not orally communicate. The treatment plan called for progressive resumption of activity. After assisting with morning care, the nurse informed the patient, "now I am going to dangle you." The patient's eyes popped open widely as he looked at the ceiling.

A more helpful statement might have been worded, "Now I would like to help you sit on the edge of the bed and dangle your feet before helping you into the chair. Moving slowly like this helps prevent feelings of dizziness that sometimes happen after surgery."

Different words can have different meanings to persons of different generations or cultures. For example, *gay* used to mean happy and lighthearted to someone who grew up in the 1960's or before; now it refers to sexual orientation. *Cool* may be a temperature or something really good. Likewise, *hot* may be a temperature or an extremely attractive person. Consider the culture, ethnicity, experiences, and perspective of the older patient in choosing your words.

INFORMAL OR SOCIAL COMMUNICATION

Simple chitchat does have a place in nurse-patient communications. If nurses talked only about things related to health treatment, they would know little about their patients. Small talk, pleasantries, and conversations about the weather, a favorite television show, or the latest news can demonstrate to the patient that you think of them as a real person, not just a patient. Likewise, older patients often like to know something about the nurses who care for them; they may ask about your family, hobbies, and interests. This is particularly true in extended-care facilities, because the nursing staff often becomes a new family for the aging person. Do not be afraid to be "human" when you are communicating with older adults, but be careful not to overdisclose information that might make the patient view you in an unprofessional light.

Be honest with your older patients. When you do not have time to visit, explain why, so that patients do not take it personally and think that they may have done something wrong. Do not be afraid to use humor appropriately, but choose the right time and place and make sure that your reply is culturally sensitive. It has been said that "laughter is the best medicine." Remember that it is okay to laugh at yourself but never at the other person. Aging does not cause people to lose their sense of humor. A humorous story or cartoon may help brighten their day.

NONVERBAL COMMUNICATION

Because so much of communication is nonverbal, it is essential that we examine each aspect of nonverbal communication to consider its effect on our interactions with the older adult (Fig. 5.1).

💬 Communication

If two people entered a room, one wearing a white laboratory coat with a stethoscope around their neck and the other wearing a clerical collar and a cross, what message would you receive? Would these people have to say anything for communication to take place? What is being communicated? The items we wear or carry (e.g., clothing, jewelry, stethoscopes, masks, gowns, and gloves) send messages; we use these symbols to communicate something about who we are. Distinctive uniforms are worn to make people identifiable. Police officers, flight attendants, clergy, and nurses wear uniforms so that they can be recognized even in a crowd.

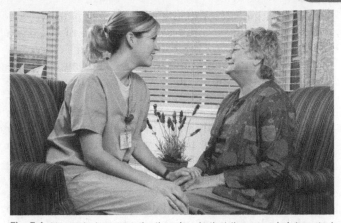

Fig. 5.1 Nonverbal communication signals that the nurse is interested in the patient and in what they are saying. (From Sorrentino, S.A., & Remmert, L.N. [2014]. *Mosby's essentials for nursing assistants*, 5th edition. Mosby.)

SYMBOLS

In the health care setting, uniform styles and colors help patients distinguish the various caregivers. Historically a white uniform and cap were symbols that helped older adults distinguish nurses from other caregivers and to distinguish the level of education attained by that nurse. Today, nurses wear scrubs in most work settings. Some settings may allow "street clothes" but will usually have guidelines for keeping a professional appearance. Although nurses may not place much importance on wearing a uniform, their attire plays an important role in communication. Whatever the dress code, it is very important that the caregiver wears a name badge that identifies their name and who they are in practice (RN, LVN, etc.) in a large enough type size that is easily readable to the older eye.

🌐 Cultural Considerations

Nonverbal Communication

- Culture and nonverbal communication play important roles in patients' perceptions. For example, immigrants who are new to a country may perceive that they are being treated differently, based on cultural misunderstandings.
- North American caregivers are often dressed in scrubs or casual clothing that does little to identify their role or status. This contrast can lead to the mistaken interpretation that the caregivers are inexperienced and do not take the patient's concerns seriously.

TONE OF VOICE

Think of the sound of a whisper, shout, or whine. Try saying, "I don't want to do that," first in a whisper, shout, and whine and then in a normal speaking voice. Was your understanding of the message the same in each situation? It probably was not. To survive, we learn early in life to understand that tone of voice is a fairly reliable way of interpreting a person's emotions. Because the nonverbal message is so strong, we typically respond to the emotion we perceive from the tone of voice and may not even hear the words. When a person shouts at us, we normally shout back. Shouting is often associated with anger or displeasure, yet many people shout when they are communicating with someone who has a hearing impairment. Shouting is not appropriate in this situation because your tone of voice may lead the hearing-impaired person to think that you are angry. It would be much more effective to speak in a low tone of voice close to the person's good ear. The use of nonverbal methods of communication, such as communication boards or gestures, can also be helpful.

 QSEN Considerations: Teamwork and Collaboration

Impact on Others

Be aware of your tone of voice and the impact of your communication style on patients, families, and other members of the health care team.

BODY LANGUAGE

You walk past a room and observe a nurse standing in the doorway with their head sticking into the room but their body still in the hallway. The verbal communication is, "Can I help you?" but the nonverbal communication is, "I'm in a hurry. You really don't want anything, do you?" We communicate many things by how we move, stand, sit, and position our bodies. In dealing with all patients, it is important that we be aware of what we communicate through our body language.

In situations where the words and body language are conveying two different messages, most people respond to the body language. By standing at the door, hurrying down the hallway, sitting behind the nurses' station, and working in the medication or treatment room, you are in each instance communicating that you are busy. Going into the rooms to talk with patients, sitting down at eye level with residents, and talking with family members are all ways of communicating nonverbally that you are truly interested and concerned.

Another part of nonverbal communication involves watching for the messages that patients are communicating through their body language. For example, patients who slump down or slouch in their chairs may be communicating many things, such as fatigue or physical weakness, lack of interest, sadness, or defiance. Turning away from the nurse could indicate anger, fear, or lack of interest. When body

language says something different from the words, believe the body language. Explore the situation using techniques such as reflective or open-ended statements. (These techniques are discussed later in the chapter.)

 Nurse Alert

Creating Barriers Through Nonverbal Communication

Be aware that our body language can communicate to patients and family members that we are busy and do not want to be bothered. If we are sitting behind the nurse's station or facing a computer screen, people may assume we are busy and may hesitate to interrupt even to report serious concerns. Nurses must be careful not to create barriers between themselves and their patients.

SPACE, DISTANCE, AND POSITION

Physical space, distance, and position are other ways in which we communicate. The study of the use of personal space in communication is referred to as *proxemics*. *Personal space* refers to how close we allow someone to be to us before we feel uncomfortable. The amount of space that separates two individuals when they communicate is significant. In traditional American culture, most people are comfortable when strangers are 12 feet or more away. This is considered "public space;" at this distance, there is no real positive or negative connection with the other person. Between 4 and 12 feet is considered "social space." This is a comfortable distance for a casual relationship, in which communication is at an impersonal level. However, if you stay this far away from your patients, you are communicating indifference. A distance of 18 inches to 4 feet is considered "personal space." This is the optimal distance for close interpersonal communication with another person. A nurse who communicates from within this space is usually viewed as concerned and interested. The space within 18 inches of the body is considered intimate space. Most people allow only trusted individuals to get this close. Entering the intimate space without permission is usually perceived as a threat.

A nurse or other caregiver may approach an older adult to provide care or treatment and, without thinking, enter this intimate space too quickly. An older adult who has poor vision or hearing, who has been sleeping, or who is not totally alert may be startled by such an approach. The person may not be able to recognize the nurse as a trusted person at first and may strike out verbally or physically from fear of physical attack. It is essential to recognize the importance of personal space and to obtain the older adult's attention and permission before attempting to perform any physical care.

GESTURES

Gestures are a specific type of nonverbal communication intended to convey ideas. Gestures are highly cultural and generational; those that are acceptable in one culture may be offensive in another. Some gestures that are accepted today as commonplace were once considered crude or insulting. Gestures that have a certain meaning in one culture may have a different meaning in another. For example, nodding the head up and down means *yes* in most cultures, but in some cultures it means *no*. Before using gestures, it is wise to determine that both parties have the same understanding of what a particular gesture means.

Gestures are helpful for people who cannot use words. After a stroke, many individuals suffer from a condition called *aphasia*. Because of brain damage, these individuals may not be able to recognize words or to "find" the words they want to use. This inability to communicate wants, needs, and feelings is often frustrating, and the use of gestures and other nonverbal forms of communication can be effective in such cases.

 Cultural Considerations

Preventing Cultural Bias in Caregiving

Culture, language, and communication are closely connected. Failure to recognize the impact of culture on communication can be a barrier to effective health care.

Health care providers, like others, often base their evaluation of a patient's words or behavior on their own culture and ethnic assumptions. To minimize cultural misunderstanding, health care providers should

- Recognize their own cultural biases and assumptions.
- Increase their knowledge and understanding of the attitudes, beliefs, and communication styles of other cultures.
- Recruit, retain, and promote health care providers from all ethnic and cultural backgrounds.
- Provide skilled interpreters, visual aids, and educational materials for predominant language groups.
- Address complaints or grievances that arise from cross-cultural misunderstandings to provide more culturally sensitive care.

FACIAL EXPRESSIONS

Facial expressions are yet another form of nonverbal communication. The human face is most expressive, and facial expressions have been shown to communicate across cultural and age barriers. Smiles, frowns, and grimaces appear to have the same meaning regardless of where you are in the world. Humans respond to facial expressions from the time they are born. We tend to mirror the expressions of the person with whom we are communicating: smiles tend to elicit smiles, and frowns elicit frowns. Fear, anger, joy, and a variety of other emotions can be conveyed by a simple change in facial expression. We must be aware of this fact and ensure that our expressions communicate what was intended. Too often, nurses are preoccupied while interacting with an older adult. A frown, inadvertently made by a nurse performing a difficult intravenous insertion, may lead the patient to think that they have done something wrong. By wrinkling their nose, particularly while cleaning up an episode of incontinence, a nurse could communicate a lack of acceptance. A smile while listening to a patient's serious concerns might make the patient wonder whether the nurse really cares about what is being said.

EYE CONTACT

Eye contact can be perceived differently by individuals. Some people consider looking another person directly in the eyes as a sign of interest, trust, and acceptance. People from other cultures may avoid eye contact because it is considered disrespectful or inappropriate, or because averting the eyes communicates respect to the person talking. When working with older adults, it is important to be sensitive to the cultural meaning of eye contact. Face-to-face, eye-to-eye contact can be helpful in communicating with older adults provided that this does not frighten or intimidate them. Face-to-face contact also maximizes the chance that an older adult with hearing problems will be able to read lips if necessary. Sitting at the bedside may facilitate eye contact. Be certain to continually assess the patient's comfort level with direct eye contact and adjust your approach accordingly.

PACE OR SPEED OF COMMUNICATION

Nurses are often younger than the aging people they serve. The resulting difference in rate of speech and movement of the nurse may convey to the older adult that they are being hurried. Do not become impatient or uneasy with silence; give the older person time to think, request what is needed, and respond when being addressed. Avoid completing sentences for patients who are organizing their thoughts; do not assume what the person was going to say. This is disrespectful and demoralizing. Provide encouragement and reassurance that those in your care will have the time they need to interact with you. Patience and active listening are important skills in working with older adults.

TIME AND TIMING

Timing is related to the pace of communication, but it has other distinct implications as well. The amount of time a person must wait after seeking attention is important. Delays in response to a call light or direct request from a person may be interpreted as a lack of concern, even if not intended. The person's response may manifest as anger, displeasure, anxiety, fear, and other feelings. Studies have shown that nurses take longer to respond to terminally ill patients. Nurses also tend to give delayed responses to demanding individuals. This sets up a vicious cycle, because the longer a person has to wait for a response, the greater their anger, fear, and anxiety will become. This only increases the demanding behaviors, which often occur in an attempt to reduce fear. If the older adult's needs are dealt with promptly, the number of demands will tend to decrease, not increase. Making older adults wait unnecessarily constitutes a subtle form of abuse.

Many older individuals have an altered sense of time. A message that is communicated too early may lead to either forgetfulness or to repeated questions such as, "Is it time yet?" A message that is communicated too late may lead to distress and frustration. Older adults often need more preparation time than younger individuals to get ready for an activity, such as going to the bathroom or getting necessary items together. Communicating an exciting message late in the evening (either good or bad news) may disturb older adults to the point that they are unable to sleep. Be aware of these issues and choose the proper time to communicate.

TOUCH

Touch is a form of communication. No words are required, and there is no need for high level sensory or cognitive functioning. When all else fails, touch is left. Caring touch is a basic need for all humans, and many older adults suffer from touch deprivation. Many older people have no one to meet this need. Research shows that patients with psychosis and older adults are touched the least by caregivers. Those who most need physical contact and the comfort provided by touch receive the least.

Use of touch as a method of communication can come naturally or be difficult for the nurse. Touching is a very personal form of communication. Affection, understanding, trust, hope, and concern can be communicated by a hand placed on a shoulder, a stroke of the forehead, or a frail hand held by another stronger one. Touch is a common method of expressing concern and caring. People who are emotionally close hold hands and touch and hug one another. High on the list of things lonely older people say they miss are hugs and touching. Empathetic use of touch is a valuable skill in working with older adults. When words do not work, touch often does (Fig. 5.2). If there is any doubt as to whether

the patient wants to be touched, the nurse can ask or watch how the person responds to touch. Touching should be done with caution when a person is experiencing pain, so as not to cause further discomfort. Cultural beliefs may dictate when, who, and how people may touch. If there is any question regarding the appropriateness of touch, clarification should be obtained beforehand.

> **! Nurse Alert**
>
> Touch, as a method of communication, can be very beneficial to older adults when used appropriately. Nurses must be aware that inappropriate touching can be destructive and should never be used to communicate anger or frustration. Rough handling, slapping, pushing, or otherwise communicating displeasure constitutes patient abuse and is completely unacceptable.

SILENCE

Saying nothing is also saying something. Being with another person and remaining silent is difficult for many people, including nurses. At times, words can be intrusive; they can interfere with true communication. Many times, older adults need more time to compose their thoughts. Silence permits them to focus on the point of a discussion, whereas continuous talking is distracting. At times, no words are necessary and silence is therapeutic. When another person is experiencing intense grief, pain, or anxiety, simply *being there* without saying or doing anything may be the most appropriate form of communication one can offer. The simple presence of another person expresses true concern and can be worth much more than words.

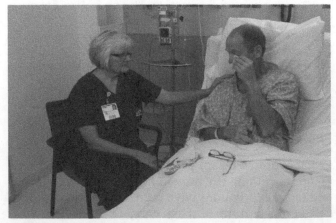

Fig. 5.2 Comfort and well-being can be promoted with eye contact and gentle touch. (From Williams, P.A. [2018]. *DeWit's fundamental concepts and skills for nursing*, 5th edition. Saunders.)

EMPATHY, ACCEPTANCE, DIGNITY, AND RESPECT IN COMMUNICATION

Empathy is defined as the willingness to attempt to understand the unique world of another person. It is the ability to put oneself in another person's place and to understand what they are feeling and thinking in that situation. Empathetic listening involves actively trying to truly understand the other person.

Effective communication starts with proper introductions. Determine how each older adult wishes to be addressed. It is presumptuous to begin communication by addressing older adults by their first names. It is better to start by using the older adult's proper title and name (e.g., Mrs. Quinn and Dr. Cortez) and then clarifying which form of address the person prefers. If someone wishes to be called by a first name or a nickname, the person will usually say so. In special situations, as when a patient has dementia or any other alterations in cognition, a first name may be most appropriate because that may be the only name the person can remember.

It is important to avoid speaking in a sing-song cadence, using inflection to make statements sound like questions, or referring to older adults by names such as "sweetie" or "honey." This type of speech is patronizing and disrespectful to older adults and is inappropriate. This type of communication is termed *elderspeak* and is a form of ageism. Elderspeak also includes incorrect use of the pronoun *we* when the correct pronoun would be *you*, as in "Are we ready to get dressed now?" Elderspeak should always be avoided because it has a subtle way of diminishing an older person's self-esteem (Zhang, Zhao, & Meng, 2020). Use a normal conversational tone of voice whenever possible. Avoid language that stereotypes or dehumanizes the older adult. Such language may be overheard by the older patient or family members, who may interpret it as disrespectful. It is best to first speak in terms of the person; for example, refer to "Ms. Drakos, who has diabetes," not "the diabetic in bed 14B." Also be mindful of the possible negative connotation that words can have to older adults or their family members; substitute appropriate terms when possible. For example:

- Instead of diapers, say briefs, pads, or use a trade name, such as Depends.
- Instead of blind or deaf, say visually or hearing impaired.
- Instead of senile or demented, say cognitively challenged or has dementia.
- Instead of nursing home, say care facility.

ACTIVE AND EMPATHETIC LISTENING

To communicate effectively, we must first learn to listen actively and empathetically. Listening is more than simply hearing. Hearing involves the ability of the ears to detect sound, whereas listening involves interpretation (i.e., determining what the sounds mean). We have not really listened until we understand for certain what was intended by the speaker. We cannot simply listen to the words; we must listen for the meaning of the words.

Active listening skills are needed in all areas of nursing but particularly when caring for older adults. Empathetic listening requires sensitivity to the strengths and limitations of the aging individual (e.g., hearing changes, vision changes, fatigue, and pain). Empathetic listening involves patience when an older adult needs extra time to voice a response or repeats the same information many times. It includes a willingness to spend time getting to know the older adult better as a human being, not just as another body in need of skilled physical care. Listening to older people reminisce about their lives can help the nurse gain better understanding of these people's values, perceptions, strengths, needs, and concerns (see Chapter 11).

Too often, nurses provide excellent physical care to people they have not taken the time to know. Nurses need to refrain from talking "over" patients while they do procedures and truly listen to older patients more often.

BARRIERS TO COMMUNICATION

To communicate effectively, we must learn to identify the barriers that can interfere with an exchange and the methods that help us to overcome these barriers. Effective communication skills require development and practice. More than just the ability to

Communication

As we attempt to build a trusting relationship with our patients, consider this: There is a reason why we have two ears and only one mouth. We are supposed to listen twice as much as we talk!

talk to someone, communication involves all of the ways in which we send messages to others, including nonverbal ways. Differences in physical abilities require different communication approaches. Communication makes use of all of the senses. Hearing and vision are the senses used most often in communication, but touch, smell, and even taste also play a part in the relay of messages. It is important to remember this when communicating with older adults because their perceptions may be altered by the normal physiologic changes of aging. Pain or extreme fatigue may make communication more challenging. It is best to limit conversation to essential topics during these times. A variety of disease processes, such as stroke and dementia, significantly affect communication processes and require specific approaches.

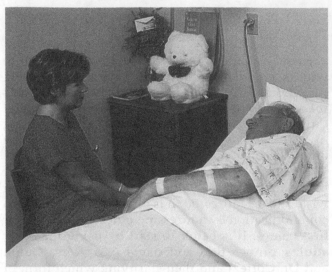

Fig. 5.3 Communication with the older adult with a vision or hearing deficit. Sit in front of the patient where your lips can be seen to communicate. (From DeWit, S. C. [2014]. *Fundamental concepts and skills for nursing*, 4th edition. Saunders.)

Box 5.1 provides additional strategies for communicating with older adults who have sensory impairments.

APHASIA

Individuals who have had a stroke or other head injuries may experience aphasia, which is a partial or total loss of the ability to use or understand words. It affects the ability to understand and express oneself through words, gestures, and writing but does not necessarily affect intellectual function. Consultation with a speech therapist can help the nurse devise approaches that will optimize function. In addition to the basic

 Communication

COVID-19 and Masks

In order to prevent the spread of COVID-19, everyone is instructed to wear a mask or face covering and to practice social distancing. Older adults who experience hearing loss may be accustomed to reading lips, which is not possible if you are wearing a mask. Those who are also vision impaired may not know that you are speaking.

Be sure to make eye contact with the person to whom you are speaking. If possible, wear a clear face mask so that your mouth can be seen. Speak slowly and in a low tone; and avoid shouting. Another useful option is video conferencing, which allows your face to be seen and the volume to be adjusted.

HEARING IMPAIRMENT

If a person in your care wears a hearing aid, make sure that it is clean, that the batteries are working, and that the device has been placed in the correct ear. Try to minimize background noise, because this can distort sounds and make hearing more difficult. Many people who are hearing impaired spontaneously begin to read lips. In addition to the basic strategies, the following actions are likely to be beneficial:

1. Stand in front of the person, at eye level.
2. Do not eat or drink while you are having a conversation.
3. Keep your hands away from your face when you are speaking.
4. Try different ways of saying the same thing, such as using various words to communicate a thought.
5. Speak more slowly and slightly louder while modulating your voice to a lower pitch.
6. Avoid exaggerated mouth motions during speech.
7. Use visual cues or written materials that support the spoken words (Fig. 5.3).

Box 5.1 | Basic Strategies for Communicating With Older Adults With Sensory Impairments

- Try not to startle the person when starting a communication.
- Identify yourself; remind the person who you are.
- Communicate when the person is most alert.
- Eliminate or reduce noise and distractions.
- Make sure you have their attention before speaking.
- Focus on the person's abilities, not disabilities.
- Select topics of interest to them.
- Use a variety of words or descriptions until meanings are clear.
- Ask clear, specific questions; one question at a time.
- Pay attention to the emotional context of conversation.
- Use pictures and gestures in addition to words.
- Have the person sit up for conversation whenever possible. Keep messages simple and repeat as needed.
- Do not interrupt. Maintain a slower pace of communication.
- Make sure they do not have any other needs before you leave.

strategies, some commonly recommended approaches include the following:

1. Keep messages simple but appropriate to the adult's developmental level; do not speak to older adults as if they were babies or children.
2. Use nonverbal modes of communication, such as picture boards, gestures, yes/no responses, and facial expressions.
3. Use visual aids for support.
4. Try increasingly specific guesses or questions to determine concerns (e.g., Is something wrong with your meal? The coffee? It's too hot? You want milk?).
5. Praise attempts to speak, and avoid correcting or criticizing errors.
6. Reassure the person that it is okay to be frustrated, but avoid empty platitudes such as "You'll be fine."

One intervention worth trying when working with an aphasic patient is singing. A different part of the brain is used for singing than is used for speaking. You may find that although speech may be hesitant and difficult for a patient with aphasia to produce, singing an old familiar song with the patient may lead to a surprisingly fluid verbal output. Researchers are studying the use of singing therapy; with it, some patients who have had a stroke have shown great progress in their speech recovery (Nania, 2020).

DEMENTIA

Dementia causes both cognitive and language deficits. The older person suffering from dementia has no control over these changes, so the responsibility for effective communication rests with the nurse. Depending on the severity of the dementia, the individual may demonstrate different levels of functioning. The abilities and limitations of each individual suffering from dementia must be evaluated so that the most effective interactions can be planned. Some characteristics of dementia include a limited attention span, inability to focus on more than one thought at a time, confusion of fact and fantasy, and the inability to follow complex instructions. In addition to the basic strategies, some recommended approaches include the following:

1. Talk about one thing or ask only one question at a time.
2. Limit choices; too many options are confusing.
3. Keep the conversation in the here and now.
4. Ask simple yes/no questions.
5. Try "filling in" or "repairing" thoughts. Rather than letting a person get upset trying to find the right words, you may offer some likely choices if you have a reasonable idea of what the person is trying to communicate. However, be careful not to finish the thoughts and sentences of patients who are not cognitively impaired.
6. Avoid asking questions that require information or recall, such as "How was your day?"

7. Use gestures or demonstrate an action so that the person can mimic your behavior.
8. Avoid the use of an intercom, which may confuse the person.
9. Avoid arguing if the person does not accept your reality.
10. Redirect the person who is acting out to an appropriate activity.
11. Share activities, such as looking at a magazine, viewing family photos, or listening to music.
12. Avoid trying too hard to communicate.
13. Watch your tone of voice, because patients with dementia are often very sensitive to nonverbal cues and may sense your frustration and become more agitated or upset.

> **! Safety Alert**
>
> **Preventing Agitation and Combativeness**
>
> According to the Alzheimer's Association, behavior is a frequent form of communication for a person with dementia. Problems with communication can result in anger, aggression, agitation, and confusion. Repetitive vocalizations, urgency, and change in tone or pace of speech can indicate an unmet need, even when the sounds are meaningless. Try to determine the meaning of the behavior rather than ignoring it as meaningless. This will often decrease a patient's agitation, which could potentially lead to aggression and combativeness (Alzheimer's Association, n.d.).

CULTURAL DIFFERENCES

People who speak languages other than English as their primary language may have varied levels of English proficiency. To communicate effectively, we need to know what language a person primarily speaks. Facilities that accept federal funds (such as Medicaid) are legally required to provide language access to all patients (Williams, 2021). To be an effective interpreter a person needs to be professionally trained and proficient in both languages, understand the clinical concepts they are expected to explain, and have been educated about the ethics of the job. Even official interpreters can make errors in communication that are potentially dangerous; however, studies note that even more mistakes are made by "unofficial" or ad hoc interpreters, such as family members (Rimmer, 2020). Family and friends of the patient do not have formal training and may have personal and emotional connections that could influence the communication or make the patient reluctant to share information. Although family members are not the most appropriate persons to interpret sensitive or technical medical information, they may be helpful in translating simple nonmedical questions or requests (Rimmer, 2020).

Some basic rules to keep in mind when working with an interpreter include the following:

- Ask short questions, and provide brief units of information so that the interpreter has time to process translation.
- Avoid excessively technical language.
- Avoid slang, idioms, or colloquial expressions.
- Encourage the interpreter to give you the response using the patient's own words, without input or paraphrasing, whenever possible.
- Focus on the patient, not the interpreter.
- Listen for emotional tone and nonverbal clues when the patient responds, even if you do not understand the words.
- Allow enough time for the interaction.
- Encourage the patient to ask questions of the staff through the interpreter.

In addition to making adaptations for language, pay close attention to nonverbal communications. Lack of recognition of cultural beliefs and practices can lead to mistakes that damage rapport. When in doubt, ask the older adult or family member if there are any special actions or behaviors that should be observed or avoided.

🌐 Cultural Considerations

Bridging Language Barriers

Many community colleges and multicultural centers offer special courses in languages for health care providers. Often, these courses are specifically designed to meet the needs of the local community. This benefits communities that speak a primary language that is not English, as well as the nurses, who are gaining a broader skill set.

❓ Critical Thinking

Culture, Ethnicity, and Communication

- Which cultural or ethnic group or groups do you consider yourself to be part of?
- List all cultural or ethnic groups with which you occasionally or regularly have contact.
- Consider the cultural or ethnic group with which you identify.
- Identify any gestures you consider acceptable.
- Is direct eye contact typical in your cultural or ethnic group? Are there times when direct eye contact is not considered appropriate?
- In your cultural or ethnic group, how close do people stand when talking to each other?
- Do people touch frequently in your cultural or ethnic group? Whom do they touch? Where or how do they touch? What type of touch is not allowed? Are there gender differences related to touching?
- How important is it in your culture to be on time and keep appointments? Does this differ between social and business situations?
- Do you feel comfortable or ill at ease when communicating with individuals from other cultures? Does your comfort level change when the interaction is one on one

or when you are in a group? Does it change if you are the only member of a specific culture or ethnicity in a group dominated by another culture or ethnicity?
- Identify two or three situations in which you felt that a person from another age, cultural, or ethnic group did not understand you or misinterpreted your nonverbal communication.
- Identify two or three situations in which you felt that you did not accurately understand the communication sent by a person from another age, cultural, or ethnic group.
- Can you think of any specific beliefs or practices from your culture that you would want a nurse caring for you to understand?

SKILLS AND TECHNIQUES

INFORMING

Informing uses direct statements regarding facts. A good information statement is clear, concise, and expressed in words the patient can understand. When the nurse is informing, the nurse is active and the patient is passive. Informing is the least effective form of communication because the patient is not actively involved. When you are giving information, ask patients to restate what they understand using their own words. A message may need to be repeated and rephrased to ensure understanding. This should be done tactfully and with care not to show personal signs of annoyance or frustration. Informing should be done in such a way that the patient is not made to feel ignorant.

DIRECT QUESTIONING

It is best to keep communication conversational and not too aggressive. Too many direct questions can overwhelm an older person and may block rather than expand communication. Direct questioning is helpful when nurses need to obtain specific information or in emergency situations, when time is precious. Direct questions tend to include the words *who*, *what*, *when*, *where*, *do you*, and *don't you*. Direct questioning is appropriate when information must be obtained quickly; however, if it is overused, patients may become defensive. Many students and new nurses approach patient assessment with a list of 50 questions that must be answered. After the first 10 questions, patients may feel frustrated and communicate only the bare minimum of information. Direct questions tend to yield brief answers and often only a *yes* or *no* response.

USING OPEN-ENDED TECHNIQUES

Open-ended communication techniques include open-ended questions, reflective statements, clarifying statements, and paraphrasing. These techniques allow the patient more leeway to respond, thus establishing a more empathetic climate. The patient is more likely to feel that you are interested in them personally and that you are not just trying to fill in blanks on a form or in the electronic health record. Examples of open-ended techniques include the following: "And after you moved to the nursing home, what happened?"; "And then?"; "That must have been frightening!"; "What I heard you say is ..."; "It sounds like you think (feel)...." Open-ended techniques allow patients to express more about their feelings and perceptions. They also allow verification that the information being relayed is accurate.

CONFRONTING

Confronting is used when there are inconsistencies in information or when verbal and nonverbal messages appear contradictory. Confrontation is an important communication technique to use and should be used based on a professional rapport that has been established. Remain objective when using confrontation. For example, you may assess that a patient reports taking an opioid medication only as directed (e.g., twice daily). However, when you complete medication reconciliation, you note that they do not have the right amount of the opioid drug left based on when it was filled. To appropriately use confrontation, you could say, "I understand that you mentioned taking your opioid medication twice daily as recommended. I'm seeing that you only have 3 pills left although your prescription was refilled last week. Can you help me understand the discrepancy?" Use of objective tone, instead of an accusatory tone, is of critical importance when using confrontation. This gives the patient the opportunity to explain the discrepancy. Then you can further assess how this answer confirms or detracts from the objective information you have reviewed.

> **! Safety Alert**
>
> **Use Confrontation Appropriately**
>
> It is never advisable to confront a highly agitated or confused person because conflict and a breakdown in communication may result. This approach may cause older adults with dementia to become combative.

COMMUNICATING WITH VISITORS AND FAMILIES

Be prepared to interact with your patient's friends, family members, and visitors. These people make up the older adult's social network and support system. Families and friends are interested and concerned about what is happening to their loved ones. They not only turn to nurses for information and reassurance but can also be a good source of information.

These *significant others*, as they are often called, can help in many ways if nurses are responsive to them. Many of the older adult's significant others are

themselves senior citizens. Communication with these individuals may also require special attention and the use of special techniques. It is important to take the time to develop good rapport with your patients' significant others. Good communication with these important people can do a great deal to facilitate care. Because they have known the patient longer and better than the nursing staff, they are often able to detect subtle changes in behavior and communication before professional nurses can.

> **? Critical Thinking**
>
> **Communication Skills**
>
> - Look at the people on each side of you in class. What is their body language communicating?
> - Think of a person you consider to be a good communicator. Next, think of a person you consider to be a poor communicator. Fold a piece of paper in half. Write "effective communicator" on one side and "ineffective communicator" on the other side. List the characteristics that make each communicator effective or ineffective. Compare and contrast your findings.
> - Compare your own communication skills with those of each side of the list that you wrote down. Which side of the list do your communication more closely align with? What can you do to become more effective in your communication ability?

DELIVERING BAD NEWS

No one likes to get bad news, and no one likes to be the bearer of bad news. Most people try to avoid this daunting task. Ideally, this task should be performed by the most experienced and knowledgeable person who knows the person best, such as the primary care provider. Occasionally, however, the nurse must be the one to break bad news to an older adult. This could be information regarding the patient's health or about someone close to the patient—for instance, announcing the death of a spouse or other loved one. The Education on Palliative and End-of-Life Care (EPEC) Project, funded by the Robert Wood Johnson Foundation, has developed guidelines for physicians that have relevance for nursing practice. Important concepts include the following:

- Prepare yourself. Make sure you have all of the information and that it is accurate.
- Think through what you want to say so that the message is compassionate and culturally sensitive.
- Establish an environment respectful of the patient's privacy.
- Determine whether anyone else (chaplain, family members, significant others, etc.) should be present when the news is delivered.
- Make sure that there is adequate time, free from interruptions, to deal with the expected emotional response.

- Determine what the person already knows and, if possible, how much they want to know.
- Recognize that ethical and cultural variations may influence the way in which information is delivered.
- Use simple, direct, but sensitive language to begin the message, such as, "The news I am about to share may be difficult to hear."
- Respond to the person's emotional reaction; for example, "I'll try to help you. Is there something I can do?" or "Do you want to talk about how you're feeling?"
- Develop a follow-up plan. Help the older person and significant others with appointments, referrals, transportation, and other activities that may be helpful based on the circumstance.
- Communicate significant information to other caregivers as part of a plan of care.

HAVING DIFFICULT CONVERSATIONS

Emotionally loaded topics are likely to generate strong emotions and often lead to conflict. Conflict is a normal and routine part of human interaction; it can occur between older adults and adult children, nurses and older adults, nurses and patients' families, nurses and other nurses, or nurses and physicians. Difficult conversations may occur in clinical areas or in home settings involving friends and family members.

Some people prefer to avoid conflict entirely; however avoidance delays solving problems that need to be addressed. The following guidelines are suggestions based on conflict resolution research:

- Pick a place that is private and a time when you and the person you need to address will be free from distractions.
- Try to focus on a single topic; do not bring up old grievances that have already been addressed.
- If a conversation is not going well, consider your own feelings and motivations. Are you reacting to this issue or to another issue that was problematic in the past?
- Express your feelings using "I" statements, such as "I get upset when ... doesn't get done" rather than "you" statements, such as "You always ignore what I ask you to do."
- Respect the right of the other person to agree or disagree.
- Keep a balance between talking and listening. Try not to dominate the conversation.
- View each communication as a new opportunity to learn something about the other person and about their unique feelings, beliefs, and perspectives. Listen to the other person, and seek clarification regarding the person's reasons and feelings.
- Do not prejudge or assume that you already know what the person is going to say. You may be wrong.

- Be aware of your own feelings regarding the issue under discussion. Keep feelings separate from facts. The fact that someone does not do what you want does not mean that the person does not like you or that they are doing it to upset you.
- Avoid blaming the other person. Look for ways to resolve disagreements.
- Accept that difficult conversations are part of life and that things do not always go right.
- Learn from both negative and positive interactions and try to improve future communication.
- Try to achieve a win-win solution.

IMPROVING COMMUNICATION BETWEEN THE OLDER ADULT AND THEIR PRIMARY CARE PROVIDER

Clear communication between the older adult and their primary care provider is essential. Most providers are aware of effective communication protocols but, because of time constraints or other factors, may not always use these techniques. Ineffective communication can result in frustration for both parties and can contribute to a lack of adherence by the patient. It is also possible that an older adult may become passive, evasive, or tentative in conversations with their primary care provider.

The nurse can often help to minimize these communication problems by (1) suggesting that the patient keep a written list of concerns and questions so that nothing will be forgotten; (2) asking the primary care provider to repeat and summarize all directions to the patient; (3) identifying printed materials that support the provider's recommendations; (4) suggesting that a trusted friend or family member be present to take notes and help the older adult express concerns; or (5) acting as a patient advocate by asking the provider to clarify questions or concerns the patient has verbalized to you.

EFFECTIVE COMMUNICATION WITH THE HEALTH CARE TEAM

The quality of communication between nurses, physicians, and other health care providers can have a significant impact on the quality of care that older patients receive. Communication problems between team members can lead to job frustration, blame, and distrust, all of which diminish the level of care provided and increase the risk for problems or errors. Conversely, good communication tends to improve job satisfaction, decrease errors, and promote quality care of the older adult patients. Mutual respect and a willingness to collaborate for the good of the older adult can form a strong basis for good interactions. The nurse can use many strategies to decrease frustrations and optimize the efficiency and effectiveness of communication (Box 5.2).

| Box 5.2 | **Additional Tips for Improving Nurse-Physician Communication** |

- Work at developing professional relationships.
- Know what you want to find out or report when calling.
- Assume that you are both on the same team.
- Have the patient's chart or health record in front of you during the call.
- At some point, try to meet face-to-face with physicians you speak with on the phone.
- Do not seek out conflict, but be prepared that it may happen occasionally.

(Modified from Burke, M., Boal, J., & Mitchell, R. [2004]. Communicating for better care: Improving nurse-physician communication. *American Journal of Nursing, 104*[40], 2004.)

 QSEN Considerations: Teamwork and Collaboration

Roles of Team Members

The roles and responsibilities of the health care team can overlap when they are caring for patients. It is important that each member function competently within their own scope of practice and, if needed, clarify their roles and accountabilities under conditions of potential overlap in team member functioning. Each member should value the perspectives and expertise of all team members.

 Coordinated Care

Communication Skills

SUPERVISION

When it is necessary to correct a subordinate for unsatisfactory performance, avoid using "you" messages, such as "You never complete your assignments." Instead, use assertive "I" messages, such as, "I am upset and disappointed when patients' needs are not thoroughly met." This is less likely to result in an argument and will more likely help to solve problems. Also be sure to praise people in public but correct them in private.

TELEPHONING PRIMARY CARE PROVIDERS

Many facilities promote the ISBAR-R communication tool for improved communication that is concise yet complete. ISBAR-R is an acronym that stands for Introduction, Situation, Background, Assessment, Recommendation, and Readback (Box 5.3).

Before you call a provider, be sure you have gathered the assessment data needed to conduct the interaction. When you make the call, begin by identifying who you are (name and title), the patient or patients you are calling about, and the specific reason for the contact. Be sure you have the patient's health record in front of you and always have a pen and paper (or the computer open to the correct section of the patient's electronic health record) ready to record new orders. Plan ahead, and have a focus for the communication. Know what you want to report or find out. Be organized, clear, precise, and complete. Provide background information. Remember, the provider is not looking at the chart and

| Box 5.3 | **An example of ISBAR-R Communication** |

Introduction: Hello, I'm May, the evening shift nurse. Mrs. Reynolds is a 57-year-old patient who is a former lawyer. She suffered a stroke and requires total care. She was admitted 2 years ago.

Situation: Three days ago, Mrs. Reynolds spoke her first two words since her stroke. Her primary care provider has ordered speech therapy to work with her twice a week. She is on a soft diet with thickened liquids. She still has her G-tube in, but we are not needing to feed her as she has a good appetite and is meeting all nutritional needs through her oral diet. We only use the G-tube to administer medications. During speech therapy, she can become upset and teary if she gets overwhelmed. Her family resides 2000 miles away and visits every 6 months. She keeps a stuffed Care Bear by her side at all times.

Background: Besides the stroke, Mrs. Reynolds has hypertension and coronary artery disease, both of which are controlled by her medications. She is Full Code, has no known drug allergies, and is a fall risk. Her husband visits every Saturday and is very involved in her care.

Assessment: Mrs. Reynolds is alert and responds to her name with eye contact. T 97.8° F, P 80 beats per minute, R 24 breaths per minute, BP 127/81 mm Hg, O_2 saturation 97% on room air. G-tube placement confirmed, patent, and flushed with 10 mL residual. Mrs. Reynolds can grasp the spoon in her left hand but requires some assistance bringing it to her mouth.

Recommendation: Monitor VS twice a shift. Check patency of G-tube before medications. Allow her to grasp items as hand exercise. Perform light ROM exercises and administer antianxiety medication before bedtime. Provide a skin check during your shift. Remind the staff on the day shift to be patient with her at meals as she eats slowly but will eat all of her food if given adequate time.

Readback: Do you have any questions about Mrs. Reynolds? I will be here another 20 minutes performing documentation if you need any additional information.

BP, Blood pressure; *G-tube*, gastrostomy tube; *P*, pulse; *R*, respirations; *ROM*, range of motion; *T*, temperature (From DeWit, S., & O'Neill, P. A. [2018]. *Fundamentals of nursing*, 5th edition. Saunders.)

may see the older adult once a month or even less frequently in the case of an independent older adult. Provide all necessary and relevant information that might be needed. Identify the patient by name, major diagnoses, medications related to currently presenting symptoms or concerns, and drug allergies. Be prepared to read back the provider's orders and clarify any data or information that the provider may request.

Compile a list of issues to be reported or discussed with the provider so that all issues can be communicated in one interaction. This will prevent repetitive interruptions for both the provider and the nurse. By identifying parameters (or guidelines) when the provider wishes to be contacted (e.g., patient's blood sugar over 200 mg/dL and blood pressure under 90 mm Hg systolic), you can minimize problems related to under- or overnotification.

Emergency situations need to be handled immediately, but these make up a small portion of nurse–provider interaction. Most communications involve either routine or somewhat urgent information and can be handled in a more methodical, planned manner. It is helpful to determine whether there is a best time and method to use when contacting the provider regarding nonemergency situations, such as by phone, fax, e-mail, HIPAA-secure texting, or other means. Planning ahead to identify the best time and methods approved by your facility will optimize communication and enhance care of the patient while minimizing frustration.

 Safety Alert

ISBAR-R

In accordance with the National Patient Safety Goals and the QSEN program, an end-of-shift report should be conducted in a standardized manner to reduce the risk of patient injuries and errors during handoff communication. The ISBAR-R format gives caregivers the opportunity to ask and respond to questions concerning patient care. This format originated from from military communication models and has been successfully used in many health care settings (Williams, 2021, p. 118).

Safety Alert

Taking Telephone Orders

To apply the ISBAR-R format to a telephone order, you should introduce yourself (including the hospital unit or facility), verify the patient's name and background, report the patient's current condition, listen to the order, write down the order, and then read it back to the provider to ensure accuracy (Williams, 2021, p. 118).

PATIENT TEACHING

Education plays an important role in promoting and maintaining the health of older adults. Teaching may take place in a one-on-one session or it may be given to a group. The ability to teach, explain, and motivate is an imperative part of the role of the nurse. To perform this role successfully, you need to know the basic principles and techniques of adult education as well as adaptations specific to older adults.

Research has shown that older adults can learn new things. It has been established that mental abilities—such as numeric tasks, word fluency, inductive reasoning, and spatial orientation—develop through the first 4 decades of life and then hold fairly stable until the 70s in most individuals, and even longer in others. Older adults can use verbal skills, experience, and judgment they have acquired over time. Learning is maximized when it can draw on the previous experiences of older adults.

Adult learners are oriented toward problem-solving, and they view learning as most desirable when it is relevant to their own lives. Teaching will be most effective when the patient recognizes and accepts the importance of learning new information or techniques. Older adults will be more willing to learn when the topic is important to them. For this reason, the nurse should try to

determine ahead of time those things the older patient thinks are most important. Prioritize teaching by starting with the area that the patient perceives to be most important and then linking that information to the other things that the nurse recognizes are necessary or important. Work in small, discrete blocks of information, proceeding from simple, more familiar concepts to more complex or difficult ones. Success breeds success: when older adults realize that they have mastered one skill or piece of information, they are more likely to have a positive attitude toward additional learning.

Choose the right place and time for teaching. The right place depends on the material the session will cover. Information that is personal or private is best taught in a quiet space away from others. More general information (such as nutrition teaching or stress reduction) may be best taught in a group, where older adults are free to share personal experiences and solutions with others. Wherever teaching takes place, the space should be adjusted for the older adult. The temperature should be set appropriately, chairs should be supportive and comfortable, lighting should be adequate and free of glare, and bathrooms should be readily accessible. Snacks and beverages are appreciated by most older adults and can make a group learning session a positive social interaction.

When selecting a teaching time, avoid times when the patient is stressed, fatigued, or in pain. All of these situations interfere with the patient's ability to process information accurately. Also avoid times when older adults may be distracted by things of higher priority to them, such as a favorite television show or anticipated visit from friends or family. In selecting a time for teaching, make sure that there is enough time to discuss the important information. Remember that older individuals may need more time to process information. Avoid trying to teach too much at one time. Break teaching into manageable blocks of concepts to allow time for reflection and learning. Whenever possible, provide printed materials to supplement and reinforce the content (Box 5.4). Practical examples or illustrations may be more effective than a quick recitation of facts. If the teaching involves a psychomotor skill, such as drawing up insulin or changing a dressing, the older adult should receive more than one demonstration of the skill and then be given ample opportunities to practice and perform the skill with supervision. Be patient and

Box 5.4	Modification in Preparing or Selecting Printed Materials for Older Adults

- Limit the amount of material on a single page.
- Allow enough white space so that material is clear and distinct.
- Use at least 12-point type for printed materials.
- Use thicker letters rather than fine print.
- Avoid elaborate fonts; stick with simple, basic lettering.
- Stick to one style of font per document.
- Use a normal mixture of capital and small letters.
- Select paper and ink of strongly contrasting colors.

supportive regardless of the amount of time needed. Remember, the goal is learning, not speed.

Modifications may be needed to compensate for common sensory changes experienced with aging. Face older individuals when speaking. Speak clearly. Try to avoid microphones or amplifiers that might distort sounds or interfere with hearing aids. Repeat information, and use audiovisual aids, such as videos, visual cues, or printed materials to reinforce a verbal message. Be sure that the type is not too small, which could be difficult for the older adult to read. Encourage hands-on practice. Use as many senses as possible, but not necessarily all at once, as this may be confusing.

Clinical Situation

Communicating With Older Adults

A physician and a clergyman happened to arrive in an older adult's room at the same time. The patient became very anxious and started to cry. The physician and the clergyman were taken aback because the patient was doing well and was ready for discharge. After much time was spent calming the patient and listening carefully, they realized that the patient responded as they did because they thought the doctor was going to tell them that they were dying and that the clergyman was there to console them.

Get Ready for the Next Generation NCLEX® Examination!

Key Points

- Keys to effective communication include knowing the other person and having respect for their culture, needs, and uniqueness.
- To develop rapport and communicate effectively with older adults, nurses must identify sensory changes that can interfere with the transmission of messages and cultural or age-related values that can result in misunderstandings. Specific approaches and adaptations are needed with older individuals experiencing sensory and cognitive changes.
- Nurses must accurately recognize and interpret verbal and nonverbal messages sent by older adults, their families, and their friends. Nurses must also be aware of the verbal and nonverbal messages they themselves are sending.
- Effective communication in nursing practice includes patience, dignity, respect, empathy, the desire to interact effectively with others, and the use of appropriate communication techniques.
- Effective communication with other members of the health care team is important for quality patient care, which ensures patient safety and improves patient outcomes.
- Communication through teaching is a nursing role related to health promotion and management. Nurses should determine the appropriate environment for teaching based on the information being taught. Determine the best time to teach by assessing factors, such as the patient's energy level, pain level, and distractions.

Additional Learning Resources

 SG Go to your Evolve website at http://evolve.elsevier.com/Williams/geriatric for the additional online resources.

Review Questions for the Next Generation NCLEX® Examination

1. The nurse is caring for an older adult in a rehabilitation unit. Which action by the nurse will most likely enhance communication with the patient? *(Select all that apply.)*

   a. Identifying yourself; remind the person who you are.
   b. Asking many questions to find out about the person.
   c. Playing music or turning on the TV to help the person relax.
   d. Address the person using friendly terms, like *sweetie*.
   e. Staying in the living area, where other people are around.
   f. Using pictures and gestures in addition to words.
   g. Being patient and not interrupting.

2. A nurse is caring for an older adult who is upset about having to move into a skilled nursing facility. Which communication technique used by the nurse would be most effective at establishing an empathetic climate?

   a. Using open-ended responses
   b. Asking direct questions
   c. Being informative
   d. Being confrontational

3. A nurse is discharging an older adult from a rehabilitation facility after a left hip replacement. The nurse designs discharge teaching based on which factor?

   a. The patient will find the topic interesting
   b. The patient will already know the information
   c. The patient needs teaching relevant to their current condition
   d. The patient selectively listens to what they want to hear

4. A 75-year-old male patient is being discharged home after being hospitalized for pneumonia. The nurse is aware that the patient suffers from presbycusis. Which technique will the nurse use when teaching this patient? *(Select all that apply.)*

   a. Standing on the affected side
   b. Speaking much more loudly
   c. Using "elderspeak"
   d. Using visual cues or written materials
   e. Repeating information as needed
   f. Facing the patient when speaking
   g. Speaking without eating or drinking
   h. Providing printed material to supplement the content
   i. Using an amplifier microphone
   j. Using many senses all at once

REFERENCES

Alzheimer's Association: Stages and behaviors (n.d.). https://www.alz.org/help-support/caregiving/stages-behaviors

Mehrabian, A. (1981). *Silent messages: Implicit communication of emotions and attitudes* (2nd ed.). Belmont, CA: Wadsworth.

Nania, R. (2020). Choir helps stroke survivors regain their voice. https://www.aarp.org/health/conditions-treatments/info-2020/music-therapy-after-stroke.html

Rimmer, A. (2020). Can patients use family members as non-professional interpreters in consultations? *British Medical Journal, 368.* https://www.bmj.com/content/368/bmj.m447.abstract

Williams, P. (2021). *Communication in nursing, in deWit's fundamental concepts and skills for nursing* (6th ed.). St. Louis: Elsevier.

Zhang, M., Zhao, H., & Meng, F.-P. (2020). Elderspeak to resident dementia patients increases resistiveness to care in health care profession. *INQUIRY: The Journal of Health Care Organization, Provision, and Financing.* doi:10.1177/0046958020948668

Maintaining Fluid Balance and Meeting Nutritional Needs

Objectives

1. Identify the various types of nutrients.
2. Discuss the components of a healthy diet for older adults.
3. Describe age-related changes in nutrition and fluid requirements.
4. Examine age-related changes that affect nutrition, digestion, and hydration.
5. Describe methods of assessing the nutritional status and practices of older adults.
6. Identify the older adults who are most at risk for problems related to nutrition and hydration.
7. Select appropriate problem statements related to nutritional or metabolic problems.
8. Identify interventions that will help older adults meet their nutrition and hydration needs.

Key Terms

anemia (ă-NĒ-mē-ă, p. 115)
basal metabolic rate (BĀ-săl mĕt-ă-BŎL-ĭk rāt, p. 112)
blood urea nitrogen (blŭd ū-RĒ-ă NĬ-trō-jĕn, p. 124)
body mass index (p. 112)
calories (KĂL-ŏ-rēs, p. 111)
carbohydrates (kăr-bō-HĬ-drāts, p. 113)
complementary proteins (p. 114)
complete proteins (p. 114)
creatinine (krē-ĂT-ĭ-nēn, p. 124)
dietary reference intakes (p. 113)
dysphagia (p. 134)
edema (ĕ-DĒ-mă, p. 131)
electrolyte (ē-LĔK-trō-līt, p. 125)

frailty syndrome (p. 119)
hematocrit (hē-MĂT-ŏ-krĭt, p. 124)
hemoglobin (HE-mō-glō-bĭn, p. 124)
interstitial (ĭn-tĕr-STĬSH-ăl, p. 130)
intracellular (ĭn-tră-SĔL-ū-lăr, p. 130)
intravascular (ĭn-tră-VĂS-cū-lăr, p. 130)
malnutrition (măl-nū-TRĬSH-ŭn, p. 119)
minerals (MĬN-ĕr-ălz, p. 117)
nasogastric (nā-zŏ-GĂS-trĭk, p. 129)
proteins (PRŌ-tēnz, p. 113)
supplement (SŬP-lĕ-mĕnt, p. 128)
trace element (p. 118)
vitamins (VĬ-tă-mĭnz, p. 115)

Nutrition plays an important role in health maintenance, rehabilitation, and the prevention and control of disease. When dealing with nutritional issues, nurses who work with older adults must consider (1) the basic components of a well-balanced diet for older adults; (2) how the normal physiologic changes of aging change nutritional needs; (3) how the normal physiologic changes of aging may interfere with the purchase, preparation, and consumption of nutrients; and (4) how cognitive, psychosocial, and pathologic changes commonly seen in aging affect one's nutritional status.

NUTRITION AND AGING

Nutritional needs do not remain static throughout life. Like other needs, the nutritional needs of older adults differ from those of younger individuals. An understanding of older adults' nutritional needs is essential to providing good nursing care to the geriatric population. To assess nutritional adequacy and select interventions that promote good nutrition, nurses must be knowledgeable about basic nutrition and diet therapy. Good nutritional practices play a vital role in health maintenance and health promotion. Good eating habits throughout life promote physical wellness and mental well-being. Inadequate intake of foods and fluids can lead to serious problems, such as malnutrition and dehydration. Poor nutritional practices can contribute to the development of osteoporosis and pressure injuries and can complicate existing conditions such as cardiovascular disease and diabetes mellitus.

CALORIC INTAKE

Calories are units of heat that are used to measure the available energy in consumed food. Because people's energy requirements differ widely, the number of calories they require also differs significantly. Many factors influence how many calories a person will use: activity patterns, gender, body size, age, body temperature, emotional status, and prevailing temperatures where the person lives. Both acute and chronic illnesses also have an impact on caloric needs. In general, when a person's caloric intake is in balance with the energy needs of the body, their weight remains constant. When caloric intake exceeds energy needs, the excess is converted into adipose (fat) tissue for storage, and the individual gains weight. When caloric intake is less than the energy needs, the person loses weight.

Various nutrients provide different amounts of calories. Fats, which can come from either plant sources (e.g., oleomargarine) or animal sources (e.g., butter), yield 9 cal/g. Proteins and carbohydrates yield 4 cal/g. Vitamins, minerals, and water yield no calories. Alcohol yields 7 cal/g and has no nutritional value.

Studies have shown that caloric needs in healthy individuals gradually decrease with age, as there is a decrease in muscle and lean tissue mass and an increase in adipose tissue. With these changes in muscle and fat, the **basal metabolic rate** (the rate at which the body uses calories) decreases. The normal decrease in physical activity commonly seen with aging further slows the rate at which the body burns calories. Healthy individuals who maintain an active lifestyle that includes exercise may see little need to change their caloric intake. Inactive individuals may need to restrict their caloric intake significantly. The lowest recommended daily intake to meet nutritional needs is 1200 calories.

When determining the adequacy of caloric intake, disease processes must be considered. Diseases that result in restricted mobility and physical activity (e.g., arthritis and stroke) are likely to decrease caloric needs. Other disease processes (e.g., cancer and critical illness) can greatly increase the body's calorie requirements because illnesses increase metabolism. Individuals with diabetes mellitus require special prescribed diets to control and treat the disease. Such a diet normally includes consistent carbohydrate intake and balanced amounts of fats and proteins.

Body mass index (BMI) is a number calculated by using a person's weight and height; it is a reliable way to measure the amount of body fat for most people. Using the BMI chart, you can determine if someone is underweight, within normal weight parameters, or obese (Fig. 6.1).

NUTRIENTS

Although caloric needs often decrease with age, the need to include all nutrients does not. Therefore foods high in nutritional value (nutrient dense) and relatively low in calories must be selected to maximize the amount of nutrients the body receives while reducing the number of calories.

$$\text{BMI (kg/m}^2\text{)} = \frac{\text{Weight (pounds)} \times 703}{\text{Height (inches)}^2}$$

Weight in Pounds

Height in Feet and Inches	120	130	140	150	160	170	180	190	200	210	220	230	240	250
4'6	29	31	34	36	39	41	43	46	48	51	53	56	58	60
4'8	27	29	31	34	36	38	40	43	45	47	49	52	54	56
4'10	25	27	29	31	34	36	38	40	42	44	46	48	50	52
5'0	23	25	27	29	31	33	35	37	39	41	43	45	47	49
5'2	22	24	26	27	29	31	33	35	37	38	40	42	44	46
5'4	21	22	24	26	28	29	31	33	34	36	38	40	41	43
5'6	19	21	23	24	26	27	29	31	32	34	36	37	39	40
5'8	18	20	21	23	24	26	27	29	30	32	34	35	37	38
5'10	17	19	20	22	23	24	26	27	29	30	32	33	35	36
6'0	16	18	19	20	22	23	24	26	27	28	30	31	33	34
6'2	15	17	18	19	21	22	23	24	26	27	28	30	31	32
6'4	15	16	17	18	20	21	22	23	24	26	27	28	29	30
6'6	14	15	16	17	19	20	21	22	23	24	25	27	28	29
6'8	13	14	15	17	18	19	20	21	22	23	24	25	26	28

Underweight · Normal weight · Overweight · Obese · Severely obese

Fig. 6.1 Body mass index (BMI) chart. (From Lewis, S. L., Bucher, L., Heitkemper, M. M., et al. [2018]. *Medical-surgical nursing: Assessment and management of clinical problems* [10th ed.]. St. Louis: Mosby.)

Vital nutrients needed by all people include carbohydrates, protein, fats, vitamins, minerals, and fluids. Because many foods contain a combination of these nutrients, various methods of determining nutritional balance have been developed. One way to measure the adequacy of a person's diet and nutritional intake is to compare their intake with accepted standards. Based on the current *Dietary Guidelines for Americans*, MyPlate is a visual representation of healthy eating habits designed by the US government (Fig. 6.2). The plate is divided into color-coded food groups, including vegetables, fruits, grains, and protein, with dairy on the

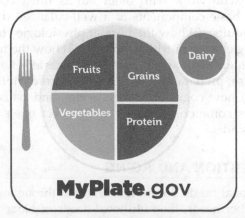

Fig. 6.2 MyPlate. (From U.S. Department of Agriculture, www.myplate.gov)

side. Regardless of the total amount of food consumed, the proportion of food from each group should remain in balance.

The plan is intended to be simple, so that people of all ages and educational background can use it. More than just a diet, MyPlate offers a health plan that encourages users to adopt healthier eating habits and increase their physical activity. Recommendations for the general population from the US Department of Agriculture (USDA) (2020) include:

- Follow a healthy eating pattern at every life stage.
- Customize and enjoy nutrient-dense food and beverage choices to reflect personal preferences, cultural traditions, and budgetary considerations.
- Focus on meeting food group needs with nutrient-dense foods and beverages, and stay within calorie limits.
- Limit foods and beverages higher in added sugars, saturated fat, and sodium, and limit alcoholic beverages.
  Other key recommendations include:
- Meet nutritional needs primarily from foods and beverages.
- Choose a variety of options from each food group.
- Pay attention to portion size.
- Consume less than 10% of calories per day from added sugars.
- Consume less than 10% of calories per day from saturated fats.
- Consume less than 2300 milligrams per day of sodium.
- If alcohol is consumed, it should be taken in moderation.
- Meet the Physical Activity Guidelines for Americans.

In addition to the guidelines for the general population, specific populations have additional recommendations. The USDA Human Nutrition Research Center on Aging has modified MyPlate to include the special needs of older adults with the addition of the MyPlate for Older Adults. Additional tips and resources, including recipes and interactive tools, are available at www.MyPlate.gov.

A modified food guide for older adults is available in Appendix C.

More precise standards for measuring the nutritional adequacy of a diet are found in the dietary reference intakes (DRIs) (see Additional Learning Resources at chapter end). These references contain specific recommendations for calories, macronutrients (protein, carbohydrate, fat), water, fiber, minerals (iron, magnesium, manganese, zinc, etc.), vitamins, and electrolytes.

Use of the DRIs requires careful weighing and measurement of portions and the use of nutritional references or complete nutrition labels that list every ingredient in detail. Older adults may consult these recommendations when they are selecting vitamins or other nutrients. Nutritional labels are commonly used by physicians, nurses, or dietitians in developing a specific therapeutic meal plan. A more general checklist that older adults can use to determine their nutritional health is shown in Fig. 6.3.

> **Health Promotion**
>
> Older adults require the same number of nutrients but fewer calories and a smaller intake. It is important to educate patients on eating a balanced, high-quality diet to ensure that they are meeting their nutritional requirements without overeating. The slogan for the *Dietary Guidelines for Americans 2020-2025* is "Make Every Bite Count."

CARBOHYDRATES

Carbohydrates include sugars and starches; these constitute approximately half of the standard American diet. Carbohydrates provide a ready source of energy for the body and are divided into two categories: simple and complex. Simple carbohydrates are used most readily by the body because their bonds are easily broken. Table sugar, honey, syrup, and candy are examples of simple carbohydrates. Complex carbohydrates must be broken down into simple sugars before they can be used by the body. This breakdown requires time and energy. Foods such as vegetables, whole grains, and fruits contain complex carbohydrates. Such foods also usually contain other nutrients (e.g., minerals and vitamins), making them more nutritious than foods containing simple carbohydrates only. The Institute of Medicine recommends that 45% to 65% of calories should come from carbohydrates, with an emphasis on complex carbohydrates (USDA, 2020). This recommendation is also appropriate for the older adult.

In addition to providing essential nutrients, complex carbohydrates usually contain significant amounts of soluble fiber, a substance that humans cannot digest, which forms bulk and aids in bowel elimination. Fiber is recommended as helpful in preventing constipation, diverticulosis, and diverticulitis. People who eat high fiber diets must also drink enough water to ensure that the fiber does not become constipating. A diet high in complex carbohydrates is recommended as part of the control of many disease processes. The soluble fiber in complex carbohydrates has been shown to reduce blood cholesterol levels, which is helpful for individuals who are at risk for coronary artery disease. Complex carbohydrates also play an important role in the control of diabetes, because they effectively meet energy needs without causing rapid increases in blood glucose levels, as simple sugars do.

PROTEINS

Proteins are composed of amino acids, which are essential for tissue repair and healing. Protein needs remain constant or may increase slightly with aging to compensate for the loss of lean body tissue (Box 6.1). According to *Dietary Guidelines for Americans* (USDA, 2020), the DRI of protein for adult women is 46 g/d;

DETERMINE YOUR NUTRITIONAL HEALTH

The Warning Signs of poor nutritional health are often overlooked. Use this checklist to find out if you or someone you know is at nutritional risk.

Read the statements below. Circle the number in the "yes" column for those that apply to you or someone you know. For each "yes" answer, score the number in the box. Total your nutritional score.

	YES
I have an illness or condition that made me change the kind and/or amount of food I eat.	2
I eat fewer than 2 meals per day.	3
I eat few fruits or vegetables or milk products.	2
I have 3 or more drinks of beer, liquor, or wine almost everyday.	2
I have tooth or mouth problems that make it hard for me to eat.	2
I don't always have enough money to buy the food I need.	4
I eat alone most of the time.	1
I take 3 or more different prescribed or over-the-counter drugs a day.	1
Without wanting to, I have lost or gained 10 pounds in the last 6 months.	2
I am not always physically able to shop, cook, and/or feed myself.	2
TOTAL	

Total Your Nutritional Score. If it's—

0–2   **Good!** Recheck your nutritional score in 6 months.

3–5   **You are at moderate nutritional risk.** See what can be done to improve your eating habits and lifestyle. Your office on aging, senior nutrition program, senior citizens' center, or health department can help. Recheck your nutritional score in 3 months.

6 or more You are at high nutritional risk. Bring this checklist the next time you see your doctor, dietitian, or other qualified health or social service professional. Talk with them about any problems you may have. Ask for help to improve your nutritional health.

Remember that warning signs suggest risk but do not represent diagnosis of any condition.

Fig. 6.3 Determine your nutritional health. Checklist of warning signs of poor nutrition. (From the Nutritional Screening Initiative, Washington, DC.)

Box 6.1   **Ways to Increase Protein Intake**

- *Add eggs.* Add extra whites to pancakes, omelets, and scrambled eggs; add hardboiled eggs to casseroles and salads.
- *Add cheese.* Sprinkle on salads, melt on sandwiches, serve on crackers, add to casseroles, use to top vegetables, blend in mashed potatoes, use in cheesecake.
- *Add milk, cream, and yogurt.* Add when baking or making pancakes. Use in hot cocoa, sauces, milk shakes, smoothies, on fruit, with cereal, as a dessert topping.
- *Add legumes and beans.* Cook these in soups and stews. Use bean curd on salads. Serve ethnic dishes made with chickpeas, such as hummus or falafel.
- *Add peanut butter.* Use in cookies, as a dip for fruit or vegetables, in sauces, and on sandwiches.

---

for adult men, the recommended daily allowance is 56 g/d. Data from the National Health and Nutrition Examination Survey reveal that 10% to 25% of women older than age 55 consume less than half of the recommended daily amount of protein. Increased protein consumption has been linked with a lower incidence of frailty (Isanejad, 2019). Protein consumption can be affected by many factors, including the ability to procure and prepare food, the cost of foods containing protein, and even the ability to chew common high-protein foods.

Tissue replacement and repair continue throughout life. Any condition in which tissue integrity is altered (e.g., surgery and pressure injuries) increases the amount of protein needed to aid in tissue repair. Red meats, poultry, fish, eggs, and dairy products are good sources of complete proteins, which contain all of the amino acids necessary for making and repairing tissues. Plant foods—such as legumes (peas and beans), nuts, and cereals (whole grains and rice)—contain smaller amounts of incomplete proteins, which do not individually contain all necessary amino acids. Complementary proteins consist of 2 or more incomplete proteins that together provide adequate amounts of essential amino acids. In the past, it was thought that incomplete proteins had to be carefully combined during meal planning. The current thinking, however, is that the body can combine complementary proteins eaten on the same day (USDA, 2020).

Some foods that are high in protein—such as steak, ham, organ meats, egg yolks, hard cheese, and whole milk—also contain large amounts of fats. Excessive consumption of proteins with a high fat content can contribute to elevated blood levels of cholesterol and triglycerides, which, in turn, contribute to plaque formation and atherosclerotic changes in the blood vessels. Atherosclerosis often results in hypertension and heart disease. For this reason, many health professionals recommend that high fat protein foods be restricted. A person who is on a fat-restricted diet should consume low fat proteins, such as fish and lean poultry, as well as protein from plant sources, such as peas and beans.

Health Promotion

The USDA (2020) recommends replacing meat with seafood at least twice a week and occasionally using legumes, nuts, and seeds in place of meat in mixed dishes. These small changes can increase or maintain the nutritional value of the foods being consumed while also decreasing the overall fat content.

FATS

It is recommended that fats be limited to approximately 20% to 35% of the total daily caloric intake. This recommendation does not change with aging. A certain amount of fat is necessary and desirable in the diet to aid in the absorption of fat-soluble vitamins and provide adequate amounts of essential fatty acids. Fat is desirable because it adds flavor to food and provides a sense of fullness with a meal. Foods with no fat would be unappealing, poor tasting, and not very satisfying.

In considering fat intake in the diet, it is important to watch the types of fats being ingested. The body incorporates fats into substances called *lipoproteins*, which contain cholesterol and proteins. There are three important types of lipoproteins: high-density lipoprotein (HDL), low-density lipoprotein (LDL), and very-low-density lipoprotein (VLDL). LDL is primarily composed of cholesterol and is believed to contribute to blood vessel disease. VLDL is primarily composed of triglycerides and may contribute to vessel disease but to a lesser extent. HDL, the so-called healthy fat, is primarily composed of protein that appears to protect against blood vessel disease.

Some individuals who have been eating high cholesterol foods for their entire lives may be reluctant to change their eating habits as they age. They may find it difficult or unpleasant to shop for and prepare foods in new ways. Others can successfully alter their dietary intake to avoid foods that are high in these substances.

QSEN Considerations: Patient-Centered Care

It is important to listen to patients regarding their dietary preferences and help them find substitutions that do not make them feel deprived. Food choices are based on a lifetime of habits, and eating has a very emotional component. Patients need help in finding ways to change their diets without taking away the enjoyment of eating. Options such as low fat milk or yogurt may provide most of the desired taste while also decreasing some of the overall fat content. There is nothing to be gained from making a plan if the patient will not adhere to it.

VITAMINS

Vitamins are organic compounds found naturally in foods. They can also be produced synthetically. Vitamins are needed for a variety of metabolic and physiologic processes. They are classified as fatsoluble or water soluble. The fat soluble vitamins include vitamins A, D, E, and K. Vitamin C and the B-complex vitamins are water soluble (Table 6.1).

The benefits of vitamins for older adults are being closely examined. Researchers who subscribe to the free radical theory of aging are studying the effects of antioxidant vitamins. It is theorized that antioxidant vitamins can block or neutralize free radicals and prevent cell damage, thereby slowing the effects of aging and preventing diseases such as cancer, heart disease, and Alzheimer disease. Although research into this area is promising, many experts are not yet convinced of the effectiveness of antioxidant vitamins or satisfied that we have an adequate understanding of their method of action, therapeutic dosage, and long-term effects. Vitamins A, C, and E, along with beta carotene, are considered antioxidants.

Vitamin deficiencies have been connected to a variety of problems experienced by older adults, including:
- Vitamin A deficiency: Poor wound healing, dry skin, and night blindness.
- Vitamin B_6 deficiency: Neurologic and immunologic problems and elevated homocysteine levels (risk factor for cardiovascular disease). Clinical manifestations of B_6 deficiency may include nausea, vomiting, loss of appetite, dermatitis, motor weakness, dizziness, depression, and sore tongue. Supplements of vitamin B_6 help to reverse these problems.
- Vitamin B_{12} deficiency: Neurologic changes that affect sensation, balance, and memory; elevated homocysteine levels. B_{12} deficiency can be related to inadequate protein consumption or physiologic changes in digestion. Normal aging changes result in the decreased production of gastric acid and pepsin, which are necessary for the digestion of protein. When less protein is digested, less B_{12} is available for absorption. Clinical manifestations of B_{12} deficiency can include vomiting, fatigue, constipation, anemia, decreased memory, and depression. If detected early and treated with supplements, symptoms may be reversible.

Table 6.1   Summary of Essential Vitamins

Fat-Soluble Vitamins	
Vitamin A	Found in milk, butter, cheese, fortified margarine, liver, green and yellow vegetables, and fruits Promotes healthy epithelium, ability to see in dim light, normal mucus formation Many older people may be deficient in vitamin A because of chronic conditions that interfere with fat absorption, such as gallbladder disease and colitis
Vitamin D	Found in fortified milk and margarine, cod liver oil, fatty fish, and eggs Promotes absorption of calcium May contribute to skeletal changes with aging
Vitamin E	Found in corn and safflower oils, margarine, seeds, nuts, and leafy green vegetables Promotes integrity of red blood cells
Vitamin K	Found in leafy green vegetables and liver; synthesized by bacteria in the colon Essential for formation of prothrombin, which is necessary for blood clotting
Water-Soluble Vitamins	
Vitamin B$_1$ (thiamine hydrochloride)	Found in organ meats, pork, legumes, and whole grains Essential for carbohydrate metabolism
Vitamin B$_2$ (riboflavin)	Found in milk, cheese, eggs, organ meats, legumes, and leafy green vegetables Essential for normal tissue maintenance and tear production
Niacin	Found in lean meats, liver, whole grains, and legumes Essential for energy release from fats, carbohydrates, and proteins
Vitamin B$_6$ (pyridoxine)	Found in whole grains, vegetables, legumes, meats, and bananas Acts in the processes of protein synthesis and amino acid metabolism May interact with levodopa (medication taken for Parkinson disease)
Folacin (folic acid)	Found in whole wheat, legumes, and green vegetables Important in hemoglobin synthesis and in metabolism of amino acids Common deficiency in older adults
Vitamin B$_{12}$ (cyanocobalamin)	Found in muscle and organ meats, eggs, shellfish, and dairy products Requires production of intrinsic factor by the stomach for absorption; inadequate absorption can result in pernicious anemia Needed for maturation of red blood cells Deficiency is commonly seen with folacin deficiency
Vitamin C (ascorbic acid)	Found in citrus fruits, tomatoes, cabbage, melons, strawberries, green peppers, and leafy green vegetables Important in the formation and maintenance of collagen structure of connective tissue Promotes healing and elasticity of capillary walls

- Vitamin C deficiency: Weakness, dry mouth, skin changes, delayed tissue healing, atherosclerosis, and decreased cognitive function.
- Vitamin D deficiency: Bone demineralization, or osteoporosis, because Vitamin D is essential for calcium absorption; depression; and immune system dysfunction. Vitamin D deficiency is more common in older adults because they generally get less exposure to the sun, their skin has a lower capacity to synthesize the vitamin, and they are likely to have less dietary intake of the vitamin. Clinical symptoms include weakness, gait disturbance, and pain. Adequate intake of vitamin D and calcium supplements can help prevent or even reverse the severity of these problems. Research shows that doses of at least 700 IU can significantly reduce the risk for falling (Kougias, 2018). Many dairy products are fortified with vitamin D because it is not found naturally in many foods.

- Vitamin K deficiency: Increased risk of fractures.
- Vitamin E deficiency: Immune dysfunction, memory problems. High doses of vitamin E (1000 IU twice daily) have been shown in studies to decrease the rate of decline in Alzheimer disease (Atri, 2019).

Older adults who consume well-balanced diets may not require supplemental vitamins. Those with increased risk factors, such as gastrointestinal (GI) disorders or inadequate nutritional intake, may benefit from selected vitamin supplements. Supplements should be used with caution and under the direction of the primary care provider or dietitian. Excess amounts of the water-soluble vitamins are quickly eliminated from the body and pose few risks. Excess amounts of the fat-soluble vitamins (A, D, E, and K) are retained in fatty tissue or stored in the liver. Overconsumption of these vitamins can lead to toxic symptoms and even permanent liver damage.

MINERALS

Minerals are inorganic chemical elements that are required for many of the body's functions. Minerals make up a small proportion of total body weight, yet a slight mineral imbalance can have serious effects.

Calcium, the most abundant mineral in the body, is necessary for the formation of bones and teeth, the transmission and conduction of nerve impulses, the contraction of muscles (including the cardiac muscles), and the clotting of blood. The main dietary sources of calcium are milk and dairy products. Calcium is normally retained in bone, with only a small amount (1%) found in the tissues and blood. With aging and immobility, the bones tend to lose calcium, resulting in osteoporosis. In certain disease states, abnormal amounts of calcium leave the bone, enter the bloodstream, and cause hypercalcemia, which is an elevated level of calcium in the blood. Hypercalcemia is seen with hyperparathyroidism, disuse atrophy, metastatic bone tumors, and vitamin D excess.

Individuals experiencing hypercalcemia may manifest symptoms including confusion, abdominal pain, muscle pain, weakness, and anorexia. These symptoms may easily be missed in older individuals because they are vague and common to many other conditions. Extremely high levels of calcium in the blood can result in shock, kidney failure, and even death. When the kidneys attempt to rid the body of excess calcium, hypercalciuria (increased calcium in the urine) results, and the risk for the formation of renal calculi (kidney stones) is increased.

An adequate calcium intake is important throughout life, but it is particularly important for those at risk for developing osteoporosis, especially postmenopausal women. Calcium may arrest the progress of osteoporosis. Vitamin D aids in the absorption of calcium. For this reason, vitamin D is added to milk products, fortified margarine, and many calcium supplements.

Phosphorus is needed for normal bone and tooth formation, activation of some B vitamins, normal neuromuscular functioning, metabolism of carbohydrates, regulation of acid-base balance, and other physiologic processes. Inadequate nutritional intake of phosphorus can result in weight loss or anemia. The typical dietary sources of phosphorus compounds are dairy products, meat, egg yolks, peas, beans, nuts, and whole grains. Because of the wide availability of phosphorus, there is normally no problem in meeting the dietary requirements for it unless a person is on a highly restricted diet.

Iron is found in the center of the heme portion of hemoglobin. Hemoglobin in the red blood cells transports oxygen to and removes carbon dioxide from the cells. Without adequate amounts of iron, the body cannot produce enough hemoglobin. When hemoglobin levels fall below normal, anemia results. Individuals with anemia may manifest many symptoms, depending on the severity of the condition: fatigue, exertional dyspnea, tachycardia, palpitations, headache, insomnia, vertigo, pallor (particularly of the mucous membranes), and cool extremities. The normal changes of aging or other disease processes may resemble these symptoms and prevent the recognition of anemia. Laboratory tests for hemoglobin levels are required to determine whether anemia is present (Table 6.2). Two forms of nutritional anemia are commonly seen in older adults: iron deficiency anemia and pernicious anemia.

Iron deficiency anemia results from inadequate intake of dietary iron. Rich sources of dietary iron include red meat, particularly organ meats, such as liver; shellfish, egg yolks, leafy green vegetables, and dried fruits. Red meat is expensive and, unless properly prepared, can be difficult for older adults to chew. Many people do not like the taste of liver and organ meats and will not eat them. In addition, organ meats and egg yolks are high in cholesterol, which is often restricted from the diet. This can make meal planning difficult. Increasing one's intake of dark green leafy vegetables, such as spinach, and eating iron-fortified cereals and pastas can help. Dried fruit, such as raisins and apricots, or beans can also be added to the diet to increase iron. In addition to increased nutritional intake of iron-rich foods, folic acid and iron supplements are commonly prescribed.

Table 6.2	Laboratory Values Used to Assess Nutritional Adequacy in Older Adults	
DIAGNOSTIC TEST	**APPROPRIATE RANGE**
Hemoglobin	14–18 g/dL (men)
	12–16 g/dL (women)
Hematocrit	42%–52% (men)
	37%–47% (women)
Blood urea nitrogen	10–20 mg/dL
	May be slightly higher in older adults
Creatinine	0.6–1.2 mg/dL (male)
	0.5–1.1 mg/dL (female)
	Slightly decreased in older adults
Albumin	3.5–5.0 g/dL
Calcium	9–10.5 mg/dL
Folic acid	5–25 mg/dL
Glucose (fasting)	Fasting 74–106 mg/dL
	Increase in normal range after age 60

Data from Pagana, K. D., & Pagana, T. J. (2021). *Mosby's diagnostic and laboratory test reference* (15th ed.). St. Louis: Mosby.

It should be remembered that a concentrated iron formulation (liquid or solid) administered orally can cause GI tract irritation, including constipation or diarrhea. To reduce GI irritation, iron supplements should be taken during or after meals. Constipation can be reduced by increasing water and fiber intake. Iron solutions can stain the teeth, so a straw should be used with liquid iron preparations. If iron is given by injection, it is important to use the Z-track method for deep intramuscular administration. Foods rich in vitamin C should be given in conjunction with iron to enhance its absorption. Patients should be told that iron will turn the stool a dark green or black color, and nurses should keep this in mind in assessing the stool of individuals receiving iron supplements.

Pernicious anemia is caused by a deficiency in intrinsic factor secreted by the stomach. Without this factor, vitamin B_{12}, which is required for the maturation of red blood cells in the bone marrow, is not absorbed. In addition, there are fewer white blood cells and there may be cellular changes in the existing cells. Individuals with pernicious anemia may manifest weakness, numbness or tingling in the extremities, anorexia, or weight loss. Treatment typically consists of cyanocobalamin injections and possibly oral folic acid and iron supplements.

Sodium is a commonly occurring mineral and is one of the important elements in the body. Sodium ions are involved in acid-base balance, fluid balance, nerve impulse transmission, and muscle contraction. Sodium is found primarily in extracellular fluid. Sodium levels are regulated by the kidneys, which retain or eliminate sodium according to the body's needs. Sodium interacts with potassium as part of the fluid exchange through cell membranes.

Sodium is naturally present in many foods. The most common, most familiar concentrated form is sodium chloride, or table salt. The typical American diet tends to be higher in sodium than is nutritionally required. Older adults often eat processed foods, such as canned or frozen items that use sodium as a preservative. Many people also salt their food before tasting it. Excessive blood levels of sodium, or hypernatremia, can cause fluid retention and hypertension and can increase the risk for osteoporosis, as excessive sodium levels lead to urinary calcium excretion. People with hypertension, kidney failure, or cardiac conditions are often placed on sodium restricted diets, and many find that food is unappetizing when prepared with less sodium. With decreased appetite, these individuals may eat less.

QSEN Considerations: Patient-Centered Care

Removing salt from the diet can be a challenge for those older adults who have salted their food throughout their lives. Provide options, such as salt substitutes (if the older adult is not taking a diuretic that would contraindicate such use) or herbs to provide flavor to food without the sodium. Many food products with reduced sodium content are also available. Checking labels for low-sodium varieties of soup, bread, and frozen foods can also help to reduce the overall amount of sodium consumed.

Potassium is the major intracellular ion in the body. Potassium ions play an important role in acid-base balance, fluid and electrolyte balance, and (with sodium) normal neuromuscular function. Potassium is less abundant in the diets of older adults than are some of the other minerals. Dietary sources of potassium include citrus fruits, milk, bananas, and apple juice. Potassium deficiency, or hypokalemia, is a common problem in older adults. Many diuretic and antihypertensive medications deplete the body of potassium, as can prolonged or frequent diarrhea. Symptoms of hypokalemia include muscle weakness, anorexia, palpitations, irritability, drowsiness, depression, and disorientation. Severe muscle weakness is the most common observation related to decreased potassium levels. Hypokalemia secondary to digitalis therapy is often a cause of cardiac arrhythmias. Because not all patients who have decreased levels of potassium demonstrate observable symptoms, nurses must check laboratory studies to verify levels of the electrolytes. Supplements are often prescribed to increase low blood potassium levels.

Zinc is a trace mineral that plays a role in protein synthesis. In adults, insufficient zinc may result in delayed wound healing, impaired immune function, lethargy, skin changes, diminished sense of smell and taste, and decreased appetite. Certain conditions—such as cirrhosis of the liver, kidney disease, cancer, and alcohol use disorder—may result in zinc deficiency. Supplemental zinc may be administered. Dietary sources of zinc include meat, shellfish, and nuts.

Trace elements—such as magnesium, copper, iodine, fluorine, chromium, selenium, nickel, and sulfur—are necessary in very small amounts for normal body functioning. Selenium is gaining importance as an antioxidant mineral, as it is believed to promote heart health; improve tissue elasticity; and decrease the risk of colorectal, lung, and prostate cancer.

FUNCTIONAL FOODS

Functional foods are foods that have been found to have overall health benefits and reduce risk factors for chronic diseases or to enhance body processes that benefit health (Ashaolu, 2020). Most have cultural origins and include soy, mushrooms, green tea, and black rice.

- Soy has been shown to decrease LDL and total cholesterol, increase HDL, increase bone density, stabilize blood glucose, and reduce breast cancer risk.
- Mushrooms can enhance immunity, guard against tumors, decrease inflammation, and improve blood lipid profiles.
- Green tea can reduce the risk for cardiovascular disease and stroke, possibly guard against cancer and Parkinson disease, and stabilize blood sugar. Even drinking three cups of ordinary tea daily has been shown to decrease stroke risk.

- Black rice is rich in phenolic compounds (antioxidants) and minerals. It has been shown to reduce BMI and body fat and increase HDL cholesterol.

WATER

Water is essential for life. Humans can survive for many days without food but not without water. Water plays a role in many aspects of normal body functioning. Water is necessary for the formation of many of the body's secretions, including tears, perspiration, and saliva. Water aids in digestion and in transportation of electrolytes and nutrients. Water facilitates elimination of waste products and plays an important role in temperature regulation.

Approximately 60% of the average adult body is composed of water, with adult men having slightly more body fluid than do women. Older individuals typically have less body fluid than do younger adults. The total amount of body fluid decreases by approximately 8% to 10% in older adults. The amount of water in the bloodstream remains relatively constant with aging, but older adults tend to have less fluid in the intracellular and interstitial spaces than do younger people. Kidney changes can affect the thirst response and decrease the amount of fluid that older adults drink. This fluid decrease results in loss of skin turgor and, along with decreased skin elasticity, leads to the wrinkled appearance common with aging. Decreased fluid increases the risk for dehydration. Inadequate fluid intake can lead to altered absorption of medications, interfere with appetite and digestion, and contribute to problems with constipation. Severe dehydration can make existing medical conditions worse and can ultimately result in death. Most adults require 2000 to 3000 mL of fluid each day. Most of this is consumed as beverages, such as water, tea, coffee, and juice. Solid foods, particularly fruits and vegetables, contain significant amounts of water.

Water is normally lost through urination, perspiration, respiration, and defecation. Abnormal fluid loss occurs with diarrhea, vomiting, diaphoresis, gastric suctioning, and wound drainage; essential minerals are often lost along with the water. The amount of fluid taken into the body should be in balance with the amount eliminated from the body. This is referred to as *fluid balance.*

MALNUTRITION AND THE OLDER ADULT

In America, where obesity is an increasing problem, undernutrition and malnutrition are significant problems for the older adult population. Statistics show that many older adults are at risk for malnutrition, whether they are living independently or are institutionalized. Malnutrition is defined as a disorder of nutrition resulting from unbalanced, insufficient, or excessive diet or from impaired absorption, assimilation,

or use of food. The risk for developing nutritional deficiencies increases with aging; however, determining nutritional status can be challenging. Older adults who appear to be healthy may have unhealthy nutritional practices. An obese older adult may be malnourished, whereas a thin person may be well nourished. Studies have shown that most older Americans believe that nutrition is important for good health but that they do not always follow good nutritional practices. Information from the National Council on Aging Nutritional Assessment Self-Test reveals that older adults have a disproportionately high risk for poor nutrition, which, in turn, has a negative effect on their health. Poorly nourished older adults are more likely to experience functional impairments, fatigue, decreased muscle strength, poor tissue healing, pressure injuries, and infections. They are likely to develop more postoperative complications, spend a longer time in the hospital, and are at increased risk for death.

Estimates of the number of malnourished older adults vary depending on the screening tool used, but they generally fall within the following ranges:
- Older adults in the community: 10% to 26.5% (Chew et al., 2020; O'Keeffe et al., 2019)
- Older adults in geriatric care facilities: 30% to 50% (O'Keeffe et al., 2019; Mullin et al., 2019)
- Hospitalized older adults: 30% to 50% (O'Keeffe et al., 2019; Mullin et al., 2019)

These data reveal the magnitude of the problems to be addressed by health care providers and demonstrate greater malnutrition as one becomes more frail and dependent on others.

Symptoms of nutritional problems include unintentional weight loss, light-headedness, disorientation, lethargy, and loss of appetite. Similar symptoms occur with a variety of illnesses, making it difficult to determine whether the primary problem is medical or nutritional in origin. Weight loss is one of the signs of frailty syndrome in older adults, which is characterized by increased susceptibility to stressors and can lead to negative health outcomes and functional impairment. Frailty is listed as a geriatric syndrome and puts the older adult at risk for gait disturbances, balance issues, poor muscle strength, cognitive changes, and lack of endurance (Magnuson et al., 2019). Nurses working in all health care settings must assess, plan, and implement strategies to maintain or improve the nutritional status of the older adults in their care.

FACTORS AFFECTING NUTRITION IN OLDER ADULTS

The nutritional status of older adults living in the community is affected by physiologic, economic, and social factors. Lack of appetite is commonly reported. The reasons for this are multiple and form the basis of risk assessment. The more risk factors present, the greater the likelihood of the older person experiencing nutritional inadequacy. Overall nutritional status will

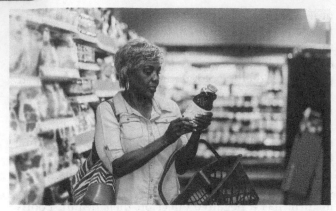

Fig. 6.4 Shopping for groceries. (Copyright © istock.com/Kali9.)

be affected if any of these problems persists for a significant period of time.

Physiologic risk factors include

- Chronic health factors, such as chronic obstructive pulmonary disease, chronic heart failure, arthritis, dementia, and many others, can interfere with obtaining and preparing adequate nutritional food. Shopping requires physical exertion. Activities that a young, healthy person does not think about, such as lifting cans from a top shelf, reaching for something near the floor, or moving groceries into and out of a store cart, can physically exhaust an infirm or older adult. Although store personnel or other shoppers would probably help with these activities (Fig. 6.4), older adults are often too embarrassed or proud to ask for help. Once food has been purchased and taken home, the task of food preparation remains. Opening cans, unsealing jars, and dealing with the ubiquitous plastic wrappers on food all present daunting obstacles to the aging individual. Think of the problems that a young, healthy person may have with current packaging, and then imagine performing the same tasks with decreased muscle strength, arthritis, or other age-related problems.
- Alcohol use disorder (formerly known as *alcoholism*) is suspected to be a risk factor in a larger percentage of older adults than is commonly recognized. Although small amounts of alcohol may stimulate the appetite, consumption of large amounts of alcohol suppresses appetite, interferes with the absorption of essential nutrients, and all too often takes the place of meals.

Health Promotion

Alcohol use disorder is a growing problem in the geriatric population. Current studies show that 10% to 15% of community-dwelling older adults meet the criteria for problem drinking. Up to 30% of older adults who are hospitalized meet the same criteria (Scott et al., 2020). Alcohol use disorder has been linked to malnutrition and the development of dementia. Assessment during regular visits is an important part of reducing the impact on this population.

- Sensory changes can cause problems with safe preparation and storage of food. Reading small print on labels can be difficult for an individual with presbyopia, cataracts, or other vision problems seen with aging. This can be problematic for someone on a restricted diet who needs to read the label to choose foods that are permitted. Older adults with altered senses of taste and smell may not be able to detect the changes that indicate spoilage. If spoiled food is eaten, the risk for GI infection or upset is increased.
- Pain, whether chronic or acute, can interfere with an older person's appetite and desire to procure, prepare, and consume food.
- Medications can cause an unpleasant change in the taste of food, suppress appetite, or cause nausea and vomiting. Many older adults complain of a "metallic taste" that interferes with the enjoyment of food. Other medications—such as antihypertensives, drugs used to treat Parkinson disease, bronchodilators, and antidepressants—can cause a dry mouth, which makes chewing and swallowing more difficult.
- Problems with chewing, swallowing, or digesting are common causes of impaired nutrition. Poor oral hygiene, lost teeth, cavities, poorly fitted dentures, and decreased oral secretions affect the taste of food and can interfere with the ability of the older person to chew foods. This is particularly a problem with protein-rich foods, such as meat, unless they are cooked to a very tender consistency or provided in a chopped or ground form. Mechanically soft food is not appetizing to look at, and patients often dislike eating food that is not visually appealing.
- Malabsorption caused by decreased production of digestive enzymes can interfere with protein breakdown and absorption of vitamin B_{12}, calcium, and folate.

Economic risk factors include

- The cost of food, which is a concern for many older adults with limited income. Foods rich in protein, such as meats and dairy products, tend to be more expensive than starchy carbohydrates. Fresh vegetables and fruits that are rich in vitamins and minerals may also be costly, depending on the season and locale. Many older adults have limited budgets and may not purchase these more expensive items, although they know the nutritional value and importance of these foods. They may skip meals or consume inadequate portions to save money.
- Difficulty getting transportation to obtain food; this is a serious problem for older adults, particularly those who live alone. The simple act of getting to a store may be difficult. Trends toward large chain supermarkets have forced many smaller neighborhood grocery stores to close. These large stores are often located in shopping plazas that are far away from home. Even if there is a nearby neighborhood grocery or convenience store, its prices must be higher for it to stay in business. Either situation presents problems for the older adult. Without a car, a

homebound older adult may find it difficult to obtain groceries, medicine, or other necessities. Many times, family members or friends drive the older adult to the store to shop or pick up groceries. As a courtesy to busy or older customers, more stores now offer call-in and delivery services for an added fee. Some communities offer scheduled transportation from senior citizen housing to grocery stores. Others provide volunteers to shop for homebound older adults.

- Obtaining an appropriate variety and sufficient amount of food; this can be difficult for older adults. Most foods are packaged in sizes appropriate for families of four or more. Although some manufacturers are responding to the needs of single adults and older adults by packaging smaller servings, the cost is often higher per serving. Older adults must decide whether thrift or variety is more important.

Social risk factors include

- Depression; this is a common reason for decreased appetite in older adults. Grief, failing health, loss of independence, and many other factors can cause depression. Malnutrition can also be a cause of depression. Often the problem is unrecognized until the person has lost significant weight or develops other health problems.
- Loneliness or being socially isolated—one of the more common risk factors for nutritional problems in older adults. Eating is usually more pleasant with company. Widowed or single older adults are less likely to prepare and consume nutritious meals than are seniors who have more social contact.
- Lack of motivation to cook; this is a common issue for older adults. Preparing food for one or two people can be more difficult. Most recipes are intended for four or more servings. Food must often be either eaten as leftovers for several days or wasted. Some older adults prepare their favorite meals and then package and freeze individual servings so that they can have variety and avoid waste. Unfortunately, not everyone has a freezer and not all foods can be frozen. Because the effort of cooking can be overwhelming for the aging person, meal after meal may consist of sandwiches or cereal. Many communities have established programs designed to help older adults meet their nutritional needs. Senior citizen meal programs provide both reasonably priced meals and companionship. Meals on Wheels programs deliver a variety of well-balanced meals to homebound individuals, allowing them to maintain some degree of independence (Fig. 6.5).

Problems related to poor nutrition are not limited to older adults residing in the community; they are also of concern for institutionalized seniors. As previously identified, up to 60% of nursing home residents may be undernourished. Although most institutions maintain well-staffed dietary departments under the supervision of trained dietitians, many older adults do not consume the nutrients that are available. This may be related to the physiologic or emotional risk factors

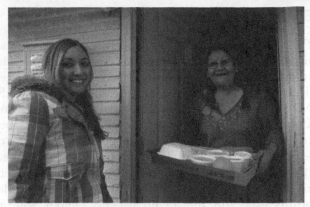

Fig. 6.5 A recipient of Meals on Wheels. (From U.S. Air Force photo/ Airman 1st Class Katrina Heikkinen.)

discussed previously or to institutional factors outside the control of the older adult. Some institutional factors that influence nutrition include

- The repetitive nature of institutional meals
- Problems maintaining the temperature and appearance of food while serving many people
- Environmental concerns, such as the type of background music being played, staff conversations, or overhead announcements
- Problems related to being fed by others
- Behavior, appearance, or odors of tablemates
- Inability of an institution to meet the specific cultural preferences or general likes and dislikes of a large number of people

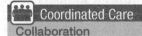

Coordinated Care
Collaboration

Nutrition

- Nursing assistants or dietary aides are most likely to be aware of the amounts and types of food consumed by older residents.
- Data that are more specific than the typical good/fair/ poor ratings or even percentages are important for good care planning.
- Assistants need to report the types of food consumed (e.g., the amount of meat and vegetables versus the amount of applesauce and dessert).

? Critical Thinking

Nutritional Assessment

An 84-year-old woman has been living in a long-term care facility for 6 months. It is noted that she has been losing weight at a rate of approximately 3 to 5 pounds a month. This was not immediately evident because she had been moderately overweight. Now her clothing is loose. She is 66 inches tall and weighs 150 pounds. She never complains about being hungry, and her health record reveals that she eats 50% to 75% of the food at each meal. Her hemoglobin is 9.6 g/dL, and her hematocrit is 32%.

- Is her weight loss desirable?
- What are possible reasons for the weight loss?
- What other information do you need to obtain?

SOCIAL AND CULTURAL ASPECTS OF NUTRITION

Food is more than a means of meeting nutritional needs. It is also used in religious ceremonies, in social interactions, and as a means of cultural expression. Throughout history, food has been linked to the gods. Many major religions—such as Islam, Judaism, and Catholicism—include some dietary restrictions. They may require the avoidance of certain foods, fasting, or special methods of food preparation for all members of the faith. Although most religions have more lenient restrictions for older adults and the infirm, many older adults, especially those who are very devout, want to comply with their religious teachings. Violating dietary rules may upset them deeply. This presents a challenge to caregivers, who are more concerned about adequate nutrition than about religious beliefs. If such a situation arises, it is appropriate to consult with a dietitian or with the rabbi, minister, priest, or spiritual leader of the specific religious group to seek clarification and guidance. Many times, the spiritual counselor can provide reassurance to the older adult and guidance to the health care team.

Cultural influences in food are also significant. The foods we eat in our homes from early in life reflect our culture. Some people are happy to eat a variety of foods; others prefer to eat only foods with which they are familiar. Various cultures ascribe certain powers to foods. The culture may dictate what, when, or how foods should be eaten. An older adult from such a cultural background may find it difficult to understand or accept mainstream American nutritional practices. Remember that good nutrition can be achieved within any culture (Table 6.3). Special planning with the dietitian is often necessary to achieve adequate nutrition and meet cultural preferences within an institutional setting. Family members and significant others from the same culture may be willing to provide special foods and assist in meeting the nutritional needs of the institutionalized older adult.

Food is often tied to social events. When people visit friends' homes, they are often served food. Food is served at parties, weddings, and wakes. People on dates go out to eat. Eating alone is often described as one of the worst things about being single or widowed. A common notion is that food eaten alone does not even taste the same. Nurses should remember this when they are working with older adults.

Many older adults like to go out to eat in restaurants. Eating out has many benefits, including a change of scenery, a wider choice of foods, and the opportunity for social interaction. Many older adults prefer restaurants with table service rather than buffets or fast-food establishments because the former tend to be less noisy and do not require a person to balance a tray. Eating out is an occasional treat for some older adults but a way of life for others. Older adults who eat out regularly should choose carefully and try to avoid the high fat, high sodium items that are common restaurant fare. Many restaurants that cater to older adults offer heart-healthy items and senior portions, often at discounted prices.

Older adults who live in long-term or assisted living settings are usually served one or more meals in a dining room. Most people tend to eat better when they are dining with others than when they are left to eat alone. Nourishing snacks served during group or social activities can supplement an older person's intake and tend to be consumed more readily (Fig. 6.6).

Independent older adults can obtain low-cost, nutritious meals and participate in social activities at congregate meal centers funded by Nutrition Services under the Older Americans Act. The purpose of this act is to reduce hunger and food insecurity as well as to promote socialization and the health and well-being of the older population (Older Americans Act, 2020). Food insecurity is defined as the lack of consistent access to enough food to support an active, healthy life (Jackson et al., 2019). Food insecurity among older adults has more than doubled in the past 20 years and is higher among adults who are frail or economically disadvantaged.

> **QSEN Considerations: Patient-Centered Care**
>
> Collaboration between the health care providers, family, and patient is essential. Cultural considerations must be identified when providing guidance on dietary changes. If the food plan is contrary to the patient's cultural beliefs, their adherence will be decreased. Look for food choices that are healthier versions of familiar foods.

❖ NURSING PROCESS/CLINICAL JUDGMENT MODEL FOR RISK FOR ALTERED NUTRITION

Changes in BMI may be an early indication of true or potential nutritional problems in older adults. BMI can be determined using a chart (see Fig. 6.1) or an online calculation tool. The height used should reflect the person's current height, not the height from a younger age commonly reported by aging individuals and recorded in the health record. If the individual appears to be well proportioned and has a BMI within recommended norms, they are probably receiving adequate calories. A slow increase or decrease in BMI indicates an imbalance between caloric intake and energy expenditure. A decrease in activity with static caloric intake normally results in a gradual increase in BMI, whereas an increase in activity with consistent caloric intake normally results in a decrease in BMI. Nurses should investigate changes in intake or activity that could account for changes in BMI.

Adequate caloric intake is not enough. It is also essential that older adults obtain enough essential nutrients. To determine whether these nutritional needs are being met, nurses must collect additional data.

Table 6.3   Popular Foods of Various Cultural and Ethnic Groups

CULTURAL OR ETHNIC GROUP OR EATING PATTERN	FOOD GROUPS				
	GRAINS	VEGETABLE	FRUIT	MILK	MEAT AND BEANS
Mexican	Tortilla Taco shell Posole (corn soup) Rice Postres (pastries)[a]	*Other vegetables:* Chayote (Mexican squash) Jicama (root vegetable) Nopales (cactus leaves) Tomato Corn	Avocado Mango Papaya Plantano (cooking banana) Zapote (sweet, yellowish fruit)	Queso blanco (white Mexican cheese) Custard (1 cup = 1 cup milk serving) Leche (milk)	Chorizo (sausage)[a] Chicken, beef, goat, or pork Beans, dried, cooked
African American soul food (Southern-style cooking)	Biscuit Cornbread Grits, rice, macaroni, or noodles Hominy Crackers Hush puppies	*Dark green:* Collard, kale, mustard, or turnip greens *Orange:* Sweet potatoes *Other:* Okra Snap, pole (green), lima, and butter beans Turnips Summer squash (yellow or zucchini) Coleslaw	Blackberries Melons Muscadines (grapes) Peaches	Buttermilk	Pork (cured ham and uncured cuts), chicken, beef, fish Peas or beans (black-eyed, crowder, purple-hull, or cream)
Vegetarian	Whole grain bread Cereal, cooked or ready-to-eat Brown rice Whole grain pasta Bagel	All	All	Milk and cheese (lacto-vegetarians) Soy milk, calcium-fortified Soy cheese	Cooked dried beans or peas Tofu (soybean curd) or tempeh (fermented soy) Nuts or seeds Peanut butter Egg (ovovegetarians)
Italian	Breadsticks, breads Gnocchi (dumplings) Polenta (cornmeal mush) Risotto (creamy rice dish) Pastas	*Dark green:* Spinach *Other:* Artichoke Eggplant Mushrooms Marinara sauce	Berries Figs Pomegranate	Cheeses (mozzarella, Parmesan, Romano, ricotta, etc.) Gelato (Italian ice cream)	Veal or beef Fish Sausage Luncheon meats[a] Lentils Squid Almonds, pistachios
Chinese	Rice or millet Rice vermicelli (thin rice pasta) Cellophane noodles (bean thread) Steamed rolls Rice congee (soup) Rice sticks	*Other:* Pea pods Yard-long beans Baby corn Bamboo shoots Straw mushrooms Eggplant Bitter melon	Guava Lychee Persimmon Pummelo Kumquat Star fruit	Soy milk	Pork, fish, chicken Shrimp, crab, lobster Tofu or tempeh

Continued

Table 6.3 Popular Foods of Various Cultural and Ethnic Groups—cont'd

CULTURAL OR ETHNIC GROUP OR EATING PATTERN	FOOD GROUPS				
	GRAINS	VEGETABLE	FRUIT	MILK	MEAT AND BEANS
Indian (south Asia)	Breads: roti (chapati), naan, paratha, batura, puris, dosa, idli Rice or rice pilau Pooha, upma, sabudana	*Dark green:* Saag (mixed greens and potatoes) Spinach *Other:* Green peppers Cabbage Eggplant Green beans Methi (fenugreek leaves) Cucumbers Chutney or vegetable pickles	Mango Dates Raisins Melons Figs Fruit juices and nectars	Yogurt	Dal (lentils, mung beans, other dried beans) Beef, chicken (some are vegetarian)
Native American[b]	Bread Fry bread Wild rice or oats Popcorn Tortilla Mush (cooked cereal)	*Orange:* Winter squash (hard outer shell) *Starchy:* Potato Corn *Other:* Rhubarb	Berries Cherries Plums Apples Peaches		Wild game (deer, rabbit, elk, beaver) Lamb Salmon and other fish Clams, mussels Crab Duck or quail
Middle Eastern	Rice or bulgur (cracked wheat) Couscous Bread Pita	*Yellow:* Pumpkin or winter squash (butternut) *Other:* Peppers Tomatoes Grape leaves Cucumbers Fava beans Eggplant	Apricots Grapes Melons Dried fruits: dates, raisins, apricots	Yogurt	Lamb, goat, fish Almonds Pistachio nuts Dried beans and peas, lentils Eggs

[a]High in fat; use sparingly.
[b]Varies widely depending on tribal grouping and locale.
Modified from Lowdermilk, D. L., Perry, S. E., Cashion, M. C., Alden, K.R.A. (2016). *Maternity & women's health care* (11th ed.). St. Louis: Elsevier.

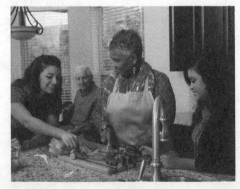

Fig. 6.6 Good nutrition at any age. (From Touhy, T. A., & Jett, K. F. [2020]. *Ebersole & Hess' toward healthy aging: Human needs and nursing response* [10th ed.]. St. Louis: Mosby.)

Laboratory values may help to support other observations. Review the hemoglobin level, hematocrit level, red blood cell (RBC) count, blood urea nitrogen (BUN) level, creatinine level, albumin level, and other nutritional indices to assess for specific nutritional deficiencies. These laboratory values do not routinely change with aging.

Hemoglobin is a complex protein-iron molecule responsible for the transport of oxygen and carbon dioxide in the bloodstream. If enough iron is not available, the hemoglobin level and the RBC count will fall below normal. Low hemoglobin levels may result from anemia or blood loss. Common forms of anemia, discussed in Chapter 3, include iron deficiency anemia and pernicious anemia. Iron deficiency anemia may result from blood loss. In older adults, this rarely takes the form of a massive hemorrhage, although a significant amount of blood may be lost from frequent nosebleeds or recent surgery. More common in older adults is subtle blood loss from bleeding gastric or duodenal ulcers, diverticulitis, tumors, or pathologic lower GI tract conditions.

A healthy person's blood glucose level changes throughout the day. It is low during periods of fasting but rises after a meal and then peaks approximately 30 to 60 minutes after eating. Within 3 hours, it returns to its normal range of 70 to 100 mg/dL. Individuals who have diabetes, are receiving steroid therapy or total parenteral nutrition, or are experiencing high levels of stress are likely to have difficulty in controlling their blood sugar levels.

Electrolyte imbalances may be due to inadequate electrolyte intake or excessive loss. Abnormal levels of calcium, sodium, and potassium are most commonly observed. Assess the diet to determine whether the patient has adequate intake of the necessary electrolytes. Medications that may cause electrolyte depletion should be considered. Vomiting, diarrhea, and gastric suction may contribute to electrolyte imbalances. Decreased kidney function also puts older adults at greater risk for problems with electrolytes.

◆ ASSESSMENT (DATA COLLECTION)

Recognize Cues
- Does the patient appear noticeably overweight or underweight?
- Does the patient's clothing appear to be abnormally loose or tight?
- What is the patient's current height and weight?
- Is the BMI within normal limits? (See Fig. 6.1.)
- Has their weight significantly increased or decreased in the past 3 to 6 months? If so, how much has it changed?
- For how long has this weight change been occurring?
- Is the weight change intentional?

◆ APPETITE CHANGES
- How does the patient describe their appetite?
- Has the patient noted changes in appetite? If yes, what are the possible reasons?
- How does food taste to the person?
- What do they like or dislike about the meals eaten (or served)?
- What would the person prefer to eat?
- Are there any cultural food preferences that are not being recognized?
- Are there any dietary restrictions? Are these understood?
- Does the patient complain of any of the following before, during, or after meals: nausea or hyperacidity?

Strange taste in the mouth? Eructation or flatulence? Chest pain?
- Do they show an unusual reaction to any foods (e.g., dairy products, nuts, and shellfish)?
- Is the patient depressed?

◆ NUTRITIONAL INTAKE
- Are the hemoglobin, hematocrit, and RBC parameters within normal limits?
- Has the blood sugar level been taken? Was this a fasting blood sugar? If taken at a nonfasting time, was it before or after a meal? How long before or after?
- Are electrolyte levels (e.g., sodium, potassium, and calcium) within normal limits?
- Is the serum albumin level within the normal range?
- Do they have a history of diabetes mellitus, anemia, or electrolyte imbalances?
- Are there any other observations, such as pallor, dizziness, or easy fatigue that may indicate anemia?
- Are there signs of hyperglycemia or hypoglycemia?
- Are there signs of electrolyte imbalance?
- Are the electrolyte levels within normal levels (especially potassium and sodium)?
- Is the patient on a prescribed meal plan that restricts sodium, calorie, sugar, or fluid intake? Are there any other dietary restrictions?
- Are calcium supplements being taken? Iron supplements?
- Does the patient drink milk and eat dairy products? (Is there lactose intolerance?)
- Are medications that can alter electrolyte levels (e.g., diuretics and cardiotonics) being taken?
- Have there been any recent episodes of vomiting?
- Are there certain foods that are never consumed? (Look particularly at meats or vegetables that may require more chewing, and compare this information with the patient's dental status.)
- What types of foods are consumed most? First? Not at all?
- What percentage of each type of food is actually consumed? How much food in general?
- What fluids are consumed during and between meals? Are the drink choices high in sugar?
- Are snacks or supplements consumed between meals? If so, are these prescribed?
- Are they sneaking snacks that are not allowed on a therapeutic meal plan?
- Does the patient receive any medications that could alter the taste of food? If so, when are these medications given?
- Are they receiving any drugs that require a restricted diet (e.g., monoamine oxidase inhibitors)?
- Is the patient receiving any medications that would affect appetite?

◆ SOCIAL AND CULTURAL FACTORS

- Do patients consume meals alone in their rooms or do they eat in the dining room?
- Do they socialize with others during meals?
- Does the family ever bring favorite foods from home?
- How do these favorite foods meet the individual's nutritional needs?
- Do the favorite foods violate any dietary restrictions (e.g., sodium or calorie restrictions)?

◆ HOME CARE OR DISCHARGE PLANNING

- What is the person's living situation: alone or with others?
- What are their health management and health maintenance abilities?
- If the person lives at home, is there adequate food in the house?
- Are there adequate financial resources to buy food?
- Can they get to a store to purchase food?
- Are there family or friends who will assist with going to the grocery store?
- Is the person's vision, stamina, and coordination good enough to enable the preparation of food?
- Do they become fatigued so easily that, by the time the food has been prepared, they are too tired to eat?
- Is there adequate equipment for refrigeration and cooking?
- Is the person aware of community resources for nutrition (e.g., Meals on Wheels and senior citizen center meal programs)?
- Do they person consume alcoholic beverages? How much? How often?

Box 6.2 lists risk factors for altered nutrition.

◆ DATA ANALYSIS/PROBLEM IDENTIFICATION

Analyze Cues and Prioritize Hypotheses: Problem statements for older adults with true or potential nutritional challenges include

Altered Nutrition
Inadequate Health Management
Potential for Altered Nutrition
Weight Above Recommended BMI
Weight Below Recommended BMI

◆ PLANNING

Generate Solutions: The nursing goals for older individuals diagnosed with some form of nutritional alteration are to (1) maintain BMI within normal limits, (2) obtain adequate nutrients to maintain healthy tissue, (3) identify internal and external cues that influence eating patterns, and (4) adhere to a prescribed therapeutic meal plan.

Box 6.2	Risk Factors Related to Altered Nutrition in Older Adults

- Metabolic disorders (diabetes, thyroid disturbances)
- Neurologic or musculoskeletal problems that interfere with food preparation, eating, or swallowing
- Disturbances of the gastrointestinal tract
- Inadequate resources to obtain food
- Loss of nutrients as a result of medications, hemorrhage, vomiting, or diarrhea
- Inadequate or excessive energy because of exercise patterns or disease processes
- Living alone
- Selective eating habits related to culture or habit
- Grief or other emotional difficulties

◆ IMPLEMENTATION

Take Action: The following nursing interventions should take place in hospitals or extended-care facilities:

1. **Assess the individual carefully to determine the causes of a problem** (e.g., dental problems, depression, cultural factors, and activity level). The types of approaches used must be tailored carefully based on the type and extent of the problem.

🌐 Cultural Considerations

Educating the Caregiver

- Because nursing assistants are typically assigned to assist older patients at mealtimes, they need to be aware of how their cultural biases influence what they communicate verbally and nonverbally.
- Home health aides who prepare meals for someone from another culture or ethnicity need additional education and training in how to prepare culturally appropriate meals that are acceptable to their aging patients.

2. **Schedule weekly weight checks.** Weight changes related to nutritional intake do not occur as rapidly as weight changes from fluid imbalance, when daily fluctuations often occur. Weighing an older person too often can cause frustration. Weekly weight checks are more reliable indicators of success. Weight checks should occur at the same time every week with the patient in similar clothing.
3. **Keep a dietary record of the amount, type, and frequency of food intake.** A careful dietary record helps determine problem areas, which helps nurses and dietitians to develop a therapeutic meal plan that is most likely to have the desired outcome. When possible, actively involve older adults in this record keeping.
4. **Explain the importance of nutrition to overall health or disease control.** Many older adults are already aware of normal nutritional needs. If the changes related to aging or disease require dietary modifications, it is important to carefully explain

the modifications and the reasons behind them. If older adults understand the rationale of dietary changes, they are more likely to cooperate with the new plan.

Culture and Food Preference

Examine your own cultural food beliefs and practices.
- What are your food preferences?
- What foods should be included in a healthy diet?
- Are there any foods that you must include or avoid in your daily diet?
- Are there foods that should not be combined or served together?
- Are any foods recommended or prohibited for special age groups across the lifespan?
- What foods are served for celebrations?
- What is your reaction when you are served foods that are culturally unfamiliar?

5. **Determine food likes and dislikes.** People tend to seek the things they like and avoid what they do not like. Food preferences should be considered when one is selecting nutritious yet acceptable foods for older adults. Many older individuals are set in their likes and dislikes and are unwilling to change.

6. **Monitor laboratory values.** RBC parameters, hematocrit, and hemoglobin values help in determining whether iron intake is adequate. Monitor electrolyte levels to verify that they are within normal limits. A low serum albumin level may indicate malnutrition.

7. **Assess the condition of the skin, hair, nails, and mucous membranes.** Signs of nutritional inadequacy can be detected by the observation of external surfaces. Cracks at the corner of the mouth, changes in the appearance of the tongue, loss or change in consistency of the hair, and slow tissue healing provide clues to nutritional status.

8. **Consult with the dietitian.** Dietitians are specially trained to assess nutritional needs, and they have in-depth knowledge of the nutritional value of foods. If an older adult has serious nutritional problems or medical conditions with nutritional implications, it is essential that the dietitian be actively involved in the nutritional plan of care.

9. **Institute measures to increase or decrease nutritional intake.** The following measures can be taken to increase the patient's intake:
   - *Provide a selection of nutritious foods.* Nurses should attempt to provide choices for those who are most in need of nutrients. Many institutions, particularly long-term care facilities, have limited menus for each meal. If the meal served does not appeal to older adults, they may eat very little, if anything. Most institutions have alternatives that do not appear on the menu, usually including simple foods such as eggs, cheese sandwiches, or soup. The older individual may not be aware of these choices or may not wish to cause additional work for the staff. It is your responsibility to explore these options with the individual.
   - *Limit excess intake of fluids during meals.* Too much low-nutritional fluid can create a sense of fullness that takes the place of more nutritious food.
   - *Supplement food intake with nutritious snacks.* It is often difficult for older adults to consume adequate calories and nutrients within the three routine daily meals. If allowed within the prescribed meal plan, offer nutritious snacks that are high in calories and nutrients (e.g., bananas, graham crackers, dried fruits, and milkshakes) between meals. Schedule these snacks so that they do not interfere with the person's appetite for regular meals. Many older individuals may stash snacks in a bedside stand or closet. Ensure that snacks are not stored where they could spoil or attract insects. Promptly discard any snacks that are not consumed promptly.
   - *Ask family members to bring the person's favorite dishes from home.* Family favorites are rarely on the menu in an institutional setting. Special favorites and foods connected with fond memories are most likely to be consumed. However, before the family brings food, be sure to discuss the care plan with them to ensure that these foods are permitted. It is frustrating for the family to make a special effort only to have the meal rejected at the institution.
   - *Serve meals in an attractive manner.* Foods that are well prepared and served in an attractive manner are more appealing. Taking plates and cups off the tray or setting a table with place mats and flowers can improve the appearance of a meal. Serving food on fancier dishes, using a special teacup, or attempting to reduce the institutional character of the meal can help to improve appetite. Foods should always be served fresh and at the appropriate temperature.
   - *Provide a social environment for meals by encouraging older adults to eat in the dining room.* The nature of meals tends to be social (Fig. 6.7). Older adults often have better appetites when they eat in groups than when they are isolated in their rooms. Alert individuals should be grouped with other alert people. Noise and distraction from confused patients can be disturbing and decrease appetite. Separate seating or rooms can provide the best environment, depending on the needs of the individual. Many older people living in institutional settings make friends with whom they prefer to sit. Older adults should have the opportunity to seek mutually agreeable seating arrangements in dining rooms without staff interference. If significant others are present at mealtime, they may want to eat with the older adult. Some institutions provide special trays for

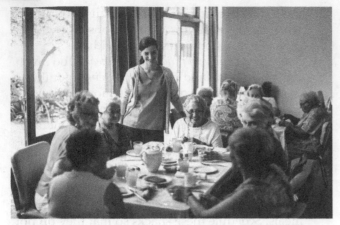

Fig. 6.7 Nursing home residents enjoy a pleasant meal in the dining room. (Copyright © istock.com/shapecharge.)

guests at a nominal charge and encourage family to share a meal in the dining room (Fig. 6.8).

- *Prepare food by opening cartons, buttering toast, or performing other activities that may be difficult for the older person.* Problems setting up food and opening cartons may lead older adults to skip or avoid certain foods. Many containers are difficult to open; even healthy young adults can have difficulty. Open these with minimal fuss so that the aging person does not feel helpless. Assist the individual to get ready to eat by cutting meats or buttering bread; perform these tasks unobtrusively.
- *Avoid hurrying the individual during meals.* If an older person eats too rapidly, indigestion, heartburn, or regurgitation may result. If rushed, many older individuals stop eating before they are truly satisfied. Avoid creating a rushed environment; allow older adults adequate time to eat at their own pace.

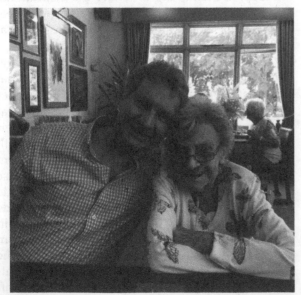

Fig. 6.8 Resident and son in the dining room. (From Williams, P. A. [2022]. *Fundamental concepts and skills for nursing* [6th ed.]. St. Louis: Mosby.)

- *Request a modification in the form of food served if the individual has difficulty chewing.* It may be difficult for older adults to chew some foods, particularly meats and undercooked vegetables. Chopped or ground meat is easier to eat for people with dentures or missing teeth. Notify the dietary department about these modifications and contact the primary care provider if an order is required. If the person is alert, avoid serving puréed foods because of their similarity to baby food (unless the individual has severe trouble chewing). If vegetables are routinely a problem, dicing or additional cooking may help. Contact the dietary department if problems are detected.
- *Provide assistive devices, such as plate sides, gripper spoons, and adaptive cups.* Older adults prefer to feed themselves whenever possible. Consult an occupational therapist regarding utensils to enable aging individuals to eat without undue difficulty (Fig. 6.9).
- *Provide oral hygiene before meals.* Normal decreases in taste and saliva production occur with aging. The decrease in saliva production reduces the normal cleansing mechanism within the mouth, leading to a buildup of debris and microorganisms that alters the taste of food and decreases the appetite. Good oral hygiene freshens the mouth and makes food taste better.
- *Assist the individual to the toilet before meals.* Many older adults have less awareness of their need to eliminate. If the need to eliminate occurs during mealtime, the person may become distracted and lose interest in the meal.
- *Provide supplemental tube feedings if ordered.* Supplemental gastric or nasogastric tube feedings are ordered for people who cannot consume adequate nutrients by eating. Administer these supplemental feedings only after the individual has had adequate opportunity for oral intake. Make all attempts at oral feeding before the supplement

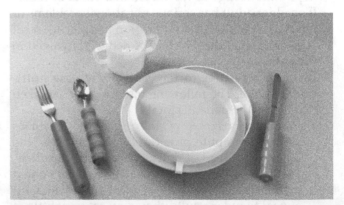

Fig. 6.9 Adaptive equipment. Clockwise from upper left: Two-handled cup with lid, plate with plate guard, utensils with splints, and utensils with enlarged handles. (From Cobbett, S., Perry A., Potter, P., Ostendorf, W., & Laplante, N. [2020]. *Canadian clinical nursing skills & techniques.* Toronto: Elsevier.)

is given. If **nasogastric** feeding is required, take all safety precautions, including checks for tube placement and positioning.

- *Time medication administration to avoid interfering with meals.* Some medications leave a bad taste in the mouth or otherwise upset the individual. If possible, these medications should be scheduled away from normal mealtimes. Other medications that may cause gastric upset may be best given after a meal.
- *Play relaxing music at mealtime.* Studies have shown that agitated behaviors decrease when quiet, melodic, peaceful music—with a steady tempo yet enough variety for interest—is played during mealtime.
- *Refer individuals for special counseling if emotional difficulties are interfering with appetite.* Individuals experiencing extreme grief or other emotional disturbances may require special nutritional approaches. Consult therapists trained to deal with eating disorders to determine the most effective interventions.

The following measures can be taken to decrease intake:

- *Assist in the selection of low-calorie foods.* Decreasing caloric intake helps the person lose weight. Foods high in bulk and low in calories, such as fresh fruits and vegetables, provide a sense of fullness without a feeling of deprivation. Involve the patient in the selection of food to find low-calorie options that seem appealing.
- *Include low-calorie snacks in the daily routine.* Snacks, such as diet beverages and unbuttered popcorn, are appropriate for older individuals unless there is a medical condition that contraindicates their inclusion. Check the sodium content of diet beverages if the person is on a sodium-restricted diet. Individuals with diverticulitis should avoid corn with husks. Planned snacks can prevent overeating at mealtimes and will help to avoid the consumption of high-calorie snacks.
- *Increase diversional activities to decrease snacking.* Some older and younger people snack when they are bored. Activities that occupy the hands and mind may reduce the urge to eat.
- *Encourage increased activity levels.* Increased activity helps burn calories. Walking is well tolerated by most older adults and is an effective means of weight reduction.

10. **Complete a thorough documentation of nutritional status, including assessment, interventions, referrals, and patient response.**

The following interventions should take place in the home:

1. **Assist the individual in obtaining resources, as by contacting Meals on Wheels, the Supplemental Nutrition Assistance Program (formerly known as food stamps), a housekeeper, or shopping services.**

Many community agencies and programs have been developed to help older adults meet their nutritional needs. Each community offers different services. Social workers often maintain directories of these agencies and can help older adults establish contact with them. Clarify and explain the available programs and provide the means for older adults or their families to contact the agencies.

Cultural Considerations

Dietary Practice

Older adults may have distinct dietary preferences based on their heritage. These preferences and practices vary widely across ethnic and cultural groups and are too extensive to enumerate in this text, but many informational sites are available on the internet. Website addresses for useful information and teaching materials include
- https://www.nal.usda.gov/sites/default/files/fnic_uploads//ethnic.pdf
- https://www.nal.usda.gov/fnic/older-individuals
- https://www.cdss.ca.gov/agedblinddisabled/res/VPTC2/9%20Food%20Nutrition%20and%20Preparation/Cultural_Consider_in_Nutrition_and_Food_Prep.pdf

2. **Involve the family in shopping and meal planning.** If the older adult is unable to meet nutritional needs without assistance, the family can often provide help. Older individuals are often too proud to ask for help, even from their own families. With help from a nurse, the older adult may be willing to accept assistance. Family members can provide transportation to the store, read labels, and assist with food preparation. Variety can be provided through meals prepared and then frozen in family members' homes for the older person's use. Teach family members about their loved one's relevant dietary restrictions so that meals do not endanger the person's well-being.
3. **Identify meal programs for the older adult that are available in the community.** Many communities offer meals at churches or senior citizen centers. These inexpensive meals are prepared by dietitians who are well versed in the nutritional needs of the aging population. These programs also provide opportunities for social interaction.
4. **Use any appropriate interventions that are used in the institutional setting.**

QSEN Considerations: Teamwork and Collaboration

Identifying resources is best done by involving all of the disciplines. If you are unaware of what community resources are available, discuss the needs with the dietary, social services, and other health care providers involved in the patient's care. Community services often go unused because the needy individuals are unaware that they exist.

❖ NURSING PROCESS/CLINICAL JUDGMENT MODEL FOR FLUID VOLUME AND POTENTIAL FOR ALTERED INTAKE

Fluid balance is not an everyday problem among healthy older adults. However, if there is a sudden change in fluid volume, an older person would be more likely than a younger one to experience significant problems. A seemingly minor problem with fluid balance can quickly become a serious concern in an aging individual. If not detected and treated, dehydration can easily become a significant problem, possibly resulting in death. People at the greatest risk for dehydration include children, people with chronic illnesses, and older adults with mobility issues who reside in nursing homes, are on multiple medications, or have dementia (Mayo Clinic, 2020).

Older adults have a lower percentage of extracellular body fluid (approximately 45% lower) than younger persons, even when they are well hydrated. Anything that restricts adequate intake of fluids or causes the body to lose water excessively can contribute to the risk for dehydration.

Common risk factors for dehydration include (1) decreased thirst sensation; (2) decreased effectiveness of the kidney at concentrating urine; (3) hormonal changes, including decreased aldosterone secretion and renin activity; (4) side effects of medications; (5) altered level of mentation; (6) altered levels of functional ability; and (7) fear of incontinence or pain, leading to inappropriate fluid restriction.

As at younger ages, older men have a higher percentage of body fluid than do older women. The decrease in the kidneys' concentrating abilities reduces the body's ability to adapt to changes in fluid volume. The aging body is less able to respond rapidly to such changes. When the many diseases that affect fluid balance are added to the normal changes of aging, the maintenance of fluid balance becomes a challenge.

Body fluids are distributed in two major compartments: intracellular and extracellular. Intracellular fluid is found within the cells and composes approximately two-thirds of the total body fluid. Extracellular fluid (ECF) makes up approximately one-third of total body fluid. ECFs are further classified as intravascular (plasma) and interstitial. ECF is in constant motion throughout the body, carrying nutrients to the cells and removing waste products. The movement of body fluids is affected by the levels of various electrolytes and proteins in the various compartments. Albumin, an important plasma protein responsible for maintaining adequate intravascular fluid levels, is often deficient, contributing to tissue edema and orthostatic hypotension.

Although the intracellular fluid is affected when the body experiences fluid imbalance, the ECF changes more rapidly and significantly. ECF deficit, or fluid volume deficit, can result in hypovolemia or dehydration.

ECF excess, or fluid volume overload, can result in hypervolemia (circulatory overload) or edema (excessive fluid in the interstitial spaces).

◆ ASSESSMENT (DATA COLLECTION)

Recognize Cues

- What are the vital signs (i.e., blood pressure, pulse, respiration, and temperature)?
- What is the appearance of the skin? Is it moist? Dry?
- Describe the skin turgor. Is the tongue dry and/or furrowed? What is the skin temperature?
- Do they individual complain of thirst? Weakness?
- Does the person manifest any mood changes, such as restlessness or confusion?
- What is the person's fluid intake per nursing shift? Per day?
- Do they receive fluids through a nonoral route, such as nasogastric feeding or intravenous fluid therapy?
- How does their fluid intake compare with the recommended intake?
- Is their weight changing rapidly? Is it increasing? Decreasing?
- Is the urine output within normal limits?
- What is the color and consistency of the urine? What is the urine specific gravity?
- Is there excessive fluid loss through hemorrhage, wound drains, gastric suction, diaphoresis, or mouth breathing?
- Do they complain about the fit of a finger ring, shoes, or clothing? Are any of these too loose or tight?
- Is the person receiving medication that is likely to cause fluid retention or loss?
- Are their laboratory values (hemoglobin, hematocrit, electrolytes, BUN, creatinine) within normal limits?

Boxes 6.3 and 6.4 list risks for fluid volume deficit or fluid volume overload in older adults.

Box 6.3	Risk Factors for Fluid Volume Deficit in Older Adults

- Altered swallow reflex (patients with stroke)
- Nausea and an unwillingness to eat or drink
- Acute emotional distress and decreased interest in personal needs
- Inability to obtain adequate fluids without assistance (bedridden patients)
- Altered cognition (Alzheimer disease or dementia) and lack of awareness of the need for fluids
- Draining wounds, open lesions, or pressure injuries
- Diuretic medications
- Kidney disease
- Tube feedings of low sodium preparations
- Diaphoresis
- Intermittent or persistent vomiting
- Intermittent or persistent diarrhea

| Box 6.4 | Risk Factors for Fluid Volume Overload in Older Adults |

- Increased fluid intake secondary to excess sodium intake, hyperglycemia, or medications
- Compulsive water drinking
- Decreased urine output secondary to kidney dysfunction
- Heart failure
- Insufficient protein intake or excessive protein loss
- Steroid therapy
- History of alcohol use disorder or liver disease
- Kidney disease

◆ FLUID VOLUME DEFICIT

Fluid volume deficit occurs when an individual has inadequate intake or excessive loss of fluids. Inadequate fluid intake can easily progress into dehydration, which, unless corrected, can result in death. A variety of conditions can contribute to fluid volume deficit in older adults. One author devised an interesting way of identifying older persons who have problems related to fluid intake. These persons were divided into three groups: (1) people who can drink but do not—that is, people who are capable of drinking but who do not know how much fluid is necessary or who have cognitive problems so that they forget to drink; (2) people who can drink but will not—they report that they never drank much or are afraid of incontinence; and (3) people who cannot drink, including those who lack the ability to access fluids independently or have impaired swallow or gag reflexes. Each group will benefit from different nursing approaches. The "don't drink" people need to be offered fluids frequently. The "can't drink" people require special approaches, including positioning, swallowing exercises, thickened fluids, and, if ordered, tube or parenteral feeding. The "won't drink" people need education regarding the importance of fluids and alternative techniques for dealing with incontinence.

Individuals experiencing fluid volume deficits are likely to manifest dry mucous membranes, thirst, decreased skin turgor (assessed over the sternum or on the inner thigh), rapid weight loss (greater than 3% of body weight), sunken eyes, weakness, and decreased volume or increased concentration of urine. Vital signs are likely to be affected. An increase in heart rate and decrease in pulse pressure can indicate a decrease in fluid volume. Hypotension, particularly orthostatic hypotension, is common. An increase in body temperature may indicate dehydration. Blood studies are likely to change with a fluid volume deficit. Hematocrit normally increases as the blood plasma volume decreases. Electrolyte levels, creatinine, and BUN are likely to be altered.

◆ FLUID VOLUME OVERLOAD

Fluid volume overload can result from the excessive intake or inadequate elimination of fluids. A primary indication of excessive fluid volume is edema, which may manifest as swelling of dependent extremities and increased abdominal girth. Pulmonary edema may result in shortness of breath, dyspnea, cough, gurgling sounds on respiration, and frothy sputum. Because fluid intake exceeds fluid output, weight gain can be sudden and dramatic. The amount of weight gained reflects the amount of fluid being retained. One liter of fluid results in a weight gain of 1 kilogram. Skin over edematous areas may appear shiny and taut. The amount and concentration of urine produced are likely to change with fluid volume overload. Hematocrit normally decreases as the blood plasma volume increases. Electrolyte levels, creatinine, and BUN are also likely to be altered. The individual may experience behavioral changes, including restlessness and anxiety.

◆ DATA ANALYSIS/PROBLEM IDENTIFICATION

Analyze Cues and Prioritize Hypotheses: Problem statements for older adults with fluid imbalances include
   Fluid Volume Deficit
   Fluid Volume Overload
   Potential for Altered Fluid Volume

◆ PLANNING

Generate Solutions: The goals for older individuals with or at risk for fluid volume deficit or fluid volume overload are to (1) manifest vital signs within normal limits or limits specified by the primary care provider; (2) demonstrate evidence of moist oral mucous membranes and good skin turgor without signs of edema; (3) maintain a stable weight within normal limits; (4) exhibit balanced fluid intake and output; (5) report no problems related to thirst or weakness; (6) exhibit blood studies (hemoglobin, hematocrit, serum electrolytes, BUN, creatinine) within normal limits; (7) verbalize an understanding of the recommended dietary and fluid intake; (8) demonstrate behaviors necessary to maintain appropriate fluid intake; (9) choose a selection of appropriate foods and fluids; (10) verbalize an understanding of prescribed medication(s), including the frequency and any precautions; and (11) verbalize signs and symptoms that should be reported to the primary care provider.

◆ IMPLEMENTATION

Take Action: The following nursing interventions should take place in hospitals or extended-care facilities:

1. **Complete a thorough assessment.** A thorough assessment is necessary to determine the presence and severity of any problems related to fluid intake.

2. **Monitor vital signs.** Vital signs can change in response to changes in fluid volume. Orthostatic hypotension is more common in individuals who have inadequate fluid intake than in those who have adequate fluid intake.

3. **Monitor intake and output (I&O).** Any individual with a true or potential alteration in fluid volume should be placed on I&O measurement. Calculate shift and daily totals and compare them with previous totals. It is essential that all individuals who provide care know how to measure I&O correctly. All caregivers should be aware that the individual is on I&O so that all fluids are recorded. If family members assist with feeding, teach them how to record fluid intake. Keep intake and output sheets in a convenient place to help ensure prompt recording. Too often, I&O monitoring is done carelessly and the data collected are meaningless.

4. **Monitor laboratory values.** Shifts in hemoglobin, hematocrit, BUN, creatinine, albumin, or electrolytes may precede or may be a result of fluid imbalance. Report changes promptly.

5. **Weigh the patient daily before breakfast.** Weights measured at a consistent time of day are the most accurate for comparison. Weigh the individual each day wearing the same clothing. Use the same scale consistently and check it for accuracy at regular intervals. Consistency is essential to eliminate errors in readings. Record daily weight checks promptly on the appropriate record.

6. **Measure changes in the girth of body parts, such as the legs and abdomen.** Take measurements at a consistent spot each day. If the person has no objections, make a small ink mark on the skin so that all staff will measure consistently. Retained fluid (edema) increases girth; fluid loss decreases girth.

7. **Maintain adequate fluid intake.** Implement the following measures to increase intake:
   - *Offer smaller amounts of fluid at more frequent intervals.* Small amounts of fluids taken frequently add up to significant fluid intake. Offer fluids, or remind the individual to take a drink, every 30 to 60 minutes throughout the day.
   - *Keep preferred beverages at the bedside.* Many older adults have distinct preferences regarding the type and temperature of beverages. Because people are most likely to consume foods and fluids that they like, determine the individual's preferences.
   - *Use smaller containers, such as medication cups or small juice glasses, when you are offering beverages.* Small beverage containers are less intimidating than large containers. An older person can often be coaxed into drinking 4 or 5 medicine cups of liquid (120 to 150 mL) far more easily than they can be persuaded to drink an entire glassful.
   - *Keep beverages easily available for individuals who are not in their rooms (e.g., in day rooms, activity rooms, lounges, or other common areas).* Low sodium, low sugar beverages are ideal because individuals on restricted meal plans can consume them. Making beverages easily accessible reminds and encourages individuals to drink. Passing a tray of assorted beverages around in an area where several older adults are congregated can encourage social interchange and provide mutual encouragement for many to participate even when they might otherwise have declined.
   - *Encourage the intake of foods with a high fluid content, such as fruits, vegetables, soups, and cooked cereals.* Significant amounts of fluid are contained in these foods. Individuals who have difficulty drinking liquids can obtain significant amounts of fluid through these alternative sources.
   - *Administer nasogastric, gastric, or parenteral fluids as ordered by the primary care provider.* Individuals who cannot drink adequate fluids may need supplemental fluids administered by other routes. All fluid given by the gastric or parenteral route must be counted as fluid intake.

Implement the following measures to decrease intake:
   - *Avoid keeping fluids at the bedside.* If fluids are easily available, older adults are likely to consume them too freely.
   - *Offer frequent oral hygiene.* When fluids are restricted, saliva production decreases and the mucous membranes feel dry and uncomfortable. Thick, tenacious secretions can build up in the mouth if not removed regularly. Provide frequent oral hygiene to compensate for the lack of oral fluids and diminished saliva production.
   - *Provide lozenges or hard candy.* Sucking on a hard lozenge stimulates the release of saliva. Offer candy and lozenges only to those who are alert enough not to swallow or choke on them. Verify that there is no dietary prohibition to additional sugar intake.
   - *Plan a schedule to distribute limited fluids throughout the day.* Plan the total fluid volume intake for the day within the prescribed limitations. Then divide the total into appropriate amounts spaced throughout the day. For example, a 600-mL restriction could be divided into 12 servings of 50 mL offered at hourly intervals between 8 AM and 8 PM. This prevents the person from consuming all of the allowance too early in the day and then having to withstand long periods of thirst or to exceed prescribed limits.
   - *Limit the quantity of foods that are high in fluid content.* Fluids contained in solid foods can contribute to excessive fluid volume and edema. Foods such as fresh fruits and vegetables have a high fluid content, whereas foods such as breads,

dried fruits, and cooked meats have a lower fluid content.

8. **Administer medications as ordered by the primary care provider.** Many individuals with alterations in fluid balance receive medication to prevent or correct this problem. Nurses must ensure that these medications are given on time and that the patient's response to the medications is assessed.

9. **Refer to the dietitian, if appropriate.** Individuals with medical conditions likely to cause excessive fluid loss or fluid retention need detailed and specific diet modifications and instructions, which are best provided by a specialist. Nurses should reinforce this teaching.

10. **Provide appropriate skin care.** Persons with fluid volume overload or fluid volume deficit require careful hygiene. Both dry, fragile skin and edematous tissue are highly susceptible to breakdown. The person's physical position should be changed frequently. Take care when moving the patient or handling the skin.

11. **Report and document significant findings promptly.** The signs and symptoms of fluid volume problems rarely occur suddenly. Rather, these problems tend to develop over time. Nurses must be sure that all changes are documented and reported promptly to the charge nurse and/or the primary care provider.

> ### 💡 QSEN Considerations: Safety
>
> Dehydration has been tied to both urinary tract infections (UTIs) and delirium. Older adults who present with recent onset confusion or other cognitive changes should be assessed for dehydration and UTIs. Delirium can mimic dementia but has a more rapid onset and is treatable. If treated, the confusion will resolve and the patient will return to their previous cognitive level. Untreated delirium can progress to stupor, coma, and death.

The following interventions should take place in the home:

1. **Complete a thorough assessment.** A thorough assessment is necessary to determine the presence and severity of any problems. It may be necessary to bring a scale, measuring tape, and sphygmomanometer to the home to complete a good assessment.

2. **Teach the individual and their family members how to monitor fluid intake.** Both the individual and family must be aware of methods used to keep track of fluid intake and loss. Teach the family to measure fluid intake using common household containers, and demonstrate how to read cartons for fluid content. It may be easier for laypersons to learn to keep track of fluid intake in ounces rather than in milliliters. Provide a specimen pan or urinal to measure output.

3. **Promote wellness by reviewing the prescribed dietary and fluid intake with the individual.** It is important that the individual understand the reason for consuming or avoiding certain foods and fluids.

The importance of adequate fluid intake, particularly during hot weather, should be stressed. Advise individuals with no acute problems to consume a minimum of 64 ounces (2000 mL) of fluid each day. Those who live alone may need reminders to consume this amount. Fluid intake reminders are particularly important during hot weather, when increased amounts of fluid are lost through perspiration.

4. **Explain methods of increasing or decreasing fluid intake.** The following measures can be taken to increase intake:
   - *Develop a schedule for fluid intake.* A planned schedule using a time list or clock helps remind older persons, as well as their spouses or caregivers, to consume fluids at regular times. It also helps them keep track of how much fluid is being consumed. Encourage them to check off or write amounts next to the times, so that they will be aware of making progress.
   - *Post signs in the kitchen and other rooms reminding the individual to drink.* Reminders help older adults remember the importance of drinking adequate amounts of fluid.
   - *Encourage friends and family to visit and share a beverage with the individual.* Social contact and sharing are natural over a cup of coffee, soda, juice, or other beverage. This is a pleasant way to promote social interaction and also encourage fluid intake.
   - *Encourage the use of fruit or other foods with a high fluid content.*

   The following measures can be taken to decrease intake:
   - Develop a schedule that spreads the limited amount of fluid throughout the day.
   - Encourage the use of hard candy or lozenges to keep the mouth moist.
   - Recommend frequent oral hygiene.
   - Discuss the importance of avoiding foods with high fluid content.

5. **Discuss signs and symptoms that should be reported promptly to the primary care provider.** Fluid imbalance may result in hospitalization and serious complications. This is particularly important for older individuals who are receiving medications that influence fluid balance. The individual should know what signs and symptoms are important. A written list of symptoms should be given to the individual and their significant others.

6. **Use any appropriate interventions that are used in the institutional setting.**

❖ NURSING PROCESS/CLINICAL JUDGMENT MODEL FOR ALTERED SWALLOWING ABILITY

Chewing and swallowing are complex processes that involve coordinated movements of the oral cavity, tongue, pharynx, larynx, and esophagus. An individual who is unable to coordinate these movements experiences difficulty swallowing, or dysphagia. Dysphagia is often a result of reduced muscle tone in the pharynx and esophagus, laxity of the ligaments and the age-related slowing of swallowing, infection, scar tissue, cancer, or dental conditions. Problems related to eating and particularly those related to swallowing are serious because they can lead to dehydration, malnutrition, or aspiration pneumonia. It is reported that 40% to 60% of older adults in long-term care facilities have dysphagia (Tagliaferri, 2019).

Swallowing problems are commonly a result of neurologic damage, or trauma that affects the cranial nerves or facial muscles; they may also be related to diseases such as Parkinson disease, Alzheimer disease, or stroke. Dysphagia can even be a sign of an emergency, such as the occurrence of an aortic aneurysm (Dejaeger et al., 2020). Recent research indicates that heart failure, diabetes, and general frailty due to age place older adults at risk for altered swallowing ability. People with an altered level of consciousness or severe fatigue are also at risk. Some individuals who are capable of swallowing may be hesitant to do so because of a lack of desire to eat or because of fear after an episode of choking, thus affecting social interactions at mealtime and decreasing the enjoyment of eating. Any of these issues can have a negative impact on nutrition.

 QSEN Considerations: Safety

Older individuals experiencing dysphagia should always be carefully assessed for possible aspiration while eating. Older adult patients with limited mobility may not demonstrate common signs of choking. When you are feeding patients with dysphagia, make sure that each bite is swallowed before offering the next bite.

◆ ASSESSMENT (DATA COLLECTION)

Recognize Cues
- Is there any history of stroke or other neurologic disease that could interfere with chewing or swallowing?
- Is the individual alert and able to follow directions?
- Is any facial drooping or difficulty chewing observed?
- Do the caregivers observe or report difficulty swallowing?
- Does the individual complain of something sticking in the throat?
- Is there coughing, choking, or drooling when eating?
- Do they complain of hoarseness or dry throat?
- Is there food stored in the person's cheek pockets?
- Is the gag reflex weak or absent?
- Can they close their lips?
- Are there problems with any particular foods or fluids?

Box 6.5 lists risk factors associated with altered swallowing ability in older adults.

Box 6.5 Risk Factors for Altered Swallowing Ability in Older Adults

- Neurologic problems resulting in paralysis or weakness of the face, mouth, or throat
- Altered level of consciousness, awareness, or sensation
- Mechanical devices, such as a tracheostomy tube or nasogastric tube
- A narrowing or obstruction of the pharynx or esophagus
- Excessive fatigue

◆ DATA ANALYSIS/PROBLEM IDENTIFICATION

Analyze Cues and Prioritize Hypotheses: Problem statement for older adults with difficulties in swallowing:
    Altered Swallowing Ability

◆ PLANNING

Generate Solutions: The patient goals for an older individual diagnosed with altered swallowing ability are to (1) pass food from mouth to the stomach without aspiration, (2) maintain adequate nutrition and hydration, and (3) maintain or achieve an appropriate BMI.

◆ IMPLEMENTATION

Take Action: The following nursing interventions should take place in hospitals or extended-care facilities:
1. **Assess the individual to determine any unique problems and needs.** Not all swallowing disorders are the same. Develop different approaches based on the individual's specific problems and needs.
2. **Consult with the speech therapist, occupational therapist, and dietitian to develop a dysphagia program.** These specialists have unique knowledge of the best techniques and methods for dealing with swallowing disorders. It is important for nurses to use their expertise when developing a feeding plan. Use special adaptive equipment (e.g., special spoons) to deliver food to the back of the throat, where it is more easily swallowed. You may also use special cups that allow the older individual to drink without tipping the head back. Teach exercises designed to strengthen the tongue to improve swallowing ability.
3. **Verify that dentures fit properly and maintain good oral hygiene.** Improperly fitted dentures can slip in the mouth, causing increased problems with swallowing. A dentist should be consulted if this is the problem. Provide good oral hygiene to enhance the appetite and remove any old food or foreign materials that may interfere with swallowing.
4. **Position the person with the head upright and chin flexed slightly forward to facilitate swallowing. Help with head control if necessary.**

Whenever possible, assist the older adult to a chair for meals. If the patient must remain in bed, raise the head of the bed as high as possible. Ensure that the head is not in malposition, as this can interfere with swallowing ability. Excessive flexion or hyperextension of the neck can interfere with the passage of food through the pharynx and into the esophagus. If a pillow is used for positioning, it should be placed behind the shoulder, not behind the head, which could interfere with swallowing. Individuals with swallowing problems should remain seated upright for at least 30 minutes after a meal to reduce the likelihood of aspiration.

5. **Encourage rest periods before meals.** Eating requires a great deal of effort from individuals with swallowing disorders. Providing rest before meals helps increase the amount of energy and strength available.

6. **Allow adequate time for meals.** Hurrying a meal increases the risk of aspiration. Older adults with swallowing difficulties are even more likely to have problems if they try to swallow too quickly.

7. **Start with small amounts of food and thickened fluids.** Provide individuals with swallowing difficulties a moderate amount of food (approximately 15 to 20 mL) at a time. This amount is enough for the individual to detect the presence of food, but it is not so much that it would be difficult to swallow. Individuals with swallowing disorders have a great deal of difficulty in controlling and swallowing liquids. Foods with a high fluid content are necessary to ensure adequate fluid intake. Many facilities add a thickening agent to flavored beverages to turn them into a gelatinous form that is more easily managed by persons with altered swallowing ability. Water is usually not given to individuals with swallowing disorders. Because water has no texture or taste, the individual may not be aware of its presence in the mouth and may aspirate it.

8. **Place foods into the unaffected or stronger side of the mouth.** The individual will be able to detect food more easily on the unaffected or stronger side.

9. **Present foods in an appealing manner.** The appearance of food affects the appetite. Even if its consistency is altered (ground or puréed), food should be served as pleasantly as possible. Do not stir foods together in an unappealing mixture. Keep each food identifiable, and serve the foods to the individual in the preferred order.

10. **Select foods based on taste, texture, temperature, and fluid content.** People with swallowing disorders may have altered senses of taste, texture, and temperature. Foods that have distinct flavors and textures, such as applesauce, are accepted more readily than are nondescript, puréed foods. Seasonings and spices can be used to enhance the flavor of many foods. The food should have some

consistency; however, foods that require chewing are not advised. Always serve food at a temperature that will not burn the mucous membranes of the mouth. Many individuals with swallowing disorders cannot sense temperature adequately. A variety of temperatures will make the person more aware of the presence of food.

11. **Make sure that the person's lips are closed by applying slight pressure or stroking.** It is almost impossible to swallow when the lips are open. To prevent aspiration, it may be necessary to close their lips mechanically.

12. **Stimulate swallowing by stroking the side of the neck, and support the weakened side if appropriate.** Stroking the neck stimulates the urge to swallow. Supporting the muscles of the affected side of the throat can enhance swallowing.

13. **Give frequent verbal cues.** Individuals with swallowing difficulties may not remember to swallow when food is in the mouth. Some are able to swallow if they are reminded to do so.

14. **Reduce distractions.** The process of eating requires the full attention of the affected individual and the caregiver. Distractions, such as television or visitors, may interfere with concentration and lead to increased problems.

15. **Keep suction equipment available in case of problems.** When giving oral feedings to an individual with a swallowing disorder, it is wise to keep a suction apparatus nearby. Most of these people also have problems with other protective reflexes, such as the gag and cough reflexes. They may be unable to clear an airway obstruction. Keep the suction machine readily available, because delay may lead to aspiration or more serious consequences.

16. **Provide oral hygiene before and after feedings.** Individuals with swallowing disorders are likely to retain food particles in the mouth, leading to altered taste. Good oral hygiene before and after meals removes debris and tenacious saliva and might improve an individual's appetite.

17. **Administer tube feedings as ordered by the primary care provider to individuals who are unable to achieve adequate oral intake.** Some individuals with swallowing disorders may not be able to eat enough to meet their nutritional needs. These individuals require feeding through either a nasogastric or gastric feeding tube. Tube feedings may be used to meet the total nutritional needs of older adults, or they may be given as a supplement for those who need additional fluid or calories. If the feeding is supplemental, administer it after the individual has had the opportunity to take as much oral nutrition as possible. These feedings are not meant as a time saving method to replace oral feedings. Use care to verify placement and absorption of nutrients before each feeding is given. Use medical asepsis in handling all nutrients and feeding

equipment to reduce the risk for contamination. Irrigation sets should be replaced every 24 hours. Use any appropriate interventions that are used in the institutional setting in the home.

❖ NURSING PROCESS/CLINICAL JUDGMENT MODEL FOR ASPIRATION RISK

Aspiration, the inhalation of solids or liquids into the upper respiratory tract, is a serious problem for many infirm older adults. Symptoms of aspiration include (1) the sudden appearance of severe coughing or cyanosis associated with eating or drinking; (2) voice changes; and (3) signs of aspiration pneumonia, including increased respiratory rate, abnormal lung sounds, fever, and behavioral changes, such as confusion or delirium. Aspiration risk is increased with dysphagia and with gastroesophageal reflux problems. Symptoms are discussed in Chapter 3.

◆ ASSESSMENT (DATA COLLECTION)

Recognize Cues

- Are the cough and gag reflexes intact?
- Is there a reduced level of consciousness?
- Does the person have a tracheostomy?
- Is the person in the supine position during feedings?
- Are feedings or medications administered through a gastric tube?
- Are there signs of abdominal distention?
- Are the stomach contents more than 150 mL before a scheduled feeding?
- Does the person breathe noisily?
- Does he or she have a productive cough? What is the consistency of the sputum?
- Are the person's pulse and respiratory rates elevated?
  Box 6.6 lists risk factors for aspiration in older adults.

◆ DATA ANALYSIS/PROBLEM IDENTIFICATION

Analyze Cues and Prioritize Hypotheses: Problem statement for older adults who are at risk for aspiration
Aspiration Risk

Box 6.6	Risk Factors for Aspiration Risk in Older Adults

- Neurologic problems, particularly those that affect the cough and/or gag reflexes
- Reduced level of consciousness
- Continuous supine positioning
- Tracheostomy tubes
- Gastric tubes
- Decreased gastric motility; excessive amounts of residual gastric contents or gas

◆ PLANNING

Generate Solutions: The patient goals for an older individual with a risk of aspiration are to (1) remain free from episodes of aspiration and (2) maintain clear, noiseless breath sounds.

◆ IMPLEMENTATION

Take Action: The following nursing interventions should take place in hospitals or extended-care facilities:

1. **Position the person appropriately.** The person should be positioned in a Fowler or semi-Fowler position before both oral and gastric tube feedings. This position should be maintained for at least 30 to 45 minutes after each feeding. Elevating the head allows solutions to flow into the stomach and reduces the chance of regurgitation. If the person must remain flat in bed, a side-lying position is better than a supine position.
2. **Assess for stomach distention.** Stomach distention can be an indication of slow gastric emptying, which can lead to regurgitation and aspiration. Monitor carefully, and report continued complaints of gastric fullness or excessive stomach gas. If these problems persist, the amount or type of feeding may need to be changed.
3. **Avoid feeding too rapidly.** Rapid ingestion of food increases the likelihood of regurgitation and aspiration. Offer oral nourishment slowly and allow adequate time for chewing and swallowing.
4. **Avoid liquids and puréed foods.** Semisolid foods are less likely to be aspirated than are liquids or puréed foods. The consistency of liquids can be modified with commercial preparations, which are available in most dietary departments.
5. **Monitor respiratory sounds and respiratory rate, and observe the amount and type of sputum produced.** Aspiration of food or fluids may result in coughing, choking, dyspnea, and respiratory distress. Increased amounts of frothy sputum are often noted. Elevated heart and respiratory rates (tachycardia and tachypnea) are usually present with aspiration.
6. **Keep suction equipment available.** Aspiration can result in respiratory distress. Keep suction equipment on hand whenever an individual with aspiration risk is being fed.
7. **Consult with specialists, such as speech therapists and dietitians.** A team approach to swallowing disorders and potential aspiration can help reduce the likelihood of problems. Speech therapists often have special training in swallowing disorders and can suggest modifications in feeding practices. Dietitians are specially trained to meet the needs of these individuals and can provide a nutritionally sound meal plan in a form modified to meet the needs of the person with aspiration risk.

The following interventions should be implemented for persons receiving tube feedings:

1. **Check placement of the nasogastric tube using the approved method.** Nasogastric tubes can become displaced into the lungs, resulting in aspiration. Tube placement should be verified before any solution is instilled. This should be done routinely according to institutional policy. If available, x-ray confirmation is recommended (Williams, 2022).

2. **Aspirate stomach contents, measure and replace before starting intermittent feeding.** Stomach distention, which is related to decreased gastric emptying time, increases the risk for regurgitation and aspiration. If possible, measure the volume of stomach contents before beginning intermittent tube feedings. This may not be possible if a small-bore tube is used because the negative pressure applied will simply cause the tube to collapse on itself, resulting in the possibly false impression that no residual is present. Follow facility policy for withholding the feeding if excessive residual volume is present. Stomach contents should be replaced through the tube to maintain electrolyte balance.

3. **Maintain clean technique for all feeding tubes, equipment, and formula.** Bacterial contamination of formula increases over time and when breaks in clean technique occur. Be sure to wash your hands before pouring formula or checking tube placement.

Wash the top of the formula can before opening. Cleanse ports before and after manipulation. Change feeding bags and irrigation sets according to agency policy, or at least every 24 hours. Clean equipment between uses and store properly. Avoid use of food dyes, which have been shown to increase the risk for contamination and even death.

The following interventions should take place in the home:

1. **Explain safety precautions to the individual and the family or caregiver.** Explain the importance of proper positioning, desired rate of feeding, and modifications to food consistency that reduce the likelihood of aspiration.

2. **Encourage enrollment in a home safety course that includes the Heimlich maneuver and cardiopulmonary resuscitation.** Aspiration of solids can sometimes be relieved by the use of the Heimlich maneuver. Respiratory distress related to aspiration may require other emergency interventions until medical assistance arrives. The family should be prepared to provide these lifesaving measures if they plan to provide care in the home.

3. **Use any appropriate interventions that are used in the institutional setting** (Nursing Care Plan 6.1).

✴ Nursing Care Plan 6.1   Aspiration Risk

Mr. Thomas, 74 years old, has recently had a stroke. His level of consciousness is decreased, he has no gag reflex, and the left side of his face shows some paralysis. His primary care provider has ordered intermittent feedings (every 4 hours) of a commercial nutrient solution through a nasogastric tube.

PROBLEM STATEMENT

Aspiration Risk

SUPPORTING ASSESSMENT DATA

- Decreased level of consciousness
- Facial paralysis
- Absence of gag reflex

PATIENT GOALS/OUTCOMES IDENTIFICATION

Mr. Thomas will remain free from episodes of aspiration.

NURSING INTERVENTIONS/IMPLEMENTATION

1. Assess for signs of stomach distention, cough, or excessive respiratory secretions during each feeding.
2. Position Mr. Thomas in Fowler position before feeding.
3. Verify placement of nasogastric tube using approved methods before each feeding.
4. Measure stomach contents before beginning feeding. Follow facility policy for withholding the feeding if excessive residual volume is present.
5. Return stomach contents through nasogastric tube.
6. Allow adequate time (approximately 30 minutes) for instillation of 250 mL.
7. Keep head elevated for 30 to 45 minutes after feeding.
8. Keep suction equipment at the bedside. Check at regular intervals to verify that equipment is functioning properly.

EVALUATION

Physical assessment reveals no signs of stomach distention. Residual stomach contents before feedings range from 25 to 70 mL. No episodes of coughing or silent tearing are noted with feedings. Lungs are clear on auscultation. Continue plan of care.

APPLYING CLINICAL JUDGMENT

The patient's family thinks that the feeding tube is unnecessary and that Mr. Thomas should be offered food and fluids by mouth.

1. How would you explain the risks to them?
2. How would you modify the plan of care if continuous feedings were ordered?

Get Ready for the Next Generation NCLEX® Examination!

Key Points

- Nutritional and fluid problems are common in the aging population.
- Knowledge of a wide range of facts and concepts about nutrition and the nutritional needs of older adults is important. This text addresses the basics only. For greater understanding, consult texts that specialize in geriatric nutrition.
- A wide range of factors increases the risk for malnutrition in the older adult population. Take these into account when assessing the nutritional status of older adults.
- Sensory or cognitive changes, weakness, activity intolerance, and loss of interest in food as a result of depression or other emotional disturbances contribute to these problems.
- Signs and symptoms of poor nutrition—such as confusion, weight loss, lethargy, and light-headedness—may be mistakenly attributed to an illness or medication reaction rather than to the underlying nutritional problem.
- Indicators of nutritional and metabolic alteration are most commonly observed in the skin, mucous membranes, hair, and nails. Assessment of these structures can tell nurses a great deal about an older adult's nutritional status and fluid balance.
- Good nutrition has been shown to be one of the most significant factors in the prevention of skin breakdown.
- Nurses play an important role in the recognition of nutritional and fluid balance problems, identification of contributing factors, and development of an appropriate plan of care.
- Nurses should recognize the importance of consultation with the dietitian and referral to community agencies that can provide nutritional support.

Additional Learning Resources

SG Go to your Evolve website at http://evolve.elsevier.com/Williams/geriatric for the additional online resources.

🌐 Online Resources

- Dietary reference intakes (DRIs): recommended intakes for individuals: https://www.nal.usda.gov/fnic/dri-tables-and-application-reports
- DRI Calculator for Healthcare Professionals: https://www.nal.usda.gov/fnic/dri-calculator/
- Older adult nutrition programs: Senior Farmers' Market Nutrition Program (SFMNP), Elderly Nutrition Program: www.nutrition.gov/food-assistance-programs/elderly-nutrition-program
- MyPlate for Older Adults: http://hnrca.tufts.edu/myplate/
- DGA Dietary Guidelines for Americans 2020-2025: https://www.dietaryguidelines.gov/sites/default/files/2020-12/Dietary_Guidelines_for_Americans_2020-2025.pdf

Review Questions for the Next Generation NCLEX® Examination

1. An older adult who resides in a long-term care facility has been refusing food and fluids for 2 days. He repeatedly says, "Leave me alone!" What is the best initial nursing intervention?
   a. Obtain an order from the primary care provider to insert a feeding tube.
   b. Assess to identify changes in the patient's physical or emotional status.
   c. Discuss the use of high nutrient supplemental shakes with the dietitian.
   d. Ask the family for assistance with feeding.

2. An older woman recently moved to the United States from the Middle East. She does not like to drink cow's milk or eat most cheeses. What is a culturally acceptable food that would best help meet her need for calcium?
   a. Yogurt
   b. Oranges
   c. Sardines
   d. Tofu

3. An older man who lives alone is placed on a sodium restricted meal plan because of heart failure. He asks you to help him make good dietary choices. Which foods should he avoid? *(Select all that apply.)*
   a. Canned tomato soup
   b. Deli bologna or ham
   c. Grilled steak
   d. Frozen spaghetti dinner
   e. Pancakes
   f. Boiled eggs

4. An 85-year-old female is being seen by her primary care provider for her annual physical. The health care provider expresses concern over an unintentional weight loss of 12 pounds and gives a probable diagnosis of malnutrition. Which other symptoms and lab result(s) would support this diagnosis? *(Select all that apply.)*
   a. Hemoglobin 10.2 g/dL
   b. Hematocrit 45%
   c. Creatinine 0.3 mg/dL
   d. Albumin 3.6 mg/dL
   e. Calcium 9.5 mg/dL
   f. Folic acid 5 mg/dL
   g. Thin, dry skin
   h. Change in balance
   i. Tearfulness
   j. Lethargy

5. An older adult is taking furosemide to reduce edema. Dietary teaching would best include increasing the intake of which food(s)? *(Select all that apply.)*
   a. Bananas
   b. Apple juice
   c. Tomatoes
   d. Oranges
   e. Grapes
   f. Milk

6. An older nursing home resident has poor skin turgor, dry mucous membranes, and very concentrated urine. Identify appropriate direction that would be given to the nursing assistant. *(Select all that apply.)*

   a. Make sure the resident eats everything served at each meal.

   b. Offer smaller amounts of fluids every hour during the day.

   c. Provide good oral hygiene.

   d. Identify the beverages that the resident prefers.

   e. Keep a large container of iced water in the resident's room.

   f. Give the resident hard candy to suck on.

REFERENCES

Ashaolu, T. J. (2020). Immune boosting functional foods and their mechanisms: A critical evaluation of probiotics and prebiotics, *Biomedicine & Pharmacotherapy*, Volume 130, 2020, 110625. https://doi.org/10.1016/j.biopha.2020.110625

Atri, A. (2019). The Alzheimer's disease clinical spectrum. *Medical Clinics of North America*, 130(2), 263–293.

Chew, S. T. H., Tan, N. C., Cheong, M., Oliver, J., Baggs, G., Choe, Y., ... Tey, S. L. (2020). Impact of specialized oral nutritional supplement on clinical, nutritional, and functional outcomes: A randomized, placebo-controlled trial in community-dwelling older adults at risk of malnutrition. *Clinical Nutrition*, S0261-5614(20), 30543–30544. doi: 10.1016/j.clnu.2020.10.015. Epub ahead of printPMID: 33268143.

Dejaeger, M., Lormans, M., Dejaeger, E., & Fagard, K. (2020). Case report: An aortic aneurysm as cause of pseudoachalasia. *BMC Gastroenterology*, 20(63). https://doi.org/10.1186/s12876-020-01198-y

Isanejad, M., Sirola, J., Rikkonen, T., Mursu, J., Kröger, H., Qazi, S. L., & Erkkilä, A. T. (2020). Higher protein intake is associated with a lower likelihood of frailty among older women: Kuopio OSTPRE-fracture prevention study. *European Journal of Nutrition*, 59(3), 1181–1189. doi: 10.1007/s00394-019-01978-7. Epub 2019 May 7. PMID: 31065844; PMCID: PMC7098934.

Jackson, J. A., Branscum, A., Tang, A., & Smit, E. (2019). Food insecurity and physical functioning limitations among older U.S. adults. *Preventive Medicine Reports*, 18(14), 100829. doi: 10.1016/j.pmedr.2019.100829 PMID: 30949424; PMCID: PMC6430734.

O'Keeffe, M., Kelly, M., O'Herlihy, E., O'Toole, P. W., Kearney, P. M., Timmons, S., ... O'Connor, E. M. (2019). MaNuEL consortium. Potentially modifiable determinants of malnutrition in older adults: A systematic review. *Clinical Nutrition*, 38(6), 2477–2498. doi: 10.1016/j.clnu.2018.12.007. Epub 2018 Dec 11. PMID: 30685297.

Older Americans Act: Nutritional Services Program, updated 2020. Downloaded from https://crsreports.congress.gov/product/pdf/IF/IF10633

Kougias, D. G., Das, T., Perez, A. B., & Pereira, S. L. (2018). A role for nutritional intervention in addressing the aging neuromuscular junction. *Nutrition Research*, 17(53), 1–14.

Magnuson, A., Sattar, S., Nightingale, G., Saracino, R., Skonecki, E., & Trevino, K. M. (2019). A practical guide to geriatric syndromes in older adults with cancer: A focus on falls, cognition, polypharmacy, and depression. *American Society of Clinical Oncology Educational Book*, 39, e96–e109. doi: 10.1200/EDBK_237641. Epub 2019 May 17. PMID: 31099668.

Mayo Clinic. (2020). Dehydration. https://www.mayoclinic.org/diseases-conditions/dehydration/symptoms-causes/syc-20354086

Mullin, G. E., Fan, L., Sulo, S., & Partridge, J. (2019). The association between oral nutritional supplements and 30-day hospital readmissions of malnourished patients at a US academic medical center. *Journal of the Academy of Nutrition and Dietetics*, 119(7), 1168–1175. doi: 10.1016/j.jand.2019.01.014. Epub 2019 Apr 4. PMID: 30954446.

Scott, D. M., Petras, H., Kalu, N., Cain, G. E., Johnson, D. B., Sloboda, Z, ... Taylor, R. E. (2020). Implementation of screening, brief intervention, and referral for treatment in the aging network of care to prevent alcohol, recreational drug, and prescription medication misuse. *Preventive Science*, 21(7), 972–978. doi: 10.1007/s11121-020-01154-y. PMID: 32803463; PMCID: PMC7429194.

Tagliaferri, S., Lauretani, F., Pelá, G., Meschi, T., & Maggio, M. (2019). The risk of dysphagia is associated with malnutrition and poor functional outcomes in a large population of outpatient older individuals. *Clinical Nutrition*, 38(6), 2684–2689. doi: 10.1016/j.clnu.2018.11.022. Epub 2018 Nov 30. PMID: 30583964.

U.S. Department of Agriculture (USDA). (2021). *Dietary guidelines for Americans, 2020-2025* (9th edition). U.S: Government Printing Office. https://www.dietaryguidelines.gov/sites/default/files/2020-12/Dietary_Guidelines_for_Americans_2020-2025.pdf

Williams, P. A. (2022). *Fundamental concepts and skills for nursing*. St. Louis: Elsevier.

Objectives

1. Identify factors that increase the risk of medication-related problems.
2. Discuss the reasons why each of these factors increases health risks for the older adult.
3. Describe how pharmacokinetics is altered with aging.
4. Discuss the pharmacodynamic changes observed in the older adult.
5. Explain specific precautions that are necessary when administering medications to older adults in an institutional setting.
6. Identify the risks related to aging and pertinent nursing observations for specific drug categories.
7. Discuss how medications fit into the nursing plan of care.
8. Describe specific nursing interventions and modifications in technique that are related to medication administration to older adults.
9. Describe the older person's rights as they relate to medication administration.
10. Identify information that should be provided to older adults regarding medications.
11. Discuss the impact of age-related changes on self-administration of medications.
12. Describe nursing interventions that can reduce problems related to self-administration of medication in the home.

Key Terms

absorption (ăb-SŎRP-shŭn, p. 141)
adverse drug event (p. 140)
distribution (dĭs-trĭ-BŬ-shŭn, p. 141)
excretion (ĕks-KRĒ-shŭn, p. 142)
first pass effect (p. 141)

geropharmacology (jĕr-ō-făr-mă-KŎL-ŏ-jē, p. 141)
half-life (p. 142)
metabolism (mĕ-TĂB-ō-lĭzm, p. 142)
pharmacokinetics (făr-mă-kō-kĭ-NĔT-ĭks, p. 141)
polypharmacy (pŏ-lē-FĂR-mă-sē, p. 142)

Problems related to medications are common in older adults, and they are costly in terms of both time and money. Medications can alter an older adult's ability to perform normal functions, can result in behavior changes, and can be life-threatening. Any injury from the use of a drug can be classified as an **adverse drug event** (ADE), and such injuries are common among older adults. Studies have revealed that about 1 in 10 hospitalizations of older persons is related to ADEs and that most of these events are likely preventable (Oscanoa et al., 2017). These ADEs are most frequently related to nonsteroidal anti-inflammatory drugs (NSAIDs). In addition, older people are more likely to develop iatrogenic (treatment-related) complications secondary to medications taken during a hospital stay. Several groups of people are known to be at greater risk for an ADE, including older adults over the age of 65, individuals with low socioeconomic status or insufficient health education, or those living in rural areas (U.S. Department of Health and Human Services, 2020). ADEs have also been linked to an increased risk

for falls and automobile accidents. Hospitalizations from ADEs cost older adults and taxpayers several billion dollars each year.

Almost all older adults take at least one prescription medication, and one-third of older adults take five (Harvard Health Letter, 2020). In addition to these prescription drugs, older adults take over-the-counter (OTC) medications and dietary supplements. Many older adults prefer to try self-treatment with OTC medications before consulting their primary care provider. Studies show that older adults purchase more than 40% of the OTCs sold (Hammond & Moseley, 2019) and that 90% of this group use OTC drugs at least occasionally. The use of combinations of prescription drugs, OTC drugs, and dietary supplements, as is common among older adults, poses the risk for dangerous drug-to-drug interactions.

Considering these numbers, it is no surprise that the use, misuse, and abuse of medications presents serious threats to the aging population. Medications are potent substances. For every desired effect, many side effects

Box 7.1	Factors That Increase the Risk for Medication-Related Problems

- Drug testing methodology
- Several health care providers
- Recent hospitalization
- Physiologic changes related to aging
- Use of multiple medications, over-the-counter medications, and herbal supplements
- Cognitive and sensory changes
- Knowledge deficits
- Financial concerns

and adverse effects are likely to occur. Although often useful or necessary to maintain health, medications present risks to people of all ages, and older adults are at even greater risk than the younger population (Box 7.1).

RISKS RELATED TO DRUG TESTING METHODS

In general, methodologies used to test drugs and to establish therapeutic dosages do not take into account the unique characteristics of older adults. Most drug testing is performed with people who are healthier, younger, and have been exposed to fewer medical interventions than the older adult who might actually be prescribed the medication. Because older adults normally have had some changes in body function and are more likely to experience at least one disease process, they are not physiologically the same as young adults. It seems obvious that an 80-year-old 94-pound woman with heart disease should not be expected to respond in the same way that a healthy 35-year-old 200-pound man would. The drugs and dosages that are appropriate for one may be unsuitable for the other. No medical professional would think of giving an adult dose of medication to a child, yet the same consideration is not always given to the unique situation presented by older adults. Geropharmacology, the study of how older adults respond to medication, is a new but growing area. Until all care providers recognize the uniqueness of older adults and modify treatment accordingly, overmedication is likely to occur.

RISKS RELATED TO THE PHYSIOLOGIC CHANGES OF AGING

People do not experience age-related physiologic changes at the same rate. When considering an older adult's response to medication, it is more important to look at the person's physiologic age than their chronologic age. The more physiologic changes experienced, the greater the risk will be of an altered response to medications. Even the most common physiologic changes of aging can have a significant effect on pharmacokinetics and pharmacodynamics (Table 7.1).

Table 7.1	Factors Affecting Drug Response in Older Adults

EFFECT	CAUSE
Absorption: altered	Decreased small bowel surface area, gastric acidity, peristalsis, and blood flow
Distribution: altered	Storing of fat-soluble drugs in fatty tissue; decreased serum albumin for binding of drugs
Metabolism: decreased	Decreased enzyme activity and blood flow in liver; decreased capacity of liver
Excretion: decreased	Decreased renal blood flow and glomerular filtration rate

Modified from: McCuistion, L. E., Vuljoin-DiMaggio, K., Winton, M. B., et al., (2021). *Pharmacology: A patient-centered nursing process approach* (10th ed.). St. Louis, MO: Elsevier.

PHARMACOKINETICS

Pharmacokinetics is the study of drug actions within the body, including absorption, distribution, metabolism, and excretion.

DRUG ABSORPTION

Most medications are taken orally and are absorbed through the gastrointestinal (GI) tract. The first pass effect is a phase of drug absorption that is altered in the older adult. In this phase, oral medications take a first pass through the liver before entering the systemic circulation, thus greatly reducing the drug's concentration. Because of decreased liver mass and blood flow, there is reduced first pass metabolism in the older adult, which can lead to a significant increase in the effects of certain medications like propranolol and labetalol. Other medications need to be "activated" by the liver, such as angiotensin-converting enzyme (ACE) inhibitors (e.g., enalapril); therefore the effect of these medications can be reduced in the older adult.

Although aging changes the absorption process in the older adult, these changes do not generally affect the amount of drug absorbed. One change in the GI system is an increase in the alkalinity (pH) of the gastric secretions, which causes irregular absorption of drugs. Peristalsis decreases, which allows enteric drugs to extend their contact with these gastric juices and allow the drugs to quickly break down. Decreased gastric motility and slower emptying of the intestines slows the onset of the drug's effect. Changes in the ability of the GI tract's cells to absorb and transport the drug can further influence its absorption. If medication is not transferred effectively through the cell membranes, absorption will be decreased.

DRUG DISTRIBUTION

With aging, there is typically a decrease in total body mass, lean body mass, and total body water and an increase in total body fat. These changes can significantly alter the distribution of medications. Because there is less total body water, water-soluble drugs—such as gentamicin, histamine receptor blockers, and lithium—tend to remain in higher concentrations in the bloodstream. This results in a increased blood concentration levels of these drugs. An older person who is dehydrated is at even greater risk for reaching excessive blood levels of water-soluble drugs.

As muscle mass decreases and the percentage of adipose tissue increases, fat-soluble drugs—such as phenobarbital and the benzodiazepines—become trapped in the fatty tissue, resulting in abnormally low blood levels. If the dosage is increased based on these blood levels, an excessive amount of medication may be administered. Because fat-soluble drugs continue to be released slowly from the fat into the bloodstream, older persons may exhibit delayed or hangover effects. A drug's half-life is the amount of time required for half of the medication to be eliminated or metabolized. The half-life of a single dose of diazepam, which is 36 hours in a young adult, may extend to as long as 100 hours in an older individual.

A decrease in hemoglobin and the plasma protein albumin is common with aging. This results in fewer available sites for protein-bound drugs such as warfarin, phenytoin, theophylline, salicylates, and tolbutamide. The danger of adverse or toxic reactions is high even with smaller doses because an unbound active drug still circulates in the bloodstream. The risk for toxicity is greater in malnourished older adults. Older adults who consume high-carbohydrate, low-protein diets are more likely to develop toxicity than are older adults who consume a well-balanced diet. Because not all of the serum drug assays can distinguish between free and bound medications, these tests may not provide reliable measures of toxicity. Because of this, nursing assessment for symptoms of toxicity becomes more important than ever.

DRUG METABOLISM

The liver is the primary site of drug metabolism. Aging often results in decreased activity of liver cells, decreased metabolic enzymes, and decreased cardiac output, all of which result in reduced blood flow to the liver. The liver of the older adult has only 40% to 45% of the perfusion of a younger adult. This reduction in perfusion decreases the liver's effectiveness in metabolizing drugs. When drugs are not metabolized effectively by the older adult's liver, the risk for toxicity increases. Toxicity is always a concern with medications commonly prescribed for older adults, including digoxin, β-blockers, calcium channel blockers, and tricyclic antidepressants.

DRUG EXCRETION

Aging kidneys are significantly less effective at removing waste products, including the by-products of medications. As the kidneys become less effective in the excretion of drugs, in part because of reduced renal perfusion, more drug remains in the circulation, leading to elevated drug levels and symptoms of drug toxicity. Because the changes in kidney function are accompanied by changes in lean body mass, serum creatinine levels often remain constant, masking the decline in function. When the risk for toxicity is assessed, the results of a creatinine clearance test will provide a more effective measure of kidney function than would be indicated by the serum creatinine level.

Some medications—such as aminoglycosides, digoxin, lithium, procainamide, and cimetidine—are likely to reach toxic levels because they are poorly excreted by the kidneys. Nonprescription drugs such as alcohol and nicotine can also affect kidney function and cause changes in drug elimination in older persons.

PHARMACODYNAMICS

Responses to medications are less predictable in the aging person; pathologic changes in target organs may affect their response. Receptor sites on the target organs may respond more or less sensitively to medications. They may respond normally to some medications but not to others. Receptors may often be more sensitive to medications, placing older adults at increased risk for toxic responses. Brain receptors are particularly sensitive; thus older adults typically respond strongly to psychotropic medications. When the receptor sites are less sensitive, the individual may require larger-than-normal doses to achieve therapeutic effects. If receptor sites in the myocardium are affected, older people may require higher doses of common medications such as propranolol and lidocaine. Administration of these higher doses increases the risk for toxicity. In addition, receptors may respond in unpredictable ways. For example, the wildly successful erectile dysfunction medication sildenafil citrate (Viagra) began as a cardiac medication; as such, it performed poorly in clinical trials for the intended effects of reducing hypertension and angina. Instead it seemed consistently to demonstrate the unusual side effect of producing penile erections in the clinical trial's participants.

POLYPHARMACY

Polypharmacy, the prescription, administration, or use of more medications than are clinically indicated, is a common problem in older adults (Fig. 7.1). As mentioned previously, older adults ingest far more medications than younger people in addition to OTC medications, herbs, and other supplements that may be taken with or without the primary care provider's recommendation or knowledge. It is estimated that older adults purchase 40% of all nonprescription medications (Gibson et al., 2020). The more medications taken—including OTCs, supplements, and herbs—the greater the risk for untoward reactions, drug interactions, and drug toxicities. Drug interactions and toxicities in

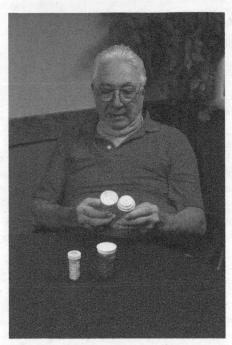

Fig. 7.1 Older adults' concurrent use of many prescription medications can lead to polypharmacy. (From Williams, P. [2021]. Fundamental concepts and skills for nursing [6th ed.]. St. Louis, MO: Elsevier.)

older adults are likely to result in behavioral or cognitive changes, often mistaken for dementia.

> **Clinical Goldmine**
>
> For an easy way to quickly discover potential drug interactions in your patient, go to http://reference.medscape.com/drug-interactionchecker. Type in the medications and supplements, one by one, and receive a list of interactions in order of severity.

Many factors contribute to the increased usage of medication among older adults. These factors include an increased likelihood of multiple acute or chronic disease conditions; increased availability of a variety of prescription medications, OTC medications, supplements, and herbs; changes in patient expectations; and changes in the health care delivery system.

Newer, better, and more potent medications are developed every day. Medical conditions of older adults that were once considered untreatable are now treated routinely using medications. Because older adults tend to have more physical complaints or diseases than younger individuals, their medication usage increases exponentially.

Older adults seek medical intervention for many reasons. Some live with their problems and seek medical attention only when they have serious concerns. By the time such people seek medical attention, their condition may have seriously deteriorated requiring the prescription of multiple medications. Other older people make frequent visits to their primary care providers,

seeking reassurance that nothing is seriously wrong. Rather than spending the time needed to reassure such older adults, some providers issue a prescription as a way of terminate the visit. Unfortunately, this practice occurs too often and can cause older adults to take unnecessary or marginally necessary medications.

Still other older people expect their primary care providers to be able to eliminate all of their problems and ailments with medications. Every website, television show, newspaper article, blog, or recommendation from a friend extolling the benefits of a new medication sends some older adults to their primary care providers' offices to request or even demand the new medicine. They expect the provider to prescribe a medication to relieve their ailments, and they often perceive that the provider is not doing anything for them unless this happens. Some older adults even go from provider to provider until they get what they want. Under these pressures, some providers prescribe medications that they otherwise would not have ordered.

Changes in health care delivery, particularly increased medical specialization, have contributed to medication-related problems. It is increasingly common for an older adult to have two or more specialists providing their care. When more than one care provider writes prescriptions, the risk for medication reactions and overmedication increases dramatically. If a care provider does not know what medications and OTC products the patient is already taking, they cannot consider those drugs when determining the safety of another prescription. Every prescribing provider must be aware of all medications that the older adult is taking, no matter who prescribed them, as well as all OTC medications, supplements, and herbs being used, as many of the popular herbs have potentially serious interactions with prescription medications (Table 7.2). Many older adults use herbs and supplements as alternatives to prescription medications, sometimes because they are less expensive and sometimes because they are marketed as "natural," which implies "safe." Remember: digoxin is an herb! It is important to carefully question older adults about supplements and herbs they are taking.

> **Pharmacology Capsule**
>
> **Medication Side Effects**
>
> A patient who was using timolol eye drops that were prescribed by an ophthalmologist for glaucoma began to experience joint pain. Not seeing any connection between his eye problems and his aching joints, the patient sought the advice of his rheumatologist. Fortunately, the rheumatologist asked the patient whether he was taking any other medications. When timolol was identified, the rheumatologist recognized the possibility of a drug-induced problem and contacted the ophthalmologist, who then changed the medication. The joint pain disappeared without further medical intervention.

Table 7.2   Selected Herbal and Supplement Considerations for Older Adults

HERB OR SUPPLEMENT	HEALTH CLAIM	OLDER ADULT CONSIDERATIONS
Black cohosh	Decreases hot flashes and other menopausal symptoms	Can cause liver damage
Ginkgo biloba	Improves memory; improves blood circulation in the brain; improves perfusion in eyes	Can cause excessive bleeding, especially if on anticoagulants or aspirin
St. John's wort	Relieves depression	Reduces the effect of some cardiac medications including digoxin; interferes with numerous other medications, including medications for transplant rejection, blood thinning, cancer, lowering blood cholesterol levels, and antidepressants
Chamomile	Calms upset stomach; helps with sleep; assists with generalized anxiety disorder	Interacts with organ transplant and blood thinner medications; may cause severe allergic reactions
Echinacea	May prevent colds	Potential for allergic reactions
Ginseng	Boosts immune system; lowers blood sugar	Can cause a severe rash known as Stevens-Johnson syndrome, liver damage, and severe allergic reaction; alters drug effectiveness for numerous medications including anticoagulants, diabetes drugs, corticosteroids, and antidepressants
Green tea	Numerous claims including prevention of cancers, prevent coronary artery disease, and many others	Can cause liver issues and injuries; may decrease blood levels of some blood pressure medications
Kava	Relieves anxiety	Can lead to liver toxicity; can impair ability to drive
Soy	Helps with high cholesterol, hypertension, and menopausal hot flashes	Might elevate the risk of endometrial hyperplasia which can be a precursor to uterine cancer
Glucosamine sulfate	Helps relieve joint pain and arthritis	Potential for interaction with blood thinning medications

National Institutes of Health. (2020). Dietary supplement fact sheets. https://ods.od.nih.gov/factsheets/list-all/#S

POTENTIALLY INAPPROPRIATE MEDICATION USE IN OLDER ADULTS

The fact that older adults respond differently to medications than younger adults do has long been recognized. Until 1991, there were no specific guidelines to aid the provider in the selection of medications least likely to cause adverse reactions. In 1991, the Beers criteria, a list of drugs that should usually be avoided by older adults, were developed. This list was improved and expanded several times over the years with the most recent revision having appeared in 2019. It is frequently used in the United States. Originally created as one list, the 2019 American Geriatrics Society Beers Criteria now consists of several lists. These identify medications best avoided by older adults both using the diagnosis and condition as the primary consideration and independent of diagnoses or conditions. The latest criteria includes the addition of a list of drugs that should be avoided or the dose adjusted based on the older adult's kidney function and a list with drug-drug interactions known to cause harm in older adults.

 Did You Know?

Over 30 medications that are potentially inappropriate for older adults are listed in the Beers criteria, as well as numerous medications and categories of medications with recommendations for lowered dosages or use in selective disorders only.

Medicare and Medicaid have developed regulations for skilled nursing facilities that are heavily based on the Beers criteria. Skilled care facilities are required to have protocols that ensure that care providers' orders are in compliance. Citations are issued to facilities that fail to comply. A mobile app is available to make prescribing providers' jobs easier in avoiding potentially inappropriate medications for older adults under their care.

Another commonly used tool used in other parts of the world is called the STOPP (Screening Tool of Older Person's Prescriptions)/START (Screening Tool to Alert doctors to Right Treatment) criteria. The STOPP/START criteria were developed in the United

Table 7.3   Examples from STOPP Criteria

PHYSIOLOGIC SYSTEM	NUMBER OF CRITERIA FOR THIS BODY SYSTEM	EXAMPLES OF THESE CRITERIA (MEDICATIONS THAT MAY BE INAPPROPRIATE UNDER CERTAIN CIRCUMSTANCES, AND PERHAPS SHOULD BE "STOPPED")
Cardiovascular system	17	• Digoxin at a long-term dose greater than 125 mcg/day in a patient with impaired kidney function • Loop diuretic for dependent ankle edema only • Thiazide diuretic in patient with gout • Beta blocker in a patient taking verapamil
Central nervous system	13	• TCAs with any of the following: dementia, glaucoma, cardiac conduction abnormalities, or constipation • Long-acting benzodiazepines for greater than 1 month
Gastrointestinal system	5	• Full-dose PPIs for peptic ulcer disease for longer than 8 weeks
Respiratory system	3	• Systemic corticosteroids for maintenance of COPD • Nebulized ipratropium in patient with glaucoma
Musculoskeletal system	8	• NSAIDs for peptic ulcer disease, unless given concurrently with H2 receptor agonist, PPI, or misoprostol • NSAIDs with moderate to severe hypertension or heart failure
Urogenital system	6	• Antimuscarinic drugs with dementia, glaucoma, chronic constipation
Endocrine system	4	• Estrogen with history of breast cancer or thromboembolism • Beta blockers in people with diabetes experiencing hypoglycemia more than once a month
Drugs that adversely affect fallers	5	• Benzodiazepines • Neuroleptic drugs
Analgesic drugs	3	• Long-term powerful opiates for first-line pain therapy • Opiates longer than 2 weeks with chronic constipation
Duplicate drug classes	1	• Any drug category with more than one medication prescribed

COPD, Chronic obstructive pulmonary disease; *NSAIDs,* nonsteroidal anti-inflammatory drugs; *PPIs,* proton-pump inhibitors; *STOPP,* Screening Tool of Older Person's Prescriptions; *TCAs,* tricyclic antidepressants.
Modified from Ryan C. (2011). The basics of the STOPP/START criteria. http://www.pcne.org/upload/ms2011d/Presentations/Ryan%20pres.pdf. Updated from O'Mahony, D., et al. (2015). STOPP/START criteria for potentially inappropriate prescribing in older people: version 2. *Age Ageing,* 44(2), 213–218.

Kingdom in 2008 in response to perceived content gaps and disagreement about the Beers content. These criteria were revised and expanded in 2013; however, several of the Beers medications continued to not be included in the European drug formularies. In 2015, the criteria were revised to create STOPP v2. Although there are still differences, the updated version is based on the same research as the Beers criteria and is now much more similar to the Beers criteria. The differences include the inclusion or omission of some symptoms (e.g., constipation) or medications and the addition of tables in the STOPP v2 criteria. Both the Beers and the STOPP criteria should be used side by side when health care providers are prescribing medications for older adults (Blanco-Reina et al., 2019). Examples of medications in the STOPP and START criteria can be found in Tables 7.3 and 7.4, respectively.

To protect older adults, physicians and others who have legal authority to prescribe medications should remember six basic guidelines: (1) start low and go slow, (2) start one drug and stop two, (3) do not use a drug if the adverse effects are worse than the disease, (4) use as few drugs as possible and use nonpharmacologic approaches whenever possible, (5) frequently assess the patient's response, and (6) consider drug holidays.

RISKS RELATED TO COGNITIVE OR SENSORY CHANGES

Cognitive and sensory limitations increase the risk for medication errors in older adults. Cognitive problems come in several forms, including a lack of the literacy skills needed to read the labels and directions, the inability to understand and comply with directions, and the inability to make correct judgments regarding medications. In severe cases of cognitive impairment, older individuals may not even recognize that they have to take medication. If they do attempt to take the medication, serious and potentially harmful errors are often made. Cognitively impaired older adults should not be responsible for medicating themselves but should be supervised by a family member or nurse.

Sensory changes, particularly visual and hearing changes, present problems for older adults in relation to the use of medications. When vision changes render an older person unable to read a medication label or to recognize the different sizes, shapes, or colors of the various medications, serious problems can arise. Many

Table 7.4   Examples from START Criteria

PHYSIOLOGIC SYSTEM	NUMBER OF CRITERIA FOR THIS BODY SYSTEM	EXAMPLES OF THESE CRITERIA (MEDICATIONS THAT OUGHT TO BE CONSIDERED, OR STARTED, IN CERTAIN SITUATIONS)
Cardiovascular system	8	• Warfarin in the presence of chronic atrial fibrillation • Antihypertensives for systolic BP chronically above 160 mm Hg • Beta blockers with chronic stable angina
Respiratory system	3	• Regular beta$_2$ agonist or anticholinergic for mild-moderate asthma or COPD • Inhaled corticosteroid for moderate-severe asthma or COPD
Central nervous system	2	• L-dopa for Parkinson disease with functional impairment • Antidepressants for moderate-severe depression greater than 3 months
Gastrointestinal system	2	• PPI for severe acid reflux or stricture • Fiber for diverticular disease with constipation
Musculoskeletal system	3	• DMARD for moderate-severe rheumatoid disease longer than 12 weeks • Bisphosphonates for patients on corticosteroids • Calcium and vitamin D for osteoporosis
Endocrine system	4	• ACE inhibitor or angiotensin receptor blocker for diabetic nephropathy

ACE, Angiotensin-converting enzyme; *BP*, blood pressure; *COPD*, chronic obstructive pulmonary disease; *DMARD*, disease-modifying antirheumatic drug; *PPI*, proton-pump inhibitor; *START*, Screening Tool to Alert doctors to Right Treatment.
Modified from Ryan C. (2011). The basics of the STOPP/START criteria. http://www.pcne.org/upload/ms2011d/Presentations/Ryan%20pres.pdf. Updated from O'Mahony, D., et al. (2015). STOPP/START criteria for potentially inappropriate prescribing in older people: version 2. *Age Ageing*, 44(2), 213–218.

older adults essentially guess what medications they are taking, often taking the wrong medication at the wrong time and in the wrong amount because they are unable to read the directions. Liquid medications, particularly injectable medications such as insulin, are commonly overdosed or underdosed because of the person's poor vision. Many of these risks can be reduced by assessing the person's ability to read labels accurately, by performing proper patient education, and by using special labels or magnifying devices that facilitate safe medication administration.

RISKS RELATED TO INADEQUATE KNOWLEDGE

Lack of knowledge about medications can result in serious problems for older adults. This knowledge deficit, which can relate to both prescription and nonprescription medications, has many causes and manifests in different ways.

One common sign of lack of knowledge involves sharing medications with friends or relatives. This practice is common and persists because many people are unaware of the dangers. When older adults find a medication that makes them feel better, they may attempt to share it with friends who have similar problems. The intention of helping friends is good, but the consequences can be serious or fatal. All people must be aware that it is not safe to take a medication prescribed for someone else. If an older adult believes that a certain medication will help, that person should get the name of the medicine and then contact their primary care provider. The care provider and not a friend will be best able to determine whether the drug will be safe and beneficial.

Many older adults have misconceptions about OTC preparations. It is estimated that over 80% of older adults use at least one OTC preparation (Hess et al., 2018). In fact, 42% of all OTC medications are consumed by older adults (Hammond & Moseley, 2019). Many do not think of OTC medications as "real" drugs because a prescription is not needed to purchase them. Because they do not consider OTC medications to be "real" drugs, older adults are not likely to consult with a physician, pharmacist, or nurse regarding their use. Many simply go to the drug or grocery store and purchase whatever preparation looks helpful. This uninformed use of OTC drugs can be hazardous to older adults, particularly those taking prescription medications. OTC medications are capable of potentiating or interfering with prescription medications, possibly resulting in serious harm. OTC drugs can also create or mask symptoms of disease. Use of these drugs can make it difficult for the primary care provider to recognize changes in an individual's health status. Older adults must be encouraged to consult with their primary care providers or pharmacists before taking any OTC medication, to carefully keep track of it, and to inform their primary care provider of all prescription and OTC medications, herbs, and supplements they take.

Alcohol is the most commonly consumed nonprescription drug used by adults. Many older adults do not think of alcohol as a drug, so they do not consider it when taking medications. Alcoholic beverages can cause adverse reactions when taken in conjunction with many prescription and OTC drugs. It is prudent to check with the primary care provider or pharmacist before drinking alcohol. Today, most prescription drugs are labeled if there is a risk for interaction with alcohol, but these labels are not always given adequate attention. In addition to OTC medications, herbal or natural remedies are being used with increased frequency; as many as 30% of Americans use herbs, and most are reluctant to tell their primary care providers (Khan et al., 2020). It is important to consider possible interactions between these substances and more traditional prescription and OTC medications.

Older adults often lack adequate knowledge regarding their prescription medications. They are often given one or more prescriptions and simply told to take them according to the directions. The directions provided may be very clear to a health care professional, but may easily be misinterpreted by an older adult. Even simple misunderstandings can lead to improper self-medication and lead to serious consequences. To reduce the risks, older adults often require additional instruction to take their prescriptions safely. Because this is a common problem among older adults, self-administration of medication is addressed in detail later in the chapter.

 Pharmacology Capsule

Polypharmacy

Mrs. Smith had been taking a medication for her high blood pressure. Because it was no longer effectively controlling her blood pressure, her primary care provider ordered a newer, more potent antihypertensive. Approximately 25 tablets of the original medication were left in the bottle, which Mrs. Smith left in her medicine cabinet. After taking the new prescription for a month, Mrs. Smith happened to check her blood pressure with one of the automatic machines located in a drugstore. She found that her blood pressure was just a little bit higher than she thought it should be. Remembering that she had another medicine for blood pressure at home, she decided (without consulting the care provider) to take a few of the "less potent" old tablets. Only when she began to feel dizzy and almost fainted did she call the care provider.

RISKS RELATED TO FINANCIAL FACTORS

Medications are expensive. A single prescription can easily cost $100 or more a month. If someone requires more than one medication, the cumulative cost can be overwhelming. To save money, older adults living on limited incomes may fail to take their medications, or they may make changes in the amount or frequency of medication in order to conserve the supply. Because these changes do not follow the recommended therapeutic schedule, a wide variety of untoward responses can occur. Even with insurance, some prescriptions may not be covered. Older adults may say, "I don't like to take pills." Others will get a prescription filled once to see whether it is "worth the price." If the benefits gained from taking the medication are not readily obvious to older adults, they may not refill the prescription.

Because medications are expensive, many frugal older adults save medications that were prescribed in the past, even if the drugs are no longer part of their therapy. Older adults are often reluctant to dispose of costly medications, holding onto them "just in case" they might be needed again. This practice can bring serious harm if the medications expire. Expired medications can undergo chemical changes that make them hazardous. Saving old medications also increases the risk for problems if the older person thinks the drug is appropriate and takes it without consulting with the primary care provider.

MEDICATION ADMINISTRATION IN AN INSTITUTIONAL SETTING

It is obvious that medications can present a wide range of problems for older adults. Nurses working with older adults must consider each of these risks in determining a plan for safe administration. Medication administration is a common part of the nursing care of older adults in hospitals, extended-care facilities, and home settings. Approaches and methods may vary according to the setting, but the safety of the older adult remains the primary concern. A significant amount of nursing time in facilities is spent on medication-related activities. Because medications play an important role in the health care of many older adults, nurses must take special precautions to ensure the safe administration of drugs.

Safe drug administration begins with a thorough knowledge and understanding of each medication. Clarify and resolve any questions regarding medication therapy before administering a medication. Information regarding medications is contained in many reference books, which should be readily available to nurses. Before administering a medication, have the following information:

- Therapeutic effects of the medication
- Reasons this individual is receiving the medication
- Normal therapeutic dosage of the medication
- Normal route or routes of administration
- Any special precautions related to administration
- Common side effects or adverse effects of the medication (see Clinical Goldmine, p. 143)
- Signs of overdose and toxicity

NURSING ASSESSMENT AND MEDICATION

Thoroughly assess the older adult before administering any medications. After administration, monitor the older adult continually to determine whether the medication is having the desired effect. Perform this after administering both scheduled and as-needed medications. Also observe for any untoward effects or significant changes in medical condition or behavior (Box 7.2).

Because normal physiologic changes and the effects of disease place the older person at increased risk for drug-related problems, be particularly watchful for any signs of overdose or toxicity. Special age-related risk factors and observations for the more common drug classifications are summarized in Table 7.5.

Cultural Considerations

Assessment and Ethnicity

Ethnicity is one factor that should be considered when you assess a patient's use of and response to medication; however, it should not be used to stereotype any group. Some ethnic variations that have been identified include the following:

- People of African descent may have a decreased response to propanolol, captopril, and warfarin.
- Antidepressants, antipsychotics, and cardiovascular drugs are not metabolized well by people of European descent. This alteration in metabolism can progress to toxicity.
- Use of herbal remedies is common in the Chinese culture. Common herbs, such as ginseng, may affect the absorption and elimination of other drugs.

Implementation of computerized records as part of the Minimum Data Set 3.0 (see Chapter 8) improves communication between nurses and pharmacists. Ideally, this interdisciplinary approach to medication will promote the early recognition of problems or areas of concern regarding the medication regimen.

MEDICATION AND THE NURSING CARE PLAN

Medications are only one part of the overall care of the older person and should be included as such. For example, the administration of laxatives should be only a part of a more comprehensive plan to assist bowel elimination, and the administration of analgesics should be only a part of an extensive nursing care plan for pain control.

Nursing interventions and precautions related to medications should be addressed in the care plan. This could include the use of safety devices, call signals, behavior monitoring, or any other specific precaution related to medications. The care plan should indicate when it is necessary to check vital signs, monitor laboratory values, or make any other special observations. All parameters specified by the prescriber should be readily identified in the care plan—for example, "Hold digoxin if apical pulse is below 60" or "Give 6 units regular insulin at bedtime if the fingerstick blood glucose is over 150."

The care plan should indicate any individual preferences of the older person. Many older adults have a particular order or method to take their medication. This information should be in the care plan so that all staff nurses can be consistent.

NURSING INTERVENTIONS RELATED TO MEDICATION ADMINISTRATION

It is often necessary to modify procedures and techniques of medication administration when working with older adults. Despite modifications, the traditional "rights" of medication administration remain essential to the process.

RIGHT PATIENT

Proper identification of the patient or resident is an essential part of safe nursing care. This simple task can be challenging for nurses who work in extended-care facilities. Whenever a large number of residents are up and about, accurate identification becomes more difficult.

The most accurate way to verify identity is to compare the medication record with the identification bracelet. A bar code system is typically used in the acute care setting (Fig. 7.2). However, not all long-term residents wear identification bracelets; if they do wear them, the bracelets are often old and blurred. When

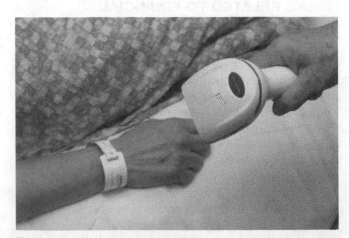

Fig. 7.2 The nurse checks the bar code on the patient's bracelet and on the medication packet. (From Williams, P. [2021]. Fundamental concepts and skills for nursing [6th ed.]. St. Louis, MO: Elsevier.)

Table 7.5 Common Drug Categories With Precautions Related to Aging

TYPE OF MEDICATION	RISK FACTORS	ASSESS FOR
Cardiac Medication		
Digoxin, propranolol	Dehydration, hypothyroidism, decreased renal excretion, and hypoxia increase the risk for toxicity.	Vision changes, headaches, fatigue, drowsiness, mental changes, altered pulse rate or regularity, loss of appetite, nausea, vomiting, diarrhea
Diuretics		
Bumetanide, furosemide	May result in dehydration. May result in altered electrolyte balance, which predisposes patient to digitalis toxicity.	Signs of dehydration, hypotension, skin changes, weight loss, electrolyte imbalances, lethargy, dizziness, light-headedness, and confusion
Antihypertensives		
Captopril, clonidine, atenolol, hydralazine, methyldopa	High doses may aggravate existing problems in cerebral, coronary, and renal circulation. Hot weather, alcohol, and exercise are likely to increase the risk for hypotension.	Bradycardia, orthostatic hypotension, weakness, headaches, dizziness, fatigue, sleeping difficulties, palpitations, nausea, vomiting, and edema
Psychotropics (Including Antianxiety Agents, Antidepressants, and Antipsychotics)		
Flurazepam, triazolam, diazepam, haloperidol, chlorpromazine, thioridazine	Older persons usually require smaller doses to achieve therapeutic response. Decreased respirations when combined with alcohol. Tardive dyskinesia is a significant risk with long-term therapy.	Apathy, confusion, drooling, lip smacking, grimacing, difficulty swallowing, decreased mobility, skin reactions, jaundice, impaired sense of balance, alteration in gait, falls, drowsiness, fainting, hypotension, palpitations, constipation, hypothermia, and complaints of feeling cold
Antibacterials		
Cephalosporins, penicillins, sulfonamides, tetracyclines	Standard dose may result in higher blood levels in older adults. Increased risk for allergic reactions or superimposed yeast infections with aging. Damage to cranial nerve VIII is particularly common in older adults.	Nausea, vomiting, diarrhea, dehydration, signs of oral or vaginal yeast infection, urticaria, and tinnitus
Nonsteroidal Anti-inflammatory Agents		
Aspirin, ibuprofen, tolmetin, naproxen	Increased risk for gastrointestinal, kidney, and central nervous system problems with aging.	Signs of gastrointestinal upset including nausea, vomiting, tarry stools, diarrhea or constipation, and occult blood loss; central nervous system side effects including dizziness, drowsiness, confusion, mood swings, depression, restlessness, and arrhythmias
Bronchodilators and Spasmolytics		
Theophylline	Increased risk for toxicity including kidney, liver, heart, or lung problems.	Tachycardia, arrhythmias, anorexia, nausea, vomiting, headaches, seizures, or insomnia
Gastrointestinal Medications		
Cimetidine, famotidine, aluminum hydroxide and magnesium hydroxide	May affect the absorption of other medications. More sensitive to the effects of these medications.	Confusion, dizziness, dry mouth, vision changes, flushing, headache, increased sweating

reliable bracelets are not available, alternative methods must be used.

A resident's picture is sometimes used as a means of identification. However, pictures that are old or bear little resemblance to the individual are useless.

Pictures used for identification must be kept up to date and must be readily available when medications are distributed.

Identification can also be accomplished by asking the resident to state their full name. Most people respond promptly and appropriately with the correct name. A response to hearing the nurse call a name that involves a head shake or a "yes" from a patient is not enough to ensure identification. Many older adults with hearing or cognitive impairment give some sort of response to any name. When an older person is not oriented to a person, bracelets or pictures must be used.

> ### QSEN Considerations: Safety
>
> Check identification, following agency policies, each time a medication is administered. Failure to do this can result in serious errors and harm to older adults.

Do not attempt to identify a resident by room and bed number because cognitively or perceptually impaired individuals often wander into the wrong room or lie down on someone else's bed. Be careful to avoid the trap of insisting that you "know the residents." Check identification with each medication pass no matter how long you have been caring for the patient. Serious mistakes can and do occur when nurses take shortcuts with safety procedures. As a method of ensuring accurate identification in accredited agencies, The Joint Commission (TJC) requires the use of two identifiers before the administration of medications.

RIGHT MEDICATION

Before administering a medication, ensure that the drug provided by the pharmacy is the correct one. This is not as easy as it seems. Because each medication has a generic name and one or more trade names and because the appearance of a medication can vary depending on the manufacturer, nurses must use a reference source to verify that the right drug is, in fact, available. Orders should be checked carefully, and the pharmacy should be contacted if any questions arise. Many drug names look or sound alike; therefore it is important to check spellings carefully.

If telephone medication orders are permitted, repeat the entire order back ("read back") to the provider, taking care to clarify the spelling of the drug to avoid the possibility of error.

RIGHT AMOUNT

The goal of drug therapy in older adults is to achieve the maximal therapeutic benefits with the smallest amount of medication necessary (see Health Promotion box, p. 51). Therefore the dosage prescribed for an older adult is often lower than what would be prescribed for a younger adult. To achieve therapeutic levels without overdosing the older adult, the primary care provider may order lower doses or less frequent administration of a medication. With lower doses, as with all medication doses, it is imperative to verify the strength of the medications (checking decimal points closely). All measurements, particularly for liquids, must be made with great care. Decreased frequency in administration can result in medications that are administered every other day or every third day. Nurses must pay close attention when administering medication to avoid administering it on a day when the drug should be withheld. Any questions regarding the dosage should be clarified with an approved reference, the pharmacist, or the prescribing care provider before the medication is administered. To prevent errors caused by misinterpretation of orders, TJC has published an official "Do Not Use" list of symbols, abbreviations, and mathematical expressions (Table 7.6). In addition to the "Do Not Use" list, it is also important to avoid certain symbols that can easily be misread when handwritten:

- The symbols > and < can easily be confused with the number 7 and capital letter L, or they may be confused with each other; instead, use the words "greater than" and "less than."
- Abbreviations for drug names: instead, use the full name.
- Apothecary units; use metric units instead.

Table 7.6   The Joint Commission's Official "Do Not Use" List[a]

DO NOT USE	POTENTIAL PROBLEM	USE INSTEAD
U, u (unit)	Mistaken for "0" (zero), "4" (four), or cc	Write "unit"
IU (international unit)	Mistaken for IV (intravenous) or the number 10 (ten)	Write "International Unit"
Q.D., QD, q.d., qd (daily)	Mistaken for each other	Write "daily"
Q.O.D., QOD, q.o.d., qod (every other day)	Period after the Q mistaken for "I" and the "O" mistaken for "I"	Write "every other day"
Trailing zero (X.0 mg)[b]	Decimal point is missed	Write X mg
Lack of leading zero (.X mg)		Write 0.X mg
MS	Can mean morphine sulfate or magnesium sulfate	Write "morphine sulfate"
MSO_4 and $MgSO_4$	Confused for one another	Write "magnesium sulfate"

[a]Applies to all orders and all medication-related documentation that is handwritten (including free-text computer entry) or on preprinted forms.
[b]Exception: A "trailing zero" may be used only where required to demonstrate the level of precision of the value being reported, such as for laboratory results, imaging studies that report size of lesions, or catheter/tube sizes. It may not be used in medication orders or other medication-related documentation. The Joint Commission, 2019. Reprinted with permission. Source: https://www.jointcommission.org/-/media/tjc/documents/fact-sheets/do-not-use-list-8-3-20.pdf

- The sign @ can be mistaken for the number 2; instead, write the word "at."
- The abbreviation cc can be mistaken for the letter "u" if poorly written; instead, use mL or milliliters.
- The abbreviation μg can be mistaken for mg, resulting in a 1000-fold dosing overdose; instead, write mcg or micrograms.

🏃 Health Promotion

Guiding Rule for Medication Administration in Older Adults

Achieve the maximal therapeutic benefits while giving the smallest necessary amount of medication: "Start low and go slow!"

RIGHT DOSAGE FORM

Problems arise when the older person is unable to swallow tablets or cannot swallow at all and relies on a gastric or nasogastric tube for nourishment. For these patients, nurses must consider safe alternatives. If the medication is available in liquid form, discuss the possibility of an order change with the provider. Because liquids might be absorbed more rapidly than solids, all changes in medication form require a new order. Many times, when the drug form is changed, the dosage is also changed. If a liquid form is not available, the tablet or capsule may have to be crushed or broken to facilitate swallowing. Not all medications can be crushed or broken because this can alter the action of the drug (Box 7.3). Consult the pharmacy if there is any question of whether or not a medication should be crushed. Lists of common medications that should not be crushed or chewed are available from many sources and should be kept on the nursing unit for reference.

RIGHT ROUTE

Most medications are prescribed for oral administration. When an oral medication is being administered, the importance of the medication, the preferences of the older person, and their capabilities must be considered.

Many older adults receive numerous medications. Administer the most important medications first, so if

Box 7.3   Medications That Should Not Be Chewed or Crushed

- Enteric coated tablets (many appear to have a "candy coating")
- Capsules (some may be opened and the contents dissolved; others may not; be sure to check with pharmacy)
- Time-release tablets or capsules (these often have names with suffixes, such as LA [long-acting], SR [sustained-release], ER [extended-release], etc.)
- Sublingual or buccal tablets
- Medications with a bitter taste
- Medications that can irritate oral mucous membranes

the person refuses to take them all, at least the most essential ones will have been administered. Whenever a person refuses to take a medication, document the event in the health record and notify the nurse in charge, as the primary care provider may need to be informed in a timely manner.

Some older adults prefer swallowing several tablets at one time to "get it over with." If they take their medications in this way without difficulty, there is no reason to try to make them change their habits. Other people prefer to take their medications one tablet at a time. If this is their preference, the nurse should oblige. Still others have trouble swallowing any solid medications.

Tablets, particularly large ones, are likely to cause the greatest problems. Dryness of the mouth related to aging often makes swallowing difficult and results in complaints of pills sticking in the throat. Encouraging older adults to take a drink of water or some other beverage before they try to swallow the tablet may make swallowing easier. Coating the tablet with a spoonful of pudding, ice cream, or applesauce might also help the patient swallow it more easily. Only small amounts of these foods should be used to facilitate swallowing. Ask the pharmacist if larger pills can be split in half; if they are scored, this will be possible (Fig. 7.3).

❓ Critical Thinking

When a Patient Refuses Medication

A 78-year-old male patient in the hospital for pneumonia has taken his medication without problems in the past. Today, he refused all oral medications, including those for his diabetes and hypertension.
- Why do you think is he refusing his medication?
- How can you determine what is going on in this situation?
- What actions should you take?

Crushed medications should not be mixed into a serving of food during mealtime. This practice is unsafe as it often results in a partial missed dose because the entire serving of food may not be consumed and also because the nursing assistant assigned to feed the patient is not qualified to administer medications. Again, use of a small amount of applesauce, pudding, or ice cream to facilitate swallowing of a crushed medication is an acceptable practice. Crushing a medication and hiding it in food to administer it to a patient

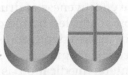

Fig. 7.3 Many tablets are scored and can be split for easier swallowing. (From McCuistion, L .E., Vuljoin DiMaggio, K., Winton, M. B., et al. [2021]. Pharmacology: A patient-centered nursing process approach [10th ed.]. St. Louis, MO: Elsevier.)

who has refused to take it violates the person's right to choose and is unethical. Administer unpleasant tasting medications after all other medications. Offer a sip of ice water before the medication or refrigerate unpleasant tasting liquid medications to make them more palatable. Facility policies should provide directions as to how to proceed when a patient refuses medications as a result of dementia or other cognitive problems.

Administration of medication through a feeding tube is often necessary and must be done correctly. Request the liquid form of a medication when available. Large particles of a medication can block the feeding tube, requiring tube replacement. To prevent blockage, finely crush each tablet and then place it in a plastic medication cup, where it should be thoroughly dissolved in a small amount of warm water. Once completely dissolved, administer the medications through the feeding tube. Administer each medication separately. Flush the feeding tube with a small amount of water before giving the first medication, again after each medication, and once more before reconnecting the tube with the feeding solution. Never mix medications together or with feeding solutions.

Transdermal delivery is a popular route for drug administration. Transdermal medications are administered using a "patch" consisting of a center that contains the medication surrounded by a skin overlay, which secures the patch to the skin. Transdermal medications are typically readily accepted by older adults because they are easy to apply and are effective for long periods of time. This route is convenient and has a high rate of adherence because it is painless, tasteless, and eliminates the need to consider the timing of application in relation to meals. Transdermal patches cause few GI problems and can help to maintain more stable plasma levels of medications, so there are fewer side effects. An additional benefit is that drug delivery can be stopped immediately by removing the patch.

The major disadvantage of the patch is skin irritation caused by either the active ingredient or the adhesive used to secure the patch. Newer techniques have reduced these problems, and the risk can be reduced by rotating the application site and cleaning the skin thoroughly following removal (Box 7.4).

The inhalation route is also used for the administration of medication. Inhalation drugs are typically administered using metered-dose inhalers and nebulizers. The older adult who has arthritis in the hands or lacks coordination may need some assistance using these devices. The effectiveness of drugs administered by inhalation is often affected by the diminished lung capacity and the decreased depth and strength of inhalation typically seen with aging.

When a parenteral medication is ordered, other precautions must be taken. Because older adults generally have less muscle mass and subcutaneous tissue than younger people, injection sites should be

---

Box 7.4 Precautions When Using Transdermal Patches

1. Check the dosage strength of the patch.
2. Verify the correct site or sites for administration.
3. Remove any protective liner so that the medication is in contact with the skin.
4. Wear gloves when applying and removing transdermal patches to avoid skin contact with the medicated portion.
5. Document where each patch is applied. Be sure to rotate sites.
6. Apply patch to dry, hairless patch of skin. Avoid areas of irritation and bony areas.
7. Remove all old patches, and clean the skin before applying a new one (pay special attention for clear patches that are difficult to see on the skin).
8. Avoid use of heat over a patch because this causes vasodilation, which increases the rate of absorption. Do not apply tape over the patch.
9. Dispose of old patches by folding sticky edges together and placing in the sharps container. If the old patch contains a controlled substance, a second nurse must witness the folding and disposal, and both will document, according to agency policy.
10. Provide patient with information on safe application, removal, and disposal of patch. Also, remind patients to report use of a patch, as well as any other medications, when seeking medical attention, particularly during emergency care or when magnetic resonance imaging (MRI) is anticipated, because many patches contain metal and can cause skin burns during the MRI procedure.

---

selected carefully. Intramuscular injections are best administered using the ventrogluteal site, which is easily accessible without excessive repositioning and is free from major nerves or blood vessels. This muscle remains large enough for injection even in very slender people. Furthermore, it is well away from areas of possible contamination if the older person is incontinent.

Choose needle length with caution, depending on the injection site. The deltoid muscle is usually a poor site for all but very infrequent administrations of very small volumes. To avoid striking the bone of an emaciated older person, a shorter needle (e.g., 1 inch instead of 1.5 inches) may be needed.

RIGHT TIME

Some medications are more effective or better tolerated if given under specific conditions. For greatest effect, medications that are ordered before meals should be given when the stomach is empty. Medications that are ordered after meals should be given only after the person has eaten.

Activities of daily living (ADLs) can be affected by medications. Medications should be administered when the drugs will interfere as little as possible with normal activities. For example, administer a diuretic medication early in the day to prevent the older person from having to get up several times at night to urinate. Administer steroids in the morning, because they can give the person an energy "boost." Steroids given in the evening can cause insomnia.

The timing of eye drop administration becomes an issue when an aging person requires more than one type of medication in the same eye. Some eye medications are compatible and can be given together, whereas others cannot. Clarify the timing and order of administration for eye drops with the pharmacy, and clearly indicate the schedule in the medication administration record.

RIGHT DOCUMENTATION

Be careful when you are documenting medications. Facilities use a variety of different forms and records to document various aspects of care, including medication administration. To ensure that all medications are administered properly, the rules of documentation must be followed.

Medications cannot be documented as having been given until they have actually been administered. This means that you must stay in the room and watch the older adult take the medication. It is not a safe practice to leave a medication at the bedside unless the resident has specific orders that permit self-medication.

Include special observations regarding the patient's or resident's response in the daily nursing notes and narrative summaries. Identify the reasons for administering "as needed" medications each time one is administered, and document the effectiveness of these medications. When a medication is refused or withheld, clearly document the reasons and notify the primary care provider so that the plan of care can be adjusted if necessary.

PATIENT RIGHTS AND MEDICATION

Older adults have the right to know what medication they are receiving and why they are receiving it. Nurses should provide this information when questioned and when a new medication is prescribed.

Older adults also have the right to refuse a medication. If a person refuses to take medication, nurses cannot use force. A positive attitude and encouragement may help encourage the individual to adhere to the treatment plan. However, when a medication is still refused, you must determine and document the reasons for refusal, notify the charge nurse, and communicate any problems to the primary care provider.

Provide privacy for the older person during injections or any other procedures. Close the doors and/or curtains. Failing to do this violates residents' rights.

Administering psychotropic drugs as chemical restraints presents a risk to the rights of older adults. Since the passage of The Nursing Home Reform Law, a part of the Omnibus Budget Reconciliation Act (OBRA) of 1987 mandating the appropriate use of physical and chemical restraints for nursing home residents, there has been a significant decrease in residents being restrained (Fashaw et al., 2020). You must follow specific guidelines carefully regarding the administration of psychotropic medications and monitoring of behavior in an older person. Each abnormal behavior that is an indication for the administration of such drugs must be individually identified in the plan of care. During each shift, you must document the number of times these identified behaviors occur. If no symptoms occur at a given dosage of psychotropic medication, the prescriber will attempt to decrease the dose. This process continues as long as the older person receives these medications.

SELF-MEDICATION AND OLDER ADULTS

IN AN INSTITUTIONAL SETTING

Under OBRA legislation, residents of care facilities should have the option of self-medication if they are capable of doing so safely. An order stating that self-medication is permitted is usually required.

Self-medication by a resident can be time-consuming because you remain responsible for monitoring the resident's adherence and response to the medications. When self-medication is anticipated, you must assess the older adult's ability to understand and adhere to the medication regimen. This assessment should include the resident's ability to read labels, follow directions, and measure dosages accurately. After it has been determined that the person can safely assume responsibility for self-medication, the nurse should develop a plan, including (1) the delivery of adequate amounts of medication, (2) safe storage of medications that will be kept at the bedside, (3) documentation of medications taken, and (4) follow-up assessments of the medications' effectiveness or side effects.

QSEN
Considerations: Teamwork and Collaboration

Delegation

MEDICATION ADMINISTRATION
Many long-term care institutions now use specially trained nursing assistants as medication assistants to administer routine oral and some topical medications to stable patients. The responsibility for for monitoring the patient's response to the medication, however, remains with the nurse.

IN THE HOME

Taking medications correctly can be a complex problem for older adults. Because medications are a significant part of the medical plan of care, older adults who live independently must learn to take them properly. The responsibility of assessing medication-taking behaviors and teaching safe self-administration often falls to the home health care nurse (see Home Health Considerations box).

 Home Health Considerations

Medications

Nurses who work in home health have a great opportunity to evaluate patients' medication knowledge and adherence to medication therapy. The number of drugs prescribed and the risks for drug-drug interactions increase when a patient is being seen by more than one specialist. Adherence issues are also likely with multiple medications. Here are some steps to increase patient awareness and adherence:

1. Explain why it is important to complete a thorough medical history and review of medications to gain the older adult's cooperation.
2. Determine what drugs (prescription, OTC, and herbal) are kept in the home. If possible, go around the home with the older adult and identify where medications are stored. Be sure to check places, such as medicine cabinets, the kitchen table, counters or cabinets, on top of and inside the refrigerator, at the bedside, and in purses.
3. Check whether there are any other "old medications" stored in a shoebox, bag, or anywhere else.
4. Gather all medications in the home and review them one at a time. Ask the patient to identify which ones are taken daily, occasionally, and as needed. If more than one older adult lives in the home, separate the medications, and evaluate each separately. Watch for drugs that do not relate to any identified health problems, for any drug duplications caused by orders under both generic and trade names, for potential drug-drug interactions (including OTC and herbs), and for inappropriate drug dosages.
5. Review each medication to determine whether the patient knows why it is being taken, when to take it, and any precautions to use regarding the drug.
6. Discuss what method (if any) the older person uses to verify that the appropriate doses of all medications are taken each day (e.g., Does the person use a daily or weekly pillbox?).
7. After obtaining the patient's consent, discard any expired drugs appropriately.

TEACHING OLDER ADULTS ABOUT MEDICATIONS

Older adults and their families or significant others should be given complete information about the prescribed medications and the proper method for taking them. Explanations should be given well in advance of the older adult's departure from the office, clinic, or hospital. If possible, nurses should select a time when the older adult's anxiety level is low, because the older adult will be more likely to remember the important points when feeling calm. If the directions are complex, extra time may be needed to ensure that they are understood completely. Commonly, older people fail to ask questions because they are afraid of being seen as ignorant or bothersome. The information should be reviewed and repeated, if necessary, at subsequent visits. Provide all information in written form in addition to the verbal instructions.

Most medications are taken orally, but increasingly drugs are administered using alternative routes. When medication is taken in any way other than the oral route, verify that the older person understands and is able to demonstrate safe self-administration. This includes transdermal patches, suppositories, eye drops or eardrops, and injections. Remember, many things that seem obvious or simple to nurses are complex for others.

In addition to providing information about their prescription medications to independent older adults, emphasize the importance of consulting with the prescribing provider or pharmacist before drinking alcoholic beverages or taking any OTC or herbal medications. Remind independent older adults never to take medication prescribed for someone else without first consulting the primary care provider.

 Patient Education

Independent Older Adults and Medications

Older adults who live independently need to know the following:

- Alcohol and nonsteroidal anti-inflammatory drugs (NSAIDs), such as ibuprofen, can increase blood pressure and interfere with the action of antihypertensive medications.
- Excessive use of acetaminophen can damage the kidneys; if the patient uses alcohol heavily, it can also damage the liver.
- Antacids do not protect the stomach from the effects of aspirin or other NSAIDs.
- Antacids, calcium supplements, and significant amounts of dairy products should be taken at least 2 hours apart from other medications.
- The combination of an NSAID with an ACE inhibitor increases the risk for kidney failure, especially when the patient is also taking a diuretic.

Each older person who lives independently should have an up-to-date record that identifies their major physical problems, their care providers, any allergies, and all current medications. This list must be updated each time a medication is added or discontinued. If the person is not capable of keeping the record up to date, the nurse or family should provide assistance. This record should be taken along each time the individual receives health care services so that all care providers have the necessary information. A written record relieves the older person of the burden of trying to remember too many details, which is particularly difficult when the person is under stress.

Nurses can assist older adults by preparing medication cards or sheets that identify and give the important information about each medication (Box 7.5). Teaching aids should be kept simple and clear; writing should be large and legible. Family members should be included in the patient education so that they are able to assist if necessary.

Box 7.5	Information to Include on Medication Teaching Sheets

- Name of the medication (trade and/or generic)
- The time or times when the medication should be taken
- Whether the medication should be taken before, with, or after meals
- Any precautions to take with medication preparation
- How much of the medication to take
- The reason why the person is receiving each medication (desired effects)
- Common side effects
- Action to take if these side effects occur
- What to do if they forget a dose of the medication
- What to do if the person experiences nausea or vomiting and is unable to take oral medication

SAFETY AND NONADHERENCE ISSUES

Nonadherence with prescribed medication regimens is common among older adults. Choosing to not take medication as prescribed can result in poorer health, adverse reactions, emergency department visits, hospitalization, and even death. The financial cost of nonadherence with medication therapy is estimated to be as high as $300 billion a year (Kim et al., 2018).

Several factors can increase the risk for nonadherence. Cognitive and sensory limitations increase the risk for medication errors. Keeping track of multiple medications can be confusing to anyone, but it is more likely to present problems for older adults. Up to 2 medications does not seem to cause many problems, but a significant number of older adults become confused and nonadherent when 3 or more medications are ordered. Special precautions and complicated time schedules compound the problems. To reduce the risk for nonadherence, encourage older adults to talk to the primary care provider and/or the pharmacist to see whether there is any safe way to reduce the number of medications or simplify the medication schedule. In addition, research has shown that depression, belief patterns, and lack of a social support system contribute to nonadherence.

Techniques that improve safety and adherence include, but are not limited to the following:

- Associating medication schedules with regular daily events, such as meals or bedtime, can help older adults remember to take their medications. Provide additional patient education if medications require special timing (e.g., before or after meals). Unless older persons are aware of the reasons and necessity for a schedule, they may not adhere to the schedule and may experience untoward effects.
- Explain the importance of preparing medication in a well-lit area. Poor lighting can further reduce vision in older adults and increase the chance of a mistake.
- Ensure that containers are properly labeled. Visually impaired older adults can continue to self-medicate if measures are taken to compensate for visual problems. Large, preferably uppercase or printed lettering should be used on all labels and teaching materials. All print or writing should be in dark, bold letters. If there is any chance of moisture on the labels, coat them in clear plastic or a wide piece of clear packing tape. This prevents blurring of the lettering, which can lead to errors.
- Apply color codes, tape strips, pictures, or textures, such as sandpaper to containers to help older adults recognize them. For example, black could indicate medicine to be taken with breakfast, red could indicate medications for lunch, and a piece of sandpaper attached to the bottle could indicate bedtime medications. Avoid yellow, because many older adults have difficulty distinguishing this color from others. Alternatively, place one strip of tape for morning administration, two strips for lunch, three strips for dinner, and four strips for bedtime. Make sure that the person understands whatever coding system is selected. Mark medication cups with dark lines or tape to improve accuracy in measuring liquids, and provide magnifiers for insulin syringes.
- Modify containers for ease of use. Impaired physical function can interfere with self-medication. Many pill bottles routinely come with safety caps that older adults cannot open. If requested, most pharmacies will provide containers that are easier to open.
- Establish measures to distinguish and separate similar containers. If the older person is receiving eardrops and eye drops, store these containers well away from each other and mark clearly with a large picture of an eye or an ear so that they are distinguishable. This is particularly important because many ear preparations can cause permanent damage to the eye.
- Provide information to older adults regarding the proper storage of medications. Medications should be stored away from direct light and moisture, which can cause chemical changes. The tiny pillboxes used by many older adults can be dangerous and should be avoided. Pills left in the boxes may undergo chemical changes. Nitroglycerine, for example, can become totally ineffective if stored improperly. Once medications have been removed from the prescription bottle, they cannot be readily identified and the older person can easily take the wrong pill. It is safest to leave medications in the pharmacy bottles even though they may be bulky.
- Obtain or devise a system to promote adherence. When older people are unable to correctly maintain their medication schedule by using the bottles provided by the pharmacy, other approaches may be necessary. There are several ways in which nurses can help older adults remember to take their medications. Medication reminder systems help some older adults remember to take medications. These systems typically consist of divided containers that sort the medications by day of the week or by time. They can be purchased inexpensively at a pharmacy. A simple check of the box will reveal whether the

medication was taken on time. Some individuals require more medication than fits into these standard containers, or they may fear that they will drop the container and mix everything up. These individuals may benefit from a system using small zip-closed plastic bags that are labeled (using masking tape) with the appropriate day and time. High-tech solutions, such as automated pill dispensing systems with alarms are available, but the cost of most of these devices is significant, and maintenance of the system may be too complex for the average older adult.

- Stress the importance of being alert when taking medications. Sleepiness can interfere with the ability to read labels. If patients are not completely awake, they can easily take the wrong medication. It is not advisable for older adults to keep any medications, particularly those taken to promote sleep, at the bedside. Because sleeping pills dull the ability to perceive things accurately, patients who have trouble getting to sleep may take extra doses of their medication and be seriously harmed.

Older adults can achieve maximal benefits from their medication when nurses pay careful attention to all aspects of medication administration. Careful assessment, good patient education, and well-planned interventions can enable many older adults to function independently.

Get Ready for the Next Generation NCLEX® Examination!

Key Points

- Most older adults take at least a single medication each day and one-third take at least 5, not including OTC preparations.
- Drug use, misuse, and abuse present serious threats to the well-being of older individuals and increase the risk for hospitalization resulting from adverse drug reactions.
- The risk for adverse reactions is increased by the normal changes of aging, pathologic changes related to the higher incidence of acute or chronic diseases, and numerous other factors.
- Polypharmacy is a significant problem for older adults; OTC medications, herbs, and supplements all need to be considered in reviewing prescription medications.
- The medical community has long recognized that children require special consideration with regard to medication, and we are now aware that the aging population also requires special consideration.
- Geropharmacology, the study of how older adults respond to medications, is an expanding area of study.
- Care providers who prescribe medication, pharmacists who dispense medication, and nurses who administer medication must continue to work together to understand the unique problems and needs of older adults with regard to these potentially dangerous substances.
- Nurses must work diligently to build a knowledge base of the medications administered to their patients or residents, know how to administer each medication safely, know how to assess the older adult's need for and response to each medication, and develop an appropriate plan of care that includes safety concerns and patient education needs.

Additional Learning Resources

SG Go to your Evolve website at http://evolve.elsevier.com/Williams/geriatric for the additional online resources.

Online Resources
- Resource for older adults to keep track of medications, herbs, and OTCs used: https://www.healthinaging.org/sites/default/files/media/pdf/HIA-MyDrug-Supplement%20Jan%202019.pdf
- Drug interaction checker: http://reference.medscape.com/drug-interactionchecker
- Beers Criteria for Potentially Inappropriate Medications: https://www.guidelinecentral.com/summaries/american-geriatrics-society-2015-updated-beers-criteria-for-potentially-inappropriate-medication-use-in-older-adults/#section-society
- Medications and older adults: http://www.healthinaging.org/medications-older-adults/

Review Questions for the Next Generation NCLEX® Examination

1. Following an appointment with the primary care provider, the nurse is performing patient education to an independent living older adult about a newly prescribed medication. Which factor is most likely to interfere with the effectiveness of this process?
   a. The patient wears a hearing aid.
   b. The patient has a history of hypothyroidism.
   c. The nurse provided written handouts.
   d. The nurse is in a hurry.

2. What is an example of a medication that can be crushed?
   a. A potassium tablet
   b. Enteric coated aspirin
   c. Sublingual nitroglycerin
   d. A calcium tablet

3. You are administering medication through a transdermal patch. What are some precautions? (Select all that apply.)
   a. Remove all old patches before applying a new patch.
   b. Use the same location each time for consistent absorption.
   c. Cleanse the skin after removing an old patch.
   d. Dispose of old patches in the toilet.
   e. Verify the dosage strength of the patch.
   f. Wear gloves.
   g. Tape over the patch to keep it secure.

4. A resident in a long-term care facility has an order for digoxin 0.25 mg every morning in tablet form. If the nurse assesses that this resident has been having difficulty swallowing, what should the nurse do?

   a. Administer the digoxin in liquid form.
   b. Crush the digoxin for administration.
   c. Withhold the digoxin and document.
   d. Discuss the possibility of an order change to liquid form with the primary care provider.

5. Older adults are more likely to experience adverse drug reactions because of which of the following? *(Select all that apply.)*

   a. The number of medications they take daily
   b. Physiologic changes in metabolism and excretion
   c. Higher percentage of body fluid
   d. Cognitive changes
   e. Interactions with foods, OTC preparations, and herbal supplements
   f. Decreased sense of taste

6. What should you include in a lesson plan for the independent living older person?

   a. Take most medications with milk or antacids to avoid stomach upset.
   b. Avoid drinking alcohol if taking acetaminophen.
   c. Keep daily medications in the kitchen cabinet near the sink.
   d. Save prescription drugs in case the care provider orders them again.

7. You are caring for a new patient who had a heart transplant 5 years ago. She takes 7 medications every day, including anti-rejection drugs, cardiac medications, and inhalers. She mentions feeling "depressed," and wants your advice about trying a new "natural" remedy she found on the internet. Which would be the best response?

   a. "That might be a good idea. I have heard good things about St. John's wort."
   b. "My Aunt Judy used to take some of those herbal remedies, and she died from liver failure."
   c. "You really should talk with your doctor first, because many things can interfere with your antirejection and heart medications, even herbs and supplements."
   d. "You're on too many pills already; you should start an exercise program instead and go outside for some fresh air to help you feel better."

8. The nurse's first appointment of the day is a 75-year old female patient for a preoperative assessment for her upcoming hip replacement surgery. The patient has hypertension and a history of thyroid cancer and deep venous thrombosis. Current medications include 40 mg lisinopril once daily, 4 mg warfarin once daily, and 85 mcg levothyroxine once daily. The nurse documents these findings as part of the assessment:

Alert and oriented
Temperature = 98.6 degrees F (37 degrees C)
Blood Pressure = 128/80 mm Hg
Respirations = 20 breaths per minute
Heart rate = 86 beats per minute and regular
Reports feeling tired in the last few days
Recent constipation
Weight increase of 10 pounds in the past 3 weeks
Skin is intact
Takes ginseng
Takes her medications with breakfast including grapefruit juice
States that her pain is currently a 2 (on a 0-10 pain intensity scale)

Highlight or place a check mark next to the assessment findings that require follow-up by the nurse.

REFERENCES

Blanco-Reina, E., Valdellés, J., Aguilar-Cano, L., et al. (2019). 2015 Beers Criteria and STOPP v2 for detecting potentially inappropriate medication in community-dwelling older people: Prevalence, profile, and risk factors. European Journal of Clinical Pharmacology, 75(10), 1459–1466, 2019.

Fashaw, S. A., Thomas, K. S., McCreedy, E., et al. (2020). Thirty-year trends in nursing home composition and quality since the passage of the Omnibus Reconciliation Act. Journal of American Medical Directors Association, 21(2), 233. 2020.

Gibson, G., Kennedy, L. H., & Balow, G. (2020). Polypharmacy in older adults. Current Psychiatry, 19(4), 40–46.

Harvard Health Publishing. (2020). Are you taking too many medications? Harvard Health Letter, 46(1), 1–7.

Hammond, L., & Moseley, K. (2019). Medication and fall safety for older adults. Nursing Made Incredibly Easy! 17(3), 16–19.

Hess, C., Linnebur, S. A., Rhyne, D. N., et al. (2018). Over-the-counter drugs to avoid in older adults with kidney impairment. CANNT Journal, 27(4), 32–44.

Kim, J., Combs, K., Downs, J., et al. (2018). Medication adherence: The elephant in the room. U.S. Pharmacist, 43(1), 30–34.

Khan, J., Zain, W. N. I. W. M., & Islam, M. N. (2020). Effect of concurrent use of herbal supplements and prescribed drugs in chronic diseases. International Medical Journal, 27(3), 277–279.

Oscanoa, T, Lizaraso, F., & Carvajal, A. (2017). Hospital admissions due to adverse drug reactions in the elderly; A meta-analysis European Journal of Clinical Pharmacology, 73(6), 759–770.

The Joint Commission. (2022). Official "Do Not Use" list, https://www.jointcommission.org/facts_about_do_not_use_list/

U.S. Department of Health and Human Services, Office of Disease Prevention and Health Promotion. (2020). National action plan for ADE prevention, https://health.gov/our-work/health-care-quality/adverse-drug-events/national-ade-action-plan/

8 | Health Assessment for Older Adults

Objectives

1. Identify different levels of assessment.
2. Compare and contrast subjective versus objective data.
3. Discuss the importance of a thorough assessment.
4. Describe appropriate methods for structuring and conducting an interview.
5. Identify approaches that facilitate a successful physical examination.
6. Discuss modifications to use when preparing an older person for a physical examination.
7. Describe techniques to use when performing a physical examination.
8. Explain adaptations to use when assessing vital signs in older adults.
9. Discuss how the Minimum Data Set affects assessments of institutionalized older adults.

Key Terms

assessment (ă-SĔS-mĕnt, p. 158)
auscultation (ăw-skŭl-TĀ-shŭn, p. 162)
inspection (ĭn-SPĔK-shŭn, p. 162)
objective data (p. 159)
orthostatic hypotension (p. 168)

palpation (păl-PĀ-shŭn, p. 162)
percussion (pĕr-KŬ-shŭn, p. 162)
pulse deficit (p. 166)
screenings (SKRĒ-nĭngs, p. 158)
subjective data (p. 159)

Health **assessment** of older adults can be done on several levels, ranging from simple screenings to complex, in-depth evaluations. To perform assessments accurately, nurses and other health care providers who interact with older adults must possess the necessary knowledge and skill to perform the assessments correctly. They must know how to use diagnostic tools and equipment safely. Furthermore, they must be knowledgeable and sensitive to the unique needs of older adults.

HEALTH SCREENING

Health **screenings** are done to identify older individuals who are in need of further, more in-depth assessment. Screenings for high blood pressure, hearing loss, foot problems, and challenges with activities of daily living (ADLs) are commonly performed at senior centers and health clinics. Screening services are often provided by medical and nursing schools or other health groups committed to helping older adults in need. Many screenings are performed by lay individuals working under the direction of professionals. Special screenings for depression and suicide risk, although less common, are recommended for the older adult population. Some health concerns are more common among certain ethnic populations, although limited use of screenings and socioeconomic status could be

contributing factors. For example, there are complex, interrelated factors contributing to different levels of cancer incidence and number of deaths among various racial, ethnic, and underserved groups. The most significant of these factors seems to be related to inadequate health care coverage and low socioeconomic status. Since the Affordable Care Act was fully implemented in 2014, this imbalance in cancer rates in various groups has decreased for all cancer deaths combined in both men and women. However, there continues to be a large racial disparity in the rates of breast cancer death among women (Riba et al., 2019). Nurses should continue to screen all populations for potential problems and promote their early identification and treatment. Today, Medicare coverage is more focused on preventive care. Annual wellness checkups and colonoscopies, for example, are two screenings covered by Medicare that should be offered to all appropriate individuals.

Screenings are not designed to provide treatment. They are intended to identify significant findings so that older individuals who are in need of care can be referred to the most appropriate health service provider (i.e., physician, social worker, dietitian, or nurse) in a timely manner. Early screenings also help to reduce frustration in older adults and the wasteful expenditure of time and resources. See Chapter 4 for common screening tests for older adults (Table 4.1).

HEALTH ASSESSMENTS

In-depth health assessments are time-consuming and must be performed by skilled professionals. Nurses perform health assessments of older adults in the community, in clinics, and in institutional settings. Health assessment includes the collection of all important health-related data using a variety of techniques. Data include all of the information gathered about a person. This information is used to identify a patient's problems and to plan their care; therefore accurate and complete data should be collected. Data can be either objective or subjective.

Objective data include information that can be gathered using the senses of vision, hearing, touch, and smell. Objective information is collected by means of direct observation, physical examination, and laboratory or diagnostic tests. Because objective data are concrete by nature, all trained observers should report similar findings about a person or that person's behavior at any given point in time. Behaviors such as crying, limping, and clutching of the abdomen can be verified by anyone who observes the patient. Rashes, skin lesions, and wound drainage are likewise observable to anyone. Objective data can be made more precise and specific by using meters, monitors, and other measuring devices. A blood pressure reading, a change in weight, the size of a wound, the volume of urine, and laboratory test results are all examples of specific objective data. Whenever possible, objective data should be stated using specific information because accurate and precise data enhance the nurse's ability to determine changes in a person's health status. For example, it is better to take a temperature reading than to touch the skin and determine that it feels warm. Both are objective observations, but one is more precise than the other.

Subjective data comprise information gathered from the older person's point of view. Fear, anxiety, frustration, and pain are examples of subjective information. Subjective data are best described in the individual's own words, such as "I'm so afraid of what is going to happen to me here," or "It hurts so much I could die!"

When nurses are performing health assessments of older adults, they may need to modify their usual approaches and techniques to make them more appropriate.

INTERVIEWING OLDER ADULTS

Interviews conducted during admission to a facility are likely to be planned and conducted in a formal manner. Other interviews may be spontaneous, informal, and based on an immediate need recognized by the nurse. Before beginning an interview with an older adult, plan ways to establish and maintain a climate that promotes comfort and develops trust. This includes preparing the physical setting, establishing rapport, and structuring the flow of the interview. During this planning phase, take into consideration the unique needs of the older person.

PREPARING THE PHYSICAL SETTING

Choose the interview environment carefully. Minimize distractions: noise from computers, televisions, radios, phones, and public address systems should not be loud enough to distract an older adult or interfere with their ability to distinguish words and understand questions. Lighting should be diffused, because bright lights or glare may make it difficult to see clearly. Furniture should be comfortable. Privacy is very important. Conduct the interview in a room where there is little chance of interruption. If such a place is not available, the patient's room may provide sufficient privacy; the curtains should be drawn and the door closed. Make sure that the room is comfortably warm and free of drafts. Many older adults experience urinary frequency or urgency, so it is advisable to either assist them to the bathroom or inform them that a bathroom is available nearby should they require it.

ESTABLISHING RAPPORT

It is most appropriate to begin the interview by greeting the older adult and introducing yourself. During this first contact, it is best to address people using their formal name (e.g., "Mr. Singh" or "Mrs. Adams"). Appropriate use of names indicates respect and helps build rapport.

 QSEN Considerations: Patient-Centered Care

Use of the individual's first name only without the person's consent is presumptuous and overly familiar. This may be resented by the older person even if it is not verbalized. If there is any doubt about someone's preference, it is best to ask the person how they wish to be addressed.

Briefly explain the purpose of the interview so that the individual will know what to expect. An explanation helps to reduce anxiety, which might otherwise interfere with understanding. Explain how long you expect the interview to last and what will happen after it is completed.

Focus on and speak directly to the older person being interviewed (Fig. 8.1). This notion may seem obvious, but it is often disregarded in practice. Often, a younger family member present during the interview "takes over" the responses for the older person. The conversation then takes place between the nurse and the family member, while the older adult remains passive. An assertive older person might speak up and say, "Let me speak for myself," whereas a nonassertive older adult may be left feeling frustrated and unimportant. The nurse should continue to direct the conversation to the older adult and, if necessary, tactfully request that the family member allow

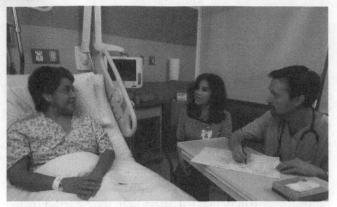

Fig. 8.1 Conducting an interview. (From Williams, P.A. [2021]. *Fundamental concepts and skills for nursing* [6th ed.]. St. Louis, MO: Elsevier.)

the older person to respond first before they add information. If the older adult is confused or nonresponsive, the family member will need to be more actively included to provide information. For an older adult who does not speak English, an interpreter will be necessary. Family members as interpreters increase the risk of information not being translated correctly, cause more medical errors, and, in some cases, break patient confidentiality policies (White et al., 2019).

 Cultural Considerations

Assessment and Culture

Different cultures approach health care and health care decisions differently. In general, Western cultures focus on self-reliance, whereas non-Western cultures tend to rely on their families. Because it is culturally appropriate to include family members, the nurse will need to determine who will answer questions and participate in the assessment process. Remember, although nurses must appreciate and acknowledge different cultures, it is important not to classify people simply by their culture.

During the physical examination, be careful to maintain the modesty standards set by each culture.

- In some cultures, it may be desirable for a family member to be present during this examination. In most cases, this should be permitted.
- Cultural values may dictate that physical contact with a nurse of the opposite gender is inappropriate. In these cases, the patient or family may request that a nurse of the same gender as the patient perform the examination.

When in doubt, consult a knowledgeable expert or an authoritative reference text about the specific cultural expectations.

Enhance rapport by first determining the problems or concerns that most trouble the patient and then focusing on those problems. This helps to reduce anxiety and increases the older adult's perception that the nurse is truly concerned about them. Begin the assessment with a look at the person as a whole before focusing on specifics.

STRUCTURING THE INTERVIEW

Plan to allow sufficient time for the interview. Older adults typically have long and complex life stories. Remember that their speed of recall and verbal responses may be slower. The individual may feel pressured or stressed if the pace of the interview is too rapid.

Try not to accomplish too much during a single interview. The effort involved in communication can be fatiguing to an older individual, particularly one with health problems. It is better to have several brief interactions lasting fewer than 30 minutes each rather than one long interview that leaves the patient exhausted.

 Nurse Alert

Stay alert for signs of fatigue (e.g., sagging head or shoulders, sighing, altered facial expression, and irritability), which indicate the need to end the interview.

During the interview, a variety of communication techniques should be used to ensure that the patient accurately understands the information. Avoid using medical terminology or abbreviations and use words that the older person is likely to understand. It is important to speak slowly and clearly, keeping messages simple without seeming to be patronizing. The fact that an older person needs extra time does not mean that the person is mentally impaired. Even if the older adult has been diagnosed with a mental impairment, they deserve to be given respectful and professional responses. Remain calm and empathetic. When the patient is speaking, do not interrupt either verbal or nonverbal messages. Some older individuals tend to ramble in conversation and may need to be brought back on track. A summary or restatement of the conversation can help. It is not appropriate to complete sentences for the older adult. Remain attentive and calm and allow patients to complete their sentences. Too often, the nurse's conclusion is considerably different from the patient's intention.

The interview should not end abruptly. A statement such as "We're almost done for now" prepares the older person for the end of the interaction. Many lonely persons will try to extend the conversation beyond the time that the nurse has available. In such cases you can set a time for further interaction by saying, "We'll talk again tomorrow morning" or "I'll set up another appointment so we can talk more;" this may help to maintain rapport. It is essential to follow through as promised or the patient may lose trust and refuse to communicate freely in the future.

OBTAINING THE HEALTH HISTORY

Before starting a physical assessment, the nurse will use interviewing techniques to obtain a health history. This history starts with basic identifying data followed by a history of past health concerns and then a review of current health issues. Some older adults are able to provide information easily, whereas others may be poor historians. Much will depend on the individual's cognitive level and the complexity of the particular medical history. When the older adult is unsure of answers, it is often wise to move on to other topics and attempt to gather the information from a family member at a later time. In addition, you may want to obtain information regarding the person's family and psychosocial status. The health history data will help the nurse to form an overall impression of the older person and help to determine those areas most in need of further exploration and assessment (Box 8.1).

PHYSICAL ASSESSMENT OF OLDER ADULTS

Once the history has been obtained, you are ready to proceed to the physical assessment. During this assessment, objective information is obtained to accompany the subjective information offered by the older adult. Objective information further helps to determine the person's abilities and limitations. It may verify the subjective information given by the older adult; it may also reveal problems that were previously unrecognized. When assessing older adults, pay close attention not only to obvious physiologic changes but also to

changes in mood or behavior that may signal a change in condition. Seemingly small pieces of information can be important to the total assessment. With aging, people experience changes in several physiologic responses. For example, a temperature change of just a few tenths of a degree—rather than rising above the reading of 100 degrees F, as would be expected in a younger person—may indicate the onset of an infection in an older adult. Other changes can be equally meaningful and may be missed or ignored if nurses are not especially careful (Table 8.1).

Perform the physical assessment in a location that promotes the physical comfort of the older adult. Often, this will be the person's room or a special examination room. Maintain privacy by keeping doors and curtains closed. Be careful not to chill the older adult while examining the body. Blankets and gowns that provide adequate warmth should be used to promptly cover the parts of the body not being assessed. If the examination is being done during physical care (e.g., during the bath), pay particular attention to prevent chilling caused by evaporation.

Collect equipment—such as a flashlight, measuring tape, scale, sphygmomanometer, stethoscope, and thermometer—before beginning the assessment. This will convey an impression of competence and enable the assessment to progress smoothly.

Box 8.1 | Health History Data

The history should include but not be limited to:

IDENTIFYING DATA
- Name
- Date of birth
- Residence
- Ethnicity and cultural preferences
- Language preferences
- Gender identity/preferred pronouns
- Religion
- Marital/significant other status
- Previous and/or current occupation
- Educational background
- Advance directives and any other relevant data

PAST HISTORY
- Perception of general health
- Frequency of medical and dental care, including screenings, such as mammography, blood pressure, etc.
- Known or suspected allergies (medicines, food, animals, etc.)
- Immunizations (type and date)
- Exposure to communicable disease, such as tuberculosis
- Serious childhood illness or injuries (rheumatic fever, fractures, etc.)
- History of serious illnesses (specify illness, date of onset, type of treatment received, resolved vs. ongoing problem)
- Hospitalizations (reason and date)
- Surgeries (type and date)

- Mental health treatment (type and date)
- Review of personal health habits, such as diet, fluid intake, exercise practices, sleep patterns, bowel and bladder routines, alcohol, caffeine and tobacco use, sexual activity, etc.

PRESENT MEDICAL HISTORY
- Major current problems or concerns (in person's own words)
- Do the problems relate to an accident or fall?
- Symptoms (location, duration, severity, etc.)
- Date of onset (sudden or gradual onset)
- What makes problem worse or better?
- What was done in response to symptoms (home remedies, visit to primary care provider or emergency room, etc.)?
- Current medications (look at bottles if possible)
- Adherence to medication regimen
- Current medical treatments or therapies (oxygen, physical therapy, etc.)

FAMILY AND PSYCHOSOCIAL HISTORY
- Living family members (spouse, children, siblings, etc.) and nature of relationships
- Friends and social activity practices (clubs, church activities, community organizations, online interactions, etc.)
- Significant deceased family members
- Hobbies and interests
- Pets

Table 8.1 Atypical Presentation of Illness

TYPE OF ILLNESS	ATYPICAL PRESENTATION
Infectious diseases	Absence of fever WBCs within normal limits Shaking chills Abdominal pain Vomiting Altered mental status
Acute abdomen	Mild abdominal discomfort Sudden anorexia, indigestion Abrupt alteration in bowel habits
Cardiac problems	Absence of chest pain Vague symptoms of fatigue or nausea Dyspnea Syncope
Pulmonary	Confusion
Thyroid disease	Hypothyroidism: Fewer and often easily ignored symptoms, including confusion, loss of appetite and/or weight, falling, loss of bladder control, and impairment in completing ADLs
Depression	Sadness, loss of hope, tearfulness, poor temperament, decline in cognitive abilities

ADLs, activities of daily living; *WBCs,* white blood cells.

Data from Barad, D. H. (2020). Pelvic pain, *Merck Manual.* https://www.merckmanuals.com/professional/gynecology-and-obstetrics/symptoms-of-gynecologic-disorders/pelvic-pain?query=abdominal%20pain%20geriatric#v1060859/

Besdine, R. W. (2019). Evaluation of the older adult, *Merck Manual.* https://www.merckmanuals.com/professional/geriatrics/approach-to-the-geriatric-patient/evaluation-of-the-older-adult?query=pulmonary%20geriatric/

Ham, R. J., Sloane, P. D., Warshaw, G. A., et al., (2014). *Primary care geriatrics: A case-based approach* (6th ed.). Saunders: Philadelphia, PA.

Complete the physical assessment in an orderly manner so that no important observations are missed (Table 8.2). Begin with an overview of the person, including their general appearance, hygiene, grooming, alertness, responsiveness, and general mobility; then proceed with more focused assessments. The most common method of physical assessment is a head-to-toe approach, in which the entire body is assessed systematically. Other approaches, such as body systems or functional approaches, are also acceptable. Later chapters provide guidelines for assessing safety needs, nutrition, skin, elimination, activity, sleep, cognitive function, and other areas in more detail.

When performing physical assessments, nurses use a variety of techniques, including inspection, palpation, auscultation, and percussion.

INSPECTION

Inspection is the most commonly used method of physical assessment; in it, the senses of vision, smell, and hearing are used to collect data. Skill at inspection improves the more often the technique is performed. Inspection requires the nurse to be completely active, alert, and aware of everything that is seen, heard, or smelled. It begins the first time we see the older adult. Even during a brief interaction, skilled nurses should be inspecting the individual, looking for anything that may indicate a change in condition.

Inspection can be both general and specific. General inspection is used to detect the need for more specific inspection. For example, if the nurse observes that the older adult is eating poorly, a more specific inspection of the oral cavity may be indicated. If body odor is

Table 8.2 Body Systems Approach to Physical Assessment*

BODY SYSTEM	HISTORY	TECHNIQUES	ASSESSMENT
Skin	Injuries, burns, infections, allergies, anemia, fluid intake levels, when and how skin change occurred, etc.	Inspection and palpation	• Color (erythema, pallor, cyanosis, jaundice, ecchymosis) • Pigment changes (hypopigmentation, hyperpigmentation) • Elasticity (turgor) • Temperature • Moisture (perspiration, oiliness) • Texture • Lesions • Primary: Macule, papule, pustule, vesicle, wheal, cyst, tumor • Secondary: Scale, scar, fissure, lichen, ulcer • Vascular: Senile purpura • Hemangioma, spider angioma • Itching/tenderness • Edema • pitting edema

Scale	Degree	Response
1+ trace	Barely detectable	Rapid
2+ mild	Less than 1/4 inch	10–15 sec
3+ moderate	1/4–1/2 inch	1–2 min
4+ severe	Greater than 1/2 inch	2–5 min

Table 8.2   Body Systems Approach to Physical Assessment*—cont'd

BODY SYSTEM	HISTORY	TECHNIQUES	ASSESSMENT
Nails	Injuries, dietary insufficiency, COPD, etc.	Inspection and palpation	• Shape • Color • Thickness • Ridges • Angle of nailbed • Surrounding tissues (paronychia)
Hair	Cosmetic use, dietary insufficiency, hormone problems, exposure to parasites	Inspection and palpation	• Color and texture • Distribution • Quantity (alopecia, hirsutism) • Condition of scalp, presence of nits
Skull, Face, and Neck	Congestion, drainage, sore throat, difficulty swallowing, dental problems, swelling, exposure to communicable disease, etc.	Inspection and palpation	• Size, shape, and symmetry (moon face) • Smile and frown (look for symmetry or drooping) • Nose (drainage, symmetry) • Sinuses (check for tenderness or pressure) • Lips (color, moisture, lesions) • Mouth, including mucous membranes, teeth, and gums • Throat and tonsils • Shape and movement of neck • Lymph nodes
Eyes	Glaucoma, cataracts, refractive problems, dry eyes, tearing, blurring, double vision, etc.	Inspection	• Placement of globes (bulging or sunken) • Eyelids (crusting, lashes, ptosis, etc.) • Conjunctiva (color, drainage, etc.) • Sclera (color) • Blinking (15 to 20 times per minute) • Pupils (PERRLA) • Dim room (so pupils dilate) • Check size and shape of pupils (should be equal and round) • Shine light into one eye (both pupils should constrict) • Have patient look at a distance then focus on a finger 4 inches (10 cm) from bridge of nose (both eyes should constrict with accommodation) • Eye movements (cardinal fields): Have the patient hold head still; then move a finger (12 inches from face) toward each field, then back to center (may elicit nystagmus) • Light reflex: Shine light 12 inches from face (should be symmetrical reflection on cornea) • Convergence: Watch as you move finger toward nose • Visual acuity: Snellen test (evaluate each eye separately, then together; evaluate first without glasses, then with close reading test—e.g., newspaper)
Ears	Difficulty hearing, etc.	Inspection	• Placement, shape, drainage • Inspection of external canal (otoscope) • Hearing acuity (whisper test, audiometry)
Respiratory	COPD, difficulty breathing, shortness of breath, lack of energy, cough, hemoptysis, tobacco use, allergies, medications, etc.	Inspection, auscultation (palpation and percussion)	• Shape of thorax (barrel, sunken) • Spinal curvatures (kyphosis, lordosis, scoliosis) • Movement of chest during respiration • Rate, rhythm, and depth of respiration • Listen to lung sounds over fields; compare side to side • Trachea (bronchial sounds) • Assess above clavicle and scapula to assess apex (bronchovesicular sounds) • Stay inside scapula when assessing midsection; move out when assessing bases (vesicular sounds) • Adventitious lung sounds

Continued

Table 8.2 Body Systems Approach to Physical Assessment*—cont'd

BODY SYSTEM	HISTORY	TECHNIQUES	ASSESSMENT
			• Crackles (rales): Fine, short, crackling sounds best heard on inspiration, commonly heard in lung bases • Wheezes: Continuous squeaky, musical sounds; best heard on expiration; may be heard all over lung fields • Gurgles (rhonchi): Continuous low-pitched sounds; coarse with snoring quality; cleared by coughing; heard over trachea and bronchi • Friction rub: Grating sound; similar to the rubbing sound made when sandpaper is used; heard on both inspiration and expiration; heard most often on lower anterior and lateral chest
Cardiovascular	History of heart disease, chest pain, lack of energy, fatigue, high BP, SOB, medications, edema, etc.	Inspection, palpation, auscultation	• Peripheral pulses (carotid, radial, brachial, pedal, popliteal, femoral) for presence, strength, symmetry • Apical pulse • Capillary refill time (normal is less than 3 sec) • Presence of varicosities • Signs of thrombophlebitis (tenderness, redness, swelling)
Gastrointestinal	GI pain, nausea, vomiting, constipation, flatulence, diarrhea, etc.	Inspection, then auscultation before palpation (empty bladder, supine with knees slightly bent)	• Shape and contour of abdomen • Presence of scars • Bowel sounds in four quadrants (use diaphragm) every 20 seconds
Musculoskeletal	Weakness, joint or muscle pain and tenderness, recent injury	Inspection and palpation	• Size and symmetry of muscles • Muscle strength bilaterally • Presence of contractures • Tremors or spasms • Swelling or deformity of joints (tenderness or pain) • Range of motion (smoothness, crepitus)
Neurologic	Any injury or illness affecting CNS or PNS, loss of consciousness, behavioral changes, loss of balance, headaches, seizures, or sensory changes	Inspection	• Orientation • Speech • Movement • Grip strength • Pupillary responses (presence and rate) • Balance or gait • Changes in smell, vision, hearing, sensation, temperature perception • Reaction to painful stimuli
Genitourinary	Voiding patterns, frequency, hesitancy, painful voiding, urgency, incontinence, history of STI, discharge or drainage from genitals, open lesions, etc.	Inspection and palpation	• Bladder fullness/distention • Amount, odor, color, and consistency of urine

BP, blood pressure; *CNS*, central nervous system; *COPD*, chronic obstructive pulmonary disease; *PERRLA*, pupils equal, round, reactive to light, accommodation; *PNS*, peripheral nervous system; *SOB*, shortness of breath; *STI*, sexually transmitted infection.

*This approach is useful for focused assessments.

detected, a more specific inspection of the skin may be indicated. If the nurse hears noisy breathing, a more specific inspection of the lungs may be necessary. If gait is abnormal, a more complete assessment of the joints, muscles, feet, and nervous system is indicated.

Inspection is used in assessing the overall level of function as well as when looking for specific areas of need within any particular area of function. When inspecting the older adult, it is important to pay close attention to details. Use adequate light (preferably natural light) when trying to detect subtle changes in skin color. Compare the size and mobility of body parts on one side of the body with those on the opposite side.

PALPATION

Palpation uses the sense of touch in the fingers and hands to obtain data. Palpation is used to evaluate many parts of a physical assessment, including pulses, temperature, the texture of the skin, texture and condition of the hair, presence and consistency of tumors or masses under the skin, distention of the urinary bladder, and the presence of pain or tenderness.

When palpating, use the fingertips, which are the most sensitive parts of the fingers. Warm hands and short fingernails promote comfort and reduce the risk for trauma to fragile older skin. Light touch should be used before deeper touch is attempted. When taking the pulse of an older adult, deep palpation may occlude the blood vessels. Deep pressure may also increase pain. Painful areas should be palpated last.

AUSCULTATION

Auscultation uses the sense of hearing to detect sounds produced within the body. Heart, lung, and bowel sounds are typically assessed using auscultation. Auscultation involves the use of a stethoscope or other sound amplifier (such as a Doppler) to make the sounds louder and more easily heard. Sounds are described according to their quality, pitch, intensity, and duration. *Quality* describes the sound being heard in subjective terms, such as *crackling*, *whistling*, or *snapping*. *Pitch* describes whether the sounds have a low or high tone. *Intensity* refers to the loudness or softness of the tone. *Duration* refers to the length of time for which a sound is heard. *Frequency* refers to how often a sound is heard. A sound can be continuous or intermittent. When sounds are intermittent, the number of times and the interval between occurrences should be determined.

Auscultation requires a quiet environment and special skills. Nurses should be skilled in the technique and knowledgeable regarding the significance of any findings.

PERCUSSION

Percussion is a technique whereby the size, position, and density of structures under the skin are assessed by tapping the area and listening to the resonance of the sound. Depending on the amount of vibration (sound) heard, the presence of masses, fluid, or air can be determined. This technique requires special skill and training and is used least often by nurses.

MEASURING VITAL SIGNS IN OLDER ADULTS

The measurement of vital signs involves all of the techniques previously discussed. When measuring vital signs, nurses should first complete a general inspection of the older adult to determine whether there are any subjective or objective observations that may affect the procedure or the accuracy of the readings. Because activity level, medications, eating, stress, disease processes, and the environment can all affect vital signs, the possible contributions of these factors should be considered.

Baseline vital sign readings should be obtained during the initial contact with the older adult. These readings are the basis for comparison with future readings, and they enable nurses to determine whether the person's health status is remaining constant or changing over time.

TEMPERATURE

The general inspection helps nurses to select the most appropriate route for temperature assessment. The oral (sublingual) route is used most commonly. Use an electronic thermometer or a glass thermometer that does not contain mercury to take an oral temperature. Electronic thermometers are preferred because they can give an accurate temperature in less than 1 minute instead of the recommended 3 minutes for a glass thermometer. However, using the oral route is not always possible with older adults. Those who are edentulous (without teeth) or have poor muscle control may be unable to close the mouth tightly enough for an accurate reading to be obtained. Older adults who are unable to follow directions are also poor candidates for oral temperature checks.

Although acceptable, the rectal route should be used with caution. Use of the rectal route can be psychologically traumatic to older adults, particularly if they are alert but unable to cooperate with an oral temperature. The rectal route should not be used in older persons who have undergone rectal surgery, have rectal bleeding, or are having an acute cardiac event, such as a myocardial infarction, because the taking of a rectal temperature can stimulate the vagus nerve. Rectal readings can be affected by the presence of stool in the rectum. Rectal temperature readings reflect changes in core body temperature more slowly than do oral readings and are usually slightly higher.

Use of the axillary route is not common in older adults. The use of this route is time-consuming, and the accuracy of the resulting temperature readings may be affected by environmental conditions. In addition, older adults often have decreased axillary tissue, which can lead to "air pockets" and a false low temperature reading.

Determination of body temperature using a sensor that measures the temperature of the tympanic membrane has received mixed reviews. This method has advantages and disadvantages. Use of the tympanic sensor takes only a few seconds, is not invasive, and does not require the patient's cooperation; however, the readings obtained using this method are not as accurate as originally claimed, particularly when the device is not used precisely as directed. Individual agencies need to determine whether this method of assessment is adequate for their needs.

In general, healthy, active older individuals are able to maintain core body temperature within normal limits. The accepted norm for oral temperature is 98.6 degrees F plus/minus 1 degree F (or 37 degrees C plus/minus 0.6 degree C). Studies have shown that older adults have a lower average core body temperature. The cause for this is not clear, but it may be the result of decreased subcutaneous fat, decreased blood circulation to the extremities, or less muscle mass. Environmental temperature appears to play a greater role in older adults because their thermoregulatory control systems are not as efficient are those in younger individuals.

PULSE

Before assessing the pulse, position the patient comfortably in such a way that you have access to the desired site. The position should be the same (e.g., lying, sitting, or standing) each time the pulse is checked; this will provide meaningful readings for comparison.

Pulse can be assessed at various sites on the body, including the temporal, carotid, brachial, radial, femoral, popliteal, posterior tibial, and dorsalis pedis arteries as well as at the apex of the heart (Fig. 8.2). Assess and compare the pulses on both sides of the body.

The radial artery is the site most commonly used for routine pulse assessment. The radial pulse is normally palpable at the lateral aspect of the wrist. Palpate this pulse gently in older adults because excessive pressure may occlude the blood vessel. Count the pulse rate, and note the rate, rhythm, and volume. The normal resting pulse rate in adults ranges from 60 to 90 beats per minute. Resting pulse rate declines in the "oldest old" and is associated with greater longevity. Rates outside this range or significant changes from an individual's normal readings indicate the need for further assessment. Older adults, particularly those with a history of cardiovascular problems and those receiving digitalis, require prompt, thorough assessment if there is a significant change in the pulse rate.

The arteries of older adults may feel stiff and knotty because of decreased elasticity. In older adults, it is common to observe irregularities in rhythm. These may be related to medical conditions or they may have no identified cause. Promptly report the detection of an irregular pulse in an older adult whose pulse was previously regular for further assessment. A change in pulse volume may indicate the need to assess fluid balance. Weak, thready pulses are often seen in individuals with fluid volume deficits or electrolyte imbalances; full or bounding pulses may indicate excessive fluid volume. Weakness of a radial pulse may make palpation impossible and necessitate the use of the apical route.

When assessing the apical pulse, help older adults to assume a comfortable position and drape them to prevent chilling and provide modesty. The apical site is located on the left side of the chest. The apical heartbeat is best heard by placing the stethoscope over the fifth intercostal space in line with the middle of the clavicle. Count the apical pulse for a full minute. Each "lub-dub" sound heard is counted as one heartbeat. Assess the apical pulse for regularity and the presence of any unusual sounds.

When assessing the pulse of someone with sagging breasts, lift the tissue gently and place the stethoscope at the lower edge of the breast. The apical pulse may be difficult to assess in older adults with obesity or in those who have had a change in the shape of the chest cavity.

Apical and radial readings, even when taken at the same time by two nurses, may be different. This is referred to as a pulse deficit. Inadequate force of the heart or disease of the blood vessels may prevent the transmission of blood from the heart to the peripheral vessels. Of the two, the apical pulse rate is considered more reliable.

Palpate and assess the peripheral pulses of the legs and feet to determine whether they are present and to assess the quality of the pulse. The peripheral pulse rate is not normally counted. Altered peripheral circulation may be an early indicator of decreased cardiac functioning or vascular changes. Compare pulses on one side of the body with those on the other side to determine whether changes have affected one or both sides of the body.

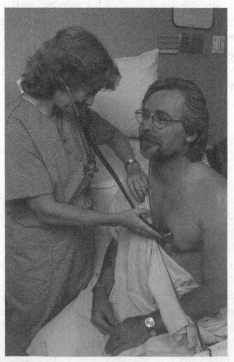

Fig. 8.2 Assessing vital signs. (From Williams, P.A. [2021]. *Fundamental concepts and skills for nursing* [6th ed.]. St. Louis, MO: Elsevier.)

Cardiovascular changes with aging, particularly arteriosclerotic changes, often result in the decrease or complete loss of palpable pulses in the lower extremities. Start with the pedal pulses. If these are not detectable, proceed upward toward the trunk and assess the popliteal and then the femoral pulses. If pulses cannot be palpated, it may be necessary to use a sound amplifier called a Doppler to evaluate circulation to the extremities.

If peripheral pulses are diminished or absent, suspect circulatory impairment and assess the extremity for capillary refill time, temperature, color changes, and the absence of hair, all of which may indicate serious medical problems.

RESPIRATION

After completing a general assessment of all of the factors that influence respiration, place the older adult in a comfortable position to maximize ease of breathing. Assess the rate, depth, and ease of breathing (Fig. 8.3). Each combination of inspiration and expiration is counted as one respiration. The normal respiratory rate for older individuals is similar to that of younger adults. A range of 12 to 20 breaths per minute is considered normal. A decrease in the resting respiratory rate is significant in the older adult. It may be an indication of impending infection and may appear before an elevation in temperature is observed. Increased respiratory rate is common with anxiety, pain, elevated temperatures, and increased activity.

The depth of respiration tends to decrease with aging. Chest expansion is often decreased because of alterations in the shape of the thoracic cavity, muscle weakness, sedentary lifestyle, or disease processes.

Slightly irregular breathing rhythms are not unusual in the aging population. However, abnormal findings—such as a highly irregular rhythm, dyspnea, or breathlessness with exertion—require further assessment to determine the cause and should be reported.

BLOOD PRESSURE

Blood pressure readings are an important part of the physical assessment. It is essential that these readings be properly obtained. To obtain the most accurate readings, position the patient so that the upper arm is at the level of the heart.

For meaningful results, all equipment should be chosen carefully. Cuff selection should be based on the patient's upper arm size. It is a common mistake to use a one-size-fits-all blood pressure cuff. Many older people, particularly those who are frail, have lost a great deal of upper arm mass. A cuff that is too wide for the size of the individual's arm provides falsely low readings. A properly sized cuff is 20% wider than the diameter of the arm at its midpoint. Once the proper cuff has been obtained, apply it gently but snugly to the arm. Be careful not to pinch the skin in the cuff, which can easily lead to bruising.

The technique used to obtain the blood pressure measurement should follow the methods approved by the American Heart Association. This includes taking the blood pressure first by palpation and then by auscultation. Do not pump the cuff to excessively high pressures, as this can result in inaccurate readings.

Blood pressure readings vary widely among older adults. Some older patients have blood pressure readings in the low-normal range; others have significantly elevated readings. Hypertension is a common problem among the older adult population because of the renal and cardiovascular changes of aging. Elevated blood pressure can also be related to emotional upset, pain, exertion, eating, or smoking. This type of elevation disappears once the precipitating event has been removed. To obtain accurate readings, attempt to reduce or minimize these factors before assessing blood pressure, and ensure that the older adult has been inactive for at least 5 minutes. Persistent elevations in blood pressure (i.e., systolic readings 130 mm Hg or higher; diastolic readings 80 mm Hg or higher; or elevations of both systolic and diastolic readings) indicate hypertension. Promptly report an elevation in blood pressure readings, particularly if they are unusual for the individual.

Many older adults take medication for hypertension. Follow through with careful blood pressure monitoring when these medications are administered, and rigorously follow all precautions related to the specific medication.

Older adults are susceptible to posture-related changes in blood pressure. Older adults who have an inactive lifestyle and those who take drugs such as vasodilators, antihypertensives, or tricyclic antidepressants are

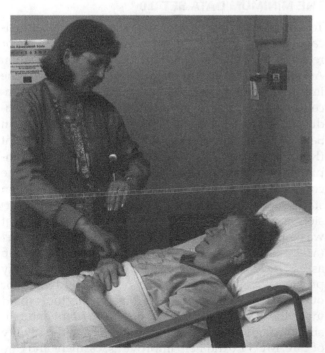

Fig. 8.3 Measuring respirations while taking pulse. (From Williams, P.A. [2021]. *Fundamental concepts and skills for nursing* [6th ed.]. St. Louis, MO: Elsevier.)

particularly prone to orthostatic hypotension, or a sudden drop in blood pressure that occurs when a person changes from a lying to a sitting or standing position. It may also occur when the person moves from sitting to standing. Those experiencing orthostatic hypotension complain of light-headedness or dizziness when changing positions. In severe cases, the person may even lose consciousness. Orthostatic hypotension is commonly observed in individuals who are on extended bed rest or receiving medication for hypertension.

To determine the existence and severity of orthostatic hypotension, the nurse must obtain several blood pressure readings in succession. Performing this assessment requires a certain amount of skill. The nurse first takes the blood pressure when the patient is at rest in bed. Then the patient sits at the edge of the bed and the nurse takes the blood pressure again in 1 to 3 minutes. The patient then stands for 1 to 3 minutes, and the nurse takes a third reading. All readings are documented, along with any subjective information provided by the patient regarding dizziness, loss of balance, or other sensations. A drop of 20 mm Hg or more in systolic or 10 mm Hg in diastolic is always significant and should be reported promptly. A standing systolic blood pressure less than 100 mm Hg should also be reported. If the individual complains of symptoms such as dizziness, safety precautions should be taken.

SENSORY ASSESSMENT OF OLDER ADULTS

Simple assessments of vision and hearing are based on empiric data (the way the individual responds to visual or auditory clues). Observe whether the person is able to read or perform close work that requires good central vision or whether they work with computers, watch television, or engage in other sight-related activities. If the older person uses eyeglasses, assess their ability to see with and without them.

Talking with older adults can reveal any difficulties with hearing. Indicators of hearing problems include difficulties getting their attention, the frequent need to repeat information, or mistakes in understanding directions. If applicable, perform the hearing aid assessment when the older person is wearing the hearing aid or aids, but only after checking for the devices' proper functioning. Special assessment by a vision or audiometric specialist can reveal more precise information regarding vision and hearing.

PSYCHOSOCIAL ASSESSMENT OF OLDER ADULTS

A psychological assessment is performed to determine whether the older person is alert and aware of the surroundings or has some level of confusion, delirium, or dementia. The differences between these conditions are discussed in detail in Chapter 10. Psychological status is best assessed by direct observation and by means of standardized assessment tools. Many assessment tools are available to assist nurses in assessing mental status in older adults. One very highly regarded tool is the Mini-Cog, a sample of which is provided in Box 8.2. This assessment can identify cognitive impairments that can be tracked over time. The test can be administered in 3 to 4 minutes, making it ideal for both hospital and routine visits. Other assessment tools may also be used. Several of these are available online in a digital format (Box 8.3).

Assessment of social function is determined by observing the amount, frequency, and type of participation in social interactions by the older person. A variety of levels and degrees of social interaction can be classified as normal as long as the individual is happy or content with that level. Chapters 11, 12, and 13 explore socialization issues further.

> ### QSEN Considerations: Evidence-Based Practice
>
> Many evidence-based assessment tools are available online from the Hartford Institute for Geriatric Nursing (https://hign.org/). According to the Hartford Institute, the goal of the *Try This: Best Practices in Care for Older Adults* series of assessment tools is to provide knowledge that is easily accessible, easily understood, and easily implemented and to encourage the use of these best practices by all direct care nurses.

SPECIAL ASSESSMENTS

THE MINIMUM DATA SET 3.0

To improve the quality of care provided in extended-care facilities, the federal government instituted major reforms through the Omnibus Budget Reconciliation Act of 1987. An important focus of this law was the improvement and standardization of assessment procedures used in these facilities. The first reform produced by the US Department of Health and Human Services was the Resident Assessment Instrument (RAI), introduced in 1990. This tool specified a comprehensive, standardized assessment that was to be completed on admission, with significant change in status, and thereafter on a yearly basis. The first version of the database used to conduct this assessment was a printed document called the *Minimum Data Set (MDS) 1.0*. This tool was designed not only to help assess residents but also to help caregivers identify problems, develop intervention plans, and monitor outcomes. It was hoped that the use of this tool would make the assessment process more consistent and reliable throughout the country and improve the quality of care. MDS 1.0 did help improve assessment and care in many cases, but information was often difficult to locate, and interdepartmental monitoring of problems

Box 8.2   **Mini-Cog© Instrument**

Step 1: Ask the person to repeat three unrelated words from one of the official versions of the instrument,*such as "*banana*," "*sunrise*," and "*chair*."

Step 2: Ask the person to draw a simple clock. Instruct the person: "First, put the numbers where they go." Once that is completed, say, "Now, set the hands to 10 past 11." Use a preprinted circle for this exercise (see below). Repeat instructions as needed, as this is not a memory test. Allow 3 minutes for completion, then move to Step 3.

Step 3: Ask the patient to recall the three words from Step 1. Say, "What were the 3 words I asked you to remember?"

SCORING

CATEGORY	DESCRIPTION	EARNED/POSSIBLE
Word Recall	Each word spontaneously recalled without cueing = 1 point	____/3
Clock Draw	Normal clock = 2 points. (Normal clock: all numbers in correct sequence with approximate correct position (e.g., 12, 3, 6, and 9 are in anchor positions) with no missing/no duplicate numbers. Hands: point to the numbers 11 and 2 (11:10). Hand length: not scored.) Inability or refusal to draw a clock (abnormal) = 0 points.	____/0 or 2
Total Score	Word Recall Score + Clock Draw Score	____/5

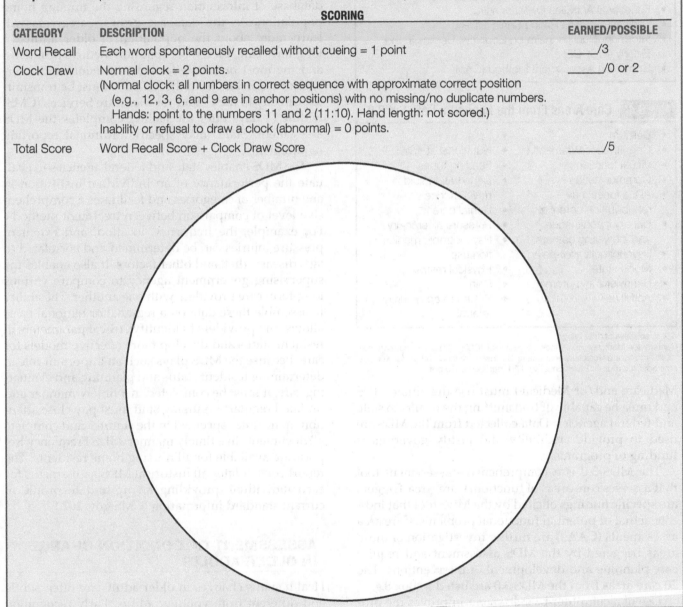

'Word pairings from the 6 different versions: Version 1: "*Banana Sunrise Chair*"; Version 2: "*Leader Season Table*"; Version 3: "*Village Kitchen Baby*"; Version 4: "*River Nation Finger*"; Version 5: "*Captain Garden Picture*"; Version 6: "*Daughter Heaven Mountain*."

From Borson, S. (2016). Mini-Cog instructions for administration & scoring. http://mini-cog.com/wp-content/uploads/2015/12/Universal-Mini-Cog-Form-011916.pdf

and outcomes was difficult because this was a paper-based assessment. The MDS 2.0 was an upgraded, computerized version of the older document. MDS 3.0 is a group of screening and assessment processes that are a piece of the RAI. The RAI reviews each long-term care resident's ability to perform activities of daily living. Using these assessments and interviews with the residents, the staff determines health issues of the residents. One of the significant goals of MDS 3.0 was to improve patient input into the assessment process by incorporating direct resident interviews into the process (the full MDS 3.0 can be found online). Design improvements in the MDS 3.0 were directed at increased reliability, enhanced accuracy, and expanded usefulness as a tool to improve clinical assessment. This new format went into effect in 2010 with a new version of the *RAI User's Manual* released in 2015 and a revised version in 2019. All health care agencies that receive

Box 8.3 **Examples of Online Psychological Assessment Tools**

- Mini-Mental State Examination (MMSE)
- General Practitioner Assessment of Cognition (GPCOG)
- Eight-item Informant Interview to Differentiate Aging and Dementia (AD8)
- Cornell Scale for Depression in Dementia
- Functional Activities Questionnaire
- Clinical Dementia Rating Scale (CDR)
- Informant Questionnaire on Cognitive Decline in the Elderly (IQCODE)
- Confusion Assessment Method (CAM)

Box 8.4 **Care Areas From the Minimum Data Set 3.0**

- Delirium
- Cognitive loss/dementia
- Visual function
- Communication
- ADLs functional/rehabilitation potential
- Urinary incontinence and indwelling catheter
- Psychosocial well-being
- Mood state
- Behavioral symptoms
- Activities
- Falls
- Nutritional status
- Feeding tubes
- Dehydration/fluid maintenance
- Dental care
- Pressure ulcer/injury
- Psychotropic medication use
- Physical restraints
- Pain
- Return to community referral

ADLs, activities of daily living.
Centers for Medicare and Medicaid Services [CMS] (2019). Long-term care facility resident assessment instrument 3.0 user's manual. https://downloads.cms.gov/files/mds-3.0-rai-manual-v1.17.1_october_2019.pdf

Medicare and/or Medicaid must use the online MDS and must be capable of transmitting the results to state and federal agencies. Data collected from the MDS are used to provide credibility and justify government funding of programs.

The MDS 3.0 is a comprehensive assessment tool that assesses core areas of function. Care Area Triggers are specific findings elicited by the MDS tool that indicate actual or potential functional problems. Care area assessments (CAAs) are further investigation of those areas triggered by the MDS assessment and require care planning and development of interventions. The 20 care areas from the MDS 3.0 are listed in Box 8.4.

Use of a computer-based system improves the process of assessment and planning. The online database helps make the process more comprehensive, more complete, and easier for the nursing staff and other departments to use once they have become familiar with the program. Computerization of records in this database enhances the flow of information between departments within a facility. For example, the pharmacy can verify that psychotropic and antidepressant medications are administered only when appropriate medical diagnoses exist, and the physicians and nurses can correlate dosage changes with observed behaviors. The dietary department can validate that appropriate meal plans are ordered based on medical diagnosis and can detect changes in weight that may

indicate the need for further intervention. Nurses can identify interventions that will be most beneficial at preventing pressure injuries, constipation, or other common problems.

The online MDS 3.0 enhances the ability to access and correlate data from every long-term care facility in the United States and provides an unprecedented database of information regarding the nursing home population. As the database grows, caregivers will learn more about the population of older adults in long-term care, their most common medical problems, and the most or least effective treatments and interventions. All data from the MDS 3.0 must be transmitted directly to the Center for Medicare Services (CMS) within 14 days after the facility completes the MDS assessment. States may specify additional reporting requirements.

The MDS enables state and federal agencies to evaluate the performance of an individual institution in any number of categories and facilitates a comprehensive level of comparison between treatment methods. For example, the frequency, location, and extent of pressure injuries can be determined and correlated to age, disease, diet, and other factors. It also enables the supervising government agency to compare various long-term care providers with one another. The ability to assemble these data on a regional or national basis allows care providers to identify critical parameters in resident status and develop more effective models for care. Because the MDS plays such an important role in determining resident status and planning and evaluating care, it must be completed in a timely manner and updated regularly. Nursing staff must pay close attention to the times specified in the statutes and complete all documents in a timely manner. MDS Frequency Reports are available for all nursing home residents. The report consolidates all historical MDS assessments for each individual, providing an up-to-date profile of current standard information (CMS.gov, 2020).

ASSESSMENT OF CONDITION CHANGE IN OLDER ADULTS

Health status changes in older adults are often subtle and different from younger adults. Early recognition and treatment of change in status can prevent serious harm for older adults. This is true in at-home care, in extended-care facilities, and in the hospital setting. A number of evidence based instruments have been developed to help the nurse perform a systematic and comprehensive assessment.

FULMER SPICES

SPICES is an acronym for six common "marker conditions" in older adults that can identify potential health-related problems. This screening tool can be used routinely during assessments to identify and/or prevent potential problems and to monitor health status over time (Fulmer, 2020). Identification of one or more of these problems indicates an increased risk for functional decline and even death. More in-depth assessments are required when a problem is identified (see appropriate chapters for assessment guidelines). This assessment is not a total list of significant problems—for example, pain and elimination are not included—but it does address the most common and relevant issues. Additional information and tools designed to help the nurse perform effective assessments of older adults are available online. Box 8.5 provides a list of some of the most helpful sites.

🏠 Nursing Tip

The Hartford Institute for Geriatric Nursing website includes a video demonstration using SPICES, defined as

S—sleep disorders
P—problems with eating or feeding
I—incontinence
C—confusion
E—evidence of falls
S—skin breakdown

See https://hign.org/consultgeri/try-this-series/fulmer-spices-overall-assessment-tool-older-adults/

FANCAPES

When the nurse suspects that an actual emergency or serious problem is present or might be developing, deep, focused assessments are appropriate and necessary. The following mnemonic can be used to organize this assessment:

F—fluid
A—aeration (oxygenation)
N—nutrition

Box 8.5	Internet Sites for Assessment of Older Adults

Many helpful geriatric assessment tools are available online. These sites contain downloadable or printable forms for use when performing both general and focused geriatric assessments.

Hartford Institute for Geriatric Nursing: https://hign.org/consultgeri/try-this/general-assessment

International Society of Geriatric Oncology: http://www.siog.org/content/comprehensive-geriatric-assessment-cga-older-patient-cancer

Merck Manual of Geriatrics: www.merckmanuals.com/professional/geriatrics

National Institute on Aging: www.nia.nih.gov/health

Primary Care Geriatrics—Functional Assessment video: www.bmj.com/content/343/bmj.d4681?keytype=ref&siteid=bmjjournals&ijkey=YKae1pWowPzkl

Stall, Robert S. MD—Senior Health Assessment: http://oldsmarts.biz/pdfs/Senior%20Health%20Assessment%20%C2%A9%20OldSmarts%20LLC.pdf

University of Maryland: /https://www.umaryland.edu/gerontology/services-and-resources/assessment-tools/

University of Missouri: http://geriatrictoolkit.missouri.edu/

C—cognition, communication
A—activity/abilities
P—pain
E—elimination
S—skin/socialization

Once the status assessment has been completed, the nurse must decide on the most appropriate action. A summary of nursing responses is presented in Table 8.3.

Table 8.3	Should I Call? Presentation and Action to Take	
PRESENTATION/ CONDITION CHANGE	**CALL MD OR APRN IMMEDIATELY IF**	**CALL 911 IF**
Vital signs	Systolic BP: greater than 200 mm Hg or less than 90 mm Hg Diastolic BP: greater than 115 mm Hg Resting pulse: greater than 130 or less than 55 beats per minute Oral temp: above 101 degrees F Rectal temp: above 102 degrees F	The vital sign changes are associated with altered and/or severe symptoms of other kinds of distress (e.g., airway obstruction or anaphylaxis)
Delirium	Any sudden onset of change in mental status	Change in mental status accompanied by suspected or possible airway obstruction Severe respiratory distress Clinical signs of shock
Edema	Sudden fluid excess noted in associated SOB, pink frothy sputum, possibly co-occurring with chest pain Abrupt onset of edema in one leg only Loss of sensation in swollen leg Associated tenderness and/or redness in affected leg	Suspicion of a cardiovascular event, such as syncope, tachycardia, or other symptoms of acute coronary syndrome
Sleeping difficulties	Only if associated with mental status changes	Not applicable
Bleeding	Uncontrolled bleeding or repeat episode (e.g., prolonged nosebleed) Emesis with frank blood Bloody stools Vaginal bleeding, profuse	Uncontrolled bleeding Bleeding with symptoms of impending shock and/or VS changes Trauma with or without evidence of overt injury

Continued

Table 8.3   Should I Call? Presentation and Action to Take—cont'd

PRESENTATION/ CONDITION CHANGE	CALL MD OR APRN IMMEDIATELY IF	CALL 911 IF
Falls	Obvious deformity of limb or alignment of same Joint or hip pain with reduced range of motion Inability to bear weight Laceration with uncontrolled bleeding	Major trauma event, such as a fall of a significant distance with associated loss of consciousness or VS changes
Chest pain	New onset or recurrent pain not relieved in 20 minutes with previously ordered nitroglycerin 3 times daily Chest pain accompanied by VS changes, dyspnea, diaphoresis, nausea/vomiting	Complaints of chest pain associated with or followed by LOC changes or obvious arrhythmia with pulse check such as severe bradycardia (HR less than 40 beats per minute) or tachycardia (HR greater than 150 beats per minute)
Medication error	Resident is symptomatic because of the error	Resident is symptomatic *and* there are VS and/or LOC changes
Constipation/ diarrhea/emesis	Severe abdominal pain Rigid abdomen or extreme tenderness on palpation Bowel sounds absent Guarding (tensing of abdominal wall to protect inflamed underlying organs)	Only when associated with other symptoms such as mental status changes or in conjunction with other cardiovascular symptoms that would necessitate transfer
Pain	Associated with a fall/trauma Noticeable and new inability to perform ROM Headache with altered vision and/or LOC	Severe, uncontrolled pain
Dehydration	More than 1 episode of vomiting in 24 hours and decreased fluid intake Less than 50% of normal fluid intake over 24 hours	VS abnormalities LOC change Suspected sepsis, such as narrowed pulse pressures, tachycardia, fever, mental status changes
Pressure injury/ skin rash	Stage 2, 3, or 4 receiving no treatment and no protocol to cover the condition Signs of wound infection: purulent discharge, erythema, odor Fever	Not applicable
Depression/suicidal ideation	Expression of suicidal ideation that contains a plan for carrying it out in the assisted living residence (e.g., "I have a lot of medications hidden away to use when I think my time has come.")	Expressed suicidal ideation with a plan and inability to monitor resident in the assisted living residence
Seizures	New onset Status epilepticus	New onset or status epilepticus *associated with* possible airway compromise, severe respiratory distress, signs of shock
Visual changes	Associated stroke symptoms (e.g., hemiparesis, slurred speech, headache, facial drooping) Complaints of seeing "halos" (a person will look at a light and see a halo or rainbow-colored circle around the light) Any abrupt onset Suspected trauma with severe pain	Suspected stroke
SOB	VS changes or suspected cardiovascular involvement Labored breathing Ashen appearance Cyanosis	Evidence of inadequate oxygenation (cyanosis, increased respiratory rate, paradoxical chest movement, diaphragmatic breathing, use of accessory muscles) despite interventions, such as oxygen via nasal cannula (0.25–4 L/min) or through simple mask (5–12 L/min)

APRN, advanced practice registered nurse; *BP,* blood pressure; *HR,* heart rate; *LOC,* level of consciousness; *MD,* medical doctor; *ROM,* range of motion; *SOB,* shortness of breath; *VS,* vital sign.

From Montgomery, J., & Mitty, E. (2008). Adapted with permission from B. Jordan, *MS, ARNP, BCPCN,* & J. Sandberg-Cook, *MS, ARNP, BCPCN.* Dartmouth-Hitchcock Medical Center, Hanover, *NH.*

Get Ready for the Next Generation NCLEX® Examination!

Key Points

- Although the initial health assessment of an older adult is important, it is only a starting point. Assessment is a continuous and ongoing process.
- As each older adult's condition changes, objective and subjective data will also change.
- MDS 3.0 helps caregivers identify problems, develop intervention plans, and monitor outcomes; it is required to be used by all facilities that receive Medicare and/or Medicaid funding.
- Nurses spend the greatest amount of time with older adults, so they have the greatest opportunity to assess and recognize significant changes.
- Nurses are responsible for continually assessing and instituting changes in care, based on those observations.

Additional Learning Resources

 Go to your Evolve website at http://evolve.elsevier.com/Williams/geriatric for the additional online resources.

Review Questions for the Next Generation NCLEX® Examination

1. Which assessment tool is most highly regarded and often used to determine the mental status of the older adult?
   - a. SPICES Assessment Tool
   - b. The Mini-Cog
   - c. Short Test for Dementia
   - d. MDS 3.0

2. When assessing the respiratory system of an older adult, the nurse hears continuous, coarse, low-pitched sounds. How would these sounds be reported?
   - a. Rales (crackles)
   - b. Wheezes
   - c. Friction rub
   - d. Gurgles (low-pitched wheezes)

3. When taking a radial pulse of an older adult, the nurse finds it difficult to count a weak and thready pulse. What should the nurse do?
   - a. Gently apply more pressure with three fingers to obtain a stronger pulse.
   - b. Take the person's blood pressure to get the heart rate reading from the machine.
   - c. Take an apical pulse instead.
   - d. Document, "Weak, thready pulse, rate N/A."

4. When performing an assessment of the gastrointestinal system of an older adult, the nurse would proceed in what order? Place the parts of a gastrointestinal system assessment in sequence from first to last.
   - a. Palpate abdomen.
   - b. Observe abdomen for scars.
   - c. Obtain a health history.
   - d. Inspect the oral cavity.
   - e. Auscultate bowel sounds.

5. When performing an interview with an older adult, the nurse should consider physical environment factors by (Select all that apply.)
   - a. Explaining what will take place during the assessment
   - b. Ensuring privacy and minimal noise levels
   - c. Selecting a room with a comfortable temperature
   - d. Ensuring bright lighting to enable the older adult to see clearly
   - e. Having the interview done by a nurse of the same gender to build rapport
   - f. Seeking a location in close proximity to a restroom

REFERENCES

American Academy of Ophthalmology (2020). Eye health information for adults 40 to 65. https://www.aao.org/eye-health/tips-prevention/midlife-adults/

American Speech-Language-Hearing Association (2020). Hearing screening, https://www.asha.org/public/hearing/hearing-screening/

Centers for Medicare & Medicaid Services (2020). Long-term care facility resident assessment instrument 3.0 user's manual, version 1.17.1. https://downloads.cms.gov/files/mds-3.0-rai-manual-v1.17.1_october_2019.pdf/

CMS.gov. (2020). Minimum data set MDS 3.0 for nursing homes and swing bed providers, Centers for Medicare & Medicaid Services. www.cms.gov/Medicare/Quality-Initiatives-Patient-Assessment-Instruments/NursingHomeQualityInits/NHQIMDS30.html/

Fulmer, T. (2020). Fulmer SPICES: An overall assessment tool for older adults, https://hign.org/consultgeri/try-this-series/fulmer-spices-overall-assessment-tool-older-adults/

Martin, E. M., & Barkley, T. W. (2016). Improving cultural competence in end-of-life pain management. Nursing, 46(1), 32–41.

Riba, L. A., Gruner, R. A., Alapati, A., et al. (2019). Association between socioeconomic factors and outcomes in breast cancer. Breast Journal, 25(3), 488–492.

U.S. Preventive Services Task Force (2020). Recommendation topics. https://www.uspreventiveservicestaskforce.org/uspstf/recommendation-topics/

White, J., Plompen, T., Tao, L, et al. (2019). What is needed in culturally competent healthcare systems? A qualitative exploration of culturally diverse patients and professional interpreters in an Australian healthcare setting. BMC Public Health, 19(8), 1096.

Objectives

1. Explore the types and extent of safety problems experienced by the aging population.
2. Describe internal and external factors that increase safety risks for older adults.
3. Discuss interventions that promote safety for older adults.
4. Examine fall prevention strategies for older adults.
5. Discuss factors that place older adults at risk for imbalanced thermoregulation.
6. Describe those older adults who are most at risk for developing problems related to imbalanced thermoregulation.
7. Identify interventions that assist older adults in maintain normal body temperature.

Key Terms

heatstroke (HĒT-strōk, p. 183)
hyperthermia (hī-pĕr-THĔR-mē-ă, p. 183)

hypothermia (hī-pō-THĔR-mē-ă, p. 182)
thermoregulation (thĕr-mō-RĔG-ū-lā-shŭn, p. 182)

Safety is a major concern when working with or providing care to older adults. The Centers for Disease Control and Prevention (CDC) reports that more than 57,000 older adults died from unintentional injury in 2018. The largest number of accidental deaths in the older adult population, by a wide margin, is due to falls, and this number is increasing (CDC, 2020a). The risk of falling peaks sharply in the ninth decade of life. Motor vehicle accidents and choking also claim many lives of older adults prematurely.

The most common safety problems for older adults involve falls and choking (as mentioned), followed by poisonings, burns, and motor vehicle accidents. Exposure to temperature extremes also places older adults at risk for injury or death. Older adults are more susceptible to accidents and injuries than are younger adults owing to both internal and external factors. Internal factors are specific to the person and include the normal physiologic changes of aging, chronic disease, use of medications, and cognitive or emotional changes. External factors are specific to the environment and include hazards such as poor lighting or slippery floors.

INTERNAL RISK FACTORS

Vision and hearing are protective senses. When the acuteness of the senses diminishes, the risk for injury increases. Changes in vision and hearing are common with aging. Diminished range of peripheral vision and changes in depth perception are common and can interfere with the ability of older adults to judge the distance and height of stairs and curbs or to determine the position and speed of motor vehicles. Night vision diminishes. In dim light or glare, older adults may be unable to see that a curb, step, or other hazard is present. They may be unable to see or read stationary road signs that provide directions or warnings. Falls or motor vehicle accidents often result from altered vision.

Changes in visual acuity make it more difficult to read labels with small print, such as those on prescription bottles. Many older adults have taken incorrect medications or wrong doses or have even consumed poisonous substances because they could not see adequately to read the labels.

Decreased auditory acuity reduces an older person's ability to detect and respond appropriately to warning calls, whistles, or alarms. For example, older adults may not hear a warning call of impending danger, may not hear a motor vehicle or siren in time to avoid an accident, or may not respond to a fire alarm in time to leave a building safely.

The senses of smell and taste also help to protect us from consuming substances that might be harmful to the body. Decreased sensitivity of these senses increases the risk for accidental food or chemical poisoning in the older adult population.

Older adults often experience one or more physiologic changes that increase their risk for falls and other accidental injuries. Any of these changes alone or in combination can reduce the older person's ability to respond quickly enough to prevent an accidental injury. When these problems are combined with chronic diseases or health problems, the risk increases dramatically. Common physiologic changes that affect

safety include
- Decreased mobility
- Decreased flexibility
- Decreased muscle strength
- Slowed reaction time
- Gait changes
- Difficulty lifting the feet
- Altered sense of balance
- Postural changes

Conditions affecting the cardiovascular, nervous, and musculoskeletal systems are most likely to contribute to safety problems. Any cardiovascular condition that decreases cardiac output and the supply of oxygen to the brain can cause older adults to experience vertigo (dizziness) or syncope (fainting). Common disorders associated with this result include anemia, cardiac arrhythmias, and orthostatic hypotension. Although often asymptomatic, orthostatic hypotension is present in 35% of older adults (Goswami et al., 2017).

Older adults with neurologic disorders such as Parkinson disease or stroke experience weakness and alterations in gait and balance, which increase fall risk. Neurologic and circulatory changes can also decrease the ability to sense painful stimuli or temperature changes, increasing the risk for tissue injuries, burns, and frostbite. Studies have shown that people of age 65 and older with diabetes, have more than a 65% risk of recurrent falls, with double the risk for injuries from the fall (Chapman & Meyer, 2017).

Musculoskeletal conditions, such as arthritis, further reduce joint mobility and flexibility, decreasing the ability of the older person to move and respond to hazards and intensifying the likelihood of accidents or injury. However, maintaining physical fitness can decrease this risk (Fig. 9.1). Box 9.1 lists injury risks for older adults.

Medications often contribute to falls and, because older adults commonly take one or more medications, their risk for untoward effects is increased. Any medication that alters sensation or perception, slows reaction time, or causes orthostatic hypotension is potentially dangerous for older adults. Common types of hazardous medications include sedatives, hypnotics, tranquilizers, diuretics, antihypertensives, and antihistamines. Alcohol, though not a prescription medication, acts as a drug in the body. Alcoholic beverages, particularly in combination with prescription drugs, increase the risk for falls and other injuries. More information regarding the safe use of medications is included in Chapter 7.

Cognitive changes or emotional disturbances and depression may be overlooked as risk factors for falls or injury. These disturbances reduce the older person's ability to recognize and process information. Distracted or preoccupied older adults are less likely to pay full attention to what is happening or what they are doing. This lack of attention and caution increases the risk for accidents and injury.

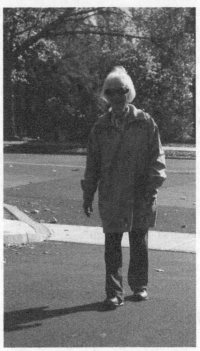

Fig. 9.1 Daily physical activity, such as walking, can maintain or improve physical function. (From Pagliarulo, M. [2016]. *Introduction to physical therapy* [5th ed.]. St. Louis, MO: Elsevier.)

Box 9.1   Injury Risks for Older Adults

- Impaired physical mobility
- Sensory deficits
- Lack of knowledge of health practices or safety precautions
- Hazardous environment
- History of accidents or injuries

FALLS

Falls are the most common safety problem among older adults. Consider the following statistics from the National Council on Aging (2018) and the CDC (2021a):
- Approximately 1 out of 4 older adults fall each year, although less than half report the fall to their primary care provider.
- Any fall is the best predictor of future falls. Falling doubles the chance of someone falling again.
- Every year 3 million older adults are treated in an emergency department for fall-related injuries.
- Falls are the leading cause of death due to injury among people older than age 65 and the most common cause of nonfatal trauma-related hospital admissions.
- Falls are the leading cause of traumatic brain injury.
- More than 95% of hip fractures are caused by falls, usually by falling sideways.
- The direct cost of falls is more than $50 billion in 2015.

Many independent older adults are reluctant to report a fall because of the implication that they are frail and dependent. Statistically, 1 in 5 older adults who fall and fracture a hip die within a year of the fall (National Council of State Legislatures, 2018), and many others do not resume their previous level of activity or independence after falling. In addition to causing bodily harm, falls take a psychological toll on the older adult; fear of falling can lead to loss of confidence, decreased mobility, and reduced physical fitness. This is unfortunate, because early recognition and interventions can reduce fall risk. Older adults living independently in the community often do not recognize hazards in their home environment; these place them at increased fall risk because they are too accustomed to their surroundings to view them as potentially hazardous. Older adults and their family members need to be aware of things they can do to reduce fall risk. Some helpful approaches are summarized in Box 9.2.

| Box 9.2 | Reducing Fall Risk |

- *Prepare safe surroundings.* Ensure there is adequate lighting, particularly in stairwells. Keep frequently needed items, such as the telephone, tissues, etc., on a table near the chair or bedside. Consider a low-rise bed (14 inches from the floor). Personal alarms and pressure sensor alarms alert nursing staff of patient movement.
- *Reduce environmental hazards and risky practices.* Ensure there are no throw rugs, uneven floors, electric wires, oxygen tubing, or other items that could cause tripping. Mop up spills in the kitchen or bathroom immediately. Avoid placing items on the floor. Encourage the older adult to not climb on anything other than an approved step stool to reach high places.
- *Allow adequate time to complete an activity or task.* Haste increases the risk of falls and other injuries. If the older adult feels dizzy or light-headed, encourage sitting for a while before standing.
- *Encourage proper-fitting footwear.* Shoes with nonslip soles and low heels are recommended, because high-heeled shoes contribute to balance problems. Shoes should have closures that are easy to manipulate. If shoes have laces, check that they do not come loose and cause tripping. Loose-fitting slippers or shoes can drop off the foot and lead to a fall.
- *Encourage assistive devices when needed.* Prescription eyeglasses enable the older adult to clearly see their environment. A cane or walker provides security with ambulation by enlarging the base of support. Keep these assistive devices close at hand to avoid leaning or reaching. The tips of the cane or walker should have solid rubber grips to prevent slipping and may need to be modified on icy surfaces to promote gripping. Provide grab bars and raised toilet seats to help with balance and support.
- *Encourage the older adult to ask for help when necessary.* Failure to seek help can lead to serious injury. Encourage older adults to recognize that good judgment is a sign of healthy aging, not a sign of weakness.
- *Provide toileting assistance at regular intervals.* Assisting the older adult every 2 hours can help reduce fall risk.

FALL PREVENTION

Fall prevention is everyone's responsibility. Outreach sessions about fall prevention designed to meet the needs of older adults, their families, and anyone who has contact with older adults could be offered at senior centers, libraries, businesses, and community colleges. Health care settings need to maintain current and complete policies and procedures for fall prevention, new employee training regarding fall prevention, a method for the prompt reporting and investigation of all falls, and scheduled multidisciplinary meetings to identify problems and plan interventions.

The CDC has created the Stopping Elderly Accidents, Deaths, and Injuries (STEADI) initiative to make fall prevention routine (CDC, 2020c). This initiative is based on clinical guidelines and provides information and resources for patients, caregivers, and all members of the health care team. Screening tools, online training, and informational brochures are provided by the STEADI initiative. The initiative is based on three steps to be included in routine office visits:
1. Ask patients if they have fallen in the past year, feel unsteady, or worry about falling.
2. Review medications and stop, switch, or reduce the dose of medications that could increase the fall risk.
3. Recommend vitamin D supplements.

Several states have passed additional legislation designed to prevent and reduce the number of falls among older adults. This legislation includes supporting older adults in their homes, communities, and clinical settings, including identification and support of the "aging in place" concept. The Joint Commission has also identified fall prevention as a priority with their Speak Up to Prevent Falls campaign established in 2019. The Speak Up campaign centers on 4 topics including awareness of health, taking extra safeguards such as the use of handrails and wearing of shoes with nonslip soles, making minor adjustments to the home, and asking for assistance in medical facilities (The Joint Commission, 2019). New research is suggesting that fall prevention programs can reduce in-home falls by nearly 40% (Everding, 2021).

Assessment begins with identifying and documenting intrinsic risk factors that place an individual at high risk for falling. These include
- A recent history of falling
- The presence of heart failure, chronic obstructive pulmonary disease, Parkinson disease, and/or anemia
- Use of assistive devices
- Cognitive impairment
- Gait, balance, or visual impairment
- Use of high-risk medications
- Lack of exercise
- Urgency and urinary incontinence
- The use of a protective device (formerly called a physical restraint)
- Walking in bare feet or with inappropriate shoes

If the patient is found to be at risk for falling, more frequent assessments must be performed and documented.

TOOLS TO ASSESS FOR FALLS

Many tools have been developed to help assess fall risk. Some of these do not require any special equipment and can easily be implemented in a home or community setting within less than 10 minutes. A summary of some common validated tests and tools can be found in Table 9.1.

SPECIFIC STRATEGIES TO PREVENT FALLS

Communicate the risk of falling to the patient, family, and staff. Fall risk should be communicated via the health record, handoff report, signs on the door or wall, and patient wristband. Once fall risk factors have been identified and documented, an individualized strategy can be developed and implemented to reduce the risk of falling. For example, studies have shown that falls are reduced when an individual engages in exercise focusing on two or more of the following elements: balance, strength, endurance, and flexibility. Exercising in a supervised group, practicing tai chi, and performing individual exercise have all proven to be effective in this manner.

Environmental modifications have been shown to be effective in reducing falls in those at high risk, such as people with severe visual deficits. The community-based older adult at risk for falls should have some sort of device enabling them to call for help in the event of a fall, such as LifeAlert.

Table 9.1   Examples of Validated Tests and Tools Available for Screening and Assessment of Fall Risk

TEST AND CRITERIA	PRACTICAL ASPECTS
Screening in the Community: Timed Up and Go Test	
Description	This test measures the time taken for a person to rise from a chair, walk 3 meters at normal pace with their usual assistive device, turn, return to the chair, and sit down
Criterion	A time of 12 seconds or longer indicates increased risk of falling.
Time to undertake test	1–2 minutes
Equipment	Chair and stopwatch or minute hand on watch
Assessment in the Community: QuickScreen	
Description	QuickScreen is a risk assessment tool designed for use by practice and rural nurses, allied health workers, and general practitioners. It allows the clinician to estimate the level of increased fall risk and determine which sensorimotor systems are impaired. The test measures previous falls, drug use, vision, peripheral sensation, lower limb strength, balance, and coordination.
Criterion	A score of 4 or more indicates an increased risk of falling.
Time to undertake test	10 minutes
Equipment	A low-contrast eye chart, a filament for measuring touch sensation, and a small step
Screening in the Emergency Department: Prevention of Falls in the Elderly Trial	
Description	Used in people presenting to the emergency department after a fall. Three simple questions identify people at increased risk of further falls: (1) Have you had any other falls over the past 12 months? (2) Have you fallen indoors? (3) Have you been unable to get up after a fall?
Criterion	If the patient answers yes to any of the questions, further assessment and intervention are needed.
Time to undertake test	1–2 minutes
Equipment	None
Screening in Hospital: Ontario Modified STRATIFY	
Description	Five-item weighted questionnaire with questions relating to falls, cognition, transfer and mobility skills, vision, and toileting practice
Criterion	A score of 9 or above identifies high-risk fallers.
Time to undertake test	1–2 minutes
Equipment	None
Screening in Nursing and Residential Care: Stay Independent	
Description	A 12-question survey with questions related to history of falls, mobility skills, fear of falling, toileting practices, and use of medications
Criterion	A score of 4 or above identifies or a score of below 4 with a fall in the past year identifies high-risk fallers.
Time to undertake test	10 minutes
Equipment	None

As noted previously, medications can increase the fall risk for an older person. Discontinuation of potentially inappropriate medications (see Chapter 7), which may include medications for sleep or pain, anxiety, or depression, has been shown to decrease falls in hospitalized older adults (Alshammari, Al-Saeed & Aslanpour, 2021). These medications, therefore, should be periodically reviewed to ensure they are truly needed.

Other individual risk factors can be medically or surgically corrected. For example, pacemaker placement will reduce the fall risk in a person with carotid sinus hypersensitivity. Cataract surgery will reduce the fall risk in an individual with cataracts. Vitamin D supplements may reduce the fall risk in someone who is deficient in vitamin D.

 QSEN Considerations: Teamwork and Collaboration

Fall Prevention

Nursing assistants are important members of the team and often have good insights into the reasons for a fall. Ask the certified nursing assistant (CNA) for suggestions for actions that might help to prevent a future fall based on their observations of the patient. Include these ideas in the plan of care. When the entire team is involved in developing the plan, cooperation and teamwork toward the common goal of fall prevention are improved. Ensure that the nursing staff and all other departments take fall prevention seriously. Report the presence of any unsafe conditions. Notify housekeeping, maintenance, or security promptly and then verify that the problem has been corrected. Another strategy is called "Catch me doing something right." Too often we are quick to blame someone when a fall occurs. It is a far better practice to praise the staff when you see call lights being answered promptly, spills being mopped up, and proper footwear or assistive devices being used. Some literature even suggests identification of a "Falls Champion"—a staff member who has additional training regarding fall prevention and who can then provide training to others, act as a mentor to new staff, and maintain a high awareness of the need for fall prevention.

 Cultural Considerations

Tai Chi for Older Adults

Tai chi is an traditional mind-body exercise and a common daily practice among older adults in China. These exercises increase balance and lower leg strength and have been shown to reduce falls in community and other older adults settings. More well controlled studies are needed to further illuminate the benefits of Tai Chi (Nyman, 2020).

EXTERNAL RISK FACTORS

Environmental hazards include everything that surrounds older adults. Potential hazards are presented by the people and the variety of objects a person comes into contact with on a daily basis. Even the climate in which a person lives can present an environmental hazard. Environmental hazards are everywhere: in the home, on the street, in public buildings, and in health care settings. Box 9.3 lists tips on preventing falls and injuries in the home. Although injuries can and do often occur in the home, a change of environment—such as hospitalization, travel, or any other move from one's familiar surroundings—can increase the risk for injury among older adults.

| Box 9.3 | **Preventing Falls and Injuries in the Home** |

- *Ensure that all rugs are firmly fixed to the floor.* Tack down loose edges, ensure that rubber skid-proofing is secure, and remove decorative scatter rugs.
- *Maintain electric safety.* Check regularly to ensure that there are no broken or frayed electric cords or plugs. Have defective electric plugs or cords repaired by an approved repair person. Discard all electric appliances that cannot be repaired. Install ground fault circuit interrupters in electric sockets near water sources to prevent accidental shocks with use of appliances.
- *Decrease clutter and other hazards.* Discard unnecessary items, such as old newspapers. Keep shoes, wastebaskets, electric cords, and charger cables out of traffic areas. Never place or store anything on stairs. Clear ice promptly from sidewalks and outside stairs. Cat litter can be used to provide traction on icy surfaces.
- *Provide adequate lighting.* This is particularly important in stairwells. Switches should be located at both the top and bottom of stairs. Use nightlights in the bedroom, bathroom, and hallways. Ensure adequate lighting in food preparation areas of the kitchen to facilitate label reading and to reduce the risk for injury when sharp objects are used.
- *Provide grip assistance wherever appropriate.* Install handrails in all stairwells to provide support for stair climbing. Grab bars alongside the toilet and in the bathtub and shower also help provide support. Lightweight cooking utensils with large handles and enlarged stove knobs make cooking easier and safer for older adults.
- *Place frequently used items at shoulder height or lower where they can be reached easily.* Keeping frequently used items available decreases the need to use climbing devices. Use only approved devices, such as step stools when reaching for items that cannot be reached easily. Ladders are not recommended for use by older adults, but if they are used, ensure that they are fully open and locked. Excessive reaching should be avoided, and another person should stand by to steady the ladder, reducing the risk for tipping.
- *Take measures to prevent burns.* Avoid smoking or the use of open flames whenever possible. Do not wear loose, long sleeves when cooking on a gas stove. Check that the hot water tank setting does not exceed 120 degrees F. Use a mixer valve to prevent sudden bursts of hot water. Have a plan for leaving the residence in case of fire.

FIRE HAZARDS

Older adults are among the highest risk groups for injury or death caused by fire. Hospitals and long-term care facilities are well aware of the danger of fire. Building codes for these institutions require safety doors, fire extinguishers, exit windows, oxygen precautions, and other safety measures. Each institution must have a fire safety plan designed to reduce the risk for fire, a quick notification system to the local fire department, protocols for fire containment, and an evacuation plan. Fortunately, these measures have made institutional fires an uncommon occurrence. Fire deaths in the community are more common than those in institutions. Overall, the number of community deaths have increased slightly over the past 10 years despite public education measures. The relative risk that an older adult will die in a home fire is 2.6 times than that for a person in the general population (U.S. Fire Administration, 2020). Residential fires injure more than 2200 older adults each year (U.S. Fire Administration, 2019). Most fire injuries stem from the use of cooking equipment, followed by heating equipment; whereas smoking materials cause the majority of fire deaths (National Fire Protection Agency, 2017). Many of these deaths could be prevented if people instituted these basic fire safety precautions in their homes:

- Make sure smoke and carbon monoxide alarms are installed. Check that the batteries are working monthly and replace the batteries twice a year. Do not disable the device if cooking fumes or steam causes it to sound. Instead, move the device or try a different type of detector.
- Use caution with cigarettes or open flames. Do not smoke in the home. Do not leave a cigarette unattended or on an unstable surface where it could fall onto a flammable floor or furniture. Empty all smoking materials into a metal container so that no smoldering materials can catch fire. Never smoke in bed.
- Make sure that there are no open flames from cigarettes, matches, candles, and so on if oxygen is in use. Oxygen does not burn, but it supports the combustion of other flammable items.
- Allow at least 3 feet of clear space around a portable heater. Residents should turn off and unplug portable heaters when they are sleeping or away from home.
- Check extension cords for fraying or loose plugs. Do not pull cords out by tugging on the wire. Be careful not to overload an outlet. Avoid using extension cords; get an electrical block with a circuit breaker instead.
- Be sure to turn off the stove or oven if you are leaving the area even for a short time. Keep baking soda and a pot lid available to smother a fire if it occurs. Do not use water, particularly if grease is involved.
- Never cook while wearing long, loose sleeves that could catch fire, causing serious burns. Secure your hair if it is long.
- If you live in a rental unit, report any fire safety hazards, such as blocked exits, cluttered hallways, malfunctioning smoke detectors, or other problems to the owner or management promptly. If these problems are not resolved, notify the fire department.
- Have an escape plan. Plan more than one escape route if possible. Practice how you would get out, particularly if you use a wheelchair or other mobility aids. Keep a flashlight, eyeglasses, and a whistle (to warn others or to help them find you) at the bedside. If the fire is in your residence, get out to safety before calling the fire department. Close the door behind you to prevent the spread of the fire. Do not try to extinguish the fire yourself.
- Do not use an elevator when there is a fire.

HOME SECURITY

People, particularly strangers, present a risk to older adults. Older adults are more vulnerable than younger persons to attack and injury from those who prey on weaker or more defenseless people, such as the infirm or older adults. Older adults need to be aware of the risks presented by strangers and learn to incorporate measures to reduce the likelihood of injury (Box 9.4).

INTERNET SAFETY

Technology is everywhere. Older adults can get news as it happens, communicate with family and friends around the world, complete financial transactions, explore details on any subject, and play a variety of games. In addition, the use of social media by older adults continues to increase. Some 27% of older adults used social networking sites in 2013, which increased to 45% of older adults in 2021 (Pew Research Center, 2022).

Along with these greater opportunities come increased risks. Internet criminals are becoming more sophisticated. Posting photos while one is on vacation can alert a criminal to an empty home from which to steal. Older adults must learn ways to protect themselves from identity theft, credit card fraud, and more (Box 9.5).

VEHICULAR ACCIDENTS

Probably the most dangerous hazards, because of their size and speed, are motor vehicles. Injuries due to motor vehicle accidents are more likely to involve the older adult, whether a pedestrian or driver.

Studies reveal facts that demonstrate the magnitude of the problem. Crossing roads is a significant problem

Box 9.4 Home Security Guidelines

- *Think and plan ahead to reduce risks to personal safety.* Unfortunately, we live in a society that is less safe than the one in which older adults grew up. Precautions that may not have been necessary in the past should now be part of each person's daily planning.
- *Identify ways an intruder could enter the home.* Defective locks on windows or doors should be replaced. Locks should be secured and checked each time the person enters and leaves. Lost or stolen keys may necessitate lock changes.
- *Maintain regular contact with friends and family.* Daily phone calls or some sort of signaling system should be used to indicate that everything is all right.
- *Use the telephone safely.* Keep a phone at the bedside and near the favorite sitting area. This eliminates the need to hurry to another room. If possible, obtain a phone with large numbers, which enables accurate dialing in a stressful situation. An autodial function with emergency numbers is also helpful. An answering machine is useful in screening unwanted or late night calls. Women living alone should never volunteer this fact to strangers. Using a male voice on the answering machine is a wise precaution.
- *Answer the door safely.* Ensure that doors are secure with a peephole at eye level for viewing visitors before opening the door. Make sure that outside lighting is available and working so that nighttime visitors can be observed. Ask for proper identification before opening the door for a stranger. Do not open the door if there is any doubt about who is there; authentic sales agents or service employees will wait and not be offended by having their identification checked with their company.
- *Bank safely.* Withdraw cash in small denomination bills. Do not carry or display large amounts of cash. Secure money immediately in a wallet, money belt, or handbag. It is wise not to put large sums of money in a shoulder or strap handbag that can be pulled away easily. It is better to keep wallets in an internal pocket or body pouch. Keep large amounts of cash and valuables in a bank or other financial institution. Vary the day and time that banking is done. When using an automated teller machine, avoid nighttime visits and whenever possible, have another person along for safety.
- *Prepare for emergencies.* Have emergency numbers posted in large, clear lettering near each telephone. If entry door locks have dead bolts, they should be left unlocked with the key in place while the older person is inside. This reduces the risk of the older person being trapped in the building in case of fire and enables emergency care providers to enter the housing unit if services are needed.

Box 9.5 Computer Safety for Older Adults

- Select a strong password
- Limit personal information when posting online
- Delay posting vacation photos until after returning home
- Keep devices in your possession
- Avoid opening attachments, clicking on links or replying to email messages from unknown senders
- Beware of any requests for personal information
- Install and routinely update security programs on your computer
- Use 2 or more credentials when logging in to your accounts, when available
- Back up data frequently
- Beware of "free" gifts or prizes

for older pedestrians. One study revealed that almost 36% of independent persons older than 70 years of age and nearly 74% of those older than 80 years of age are not able to walk fast enough to cross a street before the traffic signal changes (Eggenberger et al., 2017). The National Highway Traffic and Safety Administration (NHTSA) reports that 20% of pedestrian deaths in 2017 involved people over the age of 65 (NHTSA, 2019). Some communities with high numbers of older adults have adopted modifications that make street crossing safer. These include pedestrian-controlled timers, safety islands, and restrictions on vehicle turns at intersections. Active lobbying by seniors in other communities can help to initiate similar safety innovations.

With regard to driving, older adults are often unwilling to stop driving in spite of the serious risks to themselves and others. The need for independence is their main reason voiced by older adults for wanting to continue. A driver's license is seen as a ticket to freedom. From adolescence on, Americans' preferred method of transportation is the car. In some parts of the country, however, driving is more a necessity than a luxury. Rural and suburban areas may not offer viable alternatives other than reliance on another person to provide transportation. Currently, there are few legal measures in place to determine when an older adult's driving privileges should be terminated, but many proposals are being discussed all across the country. This is a difficult issue, often pitting younger family members against aging parents. Some states have added requirements for older adults after a certain age, such as more frequent renewals, a vision or road test, or in-person renewal. Other states offer licenses with restrictions, which allow older drivers to drive only along specific routes that they already know or only at specific times (IIHS HLDI, 2020). Health care providers are often caught in the middle of this dilemma.

Driving by older adults is a major concern in communities where many seniors reside. In 2018, almost 7700 people age 65 and older died in motor vehicle crashes, and nearly 250,000 were injured. Medical problems are twice as likely to cause driving problems for older adults than for people under age 64. Furthermore, in 2018, there were more than 45 million drivers over age 65, which is 20% of all drivers in the United States (CDC, 2020b). This number is expected to increase dramatically as the baby boom generation ages. Although it has not been shown that older drivers pose a greater risk to others in terms of injury or death, they themselves are more likely to die from injuries because of their increased susceptibility to injury and medical complications. The fatality rate for drivers over age 85 is the highest for any age group.

Several factors contribute to these statistics. Age-related vision changes result in altered depth perception, changes in night vision, and diminished ability to recover from glare. Hearing changes can interfere with the ability to recognize sirens or other auditory warnings. Decreased muscle strength, reduced flexibility, and slower reflexes reduce the ability to respond to hazards while driving a motor vehicle. Other medical conditions or medications may also have effects on driving ability. One of the growing risk factors is related to changes in cognitive functioning, particularly those caused by Alzheimer disease. Many people with early Alzheimer disease continue to drive, particularly because it is now known that Alzheimer disease is present long before dementia becomes manifest. Most states have no mandatory reporting laws for mental impairment. Some states encourage but do not require physician reporting. Only 6 states—California, Delaware, Nevada, New Jersey, Oregon, and Pennsylvania—require physician reporting (Tortorello, 2017). Some stated requirements are vague, unspecified, or address only seizure disorder/lapse of consciousness.

The National Motorists Association takes the position that those older adults who are mentally and physically fit should be able to decide when to stop driving cars. Yet advocates for people with Alzheimer disease often recommend limiting rather than terminating driving privileges in the early stages.

Community Considerations

Baby boomers represent a large segment of the market for automobiles. As this group ages, automakers are adapting their vehicles to be more friendly to older adults while still marketing a stylish image to entice baby boomers to buy their cars. Modifications include larger numbers on the instrument panel, easier-to-grip handles, adjustable pedal and seat heights, backup sensors or cameras, higher and wider bucket seats, rounded mirrors with multiple sides, and many other features. Older adults are encouraged to ask auto dealers about "senior friendly" features or options.

Although people are usually aware of the need to modify their activity levels as they age, older adults may not be equally aware of the need to make adjustments in driving. Initiating safe driving modifications can enable older adults to enjoy the freedom of

Box 9.6 Safe Driving Practices for Older Adults

DO
- Plan ahead to know where you are going
- Add extra time so that you do not feel rushed
- Limit your driving to places close to home, familiar, and easy to get to
- Avoid distractions, such as talking, playing the radio, or using a cell phone
- Wear your seat belt at all times
- Wear appropriate eyeglasses and hearing aids
- Pace trips to allow for frequent rest breaks
- Use extra caution when approaching intersections
- Drive at a safe distance behind other cars

AVOID DRIVING
- If taking medications that affect driving skills
- During rush hour
- At night, when lighting is limited, or during inclement weather
- On busy streets and in congested traffic areas
- On limited-access roads with high speed limits and complex intersections, such as freeways

movement provided by automobiles while also protecting themselves and others (Box 9.6). Sometimes these adjustments are not enough, and the difficult decision to stop driving must be made. Warning signs indicating that someone should stop driving include but are not limited to the following:
- Nervousness or lack of comfort behind the wheel
- Difficulty staying in one lane
- More "near misses"
- More dents or scrapes on the car (or hitting or scraping the garage, mailbox, etc.)
- Other drivers "honking" at them more often
- Friends or family not wanting to ride with them
- Confusing the brake and gas pedals
- Difficulty turning to look over their shoulders when they are making lane changes or reversing
- Medical conditions or medications that affect their ability to maneuver the car
- Being easily distracted or having difficulty concentrating while driving
- Getting lost
- Receiving more warnings or traffic tickets

When older adults stop driving, they need alternative means of getting around. Family and friends are often willing to provide transportation. Volunteers from churches or civic agencies may also provide rides for senior citizens. Some communities provide low-cost bus or taxi services. The local Agency on Aging (which can be found on the national website www.n4a.org) can provide information regarding services that are available in the area. Older adults may complain that alternative transportation is too costly. This can be countered by statistics by the American Automobile Association (AAA) (2020), which estimates that in 2020 the yearly expense of owning and operating a car was more than $9500. That amount would pay for quite a bit of alternative transportation.

THERMAL HAZARDS

Another external factor that presents risks to older adults is climate, with its high and low extremes. Older persons in extreme conditions (temperatures below 60 degrees F or above 90 degrees F) are at greater risk for developing problems of thermoregulation. Older persons who are sick, frail, inactive, or take medications that prevent the body from regulating temperature normally (Box 9.7) are at serious risk when exposed to even minor changes in temperature. Even active, healthy older adults are at increased risk in extremely hot or cold weather conditions.

⌂ Home Health Considerations

Hypothermia and Hyperthermia

As the cost of heating their homes increases, older adults may try to save money by lowering their thermostat settings. This can be dangerous, because a drop in environmental temperature below 65 degrees F can lead to hypothermia in those in their 80s and 90s. Likewise, air-conditioning costs are considerable, and many people may be reluctant to use their units even when they have them. The National Institute on Aging offers free "Age Pages" that provide information on how to avoid hypothermia and hyperthermia (National Institute on Aging, 2018). This information can be obtained online (https://order.nia.nih.gov/). The National Energy Assistance Referral (NEAR) project can help seniors pay their heating bills. NEAR phone operators (866-674-6327) will give callers the number of their state's Low-Income Home Energy Assistance Program (LIHEAP) office as well as referrals to local agencies that can help with the payment of energy bills. This information can also be obtained by emailing energyassistance@ncat.org.

Thermoregulation, the ability to maintain body temperature in a safe range, is controlled by the hypothalamus. The normal core body temperature is maintained between 97 degrees F and 99 degrees F. Body temperature

Box 9.7   Thermoregulation Risks for Older Adults

- Exposure to excessively cold or hot environments
- Limited financial resources to pay for heat or clothing appropriate for environmental temperature
- Neurologic, endocrine, or cardiovascular disease
- Hypometabolic or hypermetabolic disorders (diabetes, cancer, hypothyroidism, hyperthyroidism, malnutrition, obesity)
- Infection or other febrile illness
- Dehydration or electrolyte imbalances
- Inactivity or excessive activity
- Temperature-altering medications (alcohol, antidepressants, barbiturates, benzodiazepines, phenothiazines, anticholinergics)

can be affected by numerous internal and external factors. Internal factors include muscle activity, peripheral circulation, amount of subcutaneous fat, metabolic rate, amount and type of foods and fluids ingested, medications, and disease processes. External factors include humidity, environmental temperature, air movement, and amount and type of clothing or covering.

Heat is produced by metabolic processes and by muscular activity, such as shivering, and conserved by vasoconstriction. Heat is lost through vasodilation and perspiration. Anything that changes the balance of heat lost and heat retained can cause problems.

Hypothermia is defined as a core body temperature of 95 degrees F or lower. Older adults are highly susceptible to hypothermia for several reasons. Normal changes that occur with aging affect the body's ability to regulate temperature. Changes in the skin reduce the older adult's ability to perceive dangerously hot or cold environments. Decreased muscle tissue, decreased muscle activity, diminished peripheral circulation, reduced subcutaneous fat, and decreased metabolic rate affect the amount of heat produced and retained by the body. As a person ages, metabolism slows, activity decreases, and shivering diminishes. When a person is exposed to low environmental temperatures, body temperature drops further. These changes further decrease activity and heat production, allowing body temperature to decrease even further. If this cycle is not stopped, it can lead to death. The highest rates of death from hypothermia occur in adults over age 85, especially in rural settings (CDC, 2021b).

Disease processes such as hypothyroidism, hypoglycemia, and malnutrition can also cause a decrease in heat production. Medications that decrease environmental awareness—such as barbiturates, tranquilizers, and antidepressants—can increase the risk for hypothermia. Alcohol ingestion is highly dangerous because it decreases environmental awareness and simultaneously increases vasodilation, with resulting heat loss.

Although decreased body temperature is the major symptom of hypothermia, an older person may manifest other signs or symptoms (Box 9.8). One of the first signs of hypothermia in older adults is growing mental confusion that can progress from simple memory loss or changes in logical thinking to total disorientation.

Box 9.8   Signs of Hypothermia

- Mental confusion
- Decreased pulse and respiratory rate
- Decreased body temperature
- Cool/cold skin
- Pallor or cyanosis
- Swollen or puffy face
- Muscle stiffness
- Fine tremors
- Altered coordination
- Changes in gait and balance
- Lethargy, apathy, irritability, hostility, or aggression

Pulse and respiratory rate slow with hypothermia and may be difficult to detect in severe cases. The skin becomes cool or cold to the touch, and pallor or cyanosis is often present (particularly on the extremities). The face may appear swollen or puffy. Muscles appear to be stiff, and fine tremors may occur. Changes in coordination, including poor balance or gait changes, are common. Behavioral changes, such as lethargy or apathy, may occur, but irritability, hostility, and aggression are also possible responses. Shivering, an indication that the body is having difficulty maintaining adequate body temperature, may or may not be evident in older adults because this response often diminishes with aging. Because many of the signs and symptoms of hypothermia are similar to those of other disorders in older adults, they can easily be missed or mistaken for something else.

With proper precautions, hypothermia is preventable. Approaches to prevention are identified in the section on nursing interventions later in the chapter. When hypothermia is suspected, immediate intervention is necessary to prevent serious complications or death. If the person is unconscious, call 911. Special care will be required to prevent cardiovascular complications and to rewarm the person. This should be done even when the person appears to be dead because a pulse may not be palpable owing to severe vasoconstriction. If the person is conscious, move the older adult into a warmer environment. Remove cold and/or wet clothing and wrap the person with blankets or other insulating coverings. Warm blankets may be used, but heating pads, electric blankets, or immersion in a hot bath are to be avoided because they may cause cardiovascular problems and damage fragile skin. Warm, not hot, beverages are appropriate and beneficial if the person is conscious and able to drink.

Hyperthermia, a higher than normal body temperature, occurs when the body is unable to get rid of excess heat. Deaths directly or indirectly caused by hyperthermia average around 700 per year in the United States (Vaidyanathan et al., 2020). Most hyperthermia deaths occur in adults over age 50, and they affect more men than women. Hyperthermia can be caused by excessively high environmental temperatures; an inability to dissipate heat; or increased heat production caused by exercise, infection, or hyperthyroidism.

Many parts of the country experience extremely high temperatures during the summer months. When this heat is combined with high humidity, the normal cooling mechanisms of the body become ineffective. Even under moderate conditions, it takes longer for older adults to begin sweating, and—because of their diminished thirst and reduced body water—they perspire less. These factors render older adults more likely to develop heat exhaustion and heatstroke.

Hyperthermia can place a significant strain on the heart and blood vessels of older adults. Cardiovascular problems and heat are a deadly combination. Endocrine

problems, such as diabetes and psychiatric disorders, also increase the risk for hyperthermia. Medications commonly used by older adults can compromise the body's normal adaptation to heat. Diuretics prevent the body from storing fluids and can diminish superficial vasodilation. Anticholinergic medications used to treat Parkinson disease (e.g., benztropine and trihexyphenidyl) can interfere with perspiration, as do a wide range of psychotropic medications. Consumption of alcohol should be avoided because it can decrease awareness of symptoms and contribute to fluid loss.

Symptoms of hyperthermia are progressive. Mild, early signs of heat stress include feeling hot, listless, or uncomfortable. Cramps in the legs, arms, and abdomen are early indicators of elevated body temperature. Indications of a serious heat-related problem may include hot, dry skin without perspiration; tachycardia; chest pain; breathing problems; throbbing headache; dizziness; profound weakness; mental or perceptual changes; vomiting; abdominal cramps; nausea; and diarrhea.

Heat exhaustion occurs gradually and is caused by water or sodium depletion. Both active and inactive older adults can develop heat exhaustion if they do not consume adequate fluids and electrolytes when they are exposed to hot environments. If heat exhaustion is not recognized and treated, it can progress to a more severe condition called *heatstroke*.

Heatstroke, a condition in which the body temperature increases to 104 degrees F or higher, is a life-threatening emergency. It is a very real concern for active older persons, particularly those living in hot climates. Strategies that can prevent or reduce the incidence of hyperthermia are listed under Implementation in each of the Nursing Process/Clinical Judgment Model sections that follow.

SUMMARY

Psychological trauma caused by falls, assaults, motor vehicle accidents, fires, thermal events, or other injuries can be more serious than the physical trauma itself. Fear of injury often confines older adults to their homes and can cause them to lose confidence in their ability to perform even simple actions. They may restrict their activity, thereby contributing to further loss of strength, decreased mobility, social isolation, and increased dependence. If enough function is lost, institutionalization may become necessary.

❖ NURSING PROCESS/CLINICAL JUDGMENT MODEL FOR POTENTIAL FOR INJURY

◆ ASSESSMENT (DATA COLLECTION)

Recognize Cues
- Does the person have a history of falls or other injuries?

- If yes, how often have they fallen? When and where did the fall occur? What types of injuries have occurred?
- How often have they experienced injuries?
- What is the person's level of vision? Hearing? Temperature perception?
- Is there any impairment in gait or balance?
- Does the person use any assistive devices such as a cane or a walker?
- What kind of footwear is usually worn?
- Does the person have a cognitive impairment? Forgetfulness?
- Do they smoke? Light candles in the home? Use a gas stove?
- Does the home have a smoke detector? Is it working?
- Does the person live alone?
- What medications do they take?
- Does the experience dizziness or fainting?
- What are the hemoglobin and hematocrit levels?
- Are they able to follow directions?
- Does the person drive? Do they wear a seatbelt when driving or riding in a car?
- Does the person use a computer and social media?
- If the person is living at home, where are medications stored?
- Where are chemicals and cleaning supplies stored?
- Are there safety hazards in the home? Scatter rugs? Electric wires? Others?

◆ DATA ANALYSIS/PROBLEM IDENTIFICATION

Analyze Cues and Prioritize Hypotheses:
  Problem statements for older adults with potential safety concerns include
Fall Risk
Potential for Injury
Potential for Trauma
Potential for Poisoning

◆ PLANNING

Generate Solutions: The patient goals for an older person who has the potential for injury, trauma, or poisoning are to experience a decrease in the frequency and severity of injuries and to identify and correct unsafe conditions and behaviors.

◆ IMPLEMENTATION

Take Action: The following nursing interventions for those who have a potential for injury, trauma, or poisoning should take place in hospitals or extended-care facilities:

1. **Evaluate the person for fall risk.** Older adults who experience dizziness or fainting with position changes have an increased fall risk. These symptoms are often caused by a sudden drop in blood pressure (orthostatic hypotension). Instruct these individuals to move slowly and to remain seated until the dizziness passes. Episodes of orthostatic hypotension are more likely to occur early in the morning, particularly before breakfast, and may be aggravated by dehydration or medications. Promptly report any episode of dizziness to the primary care provider so that the cause can be determined. Evaluate laboratory values for the presence of anemia, which can increase fall risk. Notify the primary care provider of any abnormal values so that appropriate interventions can be initiated. Assess all new admissions for problems with balance and gait so that appropriate safety strategies can be initiated. Encourage older adults to move at a comfortable pace and not to hurry. Hurrying increases the fall risk. Encourage older adults to wear comfortable, supportive footwear. Assistive devices (e.g., canes and walkers) that improve stability by providing a wider base of support may be needed (Fig. 9.2).
  Check high-risk individuals frequently. Ensure the call light is readily available whether the person is in bed or in a chair. Lounges and bathrooms should be equipped with call lights. Answer calls from older adults promptly. If older adults have to wait too long for assistance, they may attempt to stand or walk even if they know it is unsafe.
  Provide adequate assistance based on the patient's abilities and limitations. Use lifts and other transfer devices when appropriate. Take care to prevent injury to both the patient and the caregiver.

2. **Modify the environment to reduce risks.** To prevent falls resulting from visual changes, stairwells should be well illuminated both day and night. Mark the edges of stairs, shower lips, and any other elevations using a dark or contrasting color stripe to help the aging individual recognize the edge. Hallways should have strong grip rails to provide support during ambulation (Fig. 9.3). Remove all clutter—such as newspapers, wastebaskets, shoes, and other items—from the floor. Provide nonskid footwear. Be sure to lock all devices with wheels, such as beds and wheelchairs. Use low beds or keep beds in the lowest position unless the caregiver is at the bedside. If the caregiver has to leave the person, even briefly, lower the bed. Whenever the bed is elevated, the side rail opposite the caregiver should be up to reduce the chance of falls. Electronic sensors or alarm systems designed to signal when an at-risk person attempts to stand up from a chair or get out of bed unassisted may be helpful, particularly in cases of cognitive impairment where the older adult is unaware of the fall risk. Lock and store medication carts when not in use. Never leave medications at the bedside unless permitted by the primary care provider and facility policy. Medications intended for one individual can easily be taken by a confused person who has wandered into the wrong room. Lock cleaning

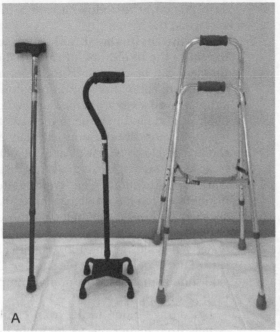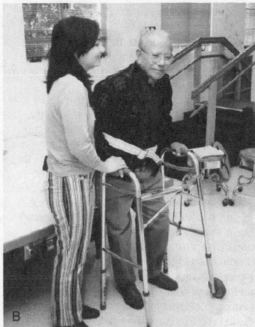

Fig. 9.2 Assistive devices promote support and safety. A, Quad cane (From Yeon-Jae Jeong, Jun-Pyo Myong, Jung-Wan Koo, Yeon-Gyu Jeong. *Gait & Posture*, Volume 41, Issue 2, February 2015, Pages 493–498.). B, Walker. (From Webb, M., Kostelnick, C., & Scott, K. [2018]. *Long-term caring* [4th ed.]. St. Louis, MO: Elsevier.)

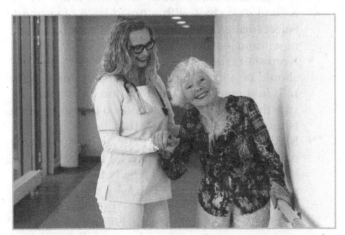

Fig. 9.3 Handrails provide support when walking. (Copyright © istock.com/Horsche.)

carts and supplies in a cabinet or closet when not in use.

> **(!) Safety**
>
> All poisonous agents, including cleaning solutions, must be stored in locked cabinets or closets, where they are out of the reach of residents. Cleaning carts should be kept within sight of staff.

Protective devices, formerly called restraints, can represent a violation of basic patient rights and may lead to injury or even death. They should be used only as a last resort. If protective devices are ever used, they must be used with caution, for a documented reason, and only after the person or guardian agrees to the use of the device. This includes use of foot pedals, vest and waist restraints, even chair tables and safety belts. The Omnibus Budget Reconciliation Act (OBRA) regulations are very specific about when and what types of devices are permitted. A primary care provider's order is needed to use a protective device; a standing order or "prn" order cannot be used. In acute and critical care settings, protective device orders should be renewed every 4 hours and the patient should be examined by the prescribing practitioner every 24 hours while the device is in use (Bauer, 2017). Protective devices must meet the following 5 criteria to be in compliance with regulations: (1) "be necessary to treat a medical symptom; (2) not be used to discipline a resident or for staff convenience in the absence of a medical symptom; (3) not be used because of family request in the absence of a medical symptom; (4) be the least restrictive device possible in use for the least amount of time per day possible; and (5) the facility must have an active plan in place to decrease usage or for eventual removal of the restraint" (Centers for Medicare & Medicaid Services, 2020).

> **(💡) QSEN Considerations: Teamwork and Collaboration**
>
> **Use of Protective Devices**
>
> All staff, including nursing assistants, should be thoroughly trained regarding the use of each type of protective device. Close attention should be paid to when, what, how, and why these devices are used.
>
> - When: Only when other less restrictive methods have been tried first and found to be ineffective. Never use protective devices as a form of punishment. The primary care provider's orders are necessary for both physical and chemical restraints. Obtain informed consent from

the patient or legal guardian before using protective devices.

- What: The least restrictive device that allows the highest level of function but still provides protection. For example, a waist bar or lap board in a wheelchair would be preferable to a full vest device.
- How: Read all manufacturers' directions and agency policies before applying a protective device. Use the correct size device. Identify the front and back of the device before applying. When the protective device has tie straps, attach them to a part of the bed or chair that moves with the patient so that they do not become overly constricting. Use only quick-release hitch knots that are affixed in locations where the nurse but not the patient can easily reach them. Check the patient frequently. Release protective devices at least every 2 hours and inspect tissues beneath the device for signs of altered circulation or tissue damage.
- Why: Inappropriate use of protective devices is dangerous for the patient. The potential for lawsuits charging abuse or neglect increases when protective devices are in use. To reduce the risk for legal liability, document the following carefully: (1) baseline assessment of physical condition, including vital signs, infections, pain, fluid and nutritional status, elimination status, medications, vision, hearing, mental status, and typical behavior patterns; (2) specific behaviors that necessitated the need for devices, including persons or events that may have triggered the behavior; (3) the type and time the devices were used; (4) the patient's response to protective device; (5) nourishment provided; (6) identifying and allowing for the need for elimination; and (7) interventions identified as part of the plan of care designed to prevent recurrences of the need for protective devices.

? Critical Thinking

Protective Devices

Identify as many alternatives to using protective devices as you can.
- Why do you think that these alternative actions will decrease the need for protective devices?
- How many of these actions have you seen used in care settings?
- Have you tried any yourself? How effective was the alternative intervention?

Complementary Health Approaches

Music Therapy

Research has found that older patients who listen to music enjoy exhibit significantly more positive behaviors than do older patients who are not exposed to music. No single type of music is right for everyone. Family members may be helpful in identifying favorite music, or the staff may try different types of music and observe the patient's response. Some may prefer classical, others like jazz, still others love gospel music. Considering the demographics, the music of the baby boomers (e.g., Elvis, James Taylor, The Beatles) may soon be what is found to be effective.

Take Action: The following interventions should take place in the home:

1. **Assess the environment for hazards and modify it to reduce the likelihood of injury.** The home environment can be dangerous for older adults. To reduce the likelihood of poisoning, store all cleaning supplies well away from food or medications. If the older person has impaired judgment, it may be necessary to keep all poisonous substances in a locked cabinet or closet. Clearly label all medications in large letters so that individuals can distinguish their names and directions. Check refrigerator for spoiled or outdated food. Bathwater temperature should be checked with a thermometer by those individuals with circulatory changes. They should not add hot water when sitting in a tub or adjust the temperature of the water while in the shower. Use only nonskid shower mats. Mop up spills promptly to reduce the risk of slipping.
   - Discourage older adults from climbing because falls from higher places are more likely to cause serious injury. In general, chairs, footstools, and other pieces of furniture are unsafe. If the person needs to reach a high area, encourage use of a good step stool with a broad base of support. Select furniture that is steady and easy to get out of without assistance.
   - Keep stairs free of clutter. Handrails in stairwells should be sturdy and in good repair. Install grip rails in showers, tubs, and around toilets, making sure that they are tightly attached to the structure (studs) of the wall, not just the plaster.
   - Make sure there is adequate lighting without glare, particularly in stairwells and bathrooms. Keep a flashlight at the bedside for emergencies or when a light cannot be easily reached. Check the floor for hazards, such as clutter, scatter rugs, or loose carpet edges that, when rolled up, may trip a person. Remove or repair all hazardous items to reduce the fall risk.
   - Make sure that smoke and carbon monoxide alarms are installed and are working correctly. Change batteries twice a year in the spring and fall when clocks are changed for daylight savings time.
   - Encourage use of a MedicAlert "panic button"—an emergency call device that is worn as a necklace or bracelet. This can be activated to summon help if a fall occurs. In addition, assess the person for depressed mood. Studies have shown that the incidence of falls is 3 times higher among depressed individuals living at home.
2. **Recruit the assistance of a family member or friend to check on the older person at regular intervals.** Regular visits to the home provide a quick check of the most obvious hazards. Correct any unsafe conditions before an injury occurs. Review the most recent and any common concerns with the visitors before

the visit. Although frequent checks will not always prevent injury, they can reduce the chance of an injured older person lying helpless for extended periods. Some older persons invest in special call signal devices that can be worn on their bodies. These call signals can be activated in case of emergency to summon help. They should be purchased only after the reputation of the company who sells and services the device has been carefully checked with an agency, such as the Better Business Bureau. Many of these so-called safety systems are worthless and only provide a false sense of security to older adults.

3. **Use any appropriate interventions that are used in the institutional setting.**

❖ NURSING PROCESS/CLINICAL JUDGMENT MODEL FOR HYPOTHERMIA/HYPERTHERMIA

◆ ASSESSMENT (DATA COLLECTION)

Recognize cues

- What is the person's body temperature?
- How does it change throughout the day?
- Is the person inactive or excessively active?
- Do they show any signs of infection, including behavioral changes?
- Does the person complain of feeling hot or cold?
- Do they have any disease conditions that increase the risk for altered thermoregulation?
- Does the person have an electrolyte imbalance?
- Do they consume alcohol or other temperature-altering medications?
- Does the person have dementia, depression, or other conditions that decrease awareness?
- Do they have adequate financial resources to pay for housing that has adequate heat and ventilation?
- Does the individual have clothing suitable for the environmental conditions?

See Box 9.7 for a list of thermoregulation risks for older adults.

◆ DATA ANALYSIS/PROBLEM IDENTIFICATION

Analyze Cues and Prioritize Hypotheses: Problem statements for older adults at risk for imbalanced thermoregulation include

Altered Thermoregulation
Potential for Altered Body Temperature

◆ PLANNING

Generate Solutions: The patient goals for an older person with altered thermoregulation or potential for altered body temperature are to maintain core body temperature within the normal range and to state the appropriate modifications in dress, activity, and environment needed to maintain body temperature within the normal limits.

◆ IMPLEMENTATION

Take Action: The following nursing interventions should take place in hospitals or extended-care facilities:

1. **Monitor the environmental temperature, humidity, and air movement.** Maintain room temperature at a comfortable level between 70 degrees F and 75 degrees F. A relative humidity between 40% and 60% is comfortable for most people. Ventilation should provide an exchange of air without drafts, which may cause chilling. Limit the time an older adult is exposed to extreme temperatures, either hot or cold.

2. **Monitor body temperature at regular intervals.** Regularly monitor the temperature of any person at risk for hyperthermia or hypothermia. In many cases, a thermometer that registers temperatures below 95 degrees F is needed for accurate measurement. Electronic thermometers or thermal ear sensors provide accurate temperatures when used correctly.

3. **Provide clothing and bed covers that are suitable for the environment.** Extra clothing and blankets may be necessary for inactive persons. Knit undergarments, layered clothing, bed socks, nightcaps, and flannel sheets or blankets are particularly effective at retaining body heat. Make sure to use adequate covers or an adequately warmed room when bathing a frail older adult. In the summer, clothing should be lightweight, loose, and nonconstricting to allow adequate movement of air over the body.

4. **Promote adequate fluid and food intake.** In cold weather, a diet rich in protein and additional snacks can help maintain the subcutaneous fat needed for insulation and promote muscle mass needed to sustain heat production. In hot weather, older adults should have fresh fluids at the bedside at all times. Provide pitchers of a cool sugar-free beverage in day rooms, activity centers, and lounges. Because older adults may have a diminished sense of thirst, frequent reminders to drink may be necessary.

5. **Monitor activity level in accordance with environmental temperature.** Increased physical activity helps older adults keep warm in cool weather. Excessive activity should be avoided during hot weather, particularly during daytime hours when the temperature is highest.

The following interventions should take place in the home:

1. **Verify that the residence has adequate heat in cold weather and adequate ventilation in hot weather.** Many older adults, particularly those who live alone and those with limited financial resources, live in marginal or substandard housing. There is often inadequate heat to provide warmth in winter or inadequate ventilation to keep cool in the summer. If the home is poorly heated, encourage the person to stay active and dress warmly. If the home is too hot or is poorly ventilated, encourage the person to reduce

activity and dress in cool clothing. If air-conditioned public buildings—such as shopping plazas, libraries, or senior centers—are accessible, encourage older adults to spend the hottest times of day in such facilities.

2. **Identify community resources that can help older adults to maintain a safe environment.** Many public utility companies have special programs designed to ensure that older adults have adequate heat in winter. Some also provide fans or air conditioners in the summer for older adults at reduced prices. Special payment plans that spread the cost of heating or air-conditioning over the year are also available in most areas of the country. Such plans can enable older adults to budget their limited resources, while maintaining a safe thermal environment.
3. **Review healthy habits.**
4. **Use any appropriate interventions that are used in the institutional setting.**

TO PREVENT HYPERTHERMIA

(1) Decrease physical activity during the daytime. (2) Do heavy chores, such as laundry, early in the morning or in the evening. (3) Perform outdoor activities after sunset. (4) Dress in light-colored, loose-fitting cotton clothing. (5) Keep out of direct sunlight—use hats, umbrellas, awnings, or other types of sunscreens to reduce sun exposure. (6) In excessive heat, take cool baths or showers several times a day, or apply cool, wet towels or ice packs to the axillae and groin. (7) Drink a minimum of 8 to 10 glasses of water or cool beverages each day regardless of thirst. When there are medical restrictions on fluid intake, the primary care provider should be consulted regarding the recommended amount of intake. (8) Avoid drinking hot beverages and alcohol. (9) Eat several small meals instead of a few large ones.

TO PREVENT HYPOTHERMIA

(1) Keep the heat within the safe temperature range of 70 degrees F to 75 degrees F. (2) Stay active. (3) Wear several layers of clothing rather than one heavy layer. Wool, knits, and flannel are particularly warm. (4) Drink 8 to 10 glasses of fluid daily, including warm beverages. Check for any fluid restrictions arising from medical conditions. (5) Avoid consuming alcohol. (6) Eat several small warm meals throughout the day.

Get Ready for the Next Generation NCLEX® Examination!

Key Points

- The normal physiologic changes of aging, increased incidence of chronic illness, increased use of medications, and sensory or cognitive changes place the older population vulnerable to possible injury.
- Potential for injury increases dramatically when older adults are exposed to multiple environmental hazards.
- The most common injuries experienced by older adults include falls, burns, poisoning, and automobile accidents.
- Falls are the leading death caused by injury in people older than age 65, the most common cause of nonfatal trauma-related hospital admissions, and the leading cause of traumatic brain injury.
- Nurses can play an important role by helping older adults recognize their risk factors, by planning coping strategies to promote safety, and by modifying their environment to minimize the likelihood of injury.

Additional Learning Resources

SG Go to your Evolve website at http://evolve.elsevier.com/Williams/geriatric for the additional online resources.

🌐 Online Resources

- Speak Up: Reducing Your Risk of Falling brochure available in English and Spanish from the Joint Commission: https://www.jointcommission.org/topics/speak_up_reducing_your_risk_of_falling.aspx

Review Questions for The Next Generation NCLEX® Examination

1. Which of the following factors can contribute to the development of hypothermia in older adults. *(Select all that apply.)*
   a. Decreased muscle tissue
   b. Decreased sensory perception of cold
   c. Decreased subcutaneous fat
   d. Increased metabolism
   e. Increased muscle activity

2. Which of the following manifestations indicate serious heat-related problems? *(Select all that apply.)*
   a. Cramps in the legs
   b. Vomiting
   c. Heavy perspiration
   d. Profound weakness
   e. Mental changes
   f. Throbbing headache

3. The nurse should instruct the nursing assistant who is caring for a patient who is receiving antihypertensive medication to
   a. Have at least 2 people assist with ambulation
   b. Encourage the patient to stand up slowly from a sitting or lying position
   c. Take the blood pressure if the patient complains of diplopia
   d. Provide additional salt with the patient's meals

4. The nurse is aware that the best predictor of an older adult falling is
   a. A history of previous falls
   b. Use of multiple medications
   c. Sensory deficits
   d. Alterations in balance

5. Your team is developing a fall reduction program on your unit. Which intervention(s) would be important to remember when developing such a program? *(Select all that apply.)*
   a. Assess patients for for fall risk factors upon admission and any change in patient condition
   b. Identify and remove environmental hazards.
   c. Avoid placing signage identifying patient with fall risk to protect privacy.
   d. Encourage patient participation in supervised group exercise program.
   e. Perform regular medication reviews.
   f. Use protective devices on patients with a high fall risk.

6. The nurse has arrived for a first postoperative and home safety visit of a 75-year-old patient who had a total hip replacement 3 days earlier. The patient has hypertension and a history of falls, the most recent having occurred 6 months earlier. Currently the patient lives independently; his daughter visits him every 3 days to help with medications. The patient also has a house cleaner and a helper who assists with preparing some meals.

The nurse documents the following findings as part of the assessment:

- Alert and oriented
- Vital signs stable
- Grip bars present in shower and bathroom
- Poor lighting in bedroom
- Computer passwords written on financial statements on desk
- Frequent use of social media with established friendships in several groups
- Several items left on staircase
- Lamp with cord on carpet across entry to bedroom
- Medications out of original labeled containers mixed in bowl on kitchen counter
- Walker positioned near patient and used when patient ambulates in home

Highlight or place a check mark next to assessment findings that require follow up by the nurse.

REFERENCES

Alshammari, H., Al-Saeed, E., Ahmed, Z., & Aslanpour, Z. (2021). Reviewing Potentially Inappropriate Medication in Hospitalized Patients Over 65 Using Explicit Criteria: A Systematic Literature Review. *Drug, healthcare and patient safety, 13,* 183–210 https://doi.org/10.2147/DHPS.S303101

American Automobile Association (AAA) Automotive (2020). Your driving costs: How much does it really cost to own a new car? https://newsroom.aaa.com/wp-content/uploads/2020/12/Your-Driving-Costs-2020-Fact-Sheet-FINAL-12-9-20-2.pdf/

Bauer, R. N. (2017). Safety regarding restraints. *MEDSURG Nursing, 26*(5), 352–355

Centers for Disease Control and Prevention (CDC) (2021a). Home and recreational safety: Deaths from older adult falls. https://www.cdc.gov/homeandrecreationalsafety/falls/data/deaths-from-falls.html/

Centers for Disease Control and Prevention (CDC) (2021a). Facts about falls. https://www.cdc.gov/falls/facts.html

Centers for Disease Control and Prevention (CDC) (2021b). QuickStats: Death rates attributed to excessive cold or hypothermia among persons aged ≥15 years, by urban-rural status and age group—National Vital Statistics System, United States, 2019. Morb Mortal Wkly Rep, 70, 258 doi: http://dx.doi.org/10.15585/mmwr.mm7007a6

Centers for Disease Control and Prevention (CDC) (2020a). Injury prevention & control: 10 leading causes of death by age group, United States–2018. https://www.cdc.gov/injury/wisqars/pdf/leading_causes_of_death_by_age_group_2018-508.pdf/

Centers for Disease Control and Prevention (CDC) (2020b). Injury prevention & control: Older adult driver safety. https://www.cdc.gov/injury/features/older-driver-safety/index.html#:~:text=In%202018%2C%20almost%207%2C700%20older,700%20are%20injured%20in%20crashes/

Centers for Disease Control and Prevention (CDC) (2020c). STEADI: Older adult fall prevention. https://www.cdc.gov/steadi/index.html/

Centers for Medicare & Medicaid Services (CMS.gov) (2020) *State Operations Manual,* Appendix A—Survey protocol, regulations and interpretive guidelines for hospitals (2020). https://www.cms.gov/Regulations-and-Guidance/Guidance/Manuals/downloads/som107ap_a_hospitals.pdf/

Chapman, A., & Meyer, C. (2017). Falls prevention in older adults with diabetes: A clinical review of screening, assessment and management recommendations. *Diabetes & Primary Care Australia, 2,* 69–74. http://pcdsa.com.au/wp-content/uploads/2017/03/DPCA2-2_69-74_wm.pdf

Eggenberger, P., Tomovic, S., Muzer, T., et al. (2017). Older adults must hurry at pedestrian lights! A cross-sectional analysis of preferred and fast walking speed under single- and dual-task condition. *PLOS ONE, 12*(7), e0182180. https://www.ncbi.nlm.nih.gov/pmc/articles/PMC5536437/

Everding, G. (2021). Fall-prevention program can help reduce harmful in-home falls by nearly 40%. Washington University School of Medicine. https://medicine.wustl.edu/news/fall-prevention-program-can-help-reduce-dangerous-in-home-tumbles-by-nearly-40/

Goswami, N., Blaber, A. P., Hinghofer-Szalkay, H., et al. (2017). Orthostatic intolerance in older persons: Etiology and counter-measures. *Frontiers in Physiology, 8,* 803. https://pubmed.ncbi.nlm.nih.gov/29163185/

Insurance Institute for Highway Safety—Highway Loss Data Institute (IIHS HLDI). (2020). Older drivers: Driver license renewal. https://www.iihs.org/topics/older-drivers#driver-license-renewal

National Council of State Legislatures (2018). Elderly falls prevention legislation and statutes. https://www.ncsl.org/research/health/elderly-falls-prevention-legislation-and-statutes.aspx/

National Council on Aging: Falls prevention facts. https://www.ncoa.org/news/resources-for-reporters/get-the-facts/falls-prevention-facts/2018/

National Fire Protection Agency (2017). Fact sheet: Research – An overview of the U. S. fire problem. https://www.nfpa.

org/-/media/Files/News-and-Research/Fire-statistics-and-reports/Fact-sheets/FireLossFacts.ashx/

National Highway Traffic Safety Administration (NHTSA) (2019). Traffic safety facts: 2017 data, Pedestrians. https://crashstats.nhtsa.dot.gov/Api/Public/ViewPublication/812681

National Institute on Aging (2018). Cold weather safety for older adults. https://www.nia.nih.gov/health/cold-weather-safety-older-adults

Nyman, S.R. (2020). Tai Chi for the prevention of falls among older adults: A critical analysis of the evidence. *Journal of Aging and Physical Activity, 29* (2), 343–352. https://doi.org/10.1123/japa.2020-0155

Pew Research Center (2022). Social media fact sheet. https://www.pewresearch.org/internet/fact-sheet/social-media/

The Joint Commission (2019). The Joint Commission launches educational campaign on preventing falls. https://www.jointcommission.org/resources/news-and-multimedia/news/2019/07/the-joint-commission-launches-educational-campaign-on-preventing-falls/

Tortorello, M. (2017). How seniors are driving safer, driving longer. *Consumer Reports*. https://www.consumerreports.org/elderly-driving/how-seniors-are-driving-safer-driving-longer/

U.S. Fire Administration, FEMA. (2019). Topical fire report series. *Fire risk in 2017, 20*(3). https://www.usfa.fema.gov/downloads/pdf/statistics/v20i3.pdf/

U.S. Fire Administration (2020). U.S. fire deaths, fire death rates, and risk of dying in a fire. https://www.usfa.fema.gov/data/statistics/fire_death_rates.html/

Vaidyanathan, A., Malilay, J., Schramm, P., Saha, S. (2020). Heat-related deaths — United States, 2004–2018. *The Morbidity and Mortality Weekly Report, 69,* 729–734. doi: http://dx.doi.org/10.15585/mmwr.mm6924a1

Cognition and Perception

http://evolve.elsevier.com/Williams/geriatric

Objectives

1. Describe normal sensory and cognitive functions.
2. Describe how sensory perception and cognition change with aging.
3. Examine the effects of disease processes on perception and cognition.
4. Describe methods of assessing changes in perception and cognition.
5. Identify older adults who are most at risk for experiencing perceptual or cognitive problems.
6. Identify current patient problem statements related to perception and cognition.
7. Select nursing interventions that are appropriate for older individuals experiencing problems related to perception or cognition.
8. Discuss pain assessment and management as they relate to older adults.

Key Terms

aphasia (ă-FA-zĕ-ă, p. 206)
catastrophic reactions (p. 199)
cognition (KŎG-nĭ-shŭn, p. 191)
confusion (kŭn-FĔW-shŭn, p. 197)
crystallized intelligence (p. 192)
delirium (dĕ-LĬR-ē-ŭm, p. 197)
dementia (dĕ-MĔN-shē-ă, p. 199)
dysarthria (dĭs-ĂR-thrē-ă, p. 205)
dysphasia (dĭs-FĂ-jē-ă, p. 206)

hemianopsia (hĕm-ē-ŭn-ŌP-sē-ă, p. 195)
intelligence (ĭn-tĕl-ĭ-jĕns, p. 191)
memory (mĕm-ŏ-rē, p. 191)
otosclerosis (ō-tō-sklĕ-RŌ-sĭs, p. 192)
perception (pĕr-sĕp-shŭn, p. 191)
presbyopia (prĕz-bē-Ō-pē-ă, p. 192)
stimuli (STĬM-ū-lĭ, p. 191)
sundowning (SŬN-doun-ĭng, p. 199)

The cognitive-perceptual health pattern deals with the ways in which people gain information from the environment and the way they interpret and use this information. Perception includes the collection, interpretation, and recognition of stimuli, including pain. Cognition includes intelligence, memory, language, and decision-making. Cognition and perception are intimately connected to the functioning of the central nervous system and the special senses of vision, hearing, touch, smell, and taste.

NORMAL COGNITIVE-PERCEPTUAL FUNCTIONING

The environment excites or stimulates the senses. The senses, in turn, pass these stimuli on to the cerebral cortex, where recognition (perception) and interpretation (cognition) occur. Specific regions of the cerebral cortex are responsible for detecting and processing the stimuli acquired by the various senses. Malfunction of the sensory organs or of the interpretation

centers in the brain results in disturbed perception and cognition.

If the senses do not function appropriately, stimuli do not enter the brain and there is not enough information for accurate interpretation. Individuals with sensory deficits in one area often attempt to compensate for these deficits by gathering more information from those senses that function normally. People with hearing deficits often lip read or otherwise rely on visual cues. People with visual deficits rely more heavily on the senses of hearing and touch. People with multiple sensory deficits have great difficulty collecting information and often experience serious cognitive and perceptual problems. Adult hearing impairment has been associated with social isolation and depression. People with sensory deficits have a normal ability to think and learn, but for them, the process is more difficult.

As discussed in Chapter 3, numerous sensory changes occur with aging. Common visual changes include farsightedness, caused by a loss of elasticity of

Sensory Compensation Hypothesis

People with sensory deficits not only try to compensate for the missing sensory input with their remaining senses, but their brain also intensifies those remaining senses. Studies have shown that when the visual sense is disturbed, the sense of touch is enhanced (Silva, 2018). How might this information affect your care for a patient with visual impairment?

the lens and resulting decrease in the power of accommodation (presbyopia); decreased ability to respond to changes in light, resulting in night blindness; and cataracts (Fig. 10.1), which cloud the lens and result in blurred vision and sensitivity to glare. Common auditory changes include loss of hearing acuity, particularly of higher-pitched sounds (presbycusis); loss of hearing resulting from reduced transmission of sound (otosclerosis); and ringing in the ears (tinnitus), which can be caused by Ménière disease (a disorder of the inner ear), age-related changes, or medications. Older adults are increasingly susceptible to misperception and therefore misinterpretation when one or more of these changes are present.

Cognition, or thought, takes place in the cerebral cortex of the brain. Cognitive development starts at the time of birth and perhaps even earlier. When the human brain is repeatedly exposed to stimuli, connections develop between nerve fibers of the cerebral cortex. Each time stimuli are introduced to the brain, they are associated (at an unconscious level) with the facts, memories, and experiences that are stored there. Once these connections are firmly established, information is said to have been learned. Once learning has taken place, information or skills can be retrieved as needed. Memory enables people to retain and recall previously experienced sensations, ideas, concepts, impressions, and all information that has been previously learned. The human mind is extraordinary in its ability to learn and process vast amounts of information. It is able to retrieve information on demand, correlate random pieces of information, make judgments, solve problems, and create ideas.

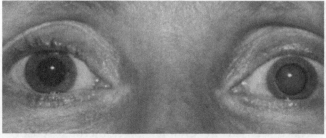

Fig. 10.1 Cataract of the left eye. (From Swartz, M. [2014]. *Textbook of physical diagnosis* [7th ed.]. Philadelphia. PA: Saunders.)

COGNITION AND INTELLIGENCE

We all have different levels of cognitive ability. People often speak of intelligence quotients (IQs) when they try to describe cognitive ability. However, IQ can be deceptive because there are different types of intelligence, and standardized testing procedures do not measure all of them.

Fluid intelligence is the ability to perform tasks or make judgments based on unfamiliar stimuli. This is sometimes referred to as the ability to "think on your feet." Crystallized intelligence (often called *wisdom*) is the ability to perform tasks and make judgments based on the knowledge and experience acquired over a lifetime. Because young people have less knowledge and experience, they must rely more on fluid intelligence. With advanced age comes an abundance of skills and knowledge that have been acquired over time, so that crystallized intelligence is used more often.

Intelligence is often measured by means of tests. Although intelligence tests are commonly used, they have distinct limitations. Most written tests measure verbal and mathematic ability. Thus a person who has had little formal education can have a high level of cognition and yet score poorly on standardized intelligence tests. Cognition is not the same as education. Cognition is the ability to think and reason. Many people have good cognitive skills but limited education.

Intelligence tests are normally timed. Because different people do not process information at the same speed, two individuals with a similar pool of knowledge and skills may be judged very differently simply because they respond at different speeds. Those with a rapid rate of information processing are typically judged as more intelligent than those who take longer to process information, even if the end result is the same. This is probably reflective of our culture, which values speed.

 QSEN Considerations: Patient-Centered Care

Because we have established that individuals process information at varying speeds, allow time for patients to process the question and then process their answer. When health care providers look impatient or frustrated with the speed of response, many older patients will try to answer faster and thus may fail to provide trustworthy answers. Provide people time to formulate their answers to ensure that their responses reflect what they truly want to say.

COGNITION AND LANGUAGE

Language is a product of cognitive function. In both spoken and written forms, language enables humans to communicate their ideas and thoughts. Language develops early in life. By age 2, the average child has a vocabulary of several hundred words. Very specific areas of the brain are dedicated to language, and they change significantly as language skills improve.

Sensory and cognitive problems can result in poor language development or loss of language skills. Damage to the language centers of the brain can result in aphasia, a condition in which people are unable to understand or express themselves through language.

Aging people commonly experience sensory changes that interfere with the collection of information. Changes in vision and hearing, taste and smell, and touch and sensation all interfere with the ability to collect accurate information from the environment (Fig. 10.2).

Many older people who are considered confused actually perceive their environment inaccurately. An older person who does not hear well (Box 10.1) or see well may walk into traffic or make mistakes about directions; these mistakes are not made because of confusion but rather because the person does not have enough sensory information to make an appropriate decision. Multiple competing stimuli can also cause problems if older adults are unable to focus on the important stimuli and disregard the nonessential stimuli.

Intelligence does not automatically decline with aging, nor does the ability to learn. Some people seem less intelligent as they age because of their tendency to be slower and more cautious in their responses. Rather than be embarrassed, older adults often take more time to be certain of their answers before they respond. This hesitancy or uncertainty may be mistaken for a lack of intelligence, which it is not.

Lack of formal schooling may make some older adults appear to be less intelligent. They may lack polish in their speech and have a more limited vocabulary than better-educated people. Many older adults who grew up in difficult times left school at a young age because they had to work to help support their families. When today's older adults entered the workforce, advanced education was not needed to earn a good living. Many continued to read and learn and often exceeded what formal schooling would have provided. Still, these older adults may be intimidated by young, well-educated caregivers.

The speed of information processing and recall by the brain changes with age. It is common for older adults to take longer to recall a specific piece of information. Short-term memory is more likely to be

affected than is long-term memory. An older person who cannot remember what they had for breakfast may be able to describe in great detail an event that occurred 50 years ago.

Some degree of forgetfulness or memory loss is common with aging. This problem can be disturbing to the alert older adult. Many begin to fear that they are "losing their minds" or developing a serious problem. Careful assessment is needed to distinguish mild memory loss from an early indication of a more serious cognitive disorder.

There is no known reason why memory loss happens, but nearly 13% of those over age 60 surveyed reported memory loss (CDC, 2020b). The more memories a person has developed throughout life, the more they will retain, so well-educated older adults tend to retain a higher level of function than do less well-educated older adults. Even without formal education, many older people are able to compensate for memory gaps by relying more on the large pool of experience gathered over a lifetime.

? Did You Know?

Use It or Lose It

Memories that are not called up from the brain and are used infrequently are more likely to be forgotten over time. *Transience*, the tendency to forget things over time, is actually the brain's way of improving efficiency by clearing unused information and making room for new memories. Unless this becomes extreme or persistent, it is considered a part of normal, healthy brain functioning (Harvard, 2020).

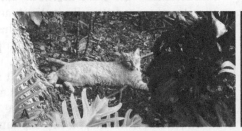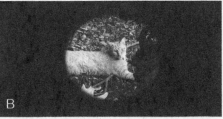

Fig. 10.2 **A,** Normal vision. **B,** Restricted visual field. (From Webb, M., Kostelnick, C., & Scott, K. [2018]. *Long-term caring* [4th ed.]. St. Louis, MO: Elsevier.)

❖ NURSING PROCESS/CLINICAL JUDGMENT MODEL FOR ALTERED SENSORY PERCEPTION

An older person can experience disturbances in any of the senses. The extent of such disturbances can range from very small changes to a total loss of sensory function. The more serious the disturbance, the greater the risks. Different nursing approaches are needed to deal with different types of sensory disturbances.

◆ ASSESSMENT (DATA COLLECTION)

Recognize Cues

- Has the person mentioned any changes in the taste or smell of food?
- Can the person detect whether something is cold or warm? Smooth or rough?
- Do they have known vision problems (e.g., glaucoma, macular degeneration, cataracts, refractive errors)?
- Does the person see small details or shadows?
- Do they frequently walk into or trip over objects?
- Can the person read? If not, why not? If yes, can they read newsprint or only large headlines?
- How close does the person sit to the television?
- Does the person wear eyeglasses? If yes, are they single lens, bifocal, or trifocal?
- When was the last vision examination?
- Does the person respond when people speak to them at a normal volume?
- Can they hear a whisper from someone behind or to the side who cannot be seen?
- Does the person turn the volume of the television or radio up very high?
- Does the person turn their head to hear? Wear a hearing aid?
- Do they respond appropriately or inappropriately to questions?
- Can the person follow directions?

Box 10.2 lists risk factors for problems related to cognition and perception in older adults.

◆ DATA ANALYSIS/PROBLEM IDENTIFICATION

Analyze Cues and Prioritize Hypotheses
Problem statements for older adults with perceptual or cognition alterations include

Altered Sensory Perception
Potential for Injury
Altered Communication Ability

◆ PLANNING

Generate Solutions: The goals for older individuals with altered sensory perception are to (1) remain free from injury, (2) demonstrate improved ability to detect changes in the environment, (3) interact appropriately

---

Box 10.2 Risk Factors Related to Cognition and Perception in Older Adults

- Vision problems (total blindness, presbyopia, macular degeneration, cataracts, hemianopsia, detached retina, diabetes, glaucoma, and significant refractive errors)
- Hearing problems (presbycusis, otosclerosis, and conductive sensorineural hearing loss)
- Dementia (including Alzheimer disease)
- Disturbed cerebral circulation (stroke, aneurysm, and head injury)
- Drugs that affect the sensorium (alcohol, narcotic analgesics, tranquilizers, sedatives, and hypnotics)
- Disturbed neurologic function resulting in decreased levels of consciousness
- Disturbed metabolic states (hypoglycemia and metabolic alkalosis)
- Environments with either inadequate or excessive sensory stimulation

---

with the environment, and (4) demonstrate the ability to compensate for deficits by using prosthetic devices and alternative senses.

◆ IMPLEMENTATION

Take Action: The following nursing interventions should take place in hospitals or extended-care facilities:

1. **Ensure that all caregivers are aware of the person's sensory problems.** The patient's records should identify and prominently display any vision or hearing problems. Inform nursing assistants and ancillary personnel about sensory problems and appropriate methods of communication before assigning them to provide care for an older individual with sensory deficits.

2. **Make appropriate sensory contact before beginning care.** If the older adult is hard of hearing, avoid startling them. Approaches should be made so that the older individual can see the nurse, or the individual should be touched gently on the hand before more personal contact is made (Fig. 10.3). If the older adult is visually impaired, speak up and introduce yourself upon entering the room. This lets the person know who is there, even if they cannot see a face clearly. Also alert the patient when you are leaving so they do not mistakenly continue a conversation after you have left.

3. **Determine the best methods for communicating with older adults.** Be patient and relaxed when working with older adults. When working with older persons whose senses are impaired, keep your messages as simple as possible, use easily understood words, and speak clearly. It may be necessary to reword a statement if the first attempt is not understood. Avoid overloading the older adult with information when you are explaining care or treatments. Use short sentences and provide directions

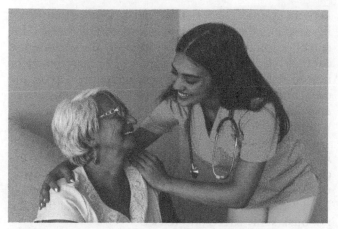

Fig. 10.3 Nurses can use touch and eye contact to enhance a patient's self-esteem. (Copyright © istock.com/dragana991)

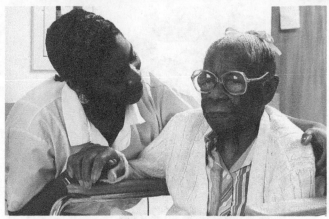

Fig. 10.4 Nurses should approach the patient who has a left sided hemiparesis from the right side. This older woman may not be able to see people to her left. (From Kostelnick, C. [2015]. *Mosby's textbook for long-term care nursing assistants* [7th ed.]. St. Louis, MO: Mosby.)

one step at a time. When writing messages, make sure that the writing is clear and large enough to be easily read.

- When working with hearing-impaired older adults, speak in a low tone of voice, because hearing losses are usually in the higher frequencies of sound. Because many hearing-impaired people compensate by lip reading, it is best to stand in good light while facing the person and to speak slowly but not unnaturally so. Do not chew gum or eat while speaking or allow anything else to cover your mouth (be aware that communication may be even more difficult when one is required to wear a mask). If one of the older person's ears is better than the other, speak into the good ear. Keep background noise from television or radio to a minimum because it may distract an older adult or interfere with verbal communication.

- Facial expressions, gestures, and other visual cues that are appropriate to the message should be used. These cues can help the person understand what the nurse is talking about. For example, if the nurse's intended message is, "Please come with me," hold out your hand and begin to walk. If it is time to groom a person's hair, show the person the brush and comb to help make the message clear. Be aware that your own nonverbal language can set the tone for the task ahead.

- Persons with hearing impairments are not likely to understand messages spoken through the call signal speakers that are used in most care settings. Instead of using the intercom, respond promptly and in person to calls from the sensorially impaired. More information regarding communication with older adults is provided in Chapter 5.

4. **Modify the environment to reduce risks. Lighting is important for older adults.** Stairs and other hazardous areas should be designed to prevent glare because it takes the aging eye longer to adjust to bright light. When an older adult has a condition in which a portion of the visual field is lost (hemianopsia), arrange the furniture to maximize the person's ability to see (Fig. 10.4). Place personal belongings toward the good side, and teach the person to turn their head and "sweep" the environment to pick up more visual cues. Do not move furniture or belongings without informing the patient.

5. **Verify that prostheses such as eyeglasses and hearing aids are functional.** Obtaining the proper corrective lenses is not a one-time requirement. As the eyes continue to change, a prescription that was once adequate may lose its effectiveness. Simply because a person wears eyeglasses does not mean that they can see clearly, particularly if they have had the eyeglasses for some time. Eye examinations should be performed regularly and prescriptions changed whenever required. Many older adults experience multiple refractive errors and require bifocals or trifocals to achieve adequate focus. Such lenses can present problems because the wearers must move their heads to shift the line of vision to the proper section, depending on what they wish to view. Some people find this so disturbing that they choose not to wear the correct prescription. Report these types of problems to the primary care provider so that an acceptable solution can be found.

- Clean eyeglasses regularly. Fingerprints and other debris can distort vision and make the glasses useless. To be of benefit, eyeglasses must also fit the person properly. Many eyeglass frames are too loose and slide down the nose; others are too snug and create uncomfortable pressure areas on the nose or ears. Check that the nose pads are present and have not fallen off. Often, older adults wear eyeglasses with broken frames that are taped together. If the eyeglasses do not help vision or are uncomfortable, older adults are likely to avoid wearing them. Nurses should arrange a consultation with an eye specialist to correct such problems.

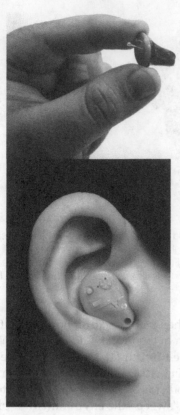

Fig. 10.5 A hearing aid in the ear canal is barely visible. (© iStock Photos.)

Hearing aids are worn by many older people. These devices do not duplicate normal hearing and are not beneficial for everyone. Hearing aids can be built in to eyeglasses or inserted into the ear canal. Some of the older units hang over the external ear; newer models are almost invisible when worn (Fig. 10.5).

Many people have difficulty adjusting to hearing aids and complain that they are bothersome. When first fitted with a hearing aid, the person may be able to tolerate it for only a few minutes a day. As the person adjusts to the device, the amount of time it is worn should be gradually increased. Older people who are adjusting to wearing a hearing aid often report that it makes them nervous or jumpy to hear so many sounds. They should be reassured that this is normal and that the jumpiness will go away as they become used to wearing the hearing aid. Many people who wear hearing aids report that the sounds they hear are "tinny" or "noisy" and that they hear feedback whistles or hums. These noises are usually caused by incorrect insertion or improper adjustment of the controls on the device. Some hearing aids have controls that can be accessed through a cell phone application. If so, ensure that the older adult is aware of how to access and use the app.

Hearing aids require a certain amount of care and maintenance. Because they are fragile, be careful not to drop them. Most are made of plastic and should be kept away from very hot or cold places. Before being inserted into the ear, hearing aids should be checked for cracks or rough edges that could injure the ear, and the ear mold should be cleaned regularly. Pay special attention to the removal of cerumen, which may plug the canal and reduce the effectiveness of the device. Check and clean batteries regularly, because the hearing aid will not work properly without a good power source. To prolong battery life, shut the hearing aid off when it is not in use. Check batteries for corrosion, and clean the contacts, particularly if the device becomes wet. Storing unused batteries in the refrigerator can prolong their life. Discard old batteries after a change so that they are not mistakenly saved and reused.

> ### QSEN Considerations: Patient-Centered Care
>
> Glasses and hearing aids are easy to lose but difficult to replace. Check that the patient has his or her prosthetics with him or her during your normal interactions. Items can be set down on food trays or in the bed sheets and may not be noticed until the patient needs them again. It is much easier to locate missing articles when their absence has been noticed quickly.

Caregivers who are not familiar with hearing aids should receive special training in how to correctly place them in the ear canal. Hearing aids are useless unless they are worn properly. Nurses should always verify that a hearing aid has been applied to the correct ear. If the person wears two aids, they should be marked so that the correct device is placed in the correct ear. If the device still does not function properly, the nurse may need to consult with an audiologist or speech therapist. If the older person is reluctant to wear the hearing aid, do a thorough assessment to determine why this is the case. A thorough reevaluation of the patient's hearing may be necessary.

The following interventions should take place in the home:

1. **Modify the home environment to compensate for sensory changes.** Modifications in the home will help older adults cope with sensory changes. Increasing the amount of light is the least expensive and most beneficial change. Lights should be positioned to avoid glare. Incandescent bulbs are better than fluorescent bulbs because they do not have a distracting flicker. Burned-out bulbs should be replaced promptly. It is even better if light bulbs are replaced when they begin to dim rather than waiting until they burn out.
   - The use of contrasting colors helps older adults see edges and borders. Apply contrasting strips to areas where there is a change in elevation, such as a shower entrance or steps. Contrasting door frames, dishes, pillows, personal care items, and toilet seats will help older adults distinguish these items more easily.

2. **Help people with impaired senses to develop techniques or acquire devices that will help compensate for their losses.**
   - *Hearing-Impaired People.* Nurses should explain ways in which hearing-impaired people can improve communications. This would include (1) telling others that they are hard of hearing, (2) focusing on the speaker and paying attention to what is being said, (3) facing the speaker or asking the speaker to face them, (4) asking the speaker to speak slowly and clearly but not to shout, and (5) asking the speaker to repeat when information is not clear.
   - Many special devices are available for hearing-impaired people. Local telephone companies can provide special equipment, such as amplifiers or video display terminals, which enable older adults to maintain contact with others. Doorbells and mats that flash a light when someone is at the door are available. Alarm clocks that vibrate rather than ring can be purchased from specialty shops or department stores. Hearing-impaired individuals with adequate vision should be made aware of closed-captioned television broadcasts, which provide typed narration of the news and many entertainment programs. Most videos on the internet are also available closed captioned; however, the accuracy of the captioning is variable and can be inaccurate if it is done by a computer. Mobile phones also have voice to text messaging, although the accuracy, again, is variable.
   - *Visually Impaired People.* Large button telephones can assist dialing. Most telephones can be programmed with commonly used numbers so that the person need push only one button to dial. Handheld or floor standing magnifying devices can help with reading or close work. Large print books and magazines can be found in most public libraries; computer settings can be altered for viewing large print. Written materials can be enlarged on photocopy machines to make reading easier. Audiobooks can be found in stores and many libraries. Talking clocks that fit into a pocket are also available.

❖ NURSING PROCESS/CLINICAL JUDGMENT MODEL FOR CHRONIC CONFUSION

Anything that damages or interferes with the normal functioning of the cerebral cortex can result in cognitive problems (i.e., in thinking and judgment). All changes in cognitive function must be given immediate attention. Prompt assessment of the type and severity of the disorder, along with identification of the cause or causes, enables the caregiver to plan the most appropriate interventions for each individual. Cognitive function can be affected by sensory changes, physiologic factors, or emotional disorders. Cognitive problems can range from mild and reversible forms of disorientation to severe and irreversible forms of dementia. Depression, hypothyroidism, and vitamin deficiencies can have symptoms similar to dementia but are actually quite treatable.

Sensory changes can result in behaviors that mimic cognitive problems but actually are not. The two should not be confused. Sensory misperception should be ruled out before further cognitive assessment is performed.

The term *confusion* is used to describe a wide range of behaviors. Both laypeople and professionals use this term far too frequently, often incorrectly and inappropriately. Confusion is defined as a mental state characterized by disorientation regarding time, place, or person that leads to bewilderment, perplexity, lack of orderly thought, and the inability to choose or act decisively and to perform the activities of daily living (ADLs). Patient problem statements that can be identified include Acute Confusion, Chronic Confusion, and Memory Impairment.

Clinical Situation

Cognition and Perception

Imagine that you are an older adult who has been hospitalized for chest pain. You have trouble seeing (you cannot reach your eyeglasses in the drawer) and are hard of hearing (you are wearing your hearing aid, but the batteries do not work). The medication you took has made you a little lightheaded, and your bladder seems to fill every 30 minutes. You activate the call light to go to the bathroom, but no one comes and you feel desperate. You attempt to get up, but the rails are in your way and you fall. Before anyone comes to help, you can wait no longer and void on the floor. By the time someone gets there, you are frightened and angry. You yell and slap the person. The next thing you know you are restrained in bed and a tube has been put in your bladder. If you could read the nurse's note, you would see this statement: "Confused, agitated, and combative. Protective device applied. Catheter inserted for incontinence." Realize that fear, anger, and anxiety have very real causes. How could this situation have been avoided?

Acute confusion, often called *delirium*, is characterized by disturbances in cognition, attention, memory, and perception. This type of confusion is usually caused by a physiologic process that affects the autonomic nervous system. Conditions that can cause delirium include uncontrolled pain, infection, metabolic disturbances, vitamin deficiencies, uremia, hypoxia, hypercalcemia, endocrine imbalance, myocardial infarction, constipation, drug toxicity, and drug withdrawal.

A mnemonic useful for focusing an assessment can be found in Table 10.1.

Acute delirium has a sudden onset of hours to days. It is characterized by rapid mood swings, disorganized sleep cycles, changes in psychomotor activity (hypoactivity, hyperactivity, or both), tremors or spasmodic activity, rapid speech patterns, loss of attention, and a

Table 10.1   Mnemonic Assessment for DELIRIUM

COMPONENT	CONSIDERATIONS
Drug use	Any recent change in medications, increase or decrease in dosage, change from specific brand to a generic. Pay special attention to sedative-hypnotics (including alcohol), antidepressants, opioids, antipsychotics, anticholinergics, anticonvulsants, antiparkinson medications, and H_2 blocking medications
Electrolyte imbalance	Abnormal levels of calcium, sodium, or magnesium often related to malnutrition or dehydration
Lack of drugs	Missed medication doses
Infection	Check for urinary tract infection (UTI), signs of inflammation, respiratory congestion, etc., remembering that the signs may be subtle in the older adult
Reduced sensory input	Visual or hearing impairment, failure to use glasses or hearing aids, social isolation
Intracranial problems	Recent head injury, history of stroke, meningitis, history of seizure
Urinary retention and/or fecal impaction	Recent anesthesia, history of benign prostatic hyperplasia, recent catheter removal
Myocardial problems	Anginal symptoms, abnormal electrocardiogram (ECG), recent cardiac surgery

wide range of cognitive changes (Tables 10.2 and 10.3). Older individuals with underlying emotional instability can exhibit a full-blown psychotic episode with delusions and auditory or visual hallucinations. The severity of symptoms may vary throughout the day, and symptoms are often worse at night. Because the cause of delirium is usually physiologic, acute confusion does not respond well to behavioral approaches, such as reorientation. Once the cause has been identified and treated, the symptoms generally disappear. Failure to identify and correct underlying physiologic problems can lead to serious physical harm or even death.

 QSEN Considerations: Patient-Centered Care

Establish a baseline, and assess any change of condition. If the family expresses concern over a sudden change in behavior, listen and look further. Even though delirium has a sudden onset, some health care providers have mistaken signs and symptoms of delirium for normal aging. The incidence of delirium in surgical populations ranges from 11% to 51%. On medical floors, delirium occurs in 18% to 40% of elderly patients (Menzenbach, 2019).

Table 10.2   Differences Between Delirium and Dementia

DELIRIUM	DEMENTIA
Rapid onset: over hours to days	Slower onset: over months to years
Reduced level of consciousness	No change in level of consciousness (initially)
Variable course over 24 hours	Stable over 24 hours
Increased or decreased psychomotor activity	Impaired memory with loss of abstract thinking, judgment, language skills (aphasia), motor skills (apraxia), and ability to recognize familiar people or objects (agnosia)
Disturbed sleep/wake patterns	
Disorientation and perceptual disturbances, possible visual and auditory hallucinations	
Memory impairment	
Decreased attention span with disorganized thinking	
In general, reversible if underlying problem is identified and treated; may recur with acute illness	In general, not reversible

Table 10.3   Nursing Interventions for Delirium and Dementia

DELIRIUM	DEMENTIA
Designed to treat underlying pathologic condition and maintain physiologic integrity	Designed to maintain or maximize level of function
Includes administration of fluids, nutrition, oxygen, antianxiety medications, and so on	Administration of medications (cholinesterase inhibitors), also making sure that intake of fluids and food is maintained
Designed to control environmental stressors, protect safety, and promote comfort	Includes environment modification, activity-based therapies, and communication strategies

Confusion can sometimes be idiopathic, or due to an unknown cause. Idiopathic confusion does not have an identifiable physiologic basis. It is most likely to occur when a person experiences a stressful disturbance in lifestyle or life patterns, such as following the death of a loved one, depression, or relocation to a hospital or new living quarters. The onset of symptoms is likely to correlate to specific occurrences or situations, although that is not always the case. The assessment of cognitive changes should always consider any recent life changes, including the loss of a loved one, a change in living situation, or financial concerns. Idiopathic confusion tends to affect memory and concentration. Affected older adults are often depressed. Common symptoms of idiopathic confusion include changes in appetite, loss of interest in activities, changes in sleep patterns, agitation, feelings of worthlessness or guilt, fatigue, or other physiologic complaints. The ability to perform routine ADLs is not usually affected, but the willingness to perform these activities might be. Individuals experiencing this form of confusion usually respond well to reorientation interventions and approaches that reduce stress levels. Symptoms may be reversible, but they may not disappear completely.

Dementia is a slow, insidious process that results in the progressive loss of cognitive function. It is caused by damage to the cerebral cortex, which is most commonly a result of disease conditions such as multiple infarcts of the cerebrum secondary to stroke or other pathologic conditions of the brain (Box 10.3). Drug intoxication, Huntington disease, Creutzfeldt-Jakob disease, Pick disease, cerebral hypoxia, hyperthyroidism, subdural hematoma, and brain tumors are less common causes. Dementia is not inevitable with advancing age. According to the CDC as many as 40% of cases of dementia can potentially be prevented or delayed (CDC, 2020a). There is strong evidence linking dementia with the long-term use of anticholinergic medications (e.g., diphenhydramine), which are consumed by 10% to 27% of older people (Gray et al., 2018). Dementia is characterized by changes in memory, judgment, language, mathematical calculation, abstract reasoning, and problem-solving ability; it is also marked by impulsive behavior, stupor, confusion, and disorientation. Changes related to dementia are progressive and irreversible. In the early stages, many cases of dementia are mistakenly seen as due to normal aging—a mistake that can lead to delayed diagnosis and treatment. Subjective cognitive decline (SCD) is one potential sign of a future diagnosis of a memory disorder. Individuals with SCD report changes to their memory or cognitive function, but when they are assessed, all tests turn out to be within the normal range (Budson, 2019). Many older adults who suffer from the early stages of dementia are able to recognize that something is wrong, but they do not know what it is. Some may be creative in the types of excuses they use to explain their problems. Friends and neighbors may fail to notice the difference

---

Box 10.3	Types of Dementia

Alzheimer disease
Vascular dementia
Dementia with Lewy bodies (DLB)
Mixed dementia
Frontotemporal lobar degeneration (FTLD)
Parkinson disease (PD)
Creutzfeldt-Jakob disease
Normal pressure hydrocephalus

From Alzheimer's Association (2018). *Alzheimer's disease facts and figures.* https://www.alz.org/media/HomeOffice/Facts%20and%20Figures/facts-and-figures.pdf/

---

because those who are affected retain their ability to engage in "small talk" or friendly chatter. In the later stages, however, their impaired cognitive function is dramatic and obvious, even to a casual observer.

Common behaviors seen with advanced dementia include wandering, excessively emotional reactions (**catastrophic reactions**), combative behaviors, suspiciousness, and hallucinations or delusions. When these agitated behaviors become worse late in the day and into the evening, they are referred to as *sundown syndrome* or *sundowning*. Affected persons often do not recognize even their closest family members and friends. These abnormal behaviors are frightening to the family as well as to anyone who cares about the affected individual.

QSEN Considerations: Patient-Centered Care

Why do patients with dementia exhibit combative behaviors and suspiciousness? Think about how you would respond if someone told you that you did something that you have no memory of (such as eating breakfast) or tried to get you do something you remember already having done (such as bathing)? Patients with dementia live in a different reality because of their lack of short-term memory. This contributes to the patient's conviction that he or she is being lied to, making them feel unsafe. Providing reassurance and avoiding arguments about what has or has not been done will make the care go much more smoothly for both the patient and the nurse.

People with dementia have increased potential for injury and personal neglect. They are unable to recognize or understand hazards in the environment. Inability for self-care in the areas of eating, bathing, grooming, and toileting are common.

In the early stages of dementia, the family may be able to provide adequate care at home. With advanced stages, full-time supervision and total physical care are often required. Dementia is likely to lead to institutional placement.

Dementia affects up to 10% of adults older than age 65 who live in the community. Approximately 5.8 million older Americans have Alzheimer disease (Box 10.4), the most common type of dementia. The incidence of dementia in those age 85 or older is estimated

Box 10.4 Facts About Alzheimer Disease

- Alzheimer disease is not a normal part of aging. It is a progressive, degenerative, irreversible disease, the last stage consisting of dementia.
- The disease was first identified in 1906 by Alois Alzheimer, a German neurologist.
- Most cases of Alzheimer disease occur in people older than 65 years of age, but it can occur as early as age 30.
- Alzheimer disease affects both men and women of all religions, races, and socioeconomic backgrounds.
- The cause of the disease remains unknown, but genetic, chemical, viral, and environmental factors are suspected. Family history and the presence of the apolipoprotein E gene appear to indicate an increased risk for development of the disease.
- Alzheimer disease causes gradual changes, such as beta-amyloid plaques outside of neurons and tau tangles inside the nerve cells of the brain; these can be detected by diagnostic imaging studies and the examination of blood or cerebrospinal fluid.
- Neurologic changes result in a loss of the ability to process information normally.
- The first signs of Alzheimer disease are subtle changes in behavior. The disease affects each individual differently;

the type and severity of symptoms, as well as the order of their appearance, differ from person to person.
- People suffering from Alzheimer disease gradually lose the ability to think, remember, understand, and make decisions. Consequently they are often unable to perform even the most basic ADLs. The ability to control basic bodily functions, such as elimination, is also lost.
- People with Alzheimer disease undergo personality changes. They lose the ability to control their moods and emotions, leading to unpredictable and often inappropriate behavior. Unusual behaviors include wandering, pacing, hiding things, swearing, disturbed sleep patterns, and repetitive actions.
- There is no known cure for Alzheimer disease. A variety of medications are being tested for use with this disease. The increasing use of biologic markers ("biomarkers"), such as beta-amyloid plaques and tau tangles, to diagnose and hopefully monitor Alzheimer disease gives promise of the development of better treatments for the disease.
- Recent research suggests that life stressors and sleep disturbances may play a role as risk factors for Alzheimer disease; a single life stressor can increase one's chance of developing Alzheimer disease, especially in minority populations (Charvat, 2020).

as high as 50%. Alzheimer disease is currently the sixth leading cause of death in the United States. The stages of Alzheimer disease are listed in Box 10.5.

 Critical Thinking

Dementia

What amount of personal connection have you had with a person who has Alzheimer disease or another form of dementia? If possible, identify one specific individual whom you can recall well.

- In what context did you interact with this person (home, hospital, extended care)?
- How much continuous time did you spend with this person?
- What behaviors did you observe?
- How did you respond to these behaviors?
- Did you find interacting with this person to be stressful? Describe.

Now imagine being a spouse or child caring for this individual in a home setting.

- How do you think this person's experiences differ from yours?
- What types of stressors do you think the person experiences?
- What could you suggest to help this person cope?
- What support services are available in your community?

Box 10.5 Stages of Alzheimer Disease

PRECLINICAL ALZHEIMER DISEASE
- Measurable biologic changes (in the brain's beta-amyloid plaque); specific biomarkers (such as the APOE gene) may include brain imaging and the examination of protein in spinal fluid
- No obvious symptoms of memory loss or confusion
- Occurs years to perhaps decades before the next stage

MILD COGNITIVE IMPAIRMENT CAUSED BY ALZHEIMER DISEASE
- Mild changes in memory, reasoning, and visual perception
- Noticeable to the person affected, friends, and family
- Person remains capable of carrying out everyday activities

DEMENTIA CAUSED BY ALZHEIMER DISEASE
- Memory impairment
- Behavioral symptoms
- Impaired ability to function in daily life

APOE, apolipoprotein E. From Williams, P. A. (2022). Common psychosocial care problems of the elderly. In *Fundamental concepts and skills for nursing* (6th ed.). St. Louis, MO: Elsevier Science.

- Does the person have difficulty remembering recent or remote events?
- Can the person grasp new ideas, or do they have difficulty with this?
- Can the person make appropriate informed decisions?
- Do they find it difficult to learn new things?
- What helps the person to learn new things?
- What is the person's dominant language?
- Do they speak other languages?

◆ ASSESSMENT (DATA COLLECTION)

Recognize cues
- Does the person mention any changes in memory?
- Do the family or significant others notice memory changes?

- What is the person's language/vocabulary level? Educational level?
- How long is the person's attention span?
- Are there significant behavior changes, including hyperactivity (agitation, excitability, distractibility) or hypoactivity (lethargy, apathy, somnolence)?
- Is the person restless, uncooperative, belligerent, angry, withdrawn, or threatening?
- Have they experienced delusions or hallucinations?
- Are there particular times of day when the person's behavior is most noticeably different?
- Do they have a history of stroke or other brain disease?
- Have there been any recent changes in the person's medication or dosage?
- Are there any signs of infection (urinary tract infection, pneumonia)?
- What is the level of hydration?
- Is the person constipated?
- What is the person's oxygen saturation?
- What are the results of the Mini-Cog? (See Chapter 8 for more details about this tool.)

◆ DATA ANALYSIS/PROBLEM IDENTIFICATION

Analyze Cues and Prioritize Hypotheses

Problem statement for older adults with impairment in cognition or perception include
Chronic Confusion

◆ PLANNING

Generate Solutions: The goals for older individuals with chronic confusion are to (1) remain free from injury, (2) assist in the ADLs to the highest degree possible, and (3) seek assistance when needed.

◆ IMPLEMENTATION

Take Action: The following nursing interventions should take place in hospitals or extended-care facilities.

1. **Assess behavior on admission and at regular intervals.** Correct identification of the type of cognitive loss is important so that appropriate medical and nursing interventions can be planned and implemented. If a sudden change in behavior is observed in a person who has had normal cognition, it is usually a physiologic problem that can be diagnosed and treated, not chronic confusion. However, for persons who already have a history of cognitive changes, it is more difficult to identify these changes. Progression from mild acute confusion to chronic confusion can occur but may be missed unless caregivers pay close attention to subtle changes in behavior.

2. **Provide assistive sensory devices.** Confusion is worse when there is inadequate or inaccurate sensory input. Nurses must ensure that older individuals wear eyeglasses, hearing aids, dentures, and other adaptive devices designed to maximize sensory perception when necessary and make sure that they are working.

3. **Orient the person to person, place, and time and provide any other important situational information, but do not force the issue, because it can lead to agitation.** Address the person by the name they respond to best. This may be their first name. Refer to calendars and clocks to provide information regarding the day, week, and month. Calendars can be used to point out important events, such as birthdays, holidays, and special activities. Remind the person of daily events; explain procedures before they happen. If the person becomes combative, do not argue. Instead, focus on the feelings that they exhibit by using reflective statements such as, "I know that this isn't what you want to do right now, but it's dinnertime and the food is here." Realize that the person may not remember events from earlier in the day because short-term memory is affected first. Be patient when you have to repeat directions or explanations over and over again. Remember that their reality (without the memories of the day) is markedly different from yours.

4. **Provide a structured environment that ensures safety yet enables the person to remain active as long as possible.** Provide an environment free from hazards that could lead to falls. Individuals who get up frequently might benefit from wearing shoes even in bed so that they have better balance and footing when they get up.

◾ Complementary Health Approaches

Light Therapy

Studies have shown that bright light therapy, also known as *phototherapy*, may improve the length of sleep and decrease some of the agitated behaviors commonly associated with sundown syndrome. In this therapy, the patient sits or works near a light therapy box, and bright light indirectly enters the patient's eyes. It is important that the patient not look directly into the therapy box, as directly looking into the light can be damaging. The therapy is prescribed for a specific length of time, from 15 minutes to 2 hours long, depending on the intensity of the light.

- Some people suffering from dementia become less active; others demonstrate pacing or other repetitive movements. To maintain strength and joint mobility, encourage inactive persons to perform some physical activity that they enjoy every day. Identify specific activities and structure time into the care plan. Activity, occupational, and physical therapists

---

Box 10.6   General Approaches for Working With Confused Older Adults

- Provide a calm, safe, and structured environment with a limited number of stimuli.
- Use a calm, gentle, one-on-one approach.
- Speak normally and informally as though the person were not confused.
- Allow plenty of time; avoid hurrying.
- Determine the confused person's reality; avoid confrontation or forced reorientation.
- Encourage reminiscence using family pictures, common activities, or objects.
- Provide familiar clothing and personal items from home.
- Redirect the person's attention or use some other form of distraction to reduce anxiety resulting from disturbing thoughts.
- Provide safe, repetitive activities within individual capabilities (e.g., winding yarn and folding towels).
- Provide continuity of care with a limited group of caregivers.
- Develop and maintain daily routines for care and activities.
- Avoid sudden changes in routine, room, or caregivers.

---

can help to develop a plan that will meet the individual's needs (Box 10.6).

- Allow individuals who pace to do so freely. Encourage people who pace to take rest periods during the day so that they do not exhaust themselves.
- People who wander may need to be housed on a care unit with controlled exits that activate alarms when anyone passes through the door. Staff can also monitor wandering by using an electronic bracelet that sounds an alarm when the wearer tries to leave the unit or building. In home or hospital settings where these controls are not practical, bed or chair alarms (weight sensitive pads that activate an alarm when the person is off the pad) can be used to notify nurses that the person has gotten out of a bed or chair. Adequate lighting is important to reduce the likelihood of falls and the fear induced by the misperception of shadows.

5. **Provide continuity.** Too many new faces or changes are frightening and disturbing to confused older adults. Whenever possible, assign care to a consistent group of caregivers who can develop a trusting relationship. The older adult should have access to familiar personal belongings such as pictures or a blanket or purse. These can provide comfort and help the person to keep some contact with reality.

6. **Administer psychotherapeutic medications as ordered.** A few medications are available to aid in the treatment of cognitive disorders such as Alzheimer disease. These do not cure or reverse existing cognitive loss but are often beneficial in improving memory, alertness, and social engagement. The five

medications approved to treat Alzheimer disease are donepezil, galantamine, memantine, rivastigmine, and combination donepezil/memantine.

7. **Avoid the use of protective devices and chemical restraints.** Keeping confused persons restrained in beds or chairs tends to increase their level of confusion. Using protective devices and chemical restraints can be harmful and can actually make the behavior worse. Protective devices are a form of imprisonment, and using them without a valid medical reason can be grounds for legal action. These devices were traditionally used to protect people from falls or other injury. Too often, however, they were used so that nursing staff would not have to take time to adequately meet the older person's needs. Rather than protecting older adults, protective devices can cause harm and lead to physical deterioration. If the person does tend to fall, it may be more appropriate to keep the bed in a low position or to place a mattress on the floor next to the bed to reduce the potential for injury.

Complementary Health Approaches

Music Therapy

Music therapy has been shown to be a beneficial tool in working with cognitively impaired older adults, including those suffering from dementia. It is hypothesized that musical stimuli activate the creative right side of the brain, which, in turn, facilitates the entry of information to the logical left side of the brain, thus enhancing cognitive function. Following are some behavioral responses to music:

- Improved mood
- Decreased depression
- Muscle relaxation
- Diminished fear and apprehension
- Improved physical movement during therapy

- Current Omnibus Budget Reconciliation Act legislation recognizes the problems involved with restraint and restricts the use of chemical restraints to specific situations. It is inappropriate to treat nonaggressive behavior with psychotropic medication. Nonaggressive individuals are more likely to respond to alternative therapies, such as music, dance, exercise, art, or other forms of activity therapy (see Complementary Health Approaches box, earlier). Verbal agitation is not typically responsive to medication. In 2008, the U.S. Food and Drug Administration ordered that a "black box" warning (the strongest advisory short of pulling a medication off the market) be placed on all antipsychotic medications when used with dementia-related psychosis because they have been associated with an increased risk of death (Rubino, 2020). Even the newer atypical antipsychotic medications, such as risperidone, have an increased risk of death and carry a black box warning for cardiovascular events. Older patients are also particularly susceptible to medication side effects, which in the case of antipsychotics increase the risk of falls, sleeplessness, and confusion (ALZ, 2021). The Centers for Medicare & Medicaid Services (CMS) established a national partnership aimed at improving dementia care in nursing homes, with an initial focus on reducing the use of antipsychotic medications. Although this partnership has been very successful, it is trying to reduce the rate further. Its larger mission is to "enhance the use of nonpharmacologic approaches and person-centered dementia care practices" (CMS, 2020). If an antipsychotic is administered, the patient must be monitored closely, and the medications should be administered at the lowest dose and for the shortest possible time.

8. **Structure participation in ADLs.** If affected people are able to perform any of their own physical care, encourage them to do so, particularly in the early stages of dementia. This helps to maintain their physical strength and range of motion and promotes self-esteem among those who are aware that they are losing functional ability. Keep routines simple. Individualize the care plan for each person and have all caregivers follow it consistently. Provide simple step-by-step directions. Keep choices to a minimum, because they tend to increase anxiety and agitation (Fig. 10.6). Keep clothing simple; modify clothing to make dressing and undressing easy, thereby reducing frustration. Clothes with elastic waistbands or Velcro can eliminate the frustration of trying to get a zipper up or down. Hair should be styled so that its care is quick and easy. Shorter styles make shampooing and grooming easier and less time consuming. Keep mealtimes as pleasant as possible. Finger foods are more easily managed than foods that require the use of silverware. Serve soup or beverages in cups with handles, as these are easier to control. To prevent burns, pay careful attention to the temperature of hot beverages or soups. Prepare trays

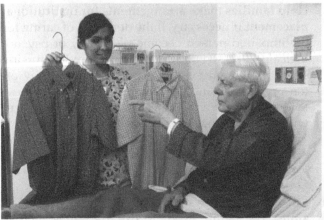

Fig. 10.6 The nurse offers simple clothing choices to the patient. (From Kostelnick, C. [2015]. *Mosby's textbook for long-term care nursing assistants* [7th ed.]. St. Louis, MO: Mosby.)

before serving to minimize delay and frustration. Cut meat into easily digested pieces because the person may forget to chew before swallowing. Reminders to swallow are necessary in some cases. Toileting schedules can help reduce episodes of incontinence. Many confused older adults become increasingly agitated when they need to eliminate, even if they do not recognize the sensation.

9. **Structure the environment to minimize disruption; avoid sudden changes of room or environment.** Frequent change of staff, large numbers of strange people, excessive noise, and excessive amounts of activity can be overly stimulating to those who suffer from dementia; therefore they should be kept to a minimum. Sudden changes of room or even rearrangement of the furniture and belongings can increase confusion, apprehension, and agitation. Whenever possible, avoid room changes. If it is necessary, the new room should be as similar to the old one as possible. Do not move personal effects unless necessary for safety.

10. **Develop a plan to deal with "acting out" behaviors.** Excessive stimulation and stress are likely to trigger catastrophic reactions or delusional behavior. Having to make decisions and respond to questions is stressful to those suffering from dementia; such pressures should be avoided if possible. Certain actions implemented by the nurses will help the person to regain control. Distractions, such as taking a walk or having a cup of tea, can serve to divert the person's attention. If this does not work, it may be necessary to take the person to their room or a quiet place free from the stimuli that caused the upset. Simple touch and reassurance, even sitting quietly with the person, may be enough to reestablish control.

QSEN Considerations: Safety

Keep Calm and Carry On

It is essential to remain calm when confused individuals act out. It is not easy for nurses to deal with repeated irritating or hostile behaviors, but it is important to remember that anger, arguments, and explanations only confuse the person and make the situation worse. Even if nurses do not say anything negative to the person, their body language may communicate a lack of acceptance. Frustration can be perceived by older persons despite their confusion. There are times when the patient may appear frustrated even when the nurse is doing their best to project acceptance. If the situation seems to be escalating, it may be best to switch staff to maintain effective care and give the nurse time away from the situation. Every care provider needs to understand their own limits and use the health care team to ensure that the patient receives proper supportive care.

11. **Use effective communication skills to can promote positive interactions with confused older adults.** Smiles, eye contact, and gentle touch should be used. Express genuine interest and warmth and

listen to the confused person, even if the words do not make sense. Allow the person adequate time to express their feelings. When giving information, keep the messages short and simple, using words that are familiar to the person, and speak in a calm, natural tone of voice.

12. **Consult with family and the multidisciplinary team.** The family may be able to provide valuable information regarding the older person's likes, dislikes, routines, and fears. When they have been providing care in the home, families may also be able to provide suggestions for approaches that have worked in the past. The care of confused older adults requires cooperation and coordination between various departments so that continuity can be maintained. Regular "staffings" that include all relevant departments and disciplines provide an opportunity to review the person's current status and revise the plan of care.

QSEN Considerations: Patient-Centered Care

How do you rinse your mouth after you brush your teeth? Do you use a cup? Do you use your hands? Do you just rinse your mouth with the wet toothbrush? Now think about your patients with dementia. Find out how they have completed their ADLs in the past. Drawing on past skills that use familiar steps can reduce a patient's agitation.

The following interventions should take place in the home:

1. **Help the family accept the diagnosis.** The diagnosis of dementia is difficult for loved ones to accept. They must be given opportunities to verbalize concerns and express feelings of anger, frustration, or helplessness. Along with concerns regarding the changes to daily life is the reality that these people are experiencing a loss. Their loved one is different and is becoming someone they do not recognize—someone who will soon not recognize them. Although their loved one has not died, the emotions are very similar, and grieving for the loss of the relationship as they had known it is normal.

2. **Help the family adjust to the demands of providing care for a cognitively impaired older person.** People with severely altered thought processes cannot be left alone. It is challenging to devise a plan that enables families to supervise impaired older adults while also allowing them to continue with their own lives. Nurses can do several things to help families cope with this situation. They can explain and demonstrate the types of behaviors, actions, and communication techniques that are likely to be effective. They can help families modify the home environment to provide optimal safety yet maintain some semblance of a normal home. Nurses can also recommend books and pamphlets that provide families more detailed and specific information. Several

good books on the care of patients with Alzheimer disease are widely available. The Alzheimer's Association has a variety of training resources and information on their website.

 Community Considerations

Silver Alert

Many states have recently enacted "Silver Alert" programs whereby local police have the authority to request the state highway patrol to send out electronic bulletins to the public, news media, and broader law enforcement when an older adult, usually with Alzheimer disease or another dementia, is reported missing and believed to be in danger. More than 35 states have enacted Silver Alert or similar programs, leading to the safe return of many older adults to their homes.

3. **Provide emotional support and help the family to identify coping strategies.** Coping with the day-to-day responsibilities of caring for a cognitively impaired older person is highly stressful. Regular visits to assess how the family is coping as well as time spent listening to their concerns can help family members to deal with their fears and anxieties. Family members may be part of the "sandwich generation," where they are also taking care of children—a situation that is stressful in itself. When dementia is added to the equation, the stress can be even more overwhelming.

4. **Identify community resources.** Support groups for the families of Alzheimer disease or other dementia sufferers are available in many communities. Nurses should keep abreast of support groups that exist in each community so that they can supply this information to concerned family members. Nurses should encourage family members to participate in these groups. Respite care programs are also available in many communities. These programs provide supervised care for a few hours and even for days at a time, so that the family members can spend time doing things they need or want to do without worrying about care responsibilities.

5. **Help families make arrangements for institutional placement if necessary.** If the demands of caring for the impaired person become physically or psychologically excessive for the spouse or family, nursing home placement may be necessary. The family often needs assistance in making contact with these facilities or with a social worker who can help them with the planning. In addition, nurses should provide emotional support to the family. The decision to move a loved one to a long-term care facility is exceedingly stressful, and the family is likely to experience feelings of helplessness or guilt.

6. **Encourage families to plan for end-of-life decisions.** The family needs to discuss issues such as implementing a guardianship or choosing a health care decision maker. They should be encouraged to

seek advice from the primary caregiver and a lawyer before severe mental deterioration occurs. In some cases, a hospice referral is appropriate and can provide valuable care for the physical needs of a patient with Alzheimer disease.

7. **Use any appropriate interventions that are used in the institutional setting** (Nursing Care Plan 10.1).

❖ NURSING PROCESS/CLINICAL JUDGMENT MODEL FOR ALTERED COMMUNICATION ABILITY

The ability to communicate by using words or language is a uniquely human skill. It is so much a part of our daily lives that we do not even consider the possibility of losing it. Yet many people are forced to live without the ability to speak or communicate through words. Individuals who experience cognitive or sensory changes commonly lose the ability to use words to communicate effectively.

Speech is the term used to refer to spoken language. Speech requires coordinated functioning of the brain, cranial nerves, pharynx, larynx, and lungs. The normal physiologic changes of aging affect the quality of speech. Normal speech in older adults tends to be slower, softer, less fluent, less rhythmic, and breathier than it is in younger individuals, and it often has a tremulous quality. Patients who suffer from neurologic damage affecting muscle control may experience more than the usual difficulty with speech articulation, a condition called *dysarthria*. Speech is only a part of language.

Language is a broad term that includes all modes of spoken or symbolic communication. Language allows us to send and receive messages from other humans. We use language to convey our ideas and make our wishes known to others. Without the ability to communicate, we are isolated from the world around us. People who lose the ability to use language or speak are likely to experience problems. Older adults with

---

 Nursing Care Plan 10.1 | Chronic Confusion

Mr. Quick has a history of neurocognitive disorder. He is not oriented to person, place, time, or situation. He often cannot remember whether he has eaten or what he should be doing at any given time. His behaviors are sometimes socially inappropriate; for example, he wanders into rooms and takes the belongings of other residents. He has a very short attention span and is unable to follow most directions. He likes to wander the halls and often laughs to himself. He sometimes sits in the dayroom if the radio is playing and taps his foot to the music.

PROBLEM STATEMENT
Chronic Confusion

SUPPORTING ASSESSMENT DATA
- Long-standing cognitive impairment
- Altered response to stimuli
- Altered personality
- Altered interpretation
- Impaired memory
- Impaired socialization

PATIENT GOALS/OUTCOMES IDENTIFICATION
Mr. Quick will sustain no harm.

NURSING INTERVENTIONS/IMPLEMENTATION
1. Address Mr. Quick by name.
2. Make eye contact before attempting to communicate.
3. Use pictures and familiar objects to orient him to his own room. Place a recognizable picture or other device at the door.
4. Provide a simple calendar or clock to help orient him to time.
5. Use simple language and short sentences.
6. Use concrete objects or other visual cues to explain things.
7. Allow adequate time for social interaction and communication.
8. Encourage participation in music therapy sessions.
9. Assess for changes in mental processes.
10. Notify primary care provider of significant changes in mental status.

EVALUATION
Mr. Quick is still not oriented to person, place, time, or situation. He continues to wander the halls when not distracted. He will sit still to fold and unfold towels or other repetitive tasks. He sings and claps along during music therapy sessions. You will continue the plan of care.

APPLYING CLINICAL JUDGMENT
1. What other activities can you identify that would be appropriate for Mr. Quick?
2. What safety precautions will be needed if he continues to wander in the halls?

altered communication ability often become depressed, agitated, and frustrated; they feel excluded from normal social interactions.

Language is a complex and not completely understood function of the brain. Both hemispheres of the cerebral cortex contribute to the process of encoding and decoding language, but two particular regions of the brain play key roles in language and speech: the Broca area, which is located in the posterior frontal lobe, and the Wernicke area, which is located in the posterior temporal lobe. If either of these areas is damaged by trauma or oxygen deprivation for prolonged periods of time due to occlusion or hemorrhage, serious language problems can arise. The most common language problem seen in older adults is called *aphasia* (or *dysphasia*).

Dysphasia should not be confused with dysphagia, which is difficulty in swallowing. Stroke or head trauma can cause both problems. Speech pathologists are an excellent resource for information about speech problems and swallowing disorders.

Aphasia has been classified in several different ways. The most common classification includes receptive aphasia, in which the person has difficulty understanding language; expressive aphasia, in which the person is unable to communicate by using language; and global aphasia, in which the person loses the ability both to understand language and to communicate using language. Each of these categories has several subclassifications.

Receptive aphasia is not the same as deafness. Communication problems in deaf people are caused by mechanical or neurologic defects that do not allow sounds to reach the nervous system. People suffering from receptive aphasia hear sounds normally but are unable to give them meaning. In some cases, this loss is complete; in others, only reception of a specific language is lost. Some people cannot understand spoken words but can understand written words. Others can repeat the spoken words but cannot give any meaning to them. Still others can understand single words but not sentences or word combinations.

Like receptive aphasia, expressive aphasia comes in more than one form. Broca aphasia is a common form in which the person is able to understand verbal and written language but unable to speak words fluently. The area of the brain that coordinates the muscles of speech is damaged. This form of aphasia is particularly frustrating because the person knows what they want to say but cannot get the words out. In Wernicke aphasia, the person is able to speak, but the words produced may be nonsensical or have little connection with reality (Table 10.4).

The term *global aphasia* is used when receptive and expressive language skills are lost. People suffering from global aphasia are profoundly affected. If any communication ability remains, it is in the form of a single sound that may be repeated with variations in pitch, rhythm, and emphasis.

Table 10.4 Comparison of Common Types of Aphasia

BROCA APHASIA	WERNICKE APHASIA
Lesion in frontal lobe	Lesion in temporal lobe
Expressive or motor	Receptive or sensory
Speech is slow, labored, hesitant, nonfluent, poorly articulated	Speech is rapid, fluent, normal in tone, clearly articulated, and long and rambling
Short sentences with little grammatical structure	May follow stereotyped patterns
Nonsense or jargon speech indicating noncomprehension	

When an older person loses the ability to talk with others, they find it difficult or impossible to maintain their normal roles and relationships. Even those who fully retain their intellectual function and understanding are viewed differently if they cannot speak clearly. Once the ability to communicate has been damaged, these older people find that they are no longer treated as capable, competent adults but are instead treated as though they were deaf or mentally impaired. Friends, family, and even health care professionals become increasingly likely to avoid such people. This avoidance is rarely deliberate; it occurs out of anxiety or ignorance. This sort of avoidance increases the affected person's feelings of frustration, depression, social isolation, and worthlessness.

QSEN Considerations: Patient-Centered Care

Working with patients with altered communication ability requires the nurse to develop advanced assessment skills. Frustration and anger can be a form of communication when words are not available. When noncommunicative patients show a behavioral change, first assess what could be problematic. Are they in pain? Are they feeling depressed? Are they unable to express something that is important to them? Think of your own frustration when you feel misunderstood. Does it affect the way you act?

◆ ASSESSMENT (DATA COLLECTION)

Recognize Cues

- Does the person have any sensory limitations? (See the assessment of altered sensory perception on page 194.)
- Has the person experienced any injury or surgery that altered the normal speech mechanisms?
- Do they have a history of stroke or cerebrovascular disease?

◆ DATA ANALYSIS/PROBLEM IDENTIFICATION

Analyze Cues and Prioritize Hypotheses

Problem statements for older adults with communication difficulties include

Altered Communication Ability

◆ **PLANNING**

The patient goals for older individuals with altered communication ability are to (1) communicate needs with minimal frustration, (2) demonstrate an increased ability to communicate needs and feelings, and (3) express satisfaction with or acceptance of alternative methods of communication.

◆ **IMPLEMENTATION**

Take Action: The following interventions should take place in hospitals, in extended-care facilities, and at home:

1. **Assess the older adult's communication abilities and difficulties.** Communication problems and abilities differ from person to person. It is important to understand the specific challenges and capabilities of each older adult so that the plan of care can be individualized to best meet the individual's needs.

2. **Identify specific approaches that are effective for each person.** Many techniques can facilitate communication; try a variety of these to determine which are most effective. In working with an older adult with altered communication ability, use the following approaches: (1) face the person when speaking, and establish eye contact; (2) speak slowly and clearly, in a low tone of voice; (3) speak in a normal way and avoid shouting; (4) allow adequate time for communication (do not hurry it); (5) pace communication to avoid fatigue; (6) keep messages simple with 1- or 2-word phrases; and (7) use touch therapeutically.

3. **Document in the care plan the selected techniques that facilitate communication.** The specific approaches or techniques that are effective should be clearly documented in the plan of care so that all caregivers can use them consistently. This will reduce frustration of both the affected person and staff.

4. **Explain effective communication techniques to family members and friends.** Explain communication techniques to visitors, including family, friends, and clergy. This promotes positive interactions and enables both the affected person and the visitors to have a good experience. If interactions are positive, there is a greater likelihood that the visitors will return regularly and interact with the affected individual. This would enable the older adult to maintain a somewhat more normal pattern of social interaction. It is wise to avoid large groups of visitors, which might interfere with the person's concentration and result in confusion, frustration, and fatigue.

5. **Teach nonverbal methods of communication to verbally impaired older adults.** If the older adult is unable to communicate verbally, provide digital tablets, flash cards, pads, pencils, picture boards, or magic slates. If they are unable to use these, encourage the use of gestures. Open-ended statements such as "Show me what you would do with (the item in question)" may help the individual describe particular needs.

6. **Consult with a speech therapist/pathologist to determine the most effective communication strategies.** Speech therapists are specially trained to identify and treat communication disorders. Whenever possible, consult with a speech therapist as soon as a communication problem is suspected. The therapist's recommendations should be incorporated into the plan of care and supported by all caregivers (Nursing Care Plan 10.2).

❖ **NURSING PROCESS/CLINICAL JUDGMENT MODEL FOR PAIN**

The origin of some stimuli, such as pain, is within the body. Either physiologic damage or psychological distress can result in the sensation we call *pain*. Pain is a subjective perception. It is what the person tells you it is. Everyone experiences pain in a unique way. Because no two people mean exactly the same thing when they say they have pain, nurses must attempt to detect and determine the severity of another person's pain through careful assessment.

Nurses can neither see pain nor measure it with a meter, but they can detect its presence by careful listening and observation. Much information regarding the severity, quality, and location of pain can be gained from listening to how the person describes it; observing the individual's level of activity; and watching body language for subtle cues, such as grimacing, guarding of a body part, or drawing away when a body part is touched. Various visual pain scales (Fig. 10.7) can help to determine the severity of pain.

Responses to pain differ from person to person. Culture, gender, spiritual beliefs, and age all play a role in what a person considers painful and how they respond to it. Some people believe that pain and suffering are punishments or ways to atone for wrongs they have done. Others believe that pain is a test of their faith.

Some cultures teach that a person should be stoic or uncomplaining or that pain should be hidden and tolerated with a minimal amount of intervention. Other cultures teach that it is acceptable to express pain by crying, moaning, and yelling. These individuals expect relief from the pain as quickly as possible. Nurses coming from one cultural perspective may be totally puzzled when they are confronted by patients from another. Nurses who think that a person who is quiet cannot be in pain often fail to look for pain in such patients. Nurses who are silent sufferers themselves often become upset with the dramatic behavior of more demonstrative people.

Older adults are at increased risk for pain because of the higher incidence of disease conditions with

Nursing Care Plan 10.2   **Altered Communication Ability**

Mr. White, age 68, has Alzheimer disease. He is able to understand simple commands and follow them. His speech is brief, hesitant, and garbled. It takes a long time for him to say anything. He often shakes his head and pauses when trying to think of words. He often repeats the phrase "Help me, help me." At times, he becomes very frustrated when he cannot make his wishes known to his family or the staff. He spends much of his time alone in his room and has been observed crying after a particularly frustrating visit with his family.

PROBLEM STATEMENT
Altered Communication Ability

SUPPORTING ASSESSMENT DATA
- Garbled speech
- Difficulty expressing thoughts verbally
- Difficulty finding words
- Difficulty forming sentences

PATIENT GOALS/OUTCOMES IDENTIFICATION
Mr. White will maintain the optimal level of interaction with family and staff.

NURSING INTERVENTIONS/IMPLEMENTATION
1. Ask yes/no questions whenever possible.
2. Observe nonverbal communication.
3. Use touch to communicate empathy.
4. Speak slowly, using short, simple sentences.
5. Repeat, rephrase, and restate messages.
6. Decrease environmental distractions.
7. Establish eye contact before starting communication.
8. Provide visual cues whenever possible.
9. Use pictures of familiar items.
10. Allow ample time for responses.
11. Explain basic communication techniques to the family.
12. Consult with a speech therapist regarding other communication techniques that may benefit Mr. White.

EVALUATION
Mr. White follows some simple 1- or 2-word directions once his attention is obtained. He points to common objects on a picture board and occasionally leads caregivers to an object when told "Show me." He continues to have episodes of crying and to make pleas of "Help me." His family states that he "seems less upset" when they sit with him in a quiet area or when they look at a family picture album. You will continue the plan of care.

APPLYING CLINICAL JUDGMENT
1. What other approaches could the nurse use to decrease Mr. White's frustration?
2. What intervention might help the family deal with Mr. White's diminishing communication ability?

---

aging. Some older adults have a decreased ability to sense pain, whereas others are highly sensitive to painful stimuli. There is no proof that pain decreases with aging. Pain influences the way older adults feel about themselves and how they interact with others. Chronic or unrelieved pain can lead to behavioral changes. Older persons who demonstrate anger, depression, or isolation from others should be evaluated for pain.

Many older adults deny pain because they fear that they will be avoided or will lose their independence. They live with pain because they think that it is a normal part of growing old. It is not. Others may deny pain out of fear of becoming "addicted" to pain medications. Most patients who take pain medications as directed, however, do not become addicted (Ball, 2021). Pain is an indicator that something is wrong

in the body. It does not have to be tolerated simply because the person is old.

Determining the presence of pain in confused older adults is difficult. If pain is not recognized and assessed, serious harm may result. Failure to recognize pain can cause delays in the treatment of serious medical conditions and in the response to a change in condition.

Confused older adults have difficulty interpreting painful stimuli, identifying the location, and communicating the nature of their distress to caregivers. They do not always respond to pain in expected ways. Changes in body language, vital signs, and level of orientation are possible indicators of pain. The presence of pain is likely to result in agitation; increased pulse, respiratory rate, and blood pressure; and a greater degree of confusion.

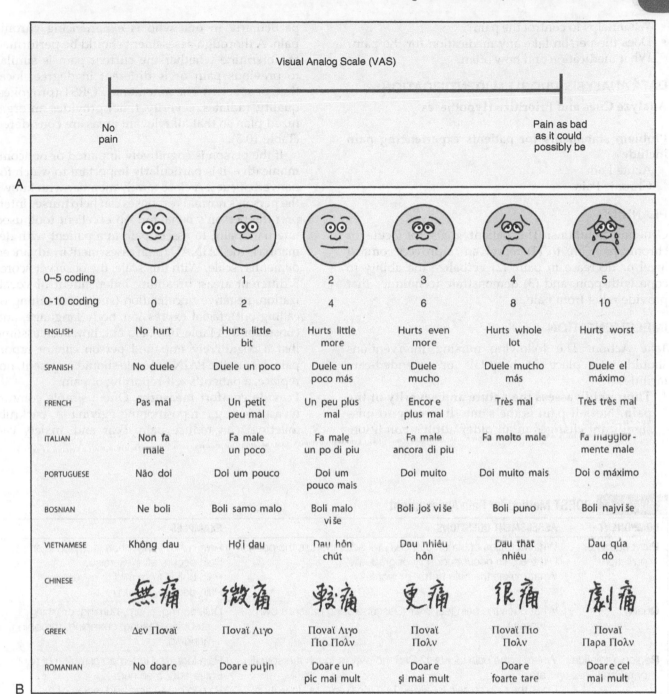

Visual Analog Scale (VAS)					

No pain ——————————————————————— Pain as bad as it could possibly be

A

0–5 coding	0	1	2	3	4	5
0-10 coding	0	2	4	6	8	10
ENGLISH	No hurt	Hurts little bit	Hurts little more	Hurts even more	Hurts whole lot	Hurts worst
SPANISH	No duele	Duele un poco	Duele un poco más	Duele mucho	Duele mucho más	Duele el máximo
FRENCH	Pas mal	Un petit peu mal	Un peu plus mal	Encore plus mal	Très mal	Très très mal
ITALIAN	Non fa male	Fa male un poco	Fa male un po di piu	Fa male ancora di piu	Fa molto male	Fa maggior-mente male
PORTUGUESE	Não doi	Doi um pouco	Doi um pouco mais	Doi muito	Doi muito mais	Doi o máximo
BOSNIAN	Ne boli	Boli samo malo	Boli malo vi še	Boli još vi še	Boli puno	Boli najvi še
VIETNAMESE	Không dau	Hởi dau	Dau hôn chút	Dau nhiêu hôn	Dau thât nhiêu	Dau qúa dô
CHINESE	無痛	微痛	較痛	更痛	很痛	劇痛
GREEK	Δεν Πoναΐ	Πoναΐ Λιγο	Πoναΐ Λιγο Πιo Πoλν	Πoναΐ Πoλν	Πoναΐ Πιo Πoλν	Πoναΐ Παρα Πoλν
ROMANIAN	No doare	Doare puţin	Doare un pic mai mult	Doare şi mai mult	Doare foarte tare	Doare cel mai mult

B

Fig. 10.7 **A,** Visual analog scale. **B,** Wong FACES Pain Rating Scale. (A, From Pasero, C., & McCaffery, M. (2011). *Pain assessment and pharmacologic management*, St. Louis, MO: Mosby.) (The scale is in the public domain. It may be duplicated for use in clinical practice.) (B, From Hockenberry, M. J., & Wilson, D. [2015] *Wong's nursing care of infants and children* [10th ed.]. St. Louis, MO: Mosby. With permission. © Mosby.)

QSEN Considerations: Patient-Centered Care

There is a reason why pain has become the fifth vital sign. Pain was typically underreported until a connection was made between the daily focus on vital signs and the lack of focus on pain. Pain was added to the vital sign list to increase the focus and ensure that each patient was assessed each time vital signs were taken. Nurses have a responsibility to demonstrate an understanding of pain and suffering and initiate steps to relieve pain in all of their patients—not just in those who are able to ask for help.

◆ ASSESSMENT (DATA COLLECTION)

Recognize cues
- Does the person complain of pain?
- Is the pain constant or intermittent? When did it start?
- Where is the pain? Is it generalized or localized?
- How does the person describe the pain (e.g., burning, stabbing, radiating, and gnawing)?
- Does the pain interfere with ADLs? With sleep?

- What helps to control the pain?
- Does the person take any medication for the pain? What medication and how often?

◆ DATA ANALYSIS/PROBLEM IDENTIFICATION

Analyze Cues and Prioritize Hypotheses

Problem statements for patients experiencing pain include
  Acute Pain
  Chronic Pain

◆ PLANNING

Generate Solutions: The patient goals for acute or chronic pain are to (1) report an improved comfort level or decrease in pain, (2) verbalize the ability to cope with pain, and (3) demonstrate techniques that provide relief from pain.

◆ IMPLEMENTATION

Take Action. The following nursing interventions should take place in hospitals or extended-care facilities:

1. **Thoroughly assess the nature and severity of the pain.** Not all pain is the same. It is easy to miss significant changes in an older adult's condition, particularly in one who is experiencing chronic pain. A thorough assessment should be performed to determine whether the current pain is similar to previous pain or is different in degree, location, or severity. The mnemonic PQRST (provokes, quality, radiates, severity, time) provides an organized plan so that all relevant areas are considered (Table 10.5).

If the person is cognitively impaired or noncommunicative, it is particularly important to watch for nonverbal cues. A close family member who knows the person's normal responses can help nurses interpret the person's behavior. An excellent tool, used internationally, to assess pain in a patient with dementia is the PAINAD (pain assessment in advanced dementia) scale. With this scale, the observer scores 5 different areas: breathing independent of vocalization, negative vocalization (such as moaning or calling out), facial expression, body language, and consolability (Table 10.6). Do not, however, assume that a cognitively impaired person cannot report pain. Use of the PAINAD scale should augment, not replace, a patient's self-reporting of pain.

2. **Provide comfort measures.** Often, simple comfort measures (e.g., repositioning, giving a backrub, toileting) can reduce pain. Fear and anxiety can

Table 10.5 PQRST Method for Pain Assessment

COMPONENT	ASSESSMENT QUESTIONS	EXAMPLES
Provocation or palliation	What activities or circumstances precede or cause the pain? Did the pain occur suddenly or gradually? What makes the pain better or worse?	Pain occurs only when stomach is empty. Pain occurs after exercise. Pain builds from mild to severe. Pain decreases with rest.
Quality	What does the pain feel like? (Describe using patient's own words.)	Dull, aching, sharp, burning, crushing, stabbing, tearing, cramping, throbbing, grinding.
Region, radiation, or referral	Where is the pain located? Can the patient touch the specific area? Does the pain remain localized to a small area or does it involve a larger area of the body? Is pain present in one or more areas of the body? Does the pain begin in one area and then move to another area? If so, where does the pain move to?	Pain localized in temporal region of skull. Entire abdomen hurts. Pain in pelvic area and region of the scapula. Pain starts in chest and radiates down left arm.
Severity	How severe is the pain on a scale of 0 to 10? Which illustration best represents pain? (Use a picture board ranging from a happy face to a face with a frown and tears.)	Pain reported at level 7.
Timing	When did the pain start? How long does the pain last? Is the pain continuous or intermittent? Does the pain occur only at certain times of the day?	Pain first noted at 7 AM. Pain has been present for 6 hours. Pain "comes and goes." Pain noticed only during evening.
Additional questions	Has the patient experienced any pain like this in the past? Is the current pain similar or different than previous episodes? Did the patient take any medication for pain? Has the medication been effective at relieving pain? How effective? How long was it effective?	History of intermittent headaches. Current headache much more severe than ever experienced previously. Acetaminophen reduces the discomfort for 2 to 3 hours but does not eliminate it.

Table 10.6	Pain Assessment in Advanced Dementia (PAINAD) Scale			
ITEMS[a]	0	1	2	SCORE
Breathing independent of vocalization	Normal	Occasional labored breathing. Short period of hyperventilation.	Noisy labored breathing. Long period of hyperventilation. Cheyne-Stokes respirations.	
Negative vocalization	None	Occasional moan or groans. Low level speech with a negative or disapproving quality.	Repeated troubled calling out. Loud moaning or groaning. Crying.	
Facial expression	Smiling or inexpressive	Sad. Frightened. Frown.	Facial grimacing.	
Body language	Relaxed	Tense. Distressed pacing. Fidgeting.	Rigid. Fists clenched. Knees pulled up. Pulling or pushing away. Striking out.	
Consolability	No need to console	Distracted or reassured by voice or touch.	Unable to console, distract or reassure.	
			Total[b]	

[a]Five-item observation tool (see the description of each item subsequently).
[b]Total scores range from 0 to 10 (based on a scale of 0 to 2 for 5 items), with a higher score indicating more severe pain (0 = no pain to 10 = severe pain).
Reproduced from Warden, V., Hurley, A. C., & Volicer, L. (2003). Development and psychometric evaluation of the Pain Assessment in Advanced Dementia (PAINAD) scale. JAMA, 4(1), 9–15, with permission from the American Medical Directors Association.

increase pain. Listening to older adults and providing emotional support can often help to reduce pain.

3. **Avoid actions that increase pain.** Simple actions, such as jarring the bed or moving an individual too rapidly, can increase pain. Because movement may increase pain, care should be used when moving, transferring, or otherwise touching people in pain. A simple touch, an explanation of what to expect, or acknowledgment of the pain can demonstrate sensitivity to the older adult's feelings.

4. **Anticipate situations likely to cause pain.** Because confused people are unable to report pain accurately, nurses need to anticipate activities or procedures that are likely to cause pain and institute measures to prevent or reduce it.

5. **Teach nonpharmacologic approaches to pain control.** Many nonpharmacologic approaches are available for pain control. Biofeedback, meditation, hypnosis, and imagery are all useful in pain control. These techniques are often not attempted with older adults because caregivers think that they will not accept or understand the techniques. Many older adults are not only capable of learning these techniques but are pleased to have some control of their pain.

6. **Administer medications as ordered.** Studies have shown that nurses tend to underestimate rather than overestimate pain in others. This leads to more suffering than necessary. Nurses are often afraid that administering medication will lead to addiction or dependence. In fact, timely administration of medication before pain becomes severe actually decreases the total amount of medication used. Administer pain medications before initiating activities or procedures that are likely to cause pain. The types and dosages of medications used to control pain in older adults are highly individualized and may differ from those used with younger adults.

The following interventions should take place in the home:

1. **Help older adults and their families develop a plan to cope with pain.** Pain, particularly the chronic pain endured by many older persons, can be physically and psychologically exhausting for the affected individuals and their loved ones. Nurses should help those living at home to develop a plan built on the interventions that are most effective for them. Older adults and their families should be shown how to incorporate these pain relief measures into their daily activities, so that pain is kept to a minimum and the person is able to lead as normal a life as possible.

2. **Apply any appropriate interventions that are used in the institutional setting.**

Get Ready for the Next Generation NCLEX® Examination!

Key Points

- Perceptual changes are among the most common problems experienced by older adults.
- Disturbed vision and hearing present multiple concerns related to safety and lifestyle.
- Pain, although not a routine problem of aging, can interfere with the older person's ability to lead a fulfilling life. Assessment of the older adults using a pain scale can be useful; the PAINAD scale is useful with cognitively impaired older adults.
- Nurses must be alert to cognitive and perceptual changes and identify ways to support as normal a lifestyle as possible.
- Delirium has a rapid onset (within hours to days) and is generally reversible; dementia has a slower onset and generally is not reversible.
- Providing care for older adults who are experiencing severe cognitive changes, particularly those with dementia, challenges the skills and capabilities of nurses, families, and other health care providers.
- Ongoing assessment of perceptual and cognitive functioning is necessary to detect subtle but potentially dangerous changes.
- Prompt recognition of problems and careful selection of appropriate interventions will allow the aging person to maintain the highest level of function possible.

Additional Learning Resources

SG Go to your Evolve website at http://evolve.elsevier.com/Williams/geriatric for the additional online resources.

https://www.alz.org/help-support/resources/care-training-resources

Review Questions for the Next Generation NCLEX® Examination

1. Hearing aids are worn by many older people. Which statement regarding hearing aids is false?

   a. Batteries should be stored in the refrigerator.
   b. Ear molds should be cleaned regularly.
   c. Most people easily adjust to hearing aid use.
   d. Hearing aids are fragile.

2. Which statement should the nurse consider when assessing pain in an older patient? *(Select all that apply.)*

   a. Chronic pain is more common with aging.
   b. Older people are able to tolerate more severe pain than are younger persons.
   c. Older people have a greater sensory perception of pain.
   d. Cognitive changes may alter a person's ability to report and describe pain.
   e. There is no useful pain assessment tool for an older adult with Alzheimer disease.
   f. Behavioral changes may be indicators of pain.

3. Which condition is progressive and irreversible?

   a. Dementia
   b. Delirium
   c. Confusion
   d. Depression

4. Which measures would be most appropriate when considering the environment for a patient with dementia?

   a. Using bright colors and textures
   b. Maintaining low lighting at all times
   c. Keeping the TV on for stimulation
   d. Placing family pictures around the room

5. What would be the most appropriate intervention for an older adult with dementia who was resisting efforts to help them reposition or ambulate?

   a. Try again in 5 minutes.
   b. Try to convince the person to perform the activity, explaining the therapeutic benefit.
   c. Call the primary care provider and ask for an antianxiety medication.
   d. Assess the person using the PAINAD scale.

6. A 75 year-old male client is being seen by his primary care provider at the request of the patient's son due to his marked behavioral changes and pain with urination. Following an assessment, the nurse notes the following selected data:

   T 102.5
   HR 120
   RR 22
   BP 100/64

   A urine sample is secured via condom catheter; it shows innumerable white cells and noticeable bacteriuria.

   Choose the most likely options for the information missing from the statements below by selecting from the list of options provided.

   The nurse recognizes that an _____ temperature and bacteria in the urine are a sign of a _____.
   The nurse knows that the behavioral changes are most likely due to _____ and will resolve after treatment. Failure to treat the underlying cause could lead to _____.

   Answer Options

OPTIONS
elevated
decreased
urinary tract infection
chronic kidney disease
urinary incontinence
fecal impaction
dementia
delirium
mild cognitive impairment
Alzheimer disease
death

REFERENCES

Alzheimer's Association (ALZ) (2021). Treatments for behavior. https://www.alz.org/alzheimers-dementia/treatments/treatments-for-behavior/

Ball, W. S. (2021). Tackling the truth about opioid addiction: 5 key tips to address patient fears. https://nurse.plus/become-anurse/tips-to-address-patient-fears-about-opioid-addiction/

Budson, A. (2019). What dementia, MCI, and subjective cognitive decline mean. https://www.psychologytoday.com/us/blog/managing-your-memory/201902/what-dementia-mci-and-subjective-cognitive-decline-mean#:~:text=%20Subjective%20cognitive%20decline%20may%20be%20a%20sign,3%20Their%20daily%20function%20is%20normal%20More%20/

Centers for Disease Control and Prevention (CDC) (2020a). The truth about aging and dementia. https://www.cdc.gov/aging/publications/features/dementia-not-normal-aging.html/.

Centers for Disease Control and Prevention (CDC) (2020b). Subjective cognitive decline — A public health issue. https://www.cdc.gov/aging/aginginfo/subjective-cognitive-decline-brief.html/

Centers for Medicare and Medicaid Services (CMS) (2020). *National partnership—dementia care resources.* https://www.cms.gov/Medicare/Provider-Enrollment-and-Certification/SurveyCertificationGenInfo/National-Partnership-Dementia-Care-Resources/

Charvat, M. (2020). Why are minorities disproportionately impacted by dementia? https://www.psychologytoday.com/us/blog/the-fifth-vital-sign/202006/why-are-minorities-disproportionately-impacted-dementia/

Gray, S. L., & Hanlon, J. T. (2018). Anticholinergic drugs and dementia in older adults. *British Medical Journal, 361,* k1722.

Harvard University (2020). *Forgetfulness—7 types of normal memory problems.* https://www.health.harvard.edu/mind-and-mood/forgetfulness-7-types-of-normal-memory -problems

Menzenbach, J., Guttenthaler, V., Kirfel, A., Ricchiuto, A., Neumann, C., Adler, L., ... Wittmann, M. (2019). PROPDESC Collaboration Group. Estimating patients' risk for postoperative delirium from preoperative routine data—Trial design of the PRe-Operative prediction of postoperative DElirium by appropriate SCreening (PROPDESC) study: A monocentre prospective observational trial. *Contemporary Clinical Trials Communications, Dec 4, 17,* 100501. doi:10.1016/j.conctc.2019.100501. D: 31890984; PMCID: PMC6926123

Rubino, A., Sanon, M., Ganz, M. L., et al. (2020). Association of the U.S. Food and Drug Administration antipsychotic drug boxed warning with medication use and health outcomes in elderly patients with dementia. *JAMA Network Open, 3*(4), e203630. doi:10.1001/jamanetworkopen.2020.3630

Silva, P. R., Farias, T., Cascio, F., Dos Santos, L., Peixoto, V., Crespo, E., & Teixeira, S (2018). Neuroplasticity in visual impairments. *Neurology International, 10*(4), 7326. doi:10.4081/ni.2018.7326. PMID: 30687464; PMCID: PMC6322049

Objectives

1. Discuss the concepts of self-perception and self-concept.
2. Examine how aging can affect self-perception and self-concept.
3. Discuss the effects of disease processes on self-perception and self-concept.
4. Identify signs of depression in later life.
5. Identify suicide risk in older adults.
6. Describe methods of assessing changes in self-perception and self-concept.
7. Identify older adults who are most at risk for problems related to self-perception and self-concept.
8. Identify problem statements related to self-perception or self-concept.
9. Describe nursing interventions designed to improve self-perception and self-concept among older adults.

Key Terms

anxiety (p. 215)
body image (p. 219)
depression (p. 215)
fear (p. 215)
feedback (p. 214)

helplessness (p. 215)
hopelessness (p. 215)
powerlessness (p. 215)
reminiscence (p. 221)
self-esteem (p. 214)

NORMAL SELF-PERCEPTION AND SELF-CONCEPT

The attitudes and perceptions people have about themselves, their abilities, and their self-worth make up what is often called *self-identity*. People form their self-identities from their values, life experiences, and interactions with others. People with good self-worth and high self-esteem share certain characteristics. They have strong personal values and believe that they have the ability to control their lives. They have had positive life experiences and have received positive feedback from others. People with poor self-worth and low self-esteem may be victims of abuse or trauma, and often feel they may have little control over their lives. They may have perceived life based on these negative experiences.

We form our self-identities by comparing ourselves and our experiences with some ideal. This can be an internal ideal drawn from our personal values or an external ideal drawn from the society around us. Many people experience problems with self-worth because they always measure themselves against external standards. Contemporary standards are communicated repeatedly by advertising and the media. People who are portrayed as young, thin, rich, successful, and attractive are idealized. Anyone who does not meet these superficial and artificial standards can be judged inferior and thus may be viewed negatively by our society. Few people are able to meet all of the idealized criteria. This results in a large number of people (of all ages) in contemporary society who suffer from negative self-esteem or poor self-identity.

In trying to meet external standards, people can lose themselves and their internal values. The more we look to the external forces, the less likely we are to have high self-esteem. The more we look internally for our self-worth, the more satisfied we will be in the long run. Shakespeare summed it up nicely in *Hamlet*: "This above all: to thine own self be true / And it must follow, as the night the day, thou canst not then be false to any man" (I, iii, 75). This issue can raise unique problems for older adults in the lesbian, gay, bisexual, and transgender population. They may be less likely to be open about their sexual orientation because of concerns about discrimination and mistreatment. The need to hide a large part of their identity can increase their feelings of social isolation and low self-esteem (Caceres, 2020).

It is easy to say that people should draw on internal ideals to maintain self-esteem, but this is difficult in light of external pressures and feedback. In today's society, people may have as many negative experiences as positive ones. Problems relating to self-perception and self-esteem are common among people of all ages. Studies have shown that self-esteem does decline in old age, particularly in very old age (Orth, et al., 2018). Not surprisingly, it was also found that health and wealth have positive effects on self-esteem. It is also important to note that self-concept can have a negative impact on health; if someone self-identifies as "old" or "frail," they tend to take on even more of the characteristics that they see as typical of the old and frail (Ravary, 2019).

QSEN Considerations: Patient-Centered Care

Actions That Caregivers Can Use to Promote Self-Esteem

- Help older adults to find interests, activities, or hobbies or to learn a new skill. Although some new skills may take longer to acquire, realize that the results could have a positive impact on the person's feelings of self-worth.
- If assisting someone to dress, provide choices that are comfortable and that they feel confident wearing. Provide time to assist with makeup, hair styling, or other personal care that they enjoy.
- Encourage volunteering, social interaction (including online communication and social media), and participation in social gatherings.
- Provide help as needed with technological devices that can keep them connected to friends and family.
- Find ways for older adults to teach tasks they have mastered—cooking, sewing, crocheting, and so on.
- Seek guidance or mentoring from older adults and listen to their advice.
- Avoid "talking down" to older adults. Remember that they have a rich history, and some of them have had to overcome hardships without modern conveniences. Keep respect at the forefront of any interaction.
- Keep older adults informed, and encourage them to maintain control of their health. See them as partners in their care, and take the time to answer questions.

Feedback from others affects our perception of ourselves. People who have caring friends and families tend to have a higher self-esteem and a strong self-identity. Positive families and friends provide support for one another. They help one another to keep things in perspective by providing meaningful feedback and buffering one another from a world that can seem very negative at times. A good family and good friends play an important part in building and maintaining our self-esteem. People who lack supportive family and friends are likely to have a poor perception of self and low self-esteem. Those who come from dysfunctional families or who are separated from loved ones are at an increased risk for development of poor self-perception and low self-esteem. Research also suggests that a negative perception of conflict may start a trajectory that brings on more conflict, thus further decreasing self-esteem (Samsudin, 2020).

A real or perceived ability to make choices plays an important role in self-perception and self-esteem. People who feel capable of controlling what happens perceive things far differently from those who feel that they have little or no control over their lives. Our sense of self-control starts with our bodies. Adults are used to having control of their bodies and bodily functions. Control of the movement of body parts and control of elimination are so basic we do not even think about them, at least not until we lose control of them for some reason. Consider how you would feel if tomorrow you woke up and could not move or could not control your bladder or bowels. Would your sense of self-worth and self-esteem change? Adults are also used to having control and making choices regarding their activities. Choices regarding activities of daily living (ADLs)—such as hygiene practices, amount and type of clothing, amount and type of food, and amount and type of exercise and sleep)—are determined by an adult's self-perception and level of self-esteem. Loss of control results in depression, powerlessness, helplessness, hopelessness, fear, and anxiety. Over a period of time, loss of control can destroy self-esteem.

Problems related to self-perception and self-esteem are not as obvious as are physical problems. By their very nature, self-perception and self-concept are subjective. Many people find it difficult to talk about their feelings, often finding themselves unable or unwilling to put their feelings into words. More often, our perceptions of self-worth and self-esteem are exhibited to others through behavior. Significant behaviors include the amount of attention paid to personal hygiene and grooming, the type and frequency of emotions exhibited, body posture, the amount and type of eye contact, and voice and speech patterns. People with very high self-esteem appear to be very much in control of themselves and their lives. They are usually well groomed, maintain an erect body posture, make eye contact with others, speak clearly in a normal tone of voice, and exhibit emotions appropriate to a given situation.

People with very low self-esteem may appear disinterested and out of control. They may appear unkempt or disheveled. They may slump or slouch, and may exhibit little purpose to their movement. Eye contact can be infrequent, although it is important to consider cultural differences about the perception of looking someone in the eye. Some cultures see direct eye contact as disrespectful. The amount of communication with others may be reduced and tends to be quiet and humble in nature, as they may believe that what they have to say in unimportant.

Most people's self-esteem and behavior fall between these two extremes. As long as behavior falls within the accepted range of normal, people tend to disregard or overlook what is going on within other people. Only when behaviors move outside of the normal range do we seriously attempt to understand what is happening in the person to cause those behaviors. This is unfortunate, because by the time behaviors become problematic, damage may have already been done to the person's self-esteem.

SELF-PERCEPTION/SELF-CONCEPT AND AGING

Erikson (see Chapter 2) has identified the major task of late life as the maintenance of ego integrity (the sense of self-worth) versus despair. Attitudes toward aging, the level of self-esteem throughout life, the extent of physical change caused by aging and illness, the presence or absence of emotional support systems, and the ability to maintain a degree of control—all of these have an impact on whether or not older adults will be successful in accomplishing this task.

? Think Critically

Erikson's Stages

Think about how Erikson's stages build on each other. He defines the task of middle adulthood (ages 40 to 65) as generativity versus stagnation and the task during late life as ego integrity versus despair. Finding a way to contribute to society or associating oneself with a cause during middle adulthood may help set the stage for successful accomplishment of tasks in later adulthood. When older people feel needed and know that they are contributing something useful, it has a positive effect on their self-worth. With this knowledge, how can nurses find ways to help older adults feel valued?

Aging individuals develop their own perceptions of aging. It is difficult to see oneself getting old. Many older adults express dismay with the realization and can even identify a particular moment when they perceived themselves as old. One older woman recently attended her 50th high school reunion. She reported having had a good time but wondered what she was doing with all of these "old people." A subtle but real change in her self-perception occurred after that incident. Before then, she did not feel old; afterward, she was more aware of her age. Successful aging is not so much a matter of years lived or health status but rather of perception and attitude. Successful aging has sometimes been described as "mind over matter." If you don't mind, it doesn't matter.

Poor self-concept, depression, and other negative feelings can be seen in the older population. Studies have shown that quality of life and life satisfaction may be linked to personality and mental health factors. Older adults who have had a poor self-concept throughout their lives are unlikely to gain self-esteem with aging. Older adults who had a healthy level of self-esteem during their younger days may experience some problems in the course of aging, but these are most often a result of circumstances or societal attitudes. Self-esteem is fostered by continuing to participate in enjoyable or meaningful activities (Fig. 11.1).

Ageism is still prevalent in many of today's western youth-oriented societies, which often portray older adults as physically and mentally inept, nonproductive, and dependent. Considering these negative

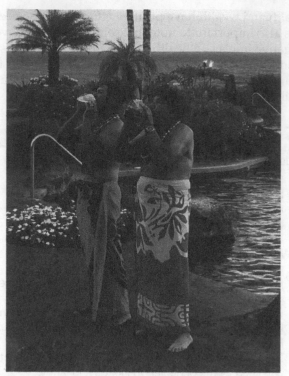

Fig. 11.1 Older adult participating in a sunset torch-lighting ceremony.

images of aging, it is easy to understand why many people do all they can to avoid the physical signs of aging. Consumers are flooded with ads for antiaging products, underscoring the perception that growing older is bad and should be stopped. One researcher commented that ageism is the most socially condoned form of prejudice in the United States (Wilson, 2019). Older adults are expected to become 22% of the world population by 2050 (World Health Organization, 2018).

Older people who accept the negative societal perceptions are likely to suffer more than those older adults who refuse to accept such stereotypes. The nurse must recognize that physical, social, and economic changes that occur with aging can result in changes in the way older adults perceive themselves and their bodies. The greater the amount of change, the more likely the person is to experience problems related to self-concept. Small changes in appearance or function (e.g., wrinkles or aches and pains) can impact an individual's self-worth. Serious illnesses (particularly those that result in obvious disfigurement or major loss of function, such as strokes) take a large toll on the older adult's perception of self. Any change to a person's ability to care for themself independently will affect their self-perception and self-worth.

Frequent and significant losses (including declining physical health; decreasing mental agility; loss of significant others; loss of pride in appearance, roles, or possessions; and loss of independence) threaten the perception of control that is important to most adults. These losses can result in a variety of problems, which often only grow worse if left unchecked.

Institutional placement further damages self-worth by stripping older adults of many of the personal belongings that make up the visible part of their identity. Facilities that are able to accommodate more than a small amount of clothing and a few mementos gathered over a lifetime are rare. The mementos amassed over perhaps 80 years of life are often reduced to whatever will fit into a small closet and bedside stand. Along with the loss of belongings is the loss of control over one's schedule. Facilities dictate times for meals, activities, and bathing based on the schedules imposed by the care providers. This can be difficult for the older adult to adjust to when transitioning homes.

Clinical Pitfall

Offering choices is one way of helping to improve a resident's self-esteem. The resident may feel powerless and want to exert independence by choosing their own time to eat and bathe. Providing choices, when available, may take longer in the short term but may lead to fewer battles in the long term.

Although the loss of physical and functional abilities is damaging to a person's self-worth, loss of the emotional support of loved ones is even more devastating. When death comes to friends or loved ones, it is a reminder to the older adult of their own mortality. The positive messages that a person is worthwhile, lovable, and loved become less frequent, and the reasons for living fade. Losses resulting from death or separation from friends and family can leave older adults without those sources of positive feedback that nourish self-worth. The term *elder orphan* describes older individuals who are thus isolated, having no known family members or care providers (Montayre, 2020). As people are living longer, this issue will require more community resources.

We cannot prevent losses due to deaths, but loss from separation is another matter. Older adults who are separated from their families and significant others are at increased risk for experiencing diminished self-worth. Breakdown of the extended family and increased geographic mobility may result in the isolation of older adults. Although a large percentage of older adults do not reside with family members, they often live alone by choice. A majority of older adults report that they continue to have regular and frequent contact with grown children either in person, by phone, or by virtual connectivity.

Separation from family is often associated with placement in an institutional setting. Although institutional placement is usually the last choice after all other alternatives have failed, older adults often feel rejected and isolated when nursing home placement has become necessary. Research shows that older adults will adjust better if they are included in the decision to move to a skilled nursing facility; if the decision is made without consulting them, the facility will never be considered "home" (Cranley, 2020).

If they were not part of the decision because they were seen as having little value or worth, it is a natural response for older adults to feel that they have been "put away." These individuals often feel unimportant, unloved, and unwanted. Even if this is completely untrue, the perception greatly decreases their sense of self-worth. If family and friends visit often and show positive concern, self-esteem can be maintained. Unfortunately, this is not always the case. It is in institutional settings, where it can be perceived that nobody cares about the inner person, that many older adults lose their remaining sense of self-esteem and self-worth. It is vital that we, the caregivers of older adults, make an effort to know and understand the person behind the aging body: the retired nurse, the world-class physicist, the retired army colonel, for example. Care for each older adult as you would want your loved ones to be cared for.

The COVID-19 pandemic of 2020 brought increased challenges related to social isolation and the older adult. Health care facilities were directed to allow only essential personnel on site, leaving families without the ability to visit their older adult relatives or friends. Loved ones who were concerned about spreading the virus were reluctant to visit older adults at home. Gyms, libraries, and restaurants were closed at various times throughout the country, and social distancing reduced opportunities for personal contact. Widespread loneliness and depression became a concern as the medical community tried to deal with the psychological and potential physical effects (e.g., hypertension, increased heart disease incidence) of isolation on the older adult and the deadly risk of the contracting the virus (Hwang, 2020).

QSEN Considerations: Patient-Centered Care

Residents in a skilled nursing facility can easily become "lost" in the sea of other residents. Remember that each resident has a unique past—one that they may be unable to communicate. Request that family members bring in pictures or mementos that personalize the resident's room with the family history. For instance, as the facility staff learn that Ms. Hrycyk was once a noted gymnast or that Mr. Jones is a veteran of WWII, it becomes easier for them to treat each resident as a valued individual.

DEPRESSION AND AGING

Depression is more common among the aging population than is generally suspected or recognized. Studies indicate the magnitude of the problem. It is estimated that among people over age 65, depression is a problem for as many as 1% to 5% of community-dwelling older adults, 13% to 15% of older adults receiving home care, 11% to 78% or more of long-term care residents, and 12% of hospitalized older adults. Research estimates that only 1 in 10 older adults who suffer from depression is recognized and treated (Depression and Bipolar Support Alliance, 2020). Depression is more difficult to recognize because typical indicators may be similar to those seen with a variety of medical disorders. For example, weight changes, changes in sleep patterns, decreased energy, and changes in psychomotor activity are signs not only of depression but also of numerous other medical problems. Sudden behavioral or personality changes are not a normal part of aging. Depression may be related to a wide range of factors, including loss of independence or loved ones or growing medical problems such as hypothyroidism, anemia, and diabetes. The use of medications—such as antihypertensives, antiarrhythmics, anticholesterolemics, cardiac glycosides, analgesics, and hormones such as corticosteroids and progesterone—is associated with a higher incidence of depression. Careful assessment is necessary to recognize depression before it leads to other, more serious problems. The National Institute of Mental Health has identified the following warning signs of depression among older adults:

- Noticeable changes in mood; feeling distant from others, flat, empty, or anxious
- Changes in energy level; feeling tired all the time but having trouble sleeping, or sleeping too much
- Difficulty carrying out daily activities for weeks at a time
- Trouble concentrating; feeling restless or on edge
- Irritability, anger, or lashing out at others
- Increased worry or stress or obsessing about minor problems or events
- Heavy use of alcohol or drugs
- Loss of interest in once pleasurable hobbies and activities, including sex
- Sadness, hopelessness, crying, or having suicidal thoughts (Kupka, 2020)

QSEN Considerations: Patient-Centered Care

Older adults may perceive a social stigma related to mental health issues. They also tend to see depression as personal weakness or may feel that they are to blame for their symptoms. Fear of discussing their symptoms may stem from memories of a relative with mental health concerns who was ostracized by the family, or worry that they will be placed on yet another medication. It is important to provide patient education on the signs and symptoms of depression and to make the environment a safe place in which to discuss feelings and concerns. By discussing depression as a medical issue rather than a personal failure, the nurse can help older adults accept that treatment (therapy and/or medication) can improve their quality of life.

SUICIDE AND AGING

Older adults make up about 13% to 15% of the total U.S. population, but they account for 18% of the suicides (AgingInPlace, 2020). The Association for Marriage and Family Therapy suggests that those statistics may be underreported by as much as 40% owing to the potential for "silent suicides," or suicides that have been incorrectly labeled as overdoses or accidents (Mendoza, 2020). Older adults at risk for suicide because of depression often present themselves to health care professionals with a variety of physical concerns. Many times, an older adult has been seen by a health professional shortly before completing suicide (38% in the week before and 64% within a month before)—a visit at which the real significance of the person's complaints was missed. Older women are more likely to experience depression, but older men who are depressed and older adults with a history of affective disorders are most at risk for attempting or completing suicide. In the general population, there is 1 death for every 20 attempts, but there is 1 death for every 4 attempts among the older adult population (AgingInPlace, 2020). Severe emotional or physical pain, a recent loss, or a stressful event (such as the diagnosis of a terminal disease) has been present in a large percentage of those who attempt suicide.

Older adults have a higher rate of suicide completion than do other age groups, and they tend to use more violent methods to end their lives. Firearms (80%), overdoses, and suffocation are common methods. Seniors are less likely to communicate their intentions, although statements regarding helplessness or hopelessness, a sudden interest in firearms, the sudden revision of a will, or talk of suicide should never be ignored. Giving away prized possessions, loss of interest in daily activities, and unexpected weight loss should also be assessed. Family members and health care professionals can help by being aware of warning signs and risk factors. If problems are suspected, prompt referral to a mental health professional would be wise.

❖ NURSING PROCESS/CLINICAL JUDGMENT MODEL FOR ALTERED SELF-PERCEPTION AND ALTERED SELF-CONCEPT

When an older adult has a poor self-concept, fear and anxiety increase. As one loses control over one's life, self-esteem plummets and the older adult falls victim to feelings of hopelessness and powerlessness, leading to depression. This, in turn, leads to isolation from others and an even poorer sense of self-worth.

◆ ASSESSMENT (DATA COLLECTION)

Recognize cues
- Does the person verbalize fears or concerns?
- Are these fears of a known or an unknown source?
- Does the person verbalize loss of control over their life?
- Have they recently experienced a significant loss?

- Has the person recently moved or been separated from significant others?
- Does the person have a support system?
- What is their general appearance and posture?
- Do they person make or avoid eye contact?
- Does the person verbalize concerns regarding changes in their appearance?
- Does the person make negative comments regarding themselves?
- Does the person avoid looking in the mirror or at altered body parts?
- Does the person question their worth as an individual?
- Does the person speak of failure? Hopelessness? Despair?
- Does the person spend most of the time alone, or do they interact with others?
- Does the person accept directions from caregivers passively? Or do they express the wish to be the one to make all decisions?
- Are there signs of aggression, anger, or demanding behaviors?
- Are there any signs of autonomic nervous system stimulation (e.g., increased pulse or respiratory rate, elevated blood pressure, diaphoresis)?
- Does the person manifest any behaviors typical of emotional upset (e.g., pacing, hand wringing, crying, repetitive motions, tics, aggressiveness)?
- Are there changes in vocal quality (e.g., quivering)?
- Does the person report ongoing headaches?
- Do they have difficulty focusing on activities, remembering things, or making decisions?
- Have there been changes in eating or sleeping patterns?
- Has the person started to give away treasured possessions?
- Do they use alcohol or other mood-altering drugs? Which drugs? How much? How often?
- Does the person verbalize the desire to end their life? If so, is there a plan?

Box 11.1 provides a list of risk factors for altered self-perception and altered self-concept in older adults.

❖ NURSING PROCESS/CLINICAL JUDGMENT MODEL FOR ALTERED BODY IMAGE

People experiencing altered body image are likely to refuse to look at or touch the affected body part. In severe disturbances, the individual may deny that the change has occurred and act as though nothing has happened. Many persons who suffer with this problem are unwilling to discuss their concerns with others for fear that they will be rejected or made to feel different. If they are willing to verbalize their concerns, they may speak of themselves in a disembodied way, as though the deformity or change were not really affecting them. They may speak of themselves negatively or

with a great deal of disgust because they are no longer who they once were. They may become preoccupied with their body function and excessively concerned about every minor change. They may need reassurance that nothing else of the sort is likely to happen to them. Many people with altered body image refuse to participate in their own care and resist any plans for rehabilitation. They are likely to verbalize feelings of worthlessness and powerlessness.

Box 11.1	Risk Factors Related to Altered Self-Perception and Altered Self-Concept in Older Adults

- Conditions that result in change of body appearance (burns, obesity, skin lesions, chemotherapy, disfiguring endocrine disorders, such as acromegaly or Cushing disease, surgical removal of body parts)
- Inability to control bodily functions
- Significant losses (of significant others, possessions, social roles, financial status)
- Recent relocation (particularly if involuntary)
- Chronic pain

ASSESSMENT (DATA COLLECTION)

Recognize cues
- See the assessment for altered self-perception and self-concept starting on p. 218.

◆ DATA ANALYSIS/PROBLEM IDENTIFICATION

Analyze Cues and Prioritize Hypotheses

Problem statements for older adults with alterations in body image include
Altered Body Image

◆ PLANNING

Generate Solutions: The patient goals for older adults with altered body image are to (1) verbalize concerns regarding changes in body appearance or function, (2) identify personal strengths, (3) acknowledge and look at the actual changes in body appearance, (4) verbalize willingness to modify lifestyle to accommodate physical changes, and (5) demonstrate readiness to participate in therapy and to use necessary assistive devices.

◆ IMPLEMENTATION

Take Action: The following interventions should take place in hospitals, in extended-care facilities, and at home:

1. **Assess the older adult's perceptions of self, including strengths and support systems.** Even with serious impairment, older adults can have strengths that will help them cope with change. Identify the unique strengths of each person so that these can

be drawn on when planning care. Discuss how they have dealt with hardships in the past.

2. **Establish a trusting relationship.** To help older adults work through and accept physical changes or deformities, demonstrate acceptance verbally and nonverbally. Actively listening to concerns and planning care to include opportunities for the patient to verbalize their feelings can help build trust. Treat this as a loss and allow the older adults to work through their grief. Do not be judgmental of their emotional responses. Comments such as "it's not that bad" can minimize their feelings and block the therapeutic relationship.

3. **Provide care in a nonjudgmental manner.** Because nurses are the people most likely to actually see any physical deformity, it is particularly important to show no sign of revulsion or disgust when you are providing care. Take particular care not to show even subtle body language or facial expressions that could be perceived by older adults as a sign of nonacceptance.

4. **Encourage the older adult to look at and touch the affected body areas.** Nurses are so used to seeing physical deformities (e.g., stomas and amputations) that they may not be aware of just how frightening these may be to the affected person. Many people need time and encouragement to even look at their affected body part. Some depersonalize the change and refer to "it," as though the deformity were something apart from themselves. Looking at and touching the deformity can help the person accept the change. Until they are able to do this, they will not be ready for patient education or self-care.

5. **Focus on abilities, not disabilities.** To become motivated, people must feel that they are capable of doing the activity. Most older adults, even those with severe deformities, are capable of doing something. Focusing on what can be done instead of on what cannot be done promotes feelings of self-worth.

6. **Assist in selecting clothing and/or dressing older adults in a manner that deemphasizes body changes.** Clothing that draws attention away from obvious deformities helps maintain body image. Sweaters, lap blankets, and properly fitted clothing can be used to make deformities less obvious.

7. **Ensure that the older adult is carefully groomed.** Change soiled clothing promptly. Always keep the face and hands clean and free from food or other debris. Little things, such as neatly combed or styled hair, a shave, or the application of a tasteful amount of makeup can make the person feel better about their appearance. How a person looks makes a difference in how they feels. Remember that an older person should never be made to look "cute." Always groom older adults appropriately for their age.

8. **Coordinate rehabilitative care with other departments.** Physical therapy, occupational therapy, speech therapy, pharmacy, and other departments may be involved in the care of individuals who have experienced significant changes in body function. Nurses spend the most time with these individuals, and they are the most aware of the total effect of various therapies. Coordinate these activities in the care plan to ensure that all groups are working toward the same goals. Monitor and document the patients' responses to the therapy and their ability to tolerate the effort required. Ensure that therapies are spaced in a way that they are effective and not overwhelming for the patient.

❖ NURSING PROCESS/CLINICAL JUDGMENT MODEL FOR POTENTIAL FOR DECREASED SELF-ESTEEM

Older adults are at risk for losing self-esteem for many reasons. Those who have decreased self-esteem are likely to display certain characteristic behaviors. Body language of people with decreased self-esteem is similar to that of individuals who are depressed. They are often observed with their head slumped on the chest or shoulder; the facial expression is one of sadness; and they usually avoid eye contact. These individuals are likely to speak of themselves in negative terms. Statements, such as "Don't waste your time on me" or "I can't do anything right," are indicative of decreased self-esteem. The speech of individuals with decreased self-esteem usually reflects sadness, loss, depression, anxiety, and anger. They can see little that is positive about their lives and may focus on negative experiences. People with decreased self-esteem may not give appropriate attention to hygiene or grooming. They may be very passive, letting caregivers control all facets of their lives. They may demonstrate extreme dependence on others, even if they are capable of doing things for themselves. They may not initiate activities, and, if they do, they are likely to leave activities unfinished. They may be resistant to positive feedback and may argue or become angry with anyone attempting to give it. Older adults with decreased self-esteem may also avoid social contact; if forced to be in contact with others, they tend to avoid interaction and stay at the edges of the group or activity.

◆ ASSESSMENT (DATA COLLECTION)

Recognize cues
- See the assessment for altered self-perception and altered self-concept on p. 219.

◆ DATA ANALYSIS/PROBLEM IDENTIFICATION

Analyze Cues and Prioritize Hypotheses: Problem statement for older adults with self-esteem issues includes
- Potential for Decreased Self-esteem

◆ PLANNING

Generate Solutions: The patient goals for older adults with potential for decreased self-esteem are to (1) identify personal strengths, (2) express feelings and concerns, and (3) practice behaviors that promote self-confidence.

◆ IMPLEMENTATION

Take Action: The following nursing interventions should take place in hospitals, in extended-care facilities, and at home:

1. **Explore feelings and concerns.** To plan effective interventions that will improve patients' sense of self-worth, nurses must be aware of their unique concerns and feelings. Allow older adults to discuss their feelings without judging or minimizing them. Nurses who try to "reassure" the patient that everything is okay sometimes create an atmosphere that make patients feel guilty for expressing themselves. Do not use any language suggesting that you think others have it worse.

2. **Demonstrate acceptance of older adults as people with value and self-worth by responding to their concerns, encouraging them to make choices, following through with their requests, and including them in care planning.** Take the time to actually listen and respond to the needs communicated by older adults; that is the best way to demonstrate acceptance. Too often, nurses "listen" and then do something completely different from what the older person had asked for. This is a subtle way of indicating that the person does not matter. If you are unable to comply with the older adult's requests, explain why, so that the reasons will be understood.

3. **Encourage participation in self-care activities.** This allows older adults to retain a sense of self-worth. Even small acts, such as washing one's own face or eating without assistance, can help make the older adult feel some control over their life (Fig. 11.2).

4. **Provide opportunities for reminiscence.** Reminiscence, sometimes called *life review*, is especially important to older adults. Nurses tend to focus on the present. Because there is so much to do, we may not take time to listen to stories of long ago. We are so busy making sure that our patients are oriented to the present that we tend to forget about their past.

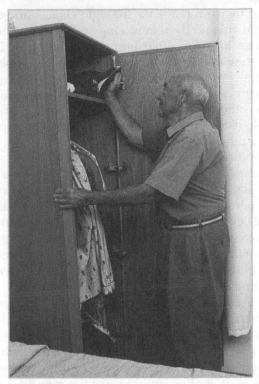

Fig. 11.2 Choosing his own clothes, this long-term resident is actively participating in his own care and is able to retain a sense of self-worth. (From Webb, M., Kostelnick, C., Scott, K. [2018]. *Long-term caring* [4th ed.]. St. Louis, MO: Elsevier.)

All people, particularly older adults, need to feel that their existence has made a difference. As death approaches, older adults need to feel that their lives have had purpose and meaning. Absence of self-worth leads to despair and hopelessness. Erikson stressed the importance of seeing value in the life stories of older adults.

People of all ages reminisce (i.e., think back to earlier times in their lives). This process helps them to work through previous problems and recognize previous successes. It helps to resolve conflicts and enables the older adult to cope with the present and future and to go on with life and living. Life review is not just looking back at the good old times; rather, it is a process of determining that one's life has had value and merit. It is a way to meet the challenges of the present and to prepare for death.

Older adults who have completed a life review, either on their own or with assistance, often gain a certain serenity. They accept that, although not perfect, their lives have been worthwhile. Some find areas of discontent that they are still able to correct: they can still find lost friends, finish incomplete personal business, and make amends. Life review is a healthy process. It is a normal and necessary way in which all individuals, particularly older adults, can maintain positive mental health.

Reminiscing can be done individually or in groups. Older adults who reminisce alone (as many do) are often highly critical of themselves, feeling that they did not make the right choices and do the right things. By reminiscing with others, the true value of a life often becomes more clear. Group sharing may feel less intense than one-on-one communication. In addition, the memories of one group member often trigger similar recollections among the others. Different perspectives on the past can help older adults see themselves and their responses in a different light.

When working with a group of older adults, nurses should ensure that the group is not too large, or some individuals will not have an opportunity to participate. Ideally, 5 to 8 people can effectively participate in a group at one time. It is essential to remain open and actively listen to all the participants. Reminiscence therapy may even be beneficial to individuals suffering from Alzheimer disease by stimulating remnants of long-term memory.

Various devices can be used to stimulate reminiscences. Items such as picture albums and old movies, magazines, newspapers, or songs can be used to start the conversation. Activities such as writing poems, assembling picture albums, making collages, or writing autobiographies may be helpful. Open statements, such as "Tell me about when you started your family" or "Tell me about your job," can be helpful as well.

5. **Encourage the family to participate in reminiscence by providing pictures or items that bring back memories of happy times.** Encourage families to take the opportunity to share their memories of their older members. Many families find boxes of old pictures among the older person's belongings. Sometimes the people and events are familiar; other times they include many unknown and unfamiliar individuals. A review of such pictures often helps trigger memories and enables older adults to show a side of themselves that their adult children and grandchildren may never have known about. Pictures of a smiling young couple kissing, dancing, taking their children to the park, or taking part in any number of other activities can help the older person to remember happy times. It can also help the family to realize that, like themselves, their parents really were young once, facing the same dreams and challenges. This knowledge can help them grow closer and more aware of the continuity of family and can provide an opening for older people and their families to share feelings that they might otherwise feel uncomfortable addressing (Fig. 11.3).

6. **Encourage families to communicate positive feelings to the older person.** Too often, especially at funerals, grief-stricken family members are heard to say, "I wish I had told my mother (or father) how much she (or he) meant to me." The best way to prevent these regrets is to say and do these things when the older person is still alive. It means a lot to all of us to hear that we are appreciated and loved.

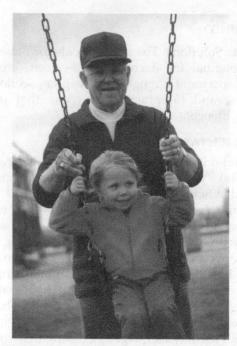

Fig. 11.3 Bringing young and old together is an important contributor to the self-esteem of older adults. (© 2010 Photos.com, a division of Getty Images. All rights reserved.)

It means even more to older adults, who may be questioning whether their lives have had meaning. Young family members may be hesitant to say positive things face-to-face because they assume that the older person knows how they feel or because they just feel awkward saying them.

The greeting card industry has capitalized on this fact by mass producing cards to help people convey feelings they cannot verbalize. Many older adults treasure greeting cards they receive because this is the closest they get to true communication of feelings from family members. Sometimes, families need to be reminded and encouraged to meet the need for support. Anything nurses can do to help families recognize the importance of positive communication will help older adults (Box 11.2).

❖ NURSING PROCESS/CLINICAL JUDGMENT MODEL FOR FEAR

Fear is a feeling of dread or apprehension regarding an identified source. Fear is not unique to older adults, but as their functional abilities decline, their fears may become more obvious. The most common fears identified in older adults include fears of change and disruption in their lives or routines, crime and victimization, loss of loved ones, disease, injury, pain and suffering, loss of independence, financial destitution, and loneliness. It is interesting to note that death is not the most feared item; in fact, many older people express less fear of death than do younger persons (Krause et al., 2018). They may state that they fear the unknown but not death itself.

| Box 11.2 | **Technology to Enhance Communication** |

Technology and computer use among older adults is increasing, and has been shown to have many benefits when encouraged. The following are some benefits that have been identified by research:
- Enhanced self-esteem
- Increased sense of productivity
- Decreased depression
- Improved social interaction
- Improved mental stimulation

The most common types of computer activities studied included word and board-type games, computer art activities, and e-mail communications.

To mediate some age-related changes in vision, hearing, and mobility, computer manufacturers are constantly improving their technology, including features such as touch screens and voice-activated commands.

Social media, including Instagram and WhatsApp, are becoming a more popular method of keeping up with family photos and events. Technology such as FaceTime, and Zoom allows older adults to communicate face to face with loved ones who may live far away. Social integration is another way to help improve older adults' quality of life and self-esteem.

Many even view death as a release from fears and an opportunity to rejoin loved ones.

Fear is closely related to anxiety. Individuals with known fears usually also experience anxiety, although anxiety can occur without a known fear. People respond to fear in different ways. Some might verbalize feelings of helplessness, whereas others might withdraw from contact with people, and still others might respond aggressively. Aggressive responses to fear are often misinterpreted by caregivers as anger. Fear can also result in physiologic symptoms resulting from stimulation of the sympathetic nervous system. Such symptoms include dilated pupils, dry mouth, trembling, elevated blood pressure, increased pulse and respiratory rate, palpitations, diaphoresis, diarrhea, and urinary frequency. The physical symptoms can mimic symptoms associated with a heart attack, which in turn increases the anxiety. Physiologic stimulation caused by high-level anxiety can be dangerous to aging individuals who are already compromised by endocrine, respiratory, cardiovascular, or neurologic disease.

◆ **ASSESSMENT (DATA COLLECTION)**

Recognize cues

See the assessment for altered self-perception and altered self-concept on p. 219.

◆ **DATA ANALYSIS/PROBLEM IDENTIFICATION**

Analyze Cues and Prioritize Hypotheses: Problem statement for older adults who are fearful includes

Fear

◆ **PLANNING**

Generate Solutions: The patient goals for fearful individuals are to (1) identify specific fears, (2) identify coping strategies that were helpful in the past and use these when fears arise, and (3) use strategies that help control fear.

◆ **IMPLEMENTATION**

Take Action: The following interventions should take place in hospitals, in extended-care facilities, and at home:

1. **Provide opportunities for older adults to express their fears.** Fear is debilitating. It stops people from being able to take positive actions. Identifying fears is the first step in dealing with them. If older adults demonstrate signs of fear during care, stop the activity and give the individual the opportunity to express their fears. These fears should then be considered when planning a strategy to reduce or eliminate them. Do not minimize or deny the person's fears. Avoid using clichés such as "Don't worry, we know what we're doing," because such statements convey the idea that the person's feelings are not valid.

2. **Remove or reduce the most common sources of fear.** Each of us is afraid of different things. Fear of falling and fear of loud noises are common from the time of birth. Falling is a very real fear to older adults who require assistance in transfers, particularly transfers that involve hydraulic devices. This fear can be reduced by ensuring that there is adequate help and by providing ongoing reassurance during the transfer.

3. **Provide explanations for all care procedures.** Fear of the unknown is common at all ages. Many activities and treatments that are familiar to nurses are extremely strange and frightening to older adults, who may fear that the procedure will cause bodily harm or pain. Take care to explain why the procedure must be done, what will happen, and what the person can do to help. Explanations do not always remove the fear, but they usually help to reduce it.

❖ **NURSING PROCESS/CLINICAL JUDGMENT MODEL FOR ANXIETY**

Anxiety is an unsettled or uneasy feeling caused by a vague or unidentified threat. Anxiety can be mild, moderate, or severe; in extreme cases, it can reach the level of panic. Anxiety can be acute or chronic. It is more prevalent among older adults than among any other age group, with studies revealing that as many as 37% of older adults report chronic, often debilitating forms of anxiety (Brenes, 2018). Mild anxiety can actually be positive for people, even older adults. A little anxiety keeps people vigilant for potential hazards.

A little anxiety provides the motivation for positive actions, such as seeking health care. A person who had never experienced anxiety would have little reason to plan ahead or take precautions in life. However, persistent or high levels of anxiety can interfere with a person's ability to perceive situations accurately and to respond to them appropriately. Stimulation of the sympathetic nervous system can result when anxiety is felt, which produces physiologic changes identical to those seen with fear.

◆ ASSESSMENT (DATA COLLECTION)

Recognize cues

See the assessment of altered self-perception and altered self-concept on p. 219.

◆ DATA ANALYSIS/PROBLEM IDENTIFICATION

Analyze Cues and Prioritize Hypotheses: Problem statement for older adults experiencing feelings of anxiety includes

Anxiety

◆ PLANNING

Generate Solutions: The patient goals for older adults with anxiety are to (1) identify methods that help reduce anxiety and (2) experience fewer episodes of anxiety.

◆ IMPLEMENTATION

Take Action: The following nursing interventions should take place in hospitals, in extended-care facilities, and at home:

1. **Encourage older adults to verbalize their thoughts and feelings.** Once thoughts and feelings are put into words, individuals are often more able to recognize the causes of their anxiety. Once the causes are recognized, strategies can be designed to help the person cope with anxiety. Nurses can often see patterns in the verbalized thoughts and feelings of anxious people. This perspective is more objective and often helps the person with anxiety gain a better understanding of themselves. Allowing the older person to verbalize anger and irritation or to cry may enable the person to calm down.
2. **Provide a quiet environment and reduce excessive stimulation.** Excessive noise or activity usually increases anxiety. A quiet room with minimal contact and stimulation may help to calm older adults. Reassurance with gentle touch and empathetic communication may also help. Stimulating beverages, such as coffee, should be avoided.
3. **Provide distraction or diversion.** Moderate anxiety may decrease if the individual becomes involved in another activity that they find pleasant. Quiet

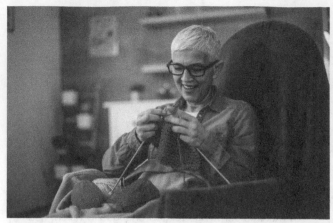

Fig. 11.4　Crafts such as knitting may help to lessen anxiety and keep older adults engaged. (Copyright © istock.com/Nikola Ilic.)

activities—such as listening to music, watching television, or working on a craft—are soothing to many older adults (Fig. 11.4).

❖ NURSING PROCESS/CLINICAL JUDGMENT MODEL FOR DECREASED HOPE

People who feel unable to solve problems or establish goals can sometimes lose hope. They feel that they have no alternatives or choices, even when they can actually control what occurs. Hopeless people express feelings of apathy in response to problems. They are often heard making statements such as "What's the use in trying? Nothing will go right anyway," or "Nothing ever goes right for me." Because people without hope cannot see any possible solutions, they may appear passive and uninterested. They may find it difficult or impossible to solve problems or make decisions. The body language of individuals with decreased hope often reflects despondency. In some cases, these persons may display few emotions (although some respond with anger). Self-destructive behaviors can occur among older adults who are feeling hopeless. Signs of decreased hope include failure to eat, failure to take prescribed medication, and failure to follow up with medical care. In extreme cases, such individuals may become suicidal. The suicide rate among older adults is higher than that in any other age group, with the highest rates among people age 85 and older (Stone et al. 2021). Any older person who demonstrates severe signs of hopelessness should be watched closely. Older adults who feel hopeless and turn to abuse of alcohol or other depressant medications are at higher-than-average risk for suicide.

◆ ASSESSMENT (DATA COLLECTION)

Recognize cues

See the assessment of altered self-perception and altered self-concept on p. 219.

◆ DATA ANALYSIS/PROBLEM IDENTIFICATION

Analyze Cues and Prioritize Hypotheses: Problem statement for older adults who may have lost hope includes

Decreased Hope

◆ PLANNING

Generate Solutions: The patient goal for older adults with decreased hope is to identify activities or interventions that promote hopefulness.

◆ IMPLEMENTATION

Take Action: The following interventions should take place in hospitals, in extended-care facilities, and at home:

1. **Visit older adults frequently, and spend time exploring the factors that contribute to feelings of decreased hope.** It is necessary to spend time with older adults to develop enough trust for them to share their concerns. Regular visits that are not related to direct physical care show that nurses are concerned with the person. This may not always be possible when nurses are tasked with many responsibilities. However, if the nurse demonstrates kindness, compassion, and personability while doing those tasks, the older adult is much more likely to feel respected. This can help patients to verbalize their feelings. Decreased hope is often related to other problems, particularly spiritual distress, grief, and depression. Unless nurses know the specific concerns, it is impossible to design approaches that will help a particular aging individual.

2. **Assess the potential for self-destructive behaviors or suicide.** Take seriously any verbalization of the wish to harm themselves or to attempt suicide. Older adults who are depressed and those who have recently experienced significant loss are at highest risk for suicidal thoughts. Older adults who live alone are more likely to try to take their own lives. Some attempt suicide passively by refusing to eat, refusing medical care, or failing to adhere to medical treatments, such as taking medications. Other older adults choose a very active form of suicide, such as drug overdose, shooting, or hanging (Boxes 11.3 and 11.4).

❖ NURSING PROCESS/CLINICAL JUDGMENT MODEL FOR LOSS OF POWER

Loss of power occurs when older adults feel that they have lost control of what happens to them. Such feelings may result from the loss of control of physical functions or body parts or from loss of a body part. A feeling of powerlessness is common with hospitalization or placement in an extended-care facility. Nurses

---

Box 11.3 Suicide and Older Adults

- At least 7500 people age 65 or older complete suicide each year.
- White men over age 85 are 6 times more likely to complete suicide as compared with the general population.
- Medical illness or chronic disability is a major contributing factor to suicide.
- Social isolation, serious depression, and a history of self-destructive behaviors increase the risk for suicide.
- Life events—such as loss of a loved one, uncontrollable pain, and major life changes such as retirement—increase the risk for suicide.

From: AgingInPlace (2020). Elderly suicide: The risks, detection, and how to help. https://aginginplace.org/ elderly-suicide-risks-detection-how-to-help/.

Box 11.4 Interventions Related to Suicide

ASSESS FOR SIGNS OF DEPRESSION
- Changes in appetite or sleep patterns
- Unexplained fatigue
- Apathy or loss of interest in life
- Trouble concentrating or indecisiveness
- Social withdrawal from family and/or friends
- Loss of interest in normal activities or hobbies
- Loss of interest in personal appearance
- Crying for no apparent reason

ASSESS FOR OTHER BEHAVIOR CHANGES
- Giving away treasured possessions
- Talking about death or suicide
- Taking unusual or unnecessary risks
- Increasing consumption of alcohol or drugs
- Failure to follow through with prescribed medication or meal plan
- Purchase of a weapon

DEMONSTRATE INTEREST AND BECOME INVOLVED WITH THE PERSON
- Take clues of suicide seriously; do not ignore them.
- Ask the person whether they are considering suicide.
- Avoid judgmental statements.
- Offer hope and help the person to find alternatives.
- Promote a safe environment by removing easy suicide methods.
- Seek help from persons or agencies that specialize in suicide prevention.

---

often contribute to feelings of powerlessness by taking over or taking charge of older adults. Doing too much for a person can be just as damaging as doing too little. By their very competence, caregivers can intimidate older adults and destroy any initiative for them to even attempt self-care. Individual dignity and control are too often sacrificed for efficiency. This is particularly true of older adults who require more time to accomplish tasks. It is easier for the staff to do something for older adults than to wait for them to do it.

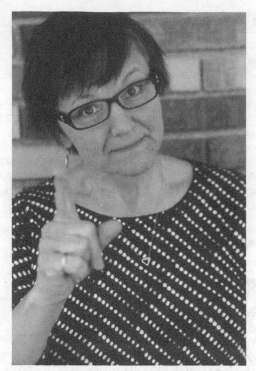

Fig. 11.5 Assertiveness. (Copyright © istock.com/ WhitneyLewisPhotography.)

Life in an institutional setting tends to be regimented and restrictive. To meet the needs of many people, it is easy to lose track of the uniqueness of the individual. The needs of the institution often take priority over the desires of the individual.

Persons who give up control are more at risk for low self-esteem, decreased hope, loss of power, and social isolation than are those who manipulate, argue, or complain to assert some control over their lives (Fig. 11.5).

◆ ASSESSMENT (DATA COLLECTION)

Recognize cues
See the assessment of altered self-perception and altered self-concept on p. 219.

◆ DATA ANALYSIS/PROBLEM IDENTIFICATION

Analyze Cues and Prioritize Hypotheses: Problem statement for older adults experiencing a loss of power includes
   Loss of Power

◆ PLANNING

Generate Solutions: The patient goals for older adults diagnosed with loss of power are to (1) identify actions in which they can exert control and (2) make decisions and have input in the plan of care.

◆ IMPLEMENTATION

Take Action: The following interventions should take place in hospitals, in extended-care facilities, and at home:

1. **Allow older adults to make choices whenever possible.** Even in institutional settings, older adults should be allowed to make choices as often as possible. Menus can be planned to include options, such as sandwiches or salad for people who do not like the main featured menu items. Display a variety of suitable clothing so that individuals can select the articles they desire. Make enough activities available so that people can find those that interests them.

2. **Encourage older adults to do as much as possible for themselves.** When people perform their own care, they feel more in control. Such control of simple things can help maintain a sense of being able to influence what happens.

3. **Adapt the environment to encourage independent activity.** Evaluate the environment, taking into consideration the strengths and limitations of older adults. Many older adults lose their sense of power because things in the environment are outside of their control. When older adults must always ask for things or call on nurses for help, they may feel that the nurses control the situation. Modifying the environment so that all necessary or desired items (e.g., walkers) are close at hand gives control back to older adults. Elevated toilets can reduce the need to call for assistance. Providing snacks and beverages in a readily accessible place, such as a lounge, provides control.

4. **Explain the reasons for any changes in the plan of care.** At times, the plan of care may need to be changed. When this is necessary, inform older adults as soon as the change is known. Explain the reasons for the change so that the person understands that the change occurred because of certain circumstances.

5. **Avoid being overprotective or directive.** Nurses and other caregivers often do not allow older adults to use their abilities. In the name of concern and caring, caregivers do too much for older adults. This can lead to one of two possible outcomes: either the older person becomes angry and tells the caregiver to leave them alone, or the older person gives up and lets the caregiver do everything. In the first case, the person may not get help when it is really needed. In the second, the person is likely to experience a rapid loss of ability. The best approach is a balanced one in which caregivers support and encourage older adults to perform as much for themselves as is safely possible. Unless the situation is harmful, nurses may have to learn to accept less than perfection and avoid redoing what the person has done for themselves. Redoing what has already been done can strip away the older person's dignity and make the person feel incapable and childlike. Therefore provide help only when it is needed and only to the extent that it is needed.

6. **Respect older adults' right to refuse.** The ultimate power held by patients is the right to refuse care. Older adults who are in control of their mental faculties retain this right, and nurses cannot force them to do anything against their wishes. When a person refuses food, care, or medication, the nurse should first determine the reasons for the refusal. Once the reasons are known, develop a plan to reduce or remove the objections. Unless the reasons for refusal are known, all approaches are likely to be unsuccessful. A good explanation of the importance of the treatment or medication can often overcome objections and relieve conflict. In other cases, minor modifications, such as changing the method or timing of medications, will work. For some individuals, consultation with the dietitian, primary health care provider, or other specialist can be helpful in solving the problem. If alert older persons continue to refuse care despite attempts to gain acceptance, accept the refusal. This does not mean that further attempts to gain adherence with the treatment plan cannot or should not be made in later on. When a person refuses some or all parts of their care, document all of the facts of the situation as well as all interventions that were tried.

If older adults are unable to make judgments because of impaired cognitive function, a different situation exists. In these cases, actively involve the families or guardians in planning care. These individuals may be able to suggest ways to get the person to cooperate. People who hold legal guardianship can speak for patients in determining what should be done. Nurses should also discuss these concerns and problems with the primary health care provider. Changes in the plan of care can often reduce or eliminate problems (Nursing Care Plan 11.1).

 Nursing Care Plan 11.1 | Loss of Power

Mrs. Green, age 90, was living independently until recently, when she suffered a fall that resulted in a broken hip. Her family is unable to provide the ongoing care she requires because they, too, are getting old, and they live in a different state. Mrs. Green is a new resident of the long-term care facility in which you work. She is very passive and allows the staff to do everything for her despite the fact that she is capable of doing many things for herself. She does not express any feelings or preferences about her care, meals, or anything else. When asked about her perceptions, she says, "It doesn't matter. You'll do whatever you want anyway." She prefers to remain in her room.

PROBLEM STATEMENT
Loss of Power

SUPPORTING ASSESSMENT DATA
- Passive behavior
- Dependence on others
- Apathetic responses
- Verbalization of lack of control
- Nonparticipation in care

PATIENT GOALS/OUTCOMES IDENTIFICATION
Mrs. Green will participate in decision-making regarding her care and identify actions within her control.

NURSING INTERVENTIONS/IMPLEMENTATION
1. Visit daily for 10 to 15 minutes to allow Mrs. Green to verbalize her feelings and concerns.
2. Respect Mrs. Green's right to private space. Allow her to choose what belongings she wants and where she wants them.
3. Actively include her in care planning, present her with options, and then follow through with her choices.
4. Explain the reasons for any changes that must be made.
5. Keep the call light handy and respond promptly when called.
6. Meet her requests promptly.
7. Encourage participation in personal care.
8. Help her to identify areas in which she can retain control.

EVALUATION
The nursing assistant reports that Mrs. Green is demonstrating more assertive behaviors, such as insisting on choosing her own clothing and stating her preferences regarding meals. She has been heard saying, "I will do that later, when I am ready." You will continue the plan of care.

APPLYING CLINICAL JUDGMENT
As her hip has healed, Mrs. Green's behavior has changed, and she is now described by the staff as being demanding and critical.
1. What do you think has caused the change in behavior?
2. How could you assess and validate your conclusions?

Get Ready for the Next Generation NCLEX® Examination!

Key Points

- Age-related and disease-related changes affect older adults' self-images; societal values and life experiences also play a role.
- Self-concept is closely related to the older person's values, beliefs, roles, and relationships.
- When older adults suffer losses in any important area of life, self-concept is threatened.
- If older adults are able to maintain a sense of self-worth and personal value, few problems occur.
- If older adults believe that they are of little value, fear, anxiety, decreased hope, and loss of power can result.
- Disturbances in self-concept and self-esteem can significantly affect the older adult's response to care.
- Nurses must listen closely to what older adults have to say about themselves.
- Measures should be taken to provide emotional support, enhance personal control, and promote self-esteem in older adults.

Additional Learning Resources

SG Go to your Evolve website at http://evolve.elsevier.com/Williams/geriatric for the additional online resources.

🌐 Internet Resources

- Evidence-Based Practices KIT: Depression and Older Adults: www.aipc.net.au/articles/what-causes-depression-in-the-elderly/
- https://www.nimh.nih.gov/health/publications/older-adults-and-depression/index.shtml
- Promoting Psychological Health and Suicide Prevention among Older Adults during COVID-19 Promoting Psychological Health and Suicide Prevention among Older Adults during COVID-19
- https://www.psychologytoday.com/us/blog/caring-the-caregivers/202002/anxiety-and-panic-in-older-people

Review Questions for the Next Generation NCLEX® Examination

1. What action(s) can the nurse take to help increase self-esteem in older adults? *(Select all that apply.)*
   a. Remind the older adult that their life wasn't as hard as they remember.
   b. Schedule time to sit and listen to older adults talk about their concerns.
   c. Develop activities that allow older adults to reminisce about their lives.
   d. Provide as much help with ADLs as possible to ensure that your patients feel some sense of control.
   e. Allow older adults to make choices during the day regarding their schedule and ADLs.

2. Which behavioral change does the nurse identify that may indicate a patient is depressed? *(Select all that apply.)*
   a. Increased alcohol consumption
   b. Changes in daily routines
   c. Agitation and irritability
   d. Isolation and withdrawal
   e. More frequent calls to family
   f. Reports of palpitations, trembling, and dry mouth

3. Which is true of suicide risk in the older adult?
   a. Older adults complete suicide less frequently and less violently than people in other age groups.
   b. Women over the age of 80 with chronic illness have the highest suicide risk.
   c. Older adults attempt suicide at a higher rate than those in other age groups but are less successful.
   d. Suicide is often triggered by pain, a recent loss, or a stressful life event affecting the older adult.

4. Which phrase spoken by an older adult warrants further assessment by the nurse of their self-perception or self-esteem?
   a. "I need help now."
   b. "I can't do anything right anymore."
   c. "I wish I were young again."
   d. "I can't do things like I used to."

5. Which intervention is appropriate for an older adult experiencing anxiety or fear?
   a. Place the resident in a populated area to make sure that they are not alone.
   b. Find a quiet activity in which to involve the person.
   c. Discourage talking about their feelings so the anxiety does not get worse.
   d. Identify coping strategies that have helped in the past.
   e. Provide explanations of any procedures that are being done.

6. A 70-year old female is being seen by her primary health care provider at the request of her daughter. Her daughter reports that her mother seems confused and depressed after the recent loss of her husband of 50 years. The patient's last exam was 2 months prior, with the following data recorded. VS: T 97.8, HR 52, R 18, BP 118/72; Weight 136 lb. Health care provider Notes: Patient seen for annual exam, immunization, and titers prior to cruise. Pt interactive and discussing trip. Pain 2/10 for chronic arthritic pain to hands.

   Highlight or place a check mark next to the assessment findings that require follow up by the nurse.
   a. Temperature = 98.2 F
   b. Heart rate = 56 bpm
   c. Respirations = 21 per minute
   d. Weight = 118 lb
   e. Pain = 2/10
   f. Patient has difficulty answering questions
   g. Patient restless and tearful
   h. Daughter reports increased use of sleep aides by the patient

REFERENCES

AgingInPlace (2020). Elderly suicide: The risks, detection, and how to help. https://aginginplace.org/elderly-suicide-risks-detection-how-to-help/

Brenes, G. A., Divers, J., Miller, M. E., & Danhauer, S. C. (2018). A randomized preference trial of cognitive-behavioral therapy and yoga for the treatment of worry in anxious older adults. *Contemporary Clinical Trials Communications, 10*, 169–176.

Caceres, B. A., Travers, J., Primiano, J. E., Luscombe, R. E., & Dorsen, C. (2020). Provider and LGBT individuals' perspectives on LGBT issues in long-term care: A systematic review. *Gerontologist, 60*(3), e169–e183. doi:10.1093/geront/gnz012. PMID: 30726910; PMCID: PMC7117618.

Cranley, L. A., Slaughter, S. E., Caspar, S., Heisey, M., Huang, M., Killackey, T., & McGilton, K. S. (2020). Strategies to facilitate shared decision-making in long-term care. *International Journal of Older People Nursing, 15*(3), e12314. doi:10.1111/opn.12314. Epub 2020 Mar 20. PMID: 32196984; PMCID: PMC7507187.

Depression and Bipolar Support Alliance (2020). Depression statistics. https://www.dbsalliance.org/education/depression/statistics/#_depression-and-the-_elderly

Hwang, T., Rabheru, K., Peisah, C., Reichman, W., & Ikeda, M. (2020). Loneliness and social isolation during the COVID-19 pandemic. *International Psychogeriatrics, 32*(10), 1217–1220. doi:10.1017/S1041610220000988

Krause, N., Pargament, K. I., & Ironson, G. (2018). In the shadow of death: Religious hope as a moderator of the effects of age on death anxiety. *The Journals of Gerontology: Series B, 73*(4), 696–703, May 2018. doi:https://doi.org/10.1093/geronb/gbw039

Kris, A. E., Henkel, L. A., & Roberto, A. (2019). Use of simulation to develop students' skills in reminiscence research. *The International Journal of Reminiscence and Life Review, 6*(1), 16–20.

Kupka, N. (2020). How to recognize and address the signs of depression in your aging parent. *Mental Health America*. https://mhanational.org/blog/how-recognize-and-address-signs-depression-your-aging-parent

Mendoza, M. A. (2020). Why do the elderly commit suicide? *Psychology Today*. https://www.psychologytoday.com/us/blog/understanding-grief/202001/why-do-the-elderly-commit-suicide

Montayre, J., Thaggard, S., & Carney, M. (2020). Views on the use of the term "elder orphans": A qualitative study. *Health & Social Care in the Community, 28*(2), 341–346. doi:10.1111/hsc.12865. Epub 2019 Oct 1. PMID: 31571322.

Orth, U., Erol, R. Y., & Luciano, E. C. (2018). Development of self-esteem from age 4 to 94 years: A meta-analysis of longitudinal studies. *Psychological Bulletin, 144*(10), 1045–1080. doi:https://doi.org/10.1037/bul0000161

Ravary, A., Stewart, E. K., & Baldwin, M. W. (2019). Insecurity about getting old: Age-contingent self-worth, attentional bias, and well-being. *Aging and Mental Health, 24*(10), 1636–1644. doi:10.1080/13607863.2019.1636202. Epub 2019 Jul 8. PMID: 31282182.

Samsudin, E. Z., Isahak, M., Rampal, S., Rosnah, I., & Zakaria, M. I. (2020). Individual antecedents of workplace victimisation: The role of negative affect, personality and self-esteem in junior doctors' exposure to bullying at work. *International Journal of Health Planning and Management, 35*(5), 1065–1082. doi:10.1002/hpm.2985. Epub 2020 May 28. PMID: 32468617.

Stone, D. M., Jones, C. M., & Mack, K. A. (2021). Changes in suicide rates—United States, 2018-2019. *Morbidity and mortality weekly report, 70*(8), 261–268. doi:https://doi.org/10.15585/mmwr.mm7008a1

Wilson, D. M., Errasti-Ibarrondo, B., & Low, G. (2021). Where are we now in relation to determining the prevalence of ageism in this era of escalating population ageing? *Ageing Research Reviews, 51*, 78–84. doi:10.1016/j.arr.2019.03.001. Epub 2019 Mar 9. PMID: 30858070.

World Health Organization (2018). *Ageing and health*. https://www.who.int/news-room/fact-sheets/detail/ageing-and-health

12 Roles and Relationships

Objectives

1. Describe normal roles and relationships.
2. Discuss how patterns of roles and relationships change with aging.
3. Describe methods of assessing changes in roles and relationships.
4. Identify older adults who are most at risk for experiencing problems related to changes in roles and relationships.
5. Describe how grief and complex grief can affect the older adult who has experienced losses.
6. Select appropriate problem statements related to role or relationship changes.
7. Describe nursing interventions that are appropriate for older adults experiencing problems related to changing roles and relationships.

Key Terms

complex grief (p. 234)
grief (p. 234)
heterogeneous (p. 231)
homogeneous (p. 231)

loneliness (p. 236)
relationships (p. 230)
role (p. 230)
social isolation (p. 236)

NORMAL ROLES AND RELATIONSHIPS

A **role** is a socially accepted behavior pattern. People tend to establish their identities and to describe themselves based on their roles in life. Man, woman, husband, wife, adult, senior citizen, parent, child, son, daughter, student, teacher, doctor, nurse, worker, and housewife are some common roles. People play many roles over a lifetime and often must attempt to play several roles simultaneously.

Roles are identified, defined, and given value by the society in which a person lives. Each member of society learns the status of various roles and learns to expect certain behaviors, symbols, and relationships that are acceptable for each role. These behaviors, symbols, and relationship patterns can differ widely, depending on the values and norms of the society in which the individual lives. The value assigned by society indicates the status of each role. Those in high status roles generally possess more privileges and receive more rewards. For example, modern society gives bosses higher status than employees; teachers higher status than students; employed persons higher status than unemployed persons; and younger, more productive members of society higher status than older, retired members.

🌐 Cultural Considerations

Asian and Pacific Islanders

- Asian and Pacific Islanders include more than 20 distinct ethnic groups.
- Many of these groups are influenced by the teachings of Confucius, which dictate the importance of the family over the individual (Kwan, 2021).
- In keeping with this, children are expected to exhibit "filial piety," a concept from Confucianism that emphasizes obedience and devotion to one's parents and ancestors, including honoring and caring for aging parents in the home (Sin, 2021).
- Belief in this concept may cause a great deal of conflict and guilt for younger family members who have become Americanized in their lifestyles.

Relationships are connections formed by the dynamic interaction of individuals who play interrelated roles. Studies have shown that if someone has a strong, positive social network it is associated with an improved quality of life (Moseley & Hammond, 2021). Most people develop a wide range of relationships within their families, at work, and during their day-to-day social activities. The way individuals occupying each role and interact with one another describes their relationships. Relationships can be short-term or long-term, personal or impersonal, intimate or superficial.

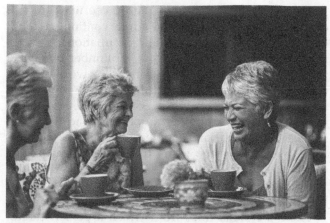

Fig. 12.1 Social networks improve quality of life. (Copyright © istock.com/PeopleImages.)

Relationships change over time and are affected by the role changes of the people involved (Fig. 12.1).

Each culture and subculture sets standards for designated roles and relationships. People in various roles or relationships are expected to behave in accord with accepted standards, which include things such as the amount and type of clothing or jewelry that are deemed appropriate. Standards specify the type of housing, the means of transportation, and even the type and amount of food consumed. Standards specify how individuals in the culture relate to each other in social and work situations. For example, the role perception for a traditional middle-class American businessman is that he is expected to wear a suit and tie with minimal jewelry, live in an apartment or house in the suburbs, drive a conventional car, eat healthful meals, show up for work on time, and demonstrate respect to the boss. If this businessman showed up late for work on a motorcycle, clad in jeans and a sweatshirt and wearing an earring, and if he was later observed eating a hamburger at his desk and telling his boss not to "bug" him, most people would be shocked. Yet this same behavior is not considered atypical for a college student, even one who is studying to be a businessman.

A simple, or homogeneous, society is one in which all members share a common historical and cultural experience. There is little confusion or conflict in a homogeneous social system because the symbols, behaviors, and relationships are perceived in the same way by all members of the society. Everyone knows the accepted roles and how people in each role are expected to relate to each other. Therefore there is little question and few problems with regard to role or relationship expectations.

A more complex, or heterogeneous, society is one in which the members of many diverse subcultures with different historical and cultural experiences must interact. These subcultures may have their origin in race, religion, ethnic heritage, or age. Because subcultures do not share the same experiences, their symbols, behaviors, roles, and relationships are not perceived in the same way by all members of the larger society. Roles and role expectations are not always clear, and this lack of shared perceptions often leads to misunderstandings, confusion, and conflict.

The American culture is very heterogeneous and is becoming even more so. Problems are likely to occur when people with different role and relationship perceptions are required to interact with each other. The greater the differences in role perceptions, role symbols, and role relationships, the greater the likelihood that cross-cultural misunderstandings will occur. This explains the confusion or stress that some people experience when they interact with individuals of different ages or from different cultural backgrounds. It also explains why a person who was raised in a specific culture might be more comfortable with similar individuals and may find it difficult to establish close relationships with people from different cultural backgrounds. Furthermore, it explains why people of different ages may have difficulty understanding each other. The diversity of the population sometimes contributes to the prevalence of role and relationship problems in contemporary American society.

However, this is not the only role or relationship issue people face. In addition to the interpersonal conflict or confusion seen in modern society, individuals can also experience internal role conflict and confusion. Problems occur when the demands of multiple roles and relationships must be met at the same time, particularly when the expectations of one role conflict with those of another. For example, a woman today is often expected to be wife, mother, and employee. She may be expected to keep up the home, prepare meals, supervise the children, be active in school or community programs, be a social and sexual companion to her spouse, and be a productive worker, capable of doing everything, while working with everyone, and always arriving on time with a smile on her face. Unless today's woman is superwoman, she is bound to fall short of all these expectations.

Because people form their self-images based on their roles and relationships, they may have difficulty accepting changes in either. Our identity and sense of self are threatened when roles are lost and the relationships associated with those roles change. The longer the role was held and the more intense the relationships, the greater the grief might be. When someone experiences role change, symbols and indicators of that role and status also change. Loss of symbols or status is often as painful as loss of the role. People may grieve a change of role or loss of relationship as much as they grieve the loss of a loved one.

ROLES, RELATIONSHIPS, AND AGING

The longer a person occupies a particular role, the more familiar and, consequently, more comfortable the person becomes with it. The more comfortable people are in their roles and relationships, the harder it might be for them to adjust to changes.

Older adults must adjust to many predictable role and relationship changes associated with aging, including retirement, altered relationships with adult children, changes in housing, loss of valued possessions, loss of friends resulting from relocation or death, loss of a spouse to death, loss of health, and loss of independence. All of these changes and losses are potentially traumatic to older adults.

Some older adults resent the fact that society forces them to retire. Age 65 was once the typical retirement age, but that is no longer the case. This change has occurred partially for financial reasons but also because many older people do not want to retire. Such people feel that they would lose too much of their identity if they retired. They say, "I don't know what I would do if I couldn't work." Older adults who do retire may adjust well or poorly, depending on the adequacy of their other roles to keep them satisfied. In general, the more roles and relationships that people develop at younger ages, the better able they will be to adjust when some of those roles and relationships are lost.

When an occupational role no longer exists, the individual often grieves its loss. Many people look forward to retirement; but once retired, they find that they miss both the status that their working role gave them and the interactions with other people that it afforded. They often resent the fact that they are no longer viewed as productive, contributing members of society. They are no longer lawyers, plumbers, nurses, or teachers; they are just retired people.

The baby boomer generation may revise this view of roles and retirement. Perhaps the fact that many have changed jobs and even careers several times during their working years has given them a different perspective on what they can do with the rest of their lives. Either from desire or necessity, a larger percentage of this cohort plans continues to work after retirement—at the highest rate seen in 50 years (Fry, 2019). Some need to continue to work because of loss of pensions or retirement investments owing to a downturn in the economy. Others want to work and "try something new" or "stay active and engaged." Many expect to never fully retire and plan to work as long as their health permits. Many people who are not interested in remaining employed after they retire make plans to volunteer, travel, or seek other outlets for their energy.

❓ Did You Know?

Early baby boomers seem to be having less difficulty adjusting to retirement than those who preceded them. Many report being highly satisfied with their lives and are in many cases developing new roles and forming new relationships. A common comment heard from this group is, "I don't know how I ever had time to work full-time. I've got too many things to do." This is more likely to be the case for those who have entered retirement in good health and with substantial economic resources. Only time will tell if this pattern continues.

To maintain a connection with those who are still employed, many retired older adults continue to think of themselves as tied to their occupation. A nurse remains a nurse throughout life, a plumber remains a plumber, and so on. Even if they have not worked in the occupation for years, older adults typically continue to identify with their previous occupational roles. This may be particularly obvious among older adult professionals (e.g., physicians, lawyers, professors, and ministers) who never stop using their titles. Many expect to retain the same status level and respect as they had when they were actively employed, and they may be highly insulted if this respect is not forthcoming.

There are some roles from which a person cannot officially "retire." Homemaker is one such role. Older persons who have spent the largest part of their lives managing a home, doing the cooking, cleaning, sewing, and other duties required of a homemaker, may feel lost when they are forced by circumstances of ill health or finances to give up the home. Some older adult homemakers have few other roles and feel a great sense of loss when they are institutionalized. Those who took the time to develop hobbies or social interests and relationships outside of the home tend to adapt better than do those who had no interests other than their homes.

Older adults do not give up the role of parent just because their children are adults. A parent is usually identified as being someone who is self-sufficient and in control. Role conflict and altered family relationships are likely to occur when older adults attempt to continue to direct their children's behavior long after the children have reached adulthood or when the parents lose the ability to function independently and are forced to become dependent on their children. Successful adjustment to changes in the parenting role is difficult and requires a great deal of patience, tact, and accommodation on the part of all family members. Families who have a history of altered parenting or poorly developed family relationships are likely to have serious problems, often leading to abuse or isolation of the older person from the family.

In addition to being the parent of adult children, many older adults are grandparents. The role of grandparent is often described as being much more pleasant than that of parent. As one grandmother said, "I can have all of the fun and enjoyment of children without the responsibility." Another grandmother replied, "Yes, it's nice when they come to visit, but it's also nice when you can send them home."

Grandparenting allows older adults to share their wisdom and experience with a new, young generation. Because grandparents are often under less daily stress and are not the primary disciplinarians of the children, they are usually more relaxed and have more time to spend on nonessential activities, such as conversation and play (Fig. 12.2). It is common for retired grandparents with time on their hands to entertain children with stories or teach the grandchildren skills,

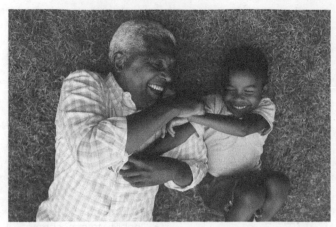

Fig. 12.2 Grandparenting. (Copyright © istock.com/monkeybusinessimages)

hobbies, or games that they learned as children. When positive interactions take place between grandparents and grandchildren, a close bond is often formed that benefits both parties (Fig. 12.3). Mobility and the resulting separation of family members often make it difficult for this relationship to develop. Divorce or separation of the child's parents can also impede the grandparent-grandchild relationship from fully developing. Whether the challenges are geographic or due to disruption of the family, it is vitally important for families to make the extra effort to foster this special grandparent-grandchild relationship. If not, both parties are usually worse off because they cannot benefit from knowing one another.

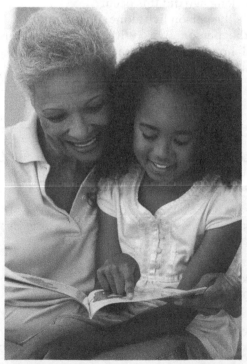

Fig. 12.3 An older woman reads with her grandchild. (Copyright © istock.com/monkeybusinessimages.)

Many older people have occupied the role of spouse for 30, 40, 50, or more years. With the death of a partner, these people are deprived of a significant role and relationship. Marriage is one of the most personal and intimate relationships. A successful long-term marriage requires a great deal of effort; the loss of this intensely personal relationship triggers a high level of emotional distress. Many widowed older adults experience severe grief and become socially isolated as a result of the loss. They describe themselves as feeling as though a part of them were missing, of feeling "half alive." Many widows and widowers find their grief to be so overwhelming that they cannot even continue to perform the normal activities of daily living (ADLs).

The loss of friends because of relocation or death also results in changed social roles and relationships. Many activities require more than one person to be fun. Many older adults have formed friendships or social groups over the years. As more and more of the members move away or die, the older person is likely to become increasingly socially isolated. Older people who outlive their families and friends often feel that their lives are without purpose.

Many older adults change housing arrangements either out of choice or necessity. The home may be too big, too expensive, or too difficult to maintain. This is particularly true when the health of one or both occupants fails or when a widowed older adult is unable to keep up the home after losing their spouse. Moving to smaller accommodations commonly necessitates the sale or distribution of personal possessions accumulated over a lifetime. This loss of possessions makes the process of moving even more traumatic for older adults. In some ways, they are "giving away" their lives.

Loss of health and loss of independence are probably the most traumatic losses because they involve changes in the very essence of who people are. When older adults lose their health and independence, they lose control over their destinies. They are at the mercy of others (either family or strangers) for care and sustenance.

As previously discussed, societies establish and define the boundaries of various roles. Individuals are judged by how well they understand and comply with their assigned roles. "Old person" is a role that has many connotations and expected behaviors. In contemporary American society, an ageist definition of the role of older adults would include adjectives such as *helpless, infirm, cranky,* and *useless.* Some older adults accept this stereotype and act the part. However, many older adults are continuing to pursue their productive roles and maintaining successful relationships well into their 80s and 90s. Indeed, it appears that the baby boomer generation is starting to reinvent aging and breaking the old stereotypes. A significant proportion of entrepreneurs are baby boomer retirees, and they are making up one of the fastest-growing segments of the online dating community, having doubled its size over the past 5 years (RetirementLiving.com, 2021). Just as they have been challenging societal norms from early youth, baby boomers are likely to redefine the meaning and intent of life's later years.

❖ NURSING PROCESS/CLINICAL JUDGMENT MODEL FOR COMPLEX GRIEF

Grief is a strong emotion. It is a combination of sorrow, loss, and confusion that one feels on losing someone or something of value. This reaction can come in response to the loss of a person, a role, a relationship, one's health, or one's independence.

Grief affects a person's thoughts, emotions, and behavior and creates a wide range of physical sensations. The normal grief response follows a somewhat predictable pattern, although the amount of time any given individual needs to work through a loss differs (Table 12.1). Dr. Elisabeth Kübler-Ross, a noted psychiatrist and pioneer in near-death studies, recognized a 5-stage grief process that may be experienced by dying patients. This grief process has also been applied to people who have lost loved ones. The 5 stages are denial, anger, bargaining, depression, and acceptance. (See Chapter 15 for further discussion of Dr. Kübler-Ross and her work.)

Grief is normal after the loss of a significant role or relationship (Box 12.1). Grieving becomes complex when the person experiences an exaggerated or prolonged period of grief. Continued sadness, anger, or denial is indicative of poorly resolved grief. Often, grief is so severe that it prevents the person from functioning normally. Older people experiencing **complex grief** may completely shut themselves off from normal support systems and feel a profound sense of detachment. They may lose interest in all activities and even fail to perform the basic ADLs.

Box 12.1 Normal Loss/Grief Reactions

PHYSICAL
- Persistent fatigue
- Tightness in chest
- Muscle weakness
- Shortness of breath
- Susceptibility to minor illnesses
- Hypersensitivity to noise
- Dry mouth
- Headaches
- Grinding teeth
- Tension
- Nausea
- Hyperacidity
- Dizziness
- Sadness
- Guilt
- Shock
- Helplessness
- Apathy

EMOTIONAL
- Anger
- Anxiety
- Ambivalence
- Depression
- Fear
- Irritability
- Loneliness
- Numbness
- Panic

COGNITIVE
- Confusion
- Forgetfulness
- Disorientation
- Disbelief
- Preoccupation
- Decreased attention
- Inability to concentrate

BEHAVIORAL
- Absentmindedness
- Crying
- Decreased motivation
- Restlessness
- Social isolation
- Inconsistency
- Irritability
- Diminished productivity
- Sleep disturbances
- Appetite disturbances

◆ ASSESSMENT (DATA COLLECTION)

Recognize cues
- What is the person's marital status (i.e., single, married, widowed, divorced)?
- If the person has lost a spouse or significant other, how long ago did this occur?
- Does the person live alone or with others?
- If the person lives with others, who are they, and how are they related? What is the family structure?

Table 12.1 Phases of Grieving

Shock and Numbness (First 2 Weeks)	
Feelings: Disbelief, denial, anger, guilt	*Behaviors*: Crying, searching, sighing, loss of appetite, sleep disturbance, limited concentration, muscle weakness, inability to make decisions, emotional outbursts
Searching and Yearning (2 Weeks to 4 Months)	
Feelings: Despair, apathy, depression, anger, guilt, hopelessness, self-doubt	*Behaviors*: Restlessness, poor memory, impatience, lack of concentration, crying, social isolation, loss of energy
Disorientation (4 to 7 Months)	
Feelings: Depression, guilt, disorganization	*Behaviors*: Resistance to seeking help or reaching out to others, trying to live as if nothing happened, restlessness, irritability
Reorganization (Up to 18 to 24 Months)	
Feelings: Sense of release, decreased sense of obsession with loss, renewed hope and optimism	*Behaviors*: Renewed energy, reorganization of eating and sleeping habits, improved judgment, renewed interest in activities and goals for the future

Grieving.com (2020). [Data from Glen Davidson MD.]. *Processing sudden loss*, Available at https://forums.grieving.com/index.php?/topic/1339-processing-loss-informative-article/

- How does the person describe relationships within the family?
- What family interactions have you or others observed?
- Does the person belong to any social groups?
- Do they have close relationships with friends?
- Is the person employed? What are the relationships at work?
- Have they person retired from work? How long ago? What are their feelings regarding retirement? What do they person do to occupy their time?
- Does the person feel a sense of belonging to the community or neighborhood?
- If in a long-term care setting, have they established relationships with other residents?
- Has the person recently relocated from home to an acute care setting? From home to an extended-care facility? From one unit or room to another?
- Do they spend a great deal of time alone?
- Does the person speak excessively with others or remain silent?
- Do they exhibit signs of withdrawal, anger, depression, sorrow, fear, or shock?
- Has the person verbalized concerns regarding the loss of persons, a job, or abilities?
- Has their sleep or eating patterns changed?
- Has their ability to concentrate changed?

Box 12.2 provides a list of risk factors for problems related to changes in roles and relationships in older adults.

◆ **DATA ANALYSIS/PROBLEM IDENTIFICATION**

Analyze Cues and Prioritize Hypotheses: Problem statement for the older adult who is grieving includes

    Complex Grief

◆ **PLANNING**

Generate Solutions: The patient goals for older individuals experiencing complex grief are to (1) verbalize their grief, (2) use available support systems, and (3) participate in ADLs.

◆ **IMPLEMENTATION**

Take Action: The following nursing interventions should take place in hospitals, in extended-care facilities, and at home:

1. **Establish a trusting relationship to encourage verbalization of feelings regarding the change or loss.** Before sharing their true feelings, older adults must develop trust in their nurses. Trust comes only when they believe that the nurses truly care about them as unique human beings and that the nurses will be understanding and sensitive to their feelings. It takes time and effort to develop trust.

Trust cannot be forced. It may take days, weeks, or even months for people experiencing grief to share their deepest feelings. Although trust cannot be forced,

 QSEN Considerations: Patient-Centered Care

Actions that promote trust:
- Spend time with the person.
- Actively listen to what they have to say.
- Address the person by name.
- Smile.
- Use a warm, friendly voice.
- Make appropriate eye contact.
- Respond honestly to questions.
- Provide consistency of care.
- Respect confidentiality.
- Follow through on commitments.

nurses can take actions to promote its development. These actions are summarized in the preceding box headed "Patient-Centered Care."

2. **Assess the source and acknowledge the reality of the grief.** Grief is very much like pain. It is a complex and personal emotion. Because most people find it difficult to deal with grief, they avoid grieving persons and avoid discussing anything that approaches the source of the grief. These behaviors leave the problem unresolved. To help with grief, it is essential that the grieving person identify and confront the loss. Nurses can help by spending time with grieving individuals and giving them an opportunity to verbalize their grief. Once older adults are able to verbalize and acknowledge their grief, nurses can use problem-solving methods to help them develop coping strategies.

3. **Encourage older adults to participate in ADLs.** Individuals experiencing complex grief are often totally preoccupied with their loss. Although this preoccupation is understandable, it is incompatible with normal living. The more such individuals are able to maintain contact with day-to-day activities, the sooner they will be able to go on with their lives. Nurses can help by providing structure to the day. A plan of care that allows for preferences while setting limits will help to provide this structure. A daily schedule that is well planned and predictable often enables grieving older adults to regain some control and to cope with the changes.

Box 12.2	**Risk Factors Related to Changes in Roles and Relationships Among Older Adults**

- Recent loss of a spouse, child, close friend, significant other, or cherished pet
- Recent loss of lifelong or valuable roles
- Recent major adjustment in living situation
- Inability to perform familiar roles owing to loss of functional abilities

To help motivate positive behaviors, provide encouragement and positive feedback for participation in daily activities.

4. **Identify sources of support.** Although nurses can provide some support to older adults experiencing grief, many other people can also help. Family, friends, spiritual advisers, counselors, therapists, and support groups are all valuable sources. Many pamphlets, books, and other materials are available to help people who are experiencing grief. Many can be found in libraries, medical offices, or other locations where older adults congregate.

❖ NURSING PROCESS/CLINICAL JUDGMENT MODEL FOR LONELINESS AND POTENTIAL FOR SOCIAL ISOLATION

Loneliness, the sense of being alone, is a common problem among older adults; it can lead to serious physical and psychosocial health problems. Studies have identified a link between loneliness and the risk of malnutrition (Besora-Moreno et al., 2020). In addition, loneliness can potentially lead to social isolation. It is estimated that between one-third and one-half of older adults in the community experience social isolation (Blazer, 2020). Such individuals are likely to be uncommunicative and withdrawn and to have few visitors or other social interactions. Social isolation is a result of many factors and can be unintentional or intentional. The more people are separated from family and friends, the greater the potential for social isolation.

Most social isolation is unintentional. Separation resulting from death is a common and unavoidable part of aging. Many older people simply outlive their families and friends. These people are likely to become isolated unless they establish new social outlets. Separation resulting from relocation is also common. Today, it is unusual for family members to remain in a single community. Young family members often move to find job opportunities; older family members may move to retirement communities.

Decreased physical mobility and limited finances can lead to potential for social isolation. Physical changes can restrict an older person's ability to move about and make social contacts. Financial limitations can lead to separation from others because of the lack of adequate money to buy appropriate clothing or transportation to social activities.

Intentional isolation is less common and is most likely to occur when older adults fear not being accepted by others. Those who suffer from grief may be too upset or absorbed in their own problems to interact with others. Older adults experiencing changes in body image from procedures such as amputation or colostomy may also isolate themselves from others. Older people who have cognitive or perceptual problems may isolate themselves because they do not understand what is going on around them.

◆ ASSESSMENT (DATA COLLECTION)

Recognize cues
See the assessment for complex grief earlier in the chapter.

◆ DATA ANALYSIS/PROBLEM IDENTIFICATION

Analyze Cues and Prioritize Hypotheses: Problem statements for older adults experiencing loneliness include
　Loneliness
　Potential for Social Isolation

◆ PLANNING

Generate Solutions: The patient goals for older individuals with loneliness and potential for social isolation are to (1) demonstrate increased participation in social activities, (2) identify actions or resources that will help reduce the potential for social isolation, and (3) maintain healthy eating habits.

◆ IMPLEMENTATION

Take Action: The following nursing interventions should take place in hospitals, in extended-care facilities, and at home:
1. **Assess the reason or reasons for the loneliness and potential for social isolation.** Because many factors can lead to potential for social isolation, nurses should identify those that affect each individual. Tailor nursing interventions toward solving specific problems.
2. **Promote social contact and interaction. Telephone calls and mail can be used to maintain contact with family and friends.** Those with computers may stay in touch using email, social media, or internet communication tools. The nurse can ensure that telephones are readily available and located so that older adults can have privacy yet comfort when using them (Fig. 12.4). Telephones should be

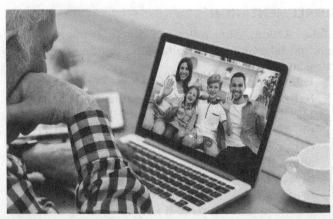

Fig. 12.4　An older adult maintaining social contact by using technology. (Copyright © istock.com/Prostock-Studio.)

equipped with amplifiers for those who are hard of hearing. Ensure that mail is delivered promptly. Offer help to visually impaired older adults in reading mail. Adjust computer screens to display large-type characters if needed.

Social rooms and lounges should be available for older adults to use for visits. If the individual is confined to bed, provide privacy to conduct visits in the room.

Information about all activities in a facility should be well communicated to older adult residents. Offer encouragement to those who are reluctant to participate in activities.

Careful planning is needed to prevent older individuals with restricted physical mobility from becoming socially isolated. Schedule care activities to allow for adequate time for social interaction. Provide for any needed assistance to enable participation in social activities.

3. **Spend one-on-one time with the lonely or isolated person.** Those who cannot or will not participate in social interaction need extra attention from the nursing staff. One-on-one interaction, even for brief intervals during the day, helps lonely or isolated people maintain some social contact. Over time, nurses can attempt to motivate these individuals to try other forms of social contact.

4. **Initiate referrals.** Often, the social worker, chaplain, or activities department can help older adults with potential for social isolation to identify acceptable social activities.

5. **Monitor nutritional status.** Ensure that the older adult experiencing loneliness and social isolation maintains adequate intake of nutritious food and does not experience a nutritional decline.

❖ NURSING PROCESS/CLINICAL JUDGMENT MODEL FOR ALTERED FAMILY FUNCTIONING

Normal changes in family dynamics were discussed in Chapter 1. When older adults or their families verbalize concern or confusion related to a change in roles or relationships, family dynamics should be assessed. Alterations in family functioning can occur at any age but are most common when an aging family member becomes dependent.

◆ ASSESSMENT (DATA COLLECTION)

Recognize cues
See the assessment for complex grief earlier in the chapter.

◆ DATA ANALYSIS/PROBLEM IDENTIFICATION

Analyze Cues and Prioritize Hypotheses: Problem statement for older adults with alterations in functioning of the family includes
Altered Family Functioning

◆ PLANNING

Generate Solutions: The patient goals for older individuals with altered family functioning are to (1) express their feelings regarding changes in roles and relationships and (2) work with family members to develop strategies for coping with changing roles and relationships.

◆ IMPLEMENTATION

Take Action: The following nursing interventions should take place in hospitals, in extended-care facilities, and at home:

1. **Assess interactions between older adults and their families.** Spend time sitting in when family members visit their aging relatives. Be alert for signs of destructive emotions, such as anger or frustration. If these are evident, suggest a rest time or coffee break to reduce the tension and allow the family members a chance to calm down. When they have been separated, attempt to explore their feelings individually and suggest coping strategies.

2. **Encourage all family members to verbalize their feelings.** It is best to explore the feelings of family members independently. People of all ages are afraid to express their real feelings in the presence of other involved parties. Spend time with older adults and individual family members in private settings. During this time, convey to concerned family members that all feelings, including those of anger and frustration, are acceptable and will be held in confidence. It is not easy for most people to express the negative emotions triggered by the stress of coping with changing roles and relationships, and it will take time. Once people's feelings have been identified, positive coping strategies can be developed.

3. **Assist family members in identifying their personal and family strengths.** Each person and each family has weaknesses and strengths. The key to maintaining or repairing family dynamics is identification of the strengths. Love, concern, and shared spiritual values can serve as a basis for positive relationships.

4. **Encourage family members to visit regularly.** When an aging family member is hospitalized or resides in an institutional setting, the family may feel useless or unnecessary. Some family members feel that their presence is not desired by the nursing staff. Nurses should recognize that family members are able to relate to older adults in unique and special ways. Rather than make the family uncomfortable, the nursing staff should do everything possible to make them feel welcome and at ease. Greet family members by name to help forge bonds of mutual caring. Respond promptly to requests and show small considerations (e.g., offering the family members coffee) to make the family feel valued.

5. **Encourage the family members to assist in caring for the older adult.** Family members are often able

and willing to help the nursing staff care for aging loved ones. Assisting with care provides the family an opportunity to show their concern for the aging person. Do not expect or demand that the family assist with care, but encourage it if the family appears willing. The amount of involvement will differ from family to family. Some family members may want to perform a great deal of the care, even bathing and feeding. Others are more comfortable helping with less technical things, such as hair grooming or shaving.

QSEN Considerations: Safety

Family Support and Consideration

Nurses can help families by providing all necessary equipment, by teaching families safe and effective ways to perform tasks, and by providing positive comments for a job well done.

6. **Assist families in identifying factors that are interfering with normal interactions.** Normal physiologic changes, illness, disability, side effects of medication, financial difficulties, and other problems can affect the behavior of older adults and interfere with normal family interactions. Perform a thorough assessment to determine the factors at play in any given situation. Once the causative factors are identified, work with older adults and their families to develop a plan that eliminates or reduces the problems and thereby facilitates more normal interactions.

7. **Explore community resources.** If the family dynamics are severely altered, nurses may be unable to meet the family's needs. Special assistance in the form of support groups, geriatric social workers, and geropsychiatric clinics are available in many communities. Be knowledgeable about available community resources and let the family members know about them (Nursing Care Plan 12.1).

 Nursing Care Plan 12.1   **Loneliness/Potential for Social Isolation**

Mrs. Hixton is an alert, generally healthy 77-year-old widow who lives alone in the home she and her husband shared until his death from cancer last year. Her daughter lives several hundred miles away and calls occasionally. The home hospice nurse who visited regularly during her husband's illness stops by as part of her routine follow-up and finds that Mrs. Hixton spends most of her time in her home with the shades drawn and goes out only to buy groceries and other necessary items. She drives to church weekly but does not speak to other church members. She speaks hesitantly to the nurse and makes little eye contact during the conversation. With tears in her eyes, she states that "Nobody cares about me anymore; they all have somebody, but I have nobody."

PROBLEM STATEMENT
Loneliness
Potential for Social Isolation

SUPPORTING ASSESSMENT DATA
- Patient statement indicating feelings of rejection and being alone
- Absence of supportive family or friends
- Withdrawal from contact with others
- Sad, dull affect
- Decreased appetite
- Lack of eye contact
- Preoccupation with own thoughts

PATIENT GOALS/OUTCOMES IDENTIFICATION
Mrs. Hixton will demonstrate increased participation in social activities and identify actions or resources that will reduce the potential for social isolation.
Mrs. Hixton will verbalize decreased sense of loneliness.
Mrs. Hixton's appetite will return to baseline.

NURSING INTERVENTIONS/IMPLEMENTATION
1. Allow Mrs. Hixton time to verbalize her feelings of sadness or depression relating to the loss of her spouse.
2. Encourage her to develop a list of family members and friends with whom she previously socialized.
3. Encourage her to make contact with her daughter by telephone on a weekly basis.
4. Identify social activities that were previously of interest to her.
5. Encourage participation in a grief counseling group.
6. Consult with her minister regarding visitations.
7. Encourage Mrs. Hixton to consider meeting an old friend for lunch or coffee.

EVALUATION

Mrs. Hixton hesitantly expressed willingness to attend one session of grief counseling. During this session, she sat quietly and listened to others explain what they were going through. At the next home visit, she told the nurse, "I think I'll go to another session. There was another woman there who's having the same problems I am. She offered to have lunch with me. It makes me feel a little less lonely." You will continue the plan of care.

APPLYING CLINICAL JUDGMENT

1. What could the nurse do to help Mrs. Hixton prepare for her next grief counseling session?
2. What could the nurse do if Mrs. Hixton had a negative experience at the group counseling session?
3. What are possible interventions the nurse could use if Mrs. Hixton refused to attend further sessions?

Get Ready for the Next Generation NCLEX® Examination!

Key Points

- People play many roles and have many integral relationships over a lifetime.
- When aging results in loss of these roles and changes in relationships, grief is a normal response.
- Grieving people are often unwilling to participate even in normal daily care or activities. With complex grief, the older person may lose all interest in life.
- To break through grief, nurses must attempt to build a trusting relationship through which the older person can work through the loss and grief. It is hoped that this will enable the person to find new meaning in life and to build new relationships.
- Older adults may become isolated from social interaction.
- An older adult can become socially isolated when there are ineffective methods of coping with grief or from impaired family dynamics.
- Roles and relationships are maintained through communication with others.
- If the ability to communicate with others is impaired (as is the case with many of the common disorders of aging, such as stroke or dementia), the ability to maintain relationships is affected.
- Older adults with impaired communication are likely to feel isolated from family and friends and from normal social interactions.
- Nurses who work with older adults should understand the effects of changes in roles and relationships.
- An understanding of the significance of these losses enables nurses to assess the behavior of older adults more effectively and to plan interventions that will be of benefit.

Additional Learning Resources

SG Go to your Evolve website at http://evolve.elsevier.com/Williams/geriatric for the additional online resources.

Review Questions for the Next Generation NCLEX® Examination

1. An older woman was widowed about a year ago. What would normal expected behavior at this stage of grieving include?
   a. Loss of appetite, sleep changes, and difficulty making decisions
   b. Improved energy, interest in new activities and goals
   c. Restlessness, poor memory, and irritability
   d. Crying, social isolation, lack of concentration

2. How do roles change as a person ages? *(Select all that apply.)*
   a. Communication becomes less important as older adults become more dependent on others for care.
   b. Relocation to new environment may separate friends, family, and possessions.
   c. Roles are lost with the death of spouse or family members.
   d. Isolation is a common expected outcome with aging.
   e. Retirement brings the loss of one's previous professional roles or status.

3. What characteristics place an older adult at increased risk for social isolation? *(Select all that apply.)*
   a. Sensory changes
   b. Decreased physical mobility
   c. Advanced age
   d. Limited financial resources
   e. Incontinence
   f. Physical deformity
   g. Belonging to an ethnic minority group

4. What is the most appropriate intervention to use for older adults who always stay in their rooms?
   a. Tell the older adult, "It's time to go out and see people."
   b. Use a wheelchair to transport the older adult to the activity room.
   c. Spend one-on-one time discussing the older adult's concerns.
   d. Call the family and request that they visit more often.

5. Which person is most likely to experience relationship issues?
   a. One who has a large pool of family and friends
   b. One who has few interests
   c. One who likes solitary activities and states, "I like to be left alone"
   d. One who has multiple chronic illnesses

6. What intervention(s) should nurses consider when an older adult is grieving the loss of a role or relationship? *(Select all that apply.)*
   a. Encourage communication with friends and family members.
   b. Build a trusting relationship.
   c. Assist with all day-to-day activities until grieving is improved.
   d. Introduce a variety of new experiences each day to encourage social interaction.
   e. Be available to discuss loss without stirring up deep emotions or feelings.
   f. Identify support groups, counselors, spiritual advisors, and family members who can provide additional support.

REFERENCES

Besora-Moreno, M., Llauradó, E., Tarro, L., & Solà, R. (2020). Social and economic factors and malnutrition or the risk of malnutrition in the elderly: A systematic review and meta-analysis of observational studies. *Nutrients, 12*, 737. https://doi.org/10.3390/nu12030737

Blazer, D. (2020). Social isolation and loneliness in older adults—A mental health/public health challenge. *JAMA Psychiatry, 77*(10), 990–991. doi:10.1001/jamapsychiatry.2020.1054.

Fry, R. (2019). Baby boomers are staying in the labor force at rates not seen in generations for people their age. *Pew Research Center.* https://www.pewresearch.org/fact-tank/2019/07/24/baby-boomers-us-labor-force/

Kwan, H. C. (2021). On family determination in reconstructionist Confucianism. In R. A. Carleo III, & Y. Huang (Eds.), *Confucian Political Philosophy.* Springer, Cham. https://doi.org/10.1007/978-3-030-70611-1_3

Moseley, K., & Hammond, L. (2021). Improving quality of life in the golden years. *Nursing Made Incredibly Easy.* 19 (3): 13–17.

RetirementLiving.com (2021). Best senior dating sites of 2021. https://www.retirementliving.com/best-senior-dating-sites#:~:text=Pew%20Research%20shows%20that%20online,have%20used%20online%20dating%20sites

Sin, W. (2021). If Confucius met Scanlon—Understanding filial piety from Confucianism and Contractualism. *Philosophy Compass, 16*(12), e12792.

Coping and Stress

13

Objectives

1. Explain the concepts of stress and coping.
2. Compare the physical, emotional, and behavioral signs of stress.
3. Describe methods for reducing stress.
4. Discuss changes in stress and coping that occur with aging.
5. Discuss methods of coping with stress and depression.
6. Describe characteristics of older adults who are most at risk for experiencing stress-related problems.
7. Identify problem statements related to stress-related factors.
8. Identify appropriate nursing interventions for older adults experiencing problems related to stress and coping.

Key Terms

coping (p. 243)
distress (p. 241)
eustress (Ū-stress, p. 241)
imaging (ĬM-ĭ-jĭng, p. 247)
mantra (MĂN-tră, p. 248)

meditation (p. 247)
proactive (p. 245)
reactive (p. 245)
relaxation (p. 245)
self-hypnosis (p. 247)

NORMAL STRESS AND COPING

Stress is a normal part of life. No one lives without it. Stress occurs when a person is faced with a real or perceived threat or experiences a significant or life-altering change. External stressors include physical threats, such as -extreme heat or cold, noise, or physical trauma; internal stressors include psychological threats (thoughts and feelings); whereas social stressors include job pressures and changing social relationships. Stress often results from a combination of these. The more stressors a person faces, the greater the level of stress; it all adds up. Stress occurs whether the threat or change is positive or negative. Stress can stem from an exciting or positive change, such as getting married or starting a new career. Dr. Hans Selye (1950) described this positive stress as *eustress*, whereas the negative stress is *distress*.

Each of us faces a steady stream of life events with which we must cope. Some are temporary or minor events, such as taking a test or giving a speech, which may cause mild stress for a short period. Major life events—such as the death of a spouse, serious injury, birth of a child, or marriage—are likely to cause significant stress that lasts for a longer period. People experiencing high levels of stress feel exhausted, anxious, and vulnerable.

Different experiences are stressful for different people. Perception plays an important role in determining what constitutes a stressor. For example, muscle pain is a stressor to most people but not to an athlete, who views it as a measure of training. Public speaking is highly stressful to most people, but not to a politician, who does it every day.

Various rating scales have been developed to quantify the amount of stress caused by common social and psychological occurrences in the lives of people (Table 13.1). The various events listed in these rating scales are based on the degree of stress involved. These scales are general guides that attempt to measure the degree stress caused by a particular event. Stress is cumulative, and a combination of several smaller stressors can have the same effect as a major stressor. The more stressors a person faces at any one time, the greater the likelihood of associated physical, cognitive, and behavioral changes such as weight gain, insomnia, and heart disease. Chronic stress has even been linked to Alzheimer disease (Lyons & Bartolomucci, 2020).

When confronted with stressful events, the body undergoes predictable physiologic responses that prepare it to withstand the threat and to maintain homeostasis. Dr. Selye's general adaptation syndrome describes the collective responses of the body to stress. According to this theory, stress activates both the sympathetic and parasympathetic components of the autonomic nervous system, initiating a series of physiologic responses (Selye, 1950).

Table 13.1 Stokes/Gordon Stress Scale: Selected Items

RANK	EVENT OR SITUATION	WEIGHT
1	Death of a son or daughter (unexpected)	100
2	Decreasing eyesight	99
2	Death of a grandchild	99
3	Death of spouse (unexpected)	97
4	Loss of ability to get around	96
4	Death of a son or daughter (expected, anticipated)	96
5	Fear of your home being invaded or robbed	93
5	Constant or recurring pain or discomfort	93
6	Illness or injury of close relative	92
7	Death of spouse (expected, anticipated)	90
7	Moving in with children or other family	90
7	Moving to an institution	90
8	Minor or major car accident	89
8	Needing to rely on a cane, wheelchair, walker, or hearing aids	89
8	Change in ability to perform personal care	89
10	Loneliness or aloneness	87
11	Having an unexpected debt	86
11	Your own hospitalization (unplanned)	86
12	Decreasing hearing	85
13	Fear of abuse from others	84
13	Being judged legally incompetent	84
13	Not feeling needed or having a purpose in life	84
14	Decreasing mental abilities	84
15	Giving up long-cherished possessions	82
15	Wishing parts of your life had been different	82
16	Using your savings for living expenses	80
17	Change in behavior of a family member	79
18	Taking a relative or friend into your home to live	78
19	Concern about elimination	77
19	Illness in public places	77
20	Feeling of remaining time being short	76
20	Giving up or losing driver's license	76
20	Change in sleeping habits	76
21	Difficulty using public transportation	75
23	Uncertainty about the future	73
25	Fear of your own or your spouse's driving	71
27	Concern for completing required forms	69
27	Death of a loved pet	69
29	Reaching a milestone year	67
32	Outstanding personal achievement	64
33	Retirement	63
35	Change in your sexual activity	59

Modified from Stokes S. A., & Gordon S. E. (1998). *User's manual,* SGSS. Pleasantville, NY: Pace University.

Table 13.2	Physical Signs of Stress
BODY SYSTEM	**CHANGES SEEN WITH STRESS**
Cardiovascular	Sensation of racing or pounding heart. Elevated pulse rate. Increased blood pressure. Cold, clammy hands and feet. Increased blood glucose level.
Respiratory	Increased respiratory rate and depth. Possible hyperventilation with a tingling sensation in the extremities, faintness, dizziness, and even seizures if the acid-base balance is seriously altered.
Musculoskeletal	Increased blood glucose level to provide energy for muscles. Increased muscle tension in the back, neck, and head. Complaint of tension headaches, teeth grinding, and backaches.
Gastrointestinal	Decreased production of digestive enzymes. Loss of appetite, nausea, abdominal distention, vomiting, and heartburn. May contribute to development of gastric or duodenal ulcers. Decreased peristalsis resulting in excess intestinal gas and constipation, but diarrhea is also quite common.
Urinary	Decreased urine production but increased urinary frequency.

The general alarm reaction, often called the *fight-or-flight response*, occurs first. In this stage, the body undergoes a predictable range of responses or physiologic changes designed to overcome the threat. If these responses are effective, the body enters a stage of resistance, during which it returns to normal functioning. If the responses are not effective, the body depletes its energy reserves and enters the stage of exhaustion, similar to aging, caused by wear and tear. In the most severe cases, this exhaustion can result in death.

PHYSICAL SIGNS OF STRESS

Physical signs of stress are similar in both young and older adults. They are summarized in Table 13.2.

COGNITIVE SIGNS OF STRESS

In addition to producing physiologic changes, stress affects the way we think, feel, and act. Although some stress is normal and necessary, even beneficial, high stress levels can be physically and mentally exhausting.

Mild stress results in a state of greater alertness. Individuals experiencing mild stress are able to pay attention to details, to learn, and to solve problems. With higher levels of stress, these abilities decrease rapidly.

Persons experiencing severe stress are likely to miss obvious details and may forget even basic information. Their problem-solving ability is severely affected. Under stress, people are likely to develop tunnel vision, focusing narrowly on one aspect of a problem and ignoring other important ones. These individuals are likely to act irrationally or impulsively and thus to make poor choices. Some become completely indecisive. Research even indicates that stress can cause physiologic changes in the brain that have an adverse effect on memory (Alzyoud et al., 2021).

EMOTIONAL SIGNS

People experiencing high levels of stress are likely to complain of fatigue, tension, and anxiety. They often report a feeling that something is wrong. They may appear distracted, irritable, short-tempered, and even angry. People living with high levels of stress often verbalize feelings of poor self-worth or low self-esteem. They may appear to be so wrapped up in their own problems that they have little ability for or interest in interacting with others. When stress becomes severe, people may experience signs of major depressive disorder or they may even verbalize suicidal thoughts.

Depression is not easily identified or diagnosed. It is often missed because it occurs in conjunction with the numerous physical and social changes that occur with aging. Depression is more than the down moods that everyone experiences now and then. For depression to be medically diagnosed, the symptoms must occur most of the day, nearly every day, for at least 2 weeks. Depression is a whole body syndrome that causes physiologic, emotional, and cognitive changes in people. The notion of mental illness is unsettling to many older people, who feel that seeking help for mental problems is a sign of a weakness that they should be able to overcome alone. Symptoms such as chronic pain, appetite loss, sleeplessness, loss of interest, and even dementia-like behavior are often attributed to other problems and the underlying depression is missed. This is unfortunate, because depression is treatable.

Depression, although common, is not a normal part of aging. In fact, studies have shown that the majority of older people are satisfied with their lives. It appears that working through the stressors of a lifetime has enabled many older people to develop a high level of self-knowledge and strong coping skills. Depression appears to be most likely to arise when older adults are under physiologic stress. Depression is also likely to occur when older adults perceive that they have lost control of a situation, that they lack the support of significant others, or that their normal coping mechanisms have been overwhelmed by the number or severity of their stressors (Boxes 13.1 and 13.2).

BEHAVIORAL SIGNS

People attempt to cope with stress in different ways. Some avoid all interactions or tasks that might increase their stress level, whereas others take on additional duties to block out the sources of their distress. In either case, performance is likely to suffer. People

Box 13.1	Symptoms of Depression

- Persistent sad, anxious, or "empty" mood
- Feelings of hopelessness or pessimism
- Irritability
- Feelings of guilt, worthlessness, or helplessness
- Loss of interest or pleasure in hobbies and activities
- Decreased energy or fatigue
- Moving or talking more slowly
- Feeling restless or having trouble sitting still
- Difficulty concentrating, remembering, or making decisions
- Difficulty sleeping, early morning awakening, or oversleeping
- Appetite and/or weight changes
- Thoughts of death or suicide, or suicide attempts
- Aches or pains, headaches, cramps, or digestive problems without a clear physical cause and/or that do not ease even with treatment

Source: National Institute of Mental Health. https://www.nimh.nih.gov/health/topics/depression/

Box 13.2	Goals of Treatment for Depression

- Decreased symptoms of depression
- Reduced risk for relapse and recurrence
- Improved quality of life
- Improved medical health status

under stress tend to be disorganized, make more errors, and leave tasks incomplete. They may appear and even sound muddled.

The thoughts, statements, and actions of stressed people often jump around in a scattered or disconnected manner. They may pace, hum, or perform other ritualistic actions, such as finger drumming, key jangling, or toe tapping. Temper tantrums, shouting, and other aggressive behaviors can occur without warning.

Self-medicating is one response to dealing with depression and other situational problems. It is certainly not a recommended method but one that is all too common among all age groups, including older adults. The substances most commonly abused include tobacco, alcohol, and prescription drugs. Some older adults also abuse illicit street drugs, and this trend has increased dramatically over the past decade. The majority of older adults are aware that tobacco has harmful effects, but they continue to use it in spite of warnings. Although it is physically damaging, tobacco does not have the same effects on the mind and behavior as do alcohol and drugs.

Although some people have abused substances from early in life onward, many addictions begin later in life. Data show that nearly 1 million older adults have a substance use disorder, including either alcohol or illicit drugs (National Institute on Drug Abuse, 2020). Drugs such as anxiolytics, tranquilizers, analgesics, and other mood-altering drugs are among the most commonly prescribed for older adults. Many

times, an older person will obtain prescriptions from several health care providers, thus increasing the availability and potential for abuse. As discussed in Chapter 7, many older adults do not adhere to the directions given on a prescription label. They alter dosage and frequency to suit themselves, thus increasing their risk for tolerance and dependence. Because alcohol is legal, socially acceptable, and readily available, it is the most often abused substance.

Alcohol tolerance changes as a result of altered physiology. Decreased lean muscle mass, changes in liver enzyme function, and increased nervous system sensitivity to alcohol decrease the safe level of intake for older adults. Older adults who have abused alcohol for many years consume larger amounts more often than do those who start abusing alcohol later in life. Long-time abusers are more likely to have classic symptoms of alcohol use disorder (formerly referred to as *alcoholism*), have disturbed family or social relationships, and experience withdrawal when alcohol consumption is stopped suddenly. People who overuse alcohol later in life are more likely to drink in response to stressful events. They suffer fewer physical symptoms, are less likely to experience withdrawal, and are more likely to have intact relationships. Both groups are likely to drink alone, at home, and in response to stressful or negative emotional perceptions.

Most health care providers overlook alcohol problems in older adults. Signs of alcohol and drug abuse are sometimes missed because they mimic age-related changes, such as bone density changes, urinary incontinence, altered sleep patterns, unsteadiness, hypertension, stomach complaints, and falls. Substance abuse should be evaluated even though it seems unlikely. Although greater numbers of older men have substance abuse problems, older widows who live alone are also a high-risk group.

Mental health resources and support groups are available in many communities to help with substance abuse. Many are tailored to meet the specific needs of older adults.

STRESS AND ILLNESS

Stress and illness are closely linked. Research has shown that both mental and physical illness cause stress, and that stress increases the risk for both mental and physical illness. A physically ill person is less able to cope with additional physical or psychological stressors, which take energy away from the individual's already depleted reserves and undermine the ability to cope. Stress can interfere with the ability to learn, function, and follow through with the plan of care. Decreasing the number of stressors or the level of stress can prevent illness or improve a person's ability to cope with existing illnesses.

Stress has been shown to have negative effects on many body systems. Because stress activates the

| Box 13.3 | Common Coping or Defense Mechanisms |

- *Repression*: The removal of anxiety-producing thoughts or experiences from conscious awareness
- *Denial*: Refusing to acknowledge some painful aspect of external reality that is obvious to others
- *Rationalization*: Creating an acceptable reason for unacceptable thoughts or actions
- *Intellectualization*: Generalizing to avoid disturbing thoughts or feelings
- *Displacement*: Transferring emotions about one situation or person onto another
- *Suppression*: Avoiding thinking about distressing situations
- *Projection*: Attributing one's own feelings to another
- *Sublimation*: Channeling negative energy into socially acceptable behaviors
- *Substitution*: Keeping so busy with activities that there is no time to think about stressors

sympathetic nervous system (arousing the fight-or-flight response), the older adult under high levels of stress is at increased risk for angina, abnormalities in heart rhythm, and even heart attack. Stress is associated with hypertension and may increase the risk for stroke. The immune system is affected because higher levels of the stress hormone cortisol are secreted, increasing the person's susceptibility to infections and potentially impairing their response to immunizations, such as the COVID-19 and pneumonia vaccines. Gastrointestinal problems—such as ulcer, gastroesophageal reflux disease, and irritable bowel disease—are more likely to occur or worsen when an older adult is under stress. Stress can exacerbate sleep problems and often triggers painful headaches or muscle spasms.

People differ in their ability to cope with stress. Those who do not cope effectively with normal day-to-day stressors cannot function normally when the stress level is high and are at risk for becoming physically or mentally ill. Those who do learn good coping strategies can maintain their ability to function despite high level stress. Many different coping or defense mechanisms are used as part of day-to-day living (Box 13.3). People who are able to cope effectively usually rely on several of these mechanisms. Coping mechanisms are neither good nor bad; they become dysfunctional only when used excessively or inappropriately as a way circumventing the stressors rather than dealing with them.

STRESS AND LIFE EVENTS

Although stress can cause physical illness, physical illness also increases stress. An older adult suffering from numerous chronic and acute conditions is under greater stress than one who is healthier. Stress can increase as a result of loss; the loss of friends, family members, and particularly a spouse can be highly stressful. Other life events, such as a change in residence or financial worries, can also cause stress.

STRESS REDUCTION AND COPING STRATEGIES

There are two basic categories of coping style: problem-focused strategies and emotion-focused strategies. Problem-focused coping strategies attempt to change or eliminate the stressful event or threat. Emotion-focused strategies attempt to change the person's response to the stressful event or threat. The type of strategy used depends on the personal significance of the event and the perceived ability to alter the outcomes.

One effective way of reducing stress is to avoid or escape the stressors. When an event has little personal significance or there is a small likelihood of its having an impact on the outcome of an event, avoidance may be the best choice. When people know that certain events are likely to increase their stress levels, the best alternative may be to avoid these situations whenever possible. It is often simpler and wiser to avoid stress than to endure it. When one is facing a major stressor, it is wise to eliminate as many smaller stressors as possible so that energy is available to cope with the major problem.

When stressors cannot be avoided, when their personal significance is high, or when the person believes that they can affect the outcome, other methods can be used. Confrontational, cognitive, and problem-solving methods are effective means of dealing with these types of stressful situations.

To use a problem-solving method, a person must first identify and examine the stressors involved. Once the stressors have been identified, the individual can determine their importance. Only then will it be possible to explore alternative actions to reduce the stress. For example, the individual can continue to face the stressor (e.g., an annoying coworker) and live with the consequences (confrontational), change jobs (escape), decrease contact with the stressor (avoidance), or consciously work to change their own attitude toward the annoying person (emotional distancing). The choice made is based on a deliberate decision. This method of taking a proactive stance (choosing an active response to control the situation) as opposed to being reactive (reacting to the situation) gives the person a sense of control and empowerment. The mere fact that the person retains control and makes a choice helps to reduce the stress level.

Many people need to be taught how to use the problem-solving method for coping with stress. Learning to use this process with small or minor stressors can help people develop the skills to cope with major stressors. Some find that physical activity helps them cope with stress. Exercise may reduce excessive levels of stress-related hormones and may allow the body to regain homeostasis. The particular physical activity chosen should be one that the stressed individual enjoys and participates in willingly. Physical activity should be carried out in moderation, not to a level of exhaustion, where it becomes another form of stress.

Relaxation techniques can be used to help people cope with stress. The most common forms of relaxation techniques include progressive relaxation, meditation, imaging, biofeedback, and self-hypnosis. In addition to these techniques, the support of friends and family will benefit most people. Talking through problems and stresses can facilitate problem solving. If the level of stress is too severe for routine stress reduction techniques, professional help from counselors, ministers, or mental health professionals may be necessary.

 Complementary Health Approaches

Geriatric Massage

- Geriatric massage is a modification of standard massage designed to meet the needs of older adults.
- Benefits of massage include improved circulation, relief of pain, increased range of motion, decreased anxiety or depression, improved sleep, and enhanced sense of well-being. These services can be provided by certified therapists available in many communities.
- Massage treatments are not covered by Medicare or Medicaid, but they may be covered by private insurance programs.
- To decrease the risk for fatigue, a typical session lasts no more than 30 minutes.
- Gentle motions designed to stimulate circulation and relax muscles are used over most of the body. Passive movement and gentle stretching with occasional stronger movements are used on larger joints in the shoulders, legs, and hips to improve joint mobility and flexibility.
- Smaller joints in the hands and feet are gently massaged to relieve pain and improve mobility.
- Massage is not a replacement for physical therapy or exercise.
- Not all older adults are candidates for full body massage. Use of this technique should be discussed with the primary care provider before initiation.

Complementary Health Approaches

Stress Reduction

- *Concentration meditation*: A variety of activities focusing on breathing, body sensation, or mantras may divert the mind from worries and concerns that increase stress.
- *Movement meditation*: Activities such as yoga, tai chi, qigong, walking, or dancing use motion and focused attention to reduce both mental and physical stress.
- *Prayer and reflection*: Prayers and reflection on sacred verses or poems, performed alone or in a group setting, can be calming and reduce stress.
- *Massage*: Focused manipulation of muscles reduces tension, decreases pain, and promotes a bond of caring, all of which reduce stress.
- *Reiki*: This Japanese technique for stress reduction and relaxation also promotes healing. It is administered by the "laying on hands" to increase the unseen "life force energy" that causes us to be alive. When this energy is low, we are more likely to feel stress; when it is high, we are more capable of being happy and healthy.

Stress is as much a fact of life for older adults as it is for the younger population. However, the amounts and types of stressors do seem to change with aging (see Table 13.1). Many negative life events have been identified as stressors in older adults; however, there can be fewer positive life events that produce stress as we age. Many of the stressors of older adults involve losses. Loss of a spouse or child, home, vision, or driver's license can result in the loss of a purpose in life and may place a severe strain on the coping abilities of older adults. Too many or too frequent stressors can overwhelm older adults, particularly those already under physiologic stress because of physical illness.

The ability to cope with stress differs widely among older adults. In general, those who have learned good coping strategies and have used them throughout life will continue to do so in old age. Those who did not learn at a younger age how to cope with stress will likely continue to experience difficulties.

Because of the unchanging nature of the many stressors seen with aging, older adults are more likely to distance themselves emotionally from situations they cannot change. They are increasingly likely to seek support in spiritual or philosophic beliefs that help them cope with these uncontrollable situations.

❖ NURSING PROCESS/CLINICAL JUDGMENT MODEL FOR LIMITED COPING ABILITY

Limited coping ability occurs when a person cannot appropriately or accurately identify stressors, responds inadequately to such stressors, or has limited knowledge of available resources. Such individuals cannot solve problems or adapt to the stressors in their lives. People experiencing limited coping ability often verbalize feelings of anxiety, anger, or sadness and can often be heard using phrases, such as "I just can't cope anymore." In addition, they may complain of changes in physical function as a result of stress. Loss of appetite, nausea, altered bowel or bladder elimination patterns, and sleep pattern disturbances are common complaints. Older adults who are having problems coping often demonstrate inadequate problem solving. In severe cases, the person may engage in destructive behavior or may withdraw from contact with others. If these individuals live independently, they may abuse tobacco, alcohol, or drugs as they attempt to cope with their stress (Box 13.4).

◆ ASSESSMENT (DATA COLLECTION)

Recognize Cues

- Does the person verbalize feelings of tension, stress, frustration, or sadness?
- Do they verbalize complaints of changes in eating habits? Sleeping patterns?
- Does the person complain of changes in bladder or bowel elimination patterns?
- Do they have difficulty making decisions or solving problems?
- Does the person appear agitated, aggressive, angry, or hostile?

Box 13.4	**Alcohol-Related Problems in Older Adults**

- The prevalence of substance use disorder in older adults is increasing; the leading substance use disorders in the older population are high-risk drinking (binge drinking) and alcohol use disorder (Seim et al., 2020).
- According to a recent survey, 11% of people over age 65 report "current" binge drinking behaviors (National Institute on Alcohol Abuse and Alcoholism, 2021).
- Alcohol-related problems often go undetected in older adults because symptoms are often mistaken for dementia or medical problems. For example, gastrointestinal problems are more likely to be correlated to anti-inflammatory medications than to alcohol consumption.
- Alcohol use in the older adult population contributes to liver disease, dementia, peripheral neuropathy, insomnia, poor nutrition, incontinence, depression, inadequate self-care, and medication reactions. Use of alcohol increases the risk for falls, hip fractures, and other accidents.
- Older men are more likely to use alcohol to cope with financial problems, whereas older women are more likely to use alcohol to cope with death or loss of relationships.

Box 13.5	**Risk Factors Related to Problems With Coping or Stress Tolerance in Older Adults**

- Recent social, physical, emotional, or financial losses
- Physical illness
- Major life changes

- Do they seem sad or withdrawn?
- Does the person smoke or consume alcohol excessively?
- Have they experienced more illness or accidents?

See Box 13.5 for a list of risk factors for problems related to coping or stress in older adults.

◆ DATA ANALYSIS/PROBLEM IDENTIFICATION

Analyze Cues and Prioritize Hypotheses: Problem statement for older adults with limited coping ability includes

Limited Coping Ability

◆ PLANNING

Generate Solutions. The patient goals for older individuals with limited coping ability are to (1) communicate feelings of stress; (2) identify personal strengths and effective methods of coping; and (3) participate in decision-making.

◆ IMPLEMENTATION

Take Action: The following nursing interventions should take place in hospitals or extended-care facilities:

1. **Maintain continuity of care to develop a stable, trusting relationship.** Before older adults will verbalize their concerns, they must develop trust in their caregivers. Gain this trust by keeping the number of caregivers to a minimum. Develop a plan of care with the individual. To reduce stress, follow this plan with minimal changes.

2. **Encourage older adults to verbalize their feelings.** Verbalization provides older adults with an opportunity to express their concerns and solve problems. Merely putting feelings into words often reduces the stress that comes from holding back anxious thoughts. Nurses should be careful to remain nonjudgmental and should allow older adults to express a full range of feelings, including fear, anger, hostility, and grief.

3. **Ensure that older adults receive adequate nutrition, rest, and pain relief.** Persons who are hungry, fatigued, or in pain are likely to have difficulty coping with other stressors. Plan care to minimize these basic physical stressors.

4. **Assist older adults to identify their personal strengths and previously successful coping strategies.** Older people typically use a variety of coping strategies throughout their lives. Unless older adults suffer from chronic mental illness, they have probably managed to cope rather successfully to have reached old age. The coping behaviors that were used throughout life can act as a basis for coping with current situations.

5. **Explain a variety of stress reduction techniques.** Stress reduction techniques can be used to help older adults manage and reduce their stress. Progressive relaxation is a simple technique that can be used by older adults. To learn to relax, the person is first taught to identify the difference between muscle tension and relaxation. Once they can identify the different sensations, they are taught to alternately tighten and relax muscles, starting at the feet and working upward through the body. This is done until the entire body is relaxed. With practice, this technique can be done quickly, effectively, and at will.

Self-hypnosis takes relaxation a step further and allows individuals to actually place themselves in a trance-like state. This technique is more complex and more difficult to learn than other relaxation techniques. Commercial audiotapes are available for teaching self-hypnosis.

Imaging is a relaxation technique in which individuals are taught to think of a calm, peaceful setting. This can be whatever setting the individual finds most relaxing. The person should visualize this setting and try to picture it in detail, taking pleasure from each aspect of the environment. Then the person imagines "being" in this environment, relaxing and enjoying the experience.

Meditation is a somewhat more difficult but highly beneficial relaxation technique. Time and effort are required to learn to meditate effectively. Individuals must learn to shut out external stimuli and focus on

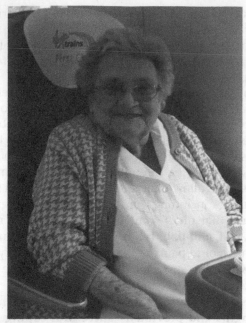

Fig. 13.1 Travel is one way in which older adults try to combat isolation.

calming their thoughts. To gain this internal focus, most meditators use a *mantra*, which is a word or sound that is repeated over and over again. To facilitate meditation, the individual should be provided with a quiet place where distractions can be minimized, and they should be assisted to assume a position that promotes comfort and relaxation.

6. **Encourage older adults to participate in activities** (Fig. 13.1). Physical and diversional activities can reduce stress by focusing excess nervous energy in productive ways, but people experiencing stress may be reluctant to participate. Encourage these individuals but never force them to attend activities, because forcing only increases stress.

7. **Consult with mental health specialists, ministers, or counselors.** Many techniques are available to help older adults cope with stress. If the problem is severe or if nurses are unable to help older adults cope with stress, consult with a specialist.

The following interventions should take place in the home:

1. **Encourage the family to provide emotional support to older adults.** It is often difficult for older adults (or anyone else) to cope with stress alone. Encourage families to spend time with older adults, listening and providing emotional support. If the family dynamics are disturbed and the family is a source of stress, it may be necessary to reduce family contact and help the older person identify other sources of emotional support, such as friends, ministers, or others.

2. **Identify community resources that can provide support to older adults and their families.** Many older adults and their families have difficulty coping on their own. Most communities have mental health clinics or older adult help lines to assist in times of stress.

3. **Use any appropriate interventions that are used in the institutional setting.**

❖ NURSING PROCESS/CLINICAL JUDGMENT MODEL FOR DISRUPTED LIVING SITUATION AND MALADAPTIVE RESPONSE TO DISRUPTED LIVING SITUATION

Disrupted living situation describes the potential physiologic or psychosocial stress that occurs when a person is transferred from one environment to another. Disrupted living situation is a common problem with aging and can occur with many types of relocation, including

- From a private home to the home of a family member
- From home to an apartment or other shared living arrangement
- From one area of the city to another
- From home to a hospital
- From home to a long-term care facility
- From home to a hospital and then to a long-term care facility
- From one unit in the hospital or long-term care facility to another unit in the same facility
- From one room to another in a hospital or long-term care facility

Older adults who are required to change residence are likely to experience losses, fears, and concerns that increase stress. Loss of independence, loss of personal possessions, loss of friends and neighbors, fear of the unknown, and concern about the future all increase stress. Stress is greatest when many losses or changes have occurred, when these changes occur in rapid succession, when the changes are unexpected, and when the individual has had little or no say in the decision-making process. In some cases, the response can be prolonged or maladaptive and lead to increased demands for care, physical regression (such as a previously continent adult becoming incontinent), changes in sleep patterns, and lack of appetite.

Older adults experiencing disrupted living situation may exhibit emotional, behavioral, and physical signs of stress. Most newly relocated older adults experience feelings of powerlessness, helplessness, and insecurity. They often verbalize unwillingness to relocate or dissatisfaction with the new living arrangements. They are likely to express feelings of grief, anger, apprehension, anxiety, loneliness, sadness, and confusion. To cope with these feelings, older adults may demonstrate a variety of behaviors (Fig. 13.2).

Some attempt to maintain control of the situation by demanding attention and verbalizing many needs. They may be more dependent on caregivers than their physical condition justifies. Others attempt to cope with the stress by becoming hostile or angry. They often deny the necessity of the change and refuse necessary

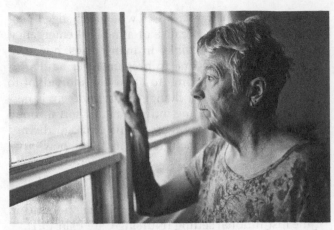

Fig. 13.2 Relocation can lead to feelings of loneliness. (Copyright © istock.com/LSOphoto.)

assistance or care. Still others cope by withdrawing and isolating themselves from contact with staff, other residents, and even family. These behaviors are usually a result of lack of trust or feelings of powerlessness in the new setting.

In addition to behavioral changes, recently relocated older adults are likely to experience physical signs of stress. Changes in eating habits, weight loss, gastrointestinal changes, changes in elimination patterns, and changes in sleep patterns are commonly seen in newly relocated older adults.

◆ ASSESSMENT (DATA COLLECTION)

Recognize Cues
See the assessment for limited coping ability earlier in the chapter.

◆ DATA ANALYSIS/PROBLEM IDENTIFICATION

Analyze Cues and Prioritize Hypotheses: Common problem statements for older adults with a disruption in their living situation include
   Disrupted Living Situation
   Maladaptive Response to Disrupted Living Situation

◆ PLANNING

Generate Solutions: The patient goals for older individuals with disrupted living situation are to (1) recognize the reasons for the move or change, (2) identify ways to maintain control and decision-making powers in the new environment, (3) verbalize concerns about new living arrangements, and (4) identify methods for coping with change.

◆ IMPLEMENTATION

Take Action: The following nursing interventions should take place in hospitals or extended-care facilities:
1. **Encourage verbalization of feelings, fears, and concerns about the move or change.** When a person holds in all fears and concerns, their stress level remains high. Allowing older adults to discuss their concerns openly and freely initiates the problem-solving process. Anger is common when older adults disagree with moving. Accept this anger as a normal and healthy response.
2. **Discuss the reasons for the move or change.** Nurses and families should be open and honest about the reasons for a move or change. Answer any questions the individual has as completely and honestly as possible. Attempting to shield older adults from the often harsh reality is likely to result in anger and loss of trust.
3. **Include older adults in care planning.** Whenever possible, encourage active participation of older adults in planning care. This allows older adults to maintain some degree of control over decisions that affect their lives.

💡 **QSEN Considerations: Patient-Centered Care**

Whenever possible, offer choices in the care planning and respect the individual's preferences.

---

4. **Encourage a positive attitude about the move or change.** Help older adults identify the benefits that will come with the change and avoid making personal or negative comments about the move.
5. **Maintain continuity of care to enhance feelings of trust.** When an older adult is newly relocated, keep the number of people providing care to a minimum and provide care in a consistent manner. Respect the individual's preferences and meet their needs promptly. This helps build a sense of trust and decreases the stress that results from rapid or unpredictable changes.
6. **Encourage the use of familiar objects and belongings.** Encourage older adults to bring as many prized personal possessions as space allows. Personal belongings enhance the sense of belonging. Seeing and using familiar items makes a new environment seem more familiar and reduces stress. Display personal possessions so that the person can easily reach or see them. Because most people feel that their personal belongings are extensions of themselves, always treat these belongings with care and respect.

Relocation to a new environment can be confusing and even disorienting to older adults. Selected items—such as calendars, clocks, night lights, and personal belongings—will help older adults make a smoother adjustment to a new environment.

The following interventions should take place in the home:
1. **Allow older adults to participate in decision-making and planning for the change.** It is important to include older adults in decisions that will have a significant impact on their lives. When a major change (e.g., a change in residence) is necessary, the older adult, their family, and possibly a social worker should make decisions together. The person should

know the reasons for the change and the available options. When choices are available, the preferences of the individual should be respected.

QSEN Considerations: Patient-Centered Care

Enabling older adults to retain control of choices and decisions about their care reduces their feelings of powerlessness and thus stress.

2. **Anticipate fears and concerns and allow adequate time to implement the change when possible.** Help older adults and their families anticipate and

plan for the change. In cases where a change in environment occurs because of a medical emergency, planning is not possible. In many cases, however, there is adequate time to prepare older adults for a change. Use this time to allow the individual to accept the fact that a change of environment is necessary. In addition, the individual can sort through their personal belongings and distribute or discard them as desired. Scheduled visits to the new environment before the actual move allow the person to become more familiar with the physical structure and people.

3. Use any appropriate interventions that are used in the institutional setting (Nursing Care Plan 13.1).

Nursing Care Plan 13.1   **Maladaptive Response to Disrupted Living Situation**

Mrs. Mack, an 81-year-old woman, recently moved into Brookline Care Center. You observe that she looks sad. She spends most of her time alone, sitting in her room looking out the window. She repeatedly asks, "Why did they have to do this to me? I was happy where I was. I just wanted to stay there until I died." Mrs. Mack makes many demands of the staff and asks many questions. She complains that she has difficulty sleeping in strange surroundings with other people so close by.

Mrs. Mack's health record reveals that she has a variety of health problems, including heart trouble and a history of high blood pressure. Until recently, she lived independently in her own apartment and required minimal help with getting to medical appointments and grocery shopping. More recently, she had become more forgetful, and her daughters were increasingly concerned about her safety and well-being living alone. Both daughters agreed that a care center would be most appropriate, and they found such a center near one of their homes that was reasonable in cost and had a vacancy. They made arrangements for the move and notified the landlord before discussing the plans with Mrs. Mack. The daughters moved a few of her personal belongings with her, but many were sold or given away to other family members.

PROBLEM STATEMENT

Maladaptive response to disrupted living situation

SUPPORTING ASSESSMENT DATA

- Sad affect
- Apprehension
- Verbalization of concern about the move
- Increased dependency
- Increased demands and verbalization of needs
- Change in sleeping patterns

PATIENT GOALS/OUTCOMES IDENTIFICATION

Mrs. Mack will verbalize an understanding of the reasons for her move, identify concerns about her new environment, and identify ways to cope with the change.

NURSING INTERVENTIONS/IMPLEMENTATION

1. Encourage Mrs. Mack to verbalize her feelings about the move.
2. Allow expressions of anger or frustration about the family's actions.
3. Encourage Mrs. Mack to discuss her feelings with her family.
4. Explain the reasons that necessitated the move.
5. Involve Mrs. Mack in decision-making and care planning.
6. Maintain stable care assignments to build trust.
7. Encourage a positive attitude about change.
8. Offer opportunities to participate in social activities.
9. Encourage the family to bring in more valued personal belongings.
10. Consult a social worker or minister as appropriate to facilitate positive family interactions.

EVALUATION

Mrs. Mack's family has brought additional family pictures, some favorite pillows, and a lap robe that had been stored in a closet. They also purchased a small color television with special earphones for listening in bed. Mrs. Mack states, "I still don't like it here, but I know that my family thinks it is best for me. They are trying to make it better, I guess." You will continue the plan of care.

APPLYING CLINICAL JUDGMENT

1. What behaviors would indicate that Mrs. Mack is adjusting to the change in her living accommodations?
2. What additional nursing interventions can you identify that might help Mrs. Mack and her family reduce their stress?

Get Ready for the Next Generation NCLEX® Examination!

Key Points

- Stress is a fact of life.
- Although the stressors may change throughout life, stress affects people of all ages. The major stressors of aging relate to losses.
- Loss of ability, loss of loved ones, loss of home, and many other losses are stressful to older adults, affecting their physical and emotional status.
- Stress can result in behavioral changes. Excessive levels of stress are harmful.
- Individuals use a variety of coping mechanisms to deal with stress.
- Any limitations of these coping strategies are of concern to nurses.
- Interventions that reduce stress and support positive coping mechanisms can be beneficial.

Additional Learning Resources

SG Go to your Evolve website at http://evolve.elsevier.com/Williams/geriatric for the additional online resources.

Review questions for the Next Generation NCLEX® examination

1. When assessing an older adult, the nurse suspects an increased level of stress while observing which physiologic data? *(Select all that apply.)*

   a. Increased urine production with retention
   b. Hyperventilation
   c. Warm hands and feet with sweating
   d. Headache
   e. Elevated pulse and blood pressure

2. What is the drug most commonly abused by older adults?

   a. Cocaine
   b. Marijuana
   c. Heroin
   d. Alcohol.

3. Which findings in the patient's history lead the nurse to suspect alcohol abuse? *(Select all that apply.)*

   a. Poor nutrition
   b. Liver disease
   c. Repeated falls
   d. Strong family relationships
   e. Peripheral neuropathy

4. An older adult tells the nurse that he feels "stressed" and asks what the nurse would recommend. What would be the nurse's best response?

   a. "See your primary care provider for an antianxiety medication."
   b. "Get more sleep and try a glass of wine with dinner."
   c. "Are you aware of the tai chi class at the recreation center?"
   d. "Just let go of whatever is bothering you."

5. Which describe characteristics of depression and the older adult? *(Select all that apply.)*

   a. Brief but intense episode of sadness
   b. Persistent feelings of sadness or "emptiness"
   c. Loss of interest in activities and hobbies
   d. Difficulty concentrating
   e. Increased energy level

6. An older adult tells the nurse that visiting her primary care provider is very stressful for her. What is the best response?

   a. Suggest that she postpone the visit and go when she is more relaxed.
   b. Tell her that she needs to work on changing her attitude.
   c. Help her develop strategies for dealing with her concerns.
   d. Stress that it is important and she needs to go and get it over with.

REFERENCES

Alzyoud, A., AlShorman, O., Masadeh, M., Alkahtani, F., & Abdelrahman, R. B. (2021). Learning and memory under stress: A review study with evaluation techniques. *Systematic Reviews in Pharmacy*, 12(1), 1602–1610

Lyons, C. E., & Bartolomucci A. (2020). Stress and Alzheimer's disease: A senescence link? *Neuroscience and Biobehavioral Reviews*, 115, 285–298. https://doi.org/10.1016/j.neubiorev.2020.05.010

National Institute on Alcohol Abuse and Alcoholism (2021). Older adults. https://www.niaaa.nih.gov/alcohols-effects-health/special-populations-co-occurring-disorders/older-adults

National Institute on Drug Abuse (2020). Substance use in older adults: Drugfacts. https://www.drugabuse.gov/publications/substance-use-in-older-adults-drugfacts#:~:text=Aging%20could%20possibly%20lead%20to,be%20more%20sensitive%20to%20drugs

Seim T, Vijapura, D., Pagali, S., & Burton, M. C. (2020). Common substance use disorders in older adults. *Hospital Practice*, 48(1), 48–55. https://doi.org/10.1080/21548331.2020.1733287

Selye H. (1950). Stress and the general adaptation syndrome. *British medical journal*, 1(4667), 1383–1392. https://doi.org/10.1136/bmj.1.4667.1383

Objectives

1. Develop an understanding of the impact of personal values and beliefs on everyday life.
2. Identify values and beliefs commonly found in today's older adult population.
3. Discuss the impact of beliefs and values on the health practices of older adults.
4. Develop an understanding of the relationship of values and beliefs to health practices.
5. Compare the spiritual practices of major religions as they relate to death.
6. Discuss how culture and ethnicity affect older adults' health beliefs and practices.
7. Describe methods of assessing beliefs and values.
8. Identify older adults at risk for experiencing problems related to values and beliefs.
9. Identify selected problem statements related to values or beliefs.
10. Describe nursing interventions appropriate for older adults who are experiencing problems related to values or beliefs.

Key Terms

agnostic (ăg-NŎS-tǐk, p. 255)
atheist (Ă-thē-ǐst, p. 255)
cultural awareness (KŬL-chŭr-ăl a-WÄR-něs, p. 253)
cultural competence (p. 253)
cultural understanding (p. 253)

faith (p. 255)
religious (p. 252)
ritual (p. 255)
spiritual (p. 255)

Values and beliefs are uniquely human concepts. As such, they are essential parts of our identity. Values and beliefs affect every aspect of our lives, including the experiences of life and death and the way we understand and manage health.

Older adults typically have an established system of values, goals, and beliefs that guide their decisions and choices. This system has developed over the older adult's lifetime of experience. One's value and belief system is a product of a dynamic interplay of a variety of sociocultural forces, such as religion, family environment, culture, and societal pressures and expectations. The foundation of the personal value system is set early in childhood. Sociologist Morris Massey (2005) has stated that people go through periods in which values are established, developed, and modified. Values carry significant implications for parents, educators, policy developers, and the larger society across the lifespan.

Values and beliefs develop in the context of a person's unique sociocultural environment. They are based on the messages communicated and reinforced by the family, friends, culture, religious institutions, school, and media while a person is growing up. The messages that are repeatedly reinforced throughout

 Cultural Considerations

IMPRINT PERIOD
We absorb the stimuli and beliefs around us, recognizing them as "true" until we are about 7 years old. During this time, the individual is learning to differentiate between right and wrong, good and bad.

MODELING PERIOD
From ages 8 through 13, we begin acting as others act and doing as others do. This is particularly true if a person finds and imitates a role model who is admired.

SOCIALIZATION PERIOD
Between the ages of 13 and 21, peers and the media have the greatest influence. We begin to identify our own values and gravitate toward others like ourselves.

Source: Changing Minds. (2021). Values Development. http://changingminds.org/explanations/values/values_development.htm

youth are likely to have the greatest influence on the person's beliefs and value system later in life. People's values reflect their unique experiences. Similar backgrounds and circumstances might result in shared values, whereas different backgrounds and circumstances may result in markedly different beliefs and value systems. This is not always true, however, especially in a mobile world with extensive virtual capability. People's experiences are not always limited to their immediate surroundings, so it is important to recognize that influences exist outside of an individual's immediate area of living.

Our beliefs and values affect our perception and experience of the world. We use them to attach meaning to life events and to evaluate other people and their actions. People have a natural tendency to view their own personal beliefs and values as "normal" or "natural." Therefore understanding people whose views are different from our own is important, as they have the same natural tendency to see their beliefs and values as normal or natural even if we are not familiar with them. Being able to honor someone else's beliefs and values significantly affects the quality and nature of interactions between individuals.

QSEN Considerations: Patient-Centered Care

This chapter examines a few aspects of different ethnicities and cultures. A patient, however, is an individual and may possess many, some, or none of the features described. A critical aspect of patient-centered care is to treat every patient as truly unique and to avoid stereotyping.

Cultural Considerations

Spirituality

Be careful not to stereotype people. Conduct a careful assessment to determine the specific beliefs, practices, and needs of each individual. Spirituality encompasses what is important to people and what gives their life meaning. For some people, religion is a portion of their spirituality. It is helpful to familiarize yourself with major branches of religion, such as Judaism, Christianity, and Islam. Recognize that each of these major faiths has specific leaders, places of worship, dietary observations, special clothing or objects, days of celebration or observation, holidays, holy books, and procedures following death. Most of all, note that you must never assume that a patient observes all of the practices and traditions associated with a particular faith.

For people who do not identify with any religion, spirituality may be felt in what they see as the meaning of life or in relating to something that they feel is larger than themselves, such as nature.

Complementary Health Approaches

Folk medicine, the treatment of a disease or condition based on tradition, may be practiced by some individuals. These types of health interventions may be deeply grounded in culture and history.

Differences in beliefs and values are a common source of communication problems. Statements such as "He just doesn't understand me" or "I just don't

understand her" usually indicate a conflict in beliefs or values, or confusion about what someone means. Think about how often you have heard parents say this about their children and vice versa. People may also make these statements when they are interacting with others of a different generation or those whose background is unfamiliar to them.

One's development, understanding, and appreciation for the values and beliefs of others comes with practice and the ongoing use of therapeutic communication. To be effective communicators, nurses must develop awareness of their own values and beliefs and the way in which they influence their perception of patients' experiences. Therapeutic communication requires openness and the ability to listen to patients without judgment. This requires an ongoing reflective evaluation of one's own beliefs. Nonjudgmental communication calls for the development of excellent communication skills.

Home Health Considerations

Cultural Understanding

Nurses must be aware of patients' cultural values and beliefs, and incorporate them into patient care whenever possible to provide care to an increasingly diverse patient population. Research shows that the patients who receive culturally congruent care are more likely to adhere to treatment, have better outcomes, and continue to use health care services. Therefore **cultural awareness** and competence are mandatory components of professional nursing practice. **Cultural competence** in nursing can be defined as a set of behaviors that includes understanding the impact of cultural values and beliefs on human experiences while maintaining awareness of one's own cultural values and their effect on the perception of self and others. **Cultural understanding** requires cultural awareness, which is knowledge and appreciation of the unique features of a cultural group. This may include recognition of components such as the history, customs, artistic expression, cuisine, and health practices of various cultures. The nurse who seeks to have cultural understanding (of the cultures of others) is more likely to successfully establish and maintain therapeutic relationships and deliver highly effective care reflective of each patients' unique needs.

The acquisition of cultural knowledge is an ongoing process. The nurse must become familiar with credible resources that can be used to facilitate that process. The following are examples of websites that contain information on cultural competence:

- https://ccnm.thinkculturalhealth.hhs.gov/
- www.tcns.org/

Developing understanding of the impact of values and beliefs on one's perceptions of self and others requires ongoing commitment to personal and professional growth. The most effective way to develop appreciation and understanding of diverse beliefs and values is through education, which can be gained through reading, participating in professional development activities, studying academics, and interacting with individuals of diverse backgrounds. Patient education and positive interactions can help people understand the way their values and beliefs influence their perception and management of health. Developing this awareness is usually the first step toward positive change toward inclusion. Nurses who develop an understanding of the beliefs and values of the groups commonly encountered in their practice can facilitate this change by providing culturally congruent care that meets the needs of their individual patients (Leininger, 1995, 2002, 2006; McFarland & Wehbe-Alamah, 2019).

COMMON VALUES AND BELIEFS OF OLDER ADULTS

The older adult population is as diverse as are younger age groups. However, they do share some values and beliefs based on the experiences of their generation. Some of these individuals developed their value systems in a world that was very different from today's world. For example, some of the older adult population spent most of their working lives before the internet and media explosion and long before mobile communication devices became a mandatory accessory. Others have actively experienced the advent and evolution of technology as well as the increasing need and desire to understand diversity. Intergenerational differences in values and beliefs may lead to misunderstanding and conflict. As the nursing workforce becomes increasingly diverse and as more young nurses enter it, it becomes increasingly important for nurses to recognize differences in beliefs in order to establish and maintain therapeutic relationships with older patients and coworkers.

ECONOMIC VALUES

Many of today's older adults, when they were children, were affected by the Depression of the 1930s. They were taught to be frugal and mindful of resources. Consequently they value independence and may have difficulties accepting monetary assistance or allowing others to manage their financial affairs. If they are not covered by Medicare, they might express concern over the cost of care and may delay seeking help or even refuse care until they are seriously ill. They might choose to forgo buying medications or take less than the amount prescribed in order to save money.

Some older adults save or hoard items, including items that present health hazards, because they value saving rather than wasting. Some older people who need to be placed in assisted living facilities face challenges and difficulty when they must part with most of their possessions. When living in a community, some older adults may have amassed a lot of clutter (excess items) in their homes, which can expose them to safety hazards and multiple health risks. Some older people may be dismayed when nurses or family members throw away food or medical supplies and may attempt to retrieve these items once they are alone.

Some of these attitudes are beginning to change as baby boomers enter late adulthood. Baby boomers grew up in a more affluent world and are more likely to value material possessions and to spend rather than save. This is likely to result in delays in retirement as older boomers remain in the workforce.

INTERPERSONAL VALUES

Today's older adults were raised in an era when interpersonal communication was more formal. Some of them may want caregivers to address them formally, using an honorific with their last name, such as "Mr. Evans" or "Mrs. Ortega." Moreover, they grew up valuing the respect given to elders and may therefore expect to be treated with deference by younger caregivers. This also applies to their relationships with their family members. Older people often cannot understand why younger family members do not automatically accept what they say and follow their directions. This can lead to misunderstanding and conflict. Nurses may need to intervene if conflicts arise or to provide support to older people who feel rejected or misunderstood by their children. The nurse's role is to act as the patient's advocate; however, it is important to refrain from acting as a mediator in the patient's personal relationships. It is often more helpful for the nurse to simply ask the family to take a break (e.g., go home to rest and refresh, or go to the cafeteria for coffee) so that the patient can get some rest. Once the family has left, the nurse can provide therapeutic support for the patient.

CULTURAL VALUES

Society in the United States is very diverse. People of many different age groups, cultural identifications, heritages, and races reside here. The proportion of people belonging to racial and ethnic minority populations who are at least 65 years of age is projected to increase by 115% by 2040 (Administration for Community Living, 2021). Nurses must be able to provide care to this increasingly diverse group.

Cultural values and beliefs can unite families, neighborhoods, and communities. Shared cultural values define an authority structure, establish norms for language and communication, and establish a basis for decision-making and lifestyle choices. Historically, society in the United States was shaped by many immigrants who arrived in search of opportunity and a better life. In addition, the cultural identity of the United States is still influenced by a troubled history of slavery and warfare with its own citizens.

Although most people express a dislike for any form of prejudice, problems still exist. The health status of minority groups still is largely inequitable due to difficulties accessing health care services and receiving less than optimal culturally congruent care. This is often due to economic and language barriers (Torres-Ruiz et al., 2018). Nurses must recognize these health disparities and work to minimize and then eradicate them by educating themselves in order to provide equitable, excellent care. Many health care organizations and agencies offer mandatory training to their clinical staff. Nursing professional organizations offer courses and other resources to support development of cultural competencies. The Transcultural Nursing Society (TCNS, 2021) offers basic and advanced certification in transcultural care.

SPIRITUAL OR RELIGIOUS VALUES

Spirituality is a deeply personal experience of connectedness with a higher entity or purpose. Some individuals find their spirituality within a specific religious community, although others ground their spirituality in social and/or natural laws. Spirituality is a deeply personal experience and can vary significantly from one person to another. Some people identify themselves as religious, whereas others state that they are agnostics or atheists. Although an atheist does not believe in the existence of a higher power, an agnostic is a person who neither believes nor denies the existence of such because it cannot be proven. Do not assume that individuals who do not practice or subscribe to a specific religion are not spiritual. People who do not identify with a certain faith may indicate that they do not subscribe to beliefs of organized religious systems, yet they still believe in a higher power. It is important for nurses to understand that all individuals have a spiritual nature, whether or not they observe a specific religion.

Spiritual beliefs have a huge impact on the way one experiences life events, including those related to health. They can inspire pleasant emotions, such as wonder, love, hope, and trust, or they can instigate unpleasant emotions, such as hatred, anger, fear, guilt, and despair. Individuals usually build their value systems and set their priorities based on their spiritual beliefs.

The need for spiritual connections grows as a person ages and death nears. Spiritual beliefs can be a source of strength, and even people who did not seem to place a high value on their spiritual development when they were younger often see a need to seek spiritual guidance or connectedness when they grow older (Fig. 14.1). Therefore incorporate spiritual assessment into the assessment of an older person and offer access to spiritual (and religious) care as requested. Respect each person's choices and never try to impose your values and beliefs on them.

Decisions regarding the end of life are greatly influenced by patients' spiritual beliefs and personal value systems. Many older adults wish to have a spiritual (or

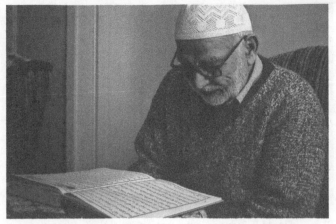

Fig. 14.1 Older adult reciting the Qur'an during Ramadan. (From Webb, M., Kostelnick, C., & Scott, K. [2018]. *Long-term caring* [4th ed.]. St. Louis, MO: Elsevier.)

religious) advisor available for guidance when making decisions about serious health matters. Caregivers must respect patients' decisions even when they are in conflict with a caregiver's beliefs and values. Survival may be less important to an older person than the violation of long-held beliefs. Older adults who are coherent have the right to make informed choices and to have them respected.

Some of today's oldest adults were brought up at a time when organized religion played an important role in society, and it may have played an important role in the formulation of their individual values and beliefs. They may be very familiar with gathering regularly to worship together. Regular attendance at places of worship has been declining in recent years. This may be partly due to transportation problems or safety concerns, such as those surrounding COVID-19, that make regular attendance difficult. Some older adults experience severe spiritual disconnection when they are no longer able to worship regularly in person because of illness, hospitalization, or relocation to an institutional setting. This is particularly important in the context of nursing care. At times of personal and/or health crisis, people often have a greater need to connect with their religious communities. Not being able to do so can adversely affect their sense of well-being.

Older adults may prefer religious observances or worship in the ways they learned as children. As society changes, so do methods and places of worship as well as qualifications for becoming a religious leader. Assess your patients to determine whether they accept contemporary practices or whether they wish to pursue traditional religious practices. This might call for adjusting care plans to reflect the older adults' beliefs.

Religious rituals are formal and observable ceremonies serving to affirm faith and provide a sense of belonging to a given community. They are part of every faith and include rituals such as prayers, chanting, cleansing, anointing, and singing religious music. They often involve the use of symbolic objects, such

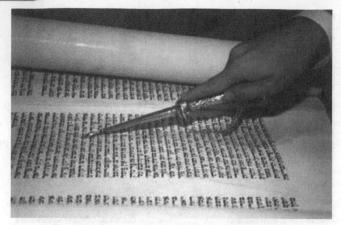

Fig. 14.2 Tradition in thought; spirituality in Judaism.

as icons, menorahs, rosaries, amulets, medals, or holy water. Religious texts—such as the Bible, Qur'an, Torah, Vedas, and Book of Mormon—are essential to the practices of their respective religions (Fig. 14.2). Many older adults find great comfort in these texts, often memorizing large segments. Older adults who are unable to read because of the changes associated with aging or illness find comfort in the mere presence of these valued texts or in having someone read these to them. Often, the family or spiritual support person will provide these symbols and texts if the older person requests them.

Complementary Health Approaches

Prayer and Meditation

Prayer is a religious ritual used in many religions to communicate with a higher power as defined by an individual's beliefs. It can be ritualized and structured or free and informal. Many times, prayers are accompanied by other religious rituals and symbols, such as candles, incense, or prayer beads. Prayer can be incorporated into the plan of care as a complementary health approach designed to meet the patient's spiritual needs.

Similar to prayer, some individuals like to use meditation to achieve relaxation, relieve stress and anxiety, or to gain a better understanding of self. Meditation has many forms, some of which are associated with specific religious practices, although others are based on nonreligious principles. The value of meditation in pain management, where it is often used, is well documented. Research has also shown that meditation can create a relaxation response, and it has been demonstrated to reduce anxiety.

Many older adults reach the end of life at peace with themselves. It is common for an older adult to say, "I'm ready to go. I've led a good life and I'm ready to meet my maker." Others may not be as peaceful, but they accept the inevitability of death. However, some older people will experience considerable anxiety and distress as the end of life approaches. The experience and reaction to the end of life is not related to a person's age. It is often related to a person's evaluation of their life in retrospect. They may experience a sense of guilt and distress because of unresolved long-standing conflict with important people in their lives or the belief that they did not resolve their personal affairs. Spiritual disconnection is characterized by hopelessness and/or failure to see one's life with a sense of peace.

Critical Thinking

Spiritual Assessment for Nurses

- Reflect on your spirituality. Do you consider yourself to be spiritual and/or religious? Why or why not?
- Develop a list of your values with the most important ones on top. Reflect on why certain values are more important than others.
- Reflect on what gives meaning to your life.
- Identify your spiritual and/or religious practices.
- Reflect on how your spiritual and/or religious beliefs impact your daily life, including your professional life.
- Identify the ways your spiritual and/or religious beliefs may affect your perception and response to patients' spiritual and/or religious needs, especially if they are different from your beliefs.

People experiencing spiritual disconnection may be fearful or angry. To be open to the spiritual needs of others and work effectively with patients experiencing spiritual disconnection, the nurse should first explore their own spiritual feelings and beliefs (see Critical Thinking box and Box 14.1).

❖ NURSING PROCESS/CLINICAL JUDGMENT MODEL FOR SPIRITUAL DISCONNECTION

◆ ASSESSMENT (DATA COLLECTION)

Recognize cues:
Ask the following questions when you are conducting a cultural and spiritual assessment:
- What is your cultural background?
- What is your preferred language?

Box 14.1 Whole Health: Change the Conversation— Spiritual Assessment Tools

Maugans' SPIRIT Mnemonic for Spiritual Assessment
- S: Spiritual belief system (religious affiliation)
- P: Personal spirituality (personal belief system)
- I: Integration into a spiritual community (sources of support)
- R: Ritualized practices (daily practices, restrictions, and their significance)
- I: Implications for medical care (spiritual aspects incorporated into care)
- T: Terminal event (end of life)

From Maugans, T. A., as presented in VA Office of Patient Centered Care and Cultural Transformation (n.d.). https://www.va.gov/WHOLEHEALTHLIBRARY/docs/M11_Spiritual_Assessment_Tools.pdf

Box 14.2   **Risk Factors for Alterations in Values and Beliefs in Older Adults**

- Major life stressors, such as severe illness or impending death
- A recent significant loss or change in role
- Values and/or beliefs different from those of caregivers or the dominant cultural values
- Removal from a familiar spiritual support system
- Loss of financial independence

- Would you like to discuss your treatment in English or in your preferred language?
- Would you like support from your family members, friends, and/or spiritual and/or religious advisors when you are making decisions about your treatment?
- How does your condition affect your life?
- What traditional remedies have you used or would like to use to treat your condition?
- Are you a member of a religious or spiritual group?
- Are there any cultural or religious practices you would like to pursue while you are in our care?
- Would you like to talk to your spiritual or religious adviser?
- Are there any foods that your prefer to avoid because of your spiritual or religious beliefs?
- Are there any religious books or symbols that you would like to have with you?
- How can we (nursing staff) support your religious practices or your spiritual needs?

Box 14.2 provides a list of risk factors for alterations in values and beliefs in older adults.

◆ DATA ANALYSIS/PROBLEM IDENTIFICATION

Analyze Cues and Prioritize Hypotheses: Problem statements for older adults with spiritual disconnectedness include the following:

Potential for Spiritual Disconnection

Spiritual Disconnection

◆ PLANNING

Generate Solutions: The patient goals for older adults suffering from spiritual disconnection are to (1) identify and verbalize sources of value conflicts, (2) specify the spiritual assistance desired, (3) discuss values and beliefs regarding spiritual practices, and (4) express feelings of spiritual comfort.

◆ IMPLEMENTATION

Take Action: The following nursing interventions should take place in hospitals or extended-care facilities:

1. **Determine whether there are special spiritual practices and/or restrictions.** Identify the unique spiritual needs of older adults. Regardless of common beliefs and practices associated with major denominations, always clarify each individual's interpretation of and compliance with these beliefs and practices. This is particularly important if a patient's spiritual or religious belief system requires or prohibits certain dietary practices or health behaviors. Whenever possible, allow the older adult to continue their habitual practices and rituals. If there is a conflict between a person's spiritual/religious values or practices and health needs, consult with the patient or family to identify acceptable strategies or compromises. Failure to consider the older adult's spiritual beliefs can arouse anger, despondency, and nonadherence to the treatment plan.

2. **Identify significant people who provide spiritual/religious support.** Many organizations recognize certain people as spiritual or religious leaders or guides who help others to learn and practice specific beliefs. Priests, rabbis, imams, ministers, deacons, and religious sisters are commonly recognized as spiritual/religious authorities who are trained to provide counsel to their own members and often to members of different faiths. Many older adults have a special closeness to a specific individual whom they trust; they will therefore appreciate a call or visit from such a person, particularly when hospitalized or in danger of death. If requested by the patient, contact this person or ask the family to initiate the contact. People often gain as much sustenance from spiritual counsel as they do from medical treatment. The spiritual counselor can also support the family experiencing a stressful situation; act as a liaison between the patient, family, and clinical staff; and aid them in dealing with spiritual practices and concerns.

3. **Determine whether there is any way nurses can aid the older adult in meeting their spiritual needs.** Conduct an assessment to determine whether any assistance is required to enable the older adult to meet their spiritual needs. Nurses are often asked to assist older adults in spiritual practices by contacting spiritual advisers, providing spiritual articles or items, or facilitating rituals.

4. **Provide opportunities for the older adult to express their spiritual needs and concerns.** Listen in a nonjudgmental manner to whatever the older adult wishes to verbalize. When problems or concerns exist, it often helps to verbalize them to someone else. In most cases, these speakers do not want to have a mutual conversation but rather to be listened to or to air their feelings openly so that they can begin to deal with them. Help the person explore issues rather than stopping the thoughts or providing false reassurance. Life review or reminiscence may be helpful in aiding the older adult through these doubts and concerns.

5. **Determine spiritual objects that have meaning to the older adult; obtain these if possible.** Place the objects that are symbolic of faith where they can be seen or touched by the older adult; they should

not be hidden or put away in a drawer. These items should be shown due respect by all caregivers.

6. **Provide opportunities for spiritual guidance with respect for privacy.** Because spiritual practices often include the sharing of private thoughts and fears, provide the older adult with opportunities to be alone to pray or meditate if desired. A chapel or quiet room free from distractions is desirable. If the person wishes to meet with a spiritual authority or to perform religious rituals, provide the opportunity to do so. This may require planning so that no interruptions (e.g., interventions or treatments) interfere at that time.

7. **Encourage contact with a spiritual counselor in times of crisis.** Privacy is important in times of spiritual crisis, such as the loss of a loved one or imminent death. Severe grief can lead to spiritual disconnection. Contact with a spiritual authority can help the older adult work through feelings of anger, resentment, or ambivalence toward their spirituality. Pay special attention to spiritual rituals related to death, such as confession, communion, or anointing. Be aware of acceptable practices before preparing the body after death.

Take Action: The following interventions should take place in the home:

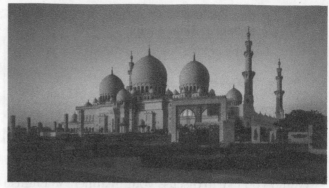

Fig. 14.3 The mosque—the main place of worship for Muslims. (From Williams, P. A. [2022]. *Fundamental concepts and skills for nursing* [6th ed.]. St. Louis, MO: Elsevier.)

1. **Make arrangements that allow the older adult to maintain their religious practices.** When possible, arrange for transportation to the place of worship or gathering (Fig. 14.3). Many organizations can find rides for members who are not able to walk or drive. If this is not possible because of severe health problems or immobility, arrange a visit from a spiritual authority if requested by the patient.

2. **Use any appropriate interventions that are used in the institutional setting** (Nursing Care Plan 14.1).

★ Nursing Care Plan 14.1 Spiritual Disconnection

Mr. Quinn, age 78, has attended Christian services regularly in his assisted living facility and has expressed a strong belief in a "merciful God." A week ago, he learned from his health care provider that he has terminal cancer and has approximately 3 months to live. After talking to the provider, he went to the chapel and cried. Since then, he has spent a great deal of time in his room reading the Bible. He angrily states to the nurse, "God hasn't shown me any mercy, and I probably will have to suffer for all I've done wrong in my life."

PROBLEM STATEMENT
Spiritual Disconnection

SUPPORTING ASSESSMENT DATA
- Expresses anger
- Verbalizes hopelessness
- Verbalizes lack of self-forgiveness
- Expresses lack of peace

PATIENT GOALS/OUTCOMES IDENTIFICATION
Mr. Quinn will recognize that illness places stress on a belief system and will express feelings of spiritual comfort.

NURSING INTERVENTIONS/IMPLEMENTATION
1. Listen to Mr. Quinn's concerns and feelings in a nonjudgmental manner.
2. Request a visit from Mr. Quinn's minister (if Mr. Quinn desires it).
3. Provide privacy for spiritual counseling and observances.
4. Keep the Bible and a prayer book readily available.
5. Assist Mr. Quinn to the chapel as requested.

EVALUATION
Mr. Quinn begins visiting the chapel daily and has a weekly visit with his minister. After each visit, he appears calmer, stating, "I still don't know why this is happening to me, but I have put my trust in God." You will continue the plan of care.

APPLYING CLINICAL JUDGMENT
1. What type of verbal or nonverbal responses from the nurse would best demonstrate nonjudgmental acceptance of Mr. Quinn's feelings?
2. What could the nurse do if Mr. Quinn states, "I don't believe in a merciful God anymore" and refuses visits from the chaplain or another spiritual counselor?

Get Ready for the Next Generation NCLEX® Examination!

Key Points

- Everyone's values and beliefs are unique. They are a product of one's culture, education, religion, and society.
- It is important to view each person as an individual and to refrain from stereotyping based on perceived culture or ethnicity.
- Values and beliefs form the basis of an older person's choices, perceptions, and behaviors.
- The values and beliefs held by older adults may significantly differ from those held by younger individuals.
- If not identified, differences in values and beliefs can result in misunderstandings, confusion, and conflict between older adults and their families or younger health care providers.
- Nurses can reduce problems related to differences in values and beliefs by openly communicating with older adults.
- Nurses have the responsibility to continue to learn about social, spiritual, and cultural diversity and to value each person's unique beliefs.

Additional Learning Resources

 SG Go to your Evolve website at http://evolve.elsevier.com/Williams/geriatric for the additional online resources.

Review Questions for the Next Generation NCLEX® Examination

1. The nurse is caring for an older adult in an extended-care facility. Which patient statement indicates possible spiritual disconnection?
   a. "I made some mistakes, but my life turned out pretty well."
   b. "I feel that God abandoned me and that I will die all alone."
   c. "My relationship with my children has not been perfect, but we fixed our differences."
   d. "My spouse died 19 years ago and is waiting for me on the other side."

2. The nurse observes an older adult who saves unopened crackers, jelly, and juice packages from the meal tray. How does the nurse interpret this behavior?
   a. The patient may want a snack later.
   b. It is not appropriate to waste items that are good and useful.
   c. Hoarding disorder is a likely diagnosis.
   d. The behavior means nothing unless it becomes compulsive.

3. An older adult patient has asked the family to bring folk remedies to the long-term care facility. Which intervention will the nurse provide?
   a. Tell the patient that these practices are harmful and should be avoided.
   b. Remind the family that only the health care provider can order treatments.
   c. Encourage the family to bring whatever is requested.
   d. Ask the patient to discuss which kind of remedies have been requested.

4. A patient says to the nurse, "I wasn't raised with any kind of religion so I guess that means I'm not spiritual." Which nursing response is appropriate?
   a. "That is correct; spirituality does not exist without religion."
   b. "Spirituality is about what you feel gives your life meaning."
   c. "Can I call a chaplain to discuss different religions with you?"
   d. "Let's talk about finding a religion that you prefer."

5. The nurse is caring for a patient who has listed "atheist" on an intake form asking about a preferred religion. Which nursing response to this notation is appropriate?
   a. "Do you have any spiritual practices we can assist you with?"
   b. "Would you like me to ask our on-call priest to help you?"
   c. "Although you don't believe, I am still praying that a higher power will heal you."
   d. "I guess you won't be needing the services of our spiritual care department."

REFERENCES

Administration for Community Living (2021). 2020 profile of older Americans. https://acl.gov/sites/default/files/Aging%20and%20Disability%20in%20America/2020Profile OlderAmericans.Final_.pdf

Jewish visiting (2021). Death and burial. http://jvisit.org.uk/death-and-burial/

Leininger, M. (1995). Teaching transcultural nursing in undergraduate and graduate programs. *Journal of Transcultural Nursing, 6*(2), 10–26. doi:10.1177/104365969500600203

Leininger, M. M., & McFarland, M. R. (Eds.). (2002). *Transcultural nursing: Concepts, theories, research, and practice* (3rd ed.). New York, NY: McGraw-Hill.

Leininger, M. M., & McFarland, M. R. (Eds.). (2006). *Culture care diversity and universality: A worldwide theory of nursing* (2nd ed.). Sudbury, MA: Jones & Bartlett.

Massey, M. (2005). *What you are is where you were when—again!* Cambridge, MA: Enterprise Media.

McFarland, M. R., & Wehbe-Alamah, H. B. (2019). Leininger's theory of culture care diversity and universality: An overview with a historical retrospective and a view toward the future. *Journal of Transcultural Nursing, 30*(6), 540–557.

National Congress of American Indians (2020). Indian country demographics. https://www.ncai.org/about-tribes/demographics#:~:text=American%20Indian%20and%20 Alaska%20Native,2.4%25%20of%20the%20U.S.%20 population

Pew Research Center (2021). Religious landscape study: Latinos. https://www.pewforum.org/religious-landscape-study/racial-and-ethnic-composition/latino/

Siler, S., Arora, K., Doyon, K., et al. (2021). Spirituality and the illness experience: Perspectives of African American older adults. *American Journal of Hospice and Palliative Medicine.* https://doi.org/10.1177/1049909120988280

Torres-Ruiz, M., Robinson-Ector, K., Attinson, D., Trotter, J., Anise, A., & Clauser, S. (2018). A portfolio analysis of culturally tailored trials to address health and healthcare disparities. *International Journal of Environmental Research and Public Health, 15.* https://doi.org/10.3390/ijerph15091859

Transcultural Nursing Society (TCNS). (2021). Certification. https://tcns.org/tcncertification/

Ulmer, K.C. (2020). Mental illness is hurting black faith communities. Prayer shouldn't be out only defense. Religious News Service. https://religionnews.com/2020/08/04/mental-illness-is-hurting-black-faith-communities-prayer-shouldnt-be-our-only-defense/

Objectives

1. Discuss personal and societal attitudes related to death and end-of-life planning.
2. Identify factors that are likely to influence end-of-life decision-making.
3. Explore caregiver attitudes toward end-of-life care.
4. Discuss the importance of effective communication at the end of life.
5. Identify cultural and spiritual considerations related to end-of-life care.
6. Describe nursing assessments and interventions appropriate to end-of-life care.
7. Discuss the role of the nurse when interacting with the bereaved.
8. Describe the stages of grief.

Key Terms

anorexia (ăn-ŏ-RĔK-sē-ă, p. 272)
cachexia (kă-KĔK-sē-ă, p. 272)
Cheyne-Stokes (chānstōks, p. 271)
ethical dilemmas (p. 263)

hospice (HŎS-pĭs, p. 264)
morgue (mörg, p. 274)
palliative (PĂL-ē-ă-tĭv, p. 265)

During the 17th century, the poet John Donne wrote, "No man is an island … any man's death diminishes me, because I am involved in mankind; and therefore never send to know for whom the bell tolls; it tolls for thee." In those days, a death was acknowledged by a solemn ringing of church bells, much the way bells are rung at many funerals today. Death was feared, but it was perceived as an inevitable part of life. Infants, children, and young adults routinely died of infection, accident, and acute illness. Death was a familiar experience to all members of society. Because most people died at home, receiving care and comfort from family members, people of all ages were exposed to the realities of death. Consequently, cultures around the world developed grieving rituals to help the deceased person's family and immediate community process and manage the experience of loss.

The end-of-life experiences are very different today. The advancements of science and technology have led to unprecedented increases in life expectancy over the past 100 years. Most deaths (over 73%) occur among people over age 65 (National Center for Health Statistics, 2018). With longer life expectancy, death is becoming increasingly associated with advanced age, usually the inevitable progression of a chronic and/or debilitating condition (Box 15.1). Typically, individuals with chronic conditions experience repetitive episodes of health crises separated by periods of relative well-being. However, even though they appear to recover between episodes, each health crisis inflicts a certain amount of irreparable damage. Eventually, the individual will run out of recuperative reserve and die.

DEATH IN WESTERN CULTURES

The experience of death in Western cultures is a reflection of an ethnocultural climate that emphasizes individualism and self-reliance. A person's family may not be readily available, and the concepts of community and family are rather flexible and open to individual interpretation. Typically, the experience of death in Western cultures involves multiple dimensions that go far beyond the loss of an individual and generates numerous psychosocial, ethical, legal, and administrative challenges. For that reason, death and dying in contemporary America are frequently subject to regulations intended to preserve individuals' autonomy and to provide necessary services and protection to all parties. However, in spite of these efforts,

Box 15.1	Common Causes of Death in Adults Ages 65 and Older

- heart disease
- malignant neoplasms
- chronic lower respiratory disease
- cerebrovascular disease
- Alzheimer disease
- diabetes mellitus
- unintentional injury
- influenza and pneumonia
- nephritis
- Parkinson disease

Source: Centers for Disease Control and Prevention (2020). https://www.cdc.gov/injury/images/lc-charts/leading_causes_of_death_by_age_group_2018_1100w850h.jpg

many older adults and their loved ones do not receive adequate service and support when faced with death and dying. All too often they are forced to make sense of the ever-changing rules and regulations entirely by themselves. This inevitably increases stress and frustration for the dying person and their loved ones. The unfortunate result is that effective end-of-life care is too often delayed for it to be of maximal benefit. Fortunately, many organizations, agencies, educators, and health care providers are working toward increasing the accessibility of the optimal end-of-life care. Organizations such as the National Hospice and Palliative Care Organization, American Geriatrics Society, the National Academy of Medicine, the American Association of Colleges of Nursing, and the Robert Wood Johnson Foundation have publications and websites providing valuable information and resources to health care professionals and consumers.

ATTITUDES TOWARD DEATH AND END-OF-LIFE PLANNING

Extended life expectancy and advancements of science have changed the average person's experiences and perceptions of death. A large number of people in Western societies have no direct experience with death and dying until middle or late adulthood. They may know someone who has died and may have attended a memorial or funeral service, but few have actually been in the presence of a dying person. However, interest in end-of-life care has been increasing in recent years. This trend was driven in large part by the baby boom generation, who were dealing with end-of-life concerns related to their parents. Now, many baby boomers make up a large part of the older adult population preparing themselves for the end of life.

In the past, health professionals often made the decisions regarding end-of-life care with minimal input from the patient and family. Physicians could unequivocally state, "We have done everything possible." This is no longer true. Today, health care consumers want to actively participate in the decision-making processes affecting their health and well-being.

 QSEN Considerations: Patient-Centered Care

There is a growing understanding among health professionals that health care consumers have a right to guide their care according to their personal beliefs and preferences. The role of health professionals has shifted from that of a decision maker to that of a service provider whose primary responsibility is to help consumers make informed decisions; this is the essence of patient-centered care. Consequently, the approach to end-of-life care has shifted from a purely medical focus to a more holistic approach that takes into consideration consumers' personal values, cultural and spiritual beliefs, and life experiences.

Some older adults and their families still prefer treatment modalities that prolong life and want to receive every treatment available. Others prefer a comfortable death in the presence of their loved ones. Many people say that they do not fear death as much as they fear how they will die.

Many people are uncomfortable talking about death. Therefore health care agencies now offer specialized services and referrals to interdisciplinary teams that provide support to individuals, families, and others making decisions about end-of-life care. Family members, nurses, and other caregivers must be able to communicate about the end of life to provide good care for older people nearing the end of their lives. These discussions are usually not as traumatic for the older adult as they are for younger people. By the time people reach advanced age, most have already experienced the death of loved ones. Parents, spouses, siblings, friends, and even children or grandchildren have died from many causes and under widely differing circumstances. These experiences generally help older adults determine what type of care they do or do not want as the reality of death approaches. Most alert older adults are quite candid in expressing their wishes if approached in a sensitive but matter-of-fact way.

Ideally, discussions regarding end-of-life care and planning for death should occur before a health crisis arises. This gives older adults enough time to make decisions when they are calm and can evaluate their situations objectively and according to their personal values. When important decisions regarding end-of-life care are avoided or delayed, family members and friends of the dying person may have to make decisions in a time of crisis. Unfortunately, they are likely to be overwhelmed by the approaching death of a loved one and may not be able to clearly identify and articulate the desires of the dying person. Consequently, their decisions may be guided by their own beliefs and values rather than the desires of the dying person.

Family members may initiate a discussion about end-of-life preferences with their loved ones after watching a show or reading a news article that deals with dying. Similarly, the discussion may be initiated during gatherings where the family reminisces about loved ones who have died or following the death of a friend or a family member. Nurses working in outpatient settings can initiate the discussion while they are reviewing patients' records. You can ask the older adults if they have advance directive documents and offer information about end-of-life care planning. Admission to an acute care setting following a health crisis offers another good opportunity to educate older adults about end-of-life care. Once the initial crisis has passed, the older adult usually has a high level of consciousness regarding death and is more likely to recognize the need to make their end-of-life care preferences known. You can assist by providing the materials needed to initiate advance directives or by offering a referral to a social worker or appropriate community resources.

ADVANCE DIRECTIVES

Specific end-of-life decisions can be expressed in advance directives and physicians orders for life sustaining treatment (POLST) (see Chapter 1). These documents specify the type and amount of intervention desired by someone. Once initiated, they remain in effect until changed. Health care consumers should provide copies of their advance directives to their primary care providers, the person holding a durable power of attorney, and any other person or health care agency who might be involved in their care. This can prevent last-minute confusion and possible violation of their wishes. If a person does not wish to be resuscitated, this must be accurately recorded in all of their health care records and communicated to anybody potentially involved in resuscitation efforts. The person can choose to wear a bracelet. Caregivers must include this information when transferring care, and if a POLST is in effect, it should be visibly posted in the home.

There is no single right plan for the end of life. The best plan is one that reflects the individual's values and beliefs. Guidance and support from physicians, clergy, nurses, social workers, and family can help a dying person make these significant decisions, but each person must ultimately make their own choices.

Decisions about end-of-life care are not unchangeable and can be altered as the situation changes. To make an informed decision about a specific intervention or treatment, a patient must have enough information, including (1) the amount of time a treatment will add to life; (2) the quality of life with this treatment; (3) the amount of pain, disability, or risk involved with the treatment; (4) the amount of time involved in the treatment; (5) the cost of treatment and whether it is covered by insurance; (6) the need for and availability of caregivers; and (7) the availability, benefits, and risks of other treatment options. This information must be provided by the practitioner providing the treatment, but patients have a right to discuss their treatment options with anybody, including their loved ones, who might help them make decisions for their treatment. If they are not satisfied with the information received from a specific health care practitioner, they have the right to request further consultation with another practitioner.

CAREGIVER ATTITUDES TOWARD END-OF-LIFE CARE

Even caregivers who routinely care for critically ill or dying patients may have difficulty accepting death. Many health care professionals have become so focused on preventing illness or curing disease that they are more likely to view death as a personal or professional failure rather than the inevitable end to the human experience. All caregivers—including nurses, physicians, social workers, family members, and others playing a role in end-of-life care—need to learn to recognize their own attitudes, feelings, values, and expectations about death. They need to explore the professional literature discussing legal, ethical, financial, and health care delivery issues related to end-of-life care. Everybody involved in the care of a dying person should collaborate to provide the dying person with holistic care that meets the patient's physical, psychological, social, and cultural needs. In addition, they need to be able to address the needs of the family, friends, and significant others as they face grief, loss, and bereavement at the end of life. Caregivers need to overcome any feelings of frustration or ineffectiveness. They need to learn when and how to shift from the aggressive medical interventions designed to cure or extend life to more palliative and holistic interventions designed to enable dying persons and their loved ones to experience a "good" death characterized by comfort, peace, dignity, and caring. The inability to facilitate a good death can become overwhelming for medical staff in times of pandemics. Many patients have been forced to die alone during the COVID-19 pandemic. Early studies have shown that health care providers on the front line showed increased insomnia, depression, anxiety, and somatization (Cabarkapa, 2020). It is important for caregivers to find an outlet for feelings of helplessness and seek assistance with their own mental health when circumstances prevent them from giving the type of care that they feel is needed.

VALUES CLARIFICATION RELATED TO DEATH AND END-OF-LIFE CARE

Beliefs, attitudes, and values regarding the experience of death and end-of-life care vary widely. Individuals' responses are influenced by their age, gender, culture, religious background, and life experiences. Caregivers should reflect on their personal values related to the end of life and identify those values that are likely to influence their decision-making processes and behavior when caring for dying patients. Ethical dilemmas relating to end-of-life care are more likely to occur when the value systems of the patient and of the care giver differ significantly. Understanding the value systems of others can help the nurse provide quality end-of-life care, even when they do not share the same values (see Critical Thinking Box above).

WHAT IS A "GOOD" DEATH?

Many groups in the United States and abroad have conducted research to identify specific end-of-life outcomes that are most valued and desired by those nearing the end of life and by their families. Themes throughout all of the studies indicate that given their choice, most people wish to be treated with respect and

Critical Thinking

Values Clarification Exercise Related to the End of Life

Complete the following statements and reflect on your answers. What do they tell you about your perceptions and values regarding end-of-life issues?

1. Death is …
2. Death means …
3. After death …
4. Decisions about my end-of-life care should be made by …
5. Talking about dying makes me feel …
6. When I am nearing the end of life, I want my family to …
7. When I am nearing the end of life, I want my caregivers to …
8. As death nears, I am afraid of …
9. I am in pain as I near the end of life …
10. I am dying and I do not want …
11. Because I am old, death …
12. After I die, I want people to …

 Critical Thinking

Personal Beliefs and Attitudes About Death

- What are your personal experiences with death?
- Have you lost a close friend, family member, or patient to death?
- How did you feel when you heard that the person had died?
- If you have had more than one experience, did you respond differently to the deaths? Why do you think you responded differently?
- Have you ever been with a person at the time of death?
- What thoughts crossed your mind as the person died?
- Were other people present?
- What was said or done?
- What spiritual or cultural rituals were performed at the time of death or burial?

 Critical Thinking

Ethical Dilemmas

This chapter has identified the most commonly identified wishes of individuals nearing the end of life.

- What should happen if one or more of these wishes conflicts with those of the caregivers?
- What if a spouse values the companionship of the dying person and wants all possible life-extending actions to be provided in conflict with the patient's advance directives?
- What if a physician or family member determines that a patient cannot cope with hearing a terminal diagnosis?
- What if the nurse thinks that the amount of pain medication ordered is excessive?
- What should be done if death seems imminent during the middle of the night when no family is present?

dignity and to die quietly and peacefully with loved ones nearby. Box 15.2 identifies the common threads identified by these studies.

Nurses need to be able to assess the needs of a dying person and plan the care accordingly to facilitate a

---

Box 15.2 Summary of Patients' Wishes Related to the End of Life

Most dying patients want to

- Be able to issue advance directives to ensure their wishes are respected
- Be afforded dignity, respect, and privacy
- Know when death is coming and what to expect
- Have access to information and options related to care
- Retain control of decision-making regarding care
- Have control over symptom and pain relief
- Have access to emotional, cultural, and spiritual support
- Retain control regarding who may be present at the end of life
- Know possible options (e.g., hospital, home care, and hospice) and have a choice regarding where and how death will occur
- Have time to say goodbye to significant others
- Leave life when ready to go without unnecessary or pointless interventions

healthy experience of death and dying. Human needs at the end of life follow the universal pattern of human needs. Psychologist Abraham Maslow introduced this well-accepted hierarchy of needs, where people are motivated to fulfill basic needs (such as physiological needs like food) before fulfilling more advanced human needs (Maslow, 1943). Fig. 15.1 summarizes the needs of the dying person using Maslow's hierarchy of needs.

WHERE PEOPLE DIE

Studies indicate that 80% of people wish to die at home (Stanford School of Medicine, 2021). In spite of that, the vast majority of deaths occur in institutional settings, with less than one-fourth of deaths occurring at home. Approximately 60% of deaths occur in hospitals, and another one-fourth occur in extended-care facilities. Death in the hospital setting is particularly problematic because hospitals are focused on curative and restorative care and may not be ideally suited for end-of-life care. The focus of care in extended-care facilities is on care, not cure. They might offer an experience that is closer to that of dying at home, but even these facilities may not be able to focus fully on the dying person's needs.

The concept of hospice care was developed in response to the challenges of providing end-of-life care. Rather than referring to a specific care setting, hospice denotes a care philosophy with the focus on humane, dignified, and compassionate care of dying persons and their loved ones (Fig. 15.2). Hospice care has been gaining recognition since 1983, when the Medicare Hospice Benefit began funding this type of care. It can be delivered in the community or in institutional settings. In 2016, an estimated 1.4 million Medicare beneficiaries in the United States received hospice care. Over 40% of patients enroll in hospice fewer than 14 days before their death (National Hospice and Palliative Care Organization, 2020). However, in spite of the growing number of hospice users, many dying people still do not receive

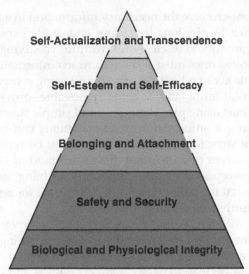

Self-Actualization and Transcendence

Self-Esteem and Self-Efficacy

Belonging and Attachment

Safety and Security

Biological and Physiological Integrity

To share and come to terms with the unavoidable future
To perceive meaning in death

To maintain respect in the face of increasing weakness
To maintain independence
To feel like a normal person, a part of life right to the end
To preserve personal identity

To talk
To be listened to with understanding
To be loved and to share love
To be with a caring person when dying

To be given the opportunity to voice hidden fears
To trust those who care for them
To feel that they are being told the truth
To be secure

To obtain relief from physical symptoms
To conserve energy
To be free from pain

Fig. 15.1 Hierarchy of the dying person's needs, based on Maslow. (From Touhy, T. A., & Jett, K. [2016]. Ebersole and Hess' toward healthy aging: Human needs and nursing response [9th ed.]. St. Louis, MO: Mosby.)

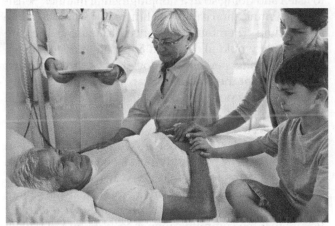

Fig. 15.2 Hospice is a philosophical concept of providing palliative or supportive care to dying people. (Copyright © istock.com/annebaek.)

adequate end-of-life care, mainly because of the failure of health professionals to initiate hospice care in a timely fashion. Nurses can facilitate the process by advocating for their patients and encouraging early referrals to hospice care when appropriate.

PALLIATIVE CARE

According to World Health Organization (2020), palliative care focuses on improving the quality of life for people facing life-threatening illness through the reduction of suffering from pain and other distressing symptoms. Palliative care neither hastens nor postpones death; it affirms life while accepting death as its normal conclusion. Interventions are designed to optimize the patient's ability to live as active and complete a life as possible until death comes. Competent adults, regardless of age, who are suffering from life-threatening diseases such as cancer or advanced chronic conditions such as emphysema or end-stage kidney disease can, and often do, make the decision that they no longer want to receive aggressive treatment, such as chemotherapy, assisted ventilation, or dialysis. This does not mean that these patients forgo all medical intervention. They will still receive treatments that support the goal of optimizing their ability to live as active and complete a life as possible until death. For example, wounds will be treated and a fracture will be placed in a cast. Individuals who choose palliative care typically choose to decline other procedures, such as cardiopulmonary resuscitation, mechanical ventilation, and artificial feeding, which may prolong the dying process. Medical treatment and nursing care focus on actions that enable the dying person to have the highest quality of life for whatever time remains.

COLLABORATIVE ASSESSMENT AND INTERVENTIONS FOR END-OF-LIFE CARE

Good end-of-life care requires a coordinated effort on the part of all caregivers. No matter who is designated as the primary caregiver, all parties—including the family, nurses, physicians, social workers, clergy, psychologists, dietitians, pharmacists, therapists, and volunteers—must work together effectively for the good of the dying person. Problem solving requires mutual respect and prompt, effective communication among all involved parties. Team members also need to recognize the physical and emotional toll on the caregivers working with dying persons and their loved ones. Providing emotional support to caregivers can help them maintain the high level of energy and well-being needed to meet the various physical and psychosocial needs of the dying.

COMMUNICATION AT THE END OF LIFE

Effective communication is a challenge at the best of times. The unique demands and emotional reactions related to end-of-life care can make communication even more challenging. Everything takes on increased importance in this once-in-a-lifetime experience. There is no chance to do things over, so it is essential that everything be done right.

One of the most important things caregivers can do is to spend more time with the dying person and to encourage family members to do the same. This might be difficult for nurses who typically care for multiple patients and have to manage competing priorities. To adequately prioritize care, nurses must understand the importance of therapeutic communication with the dying person and their loved ones. Most people do not wish to die alone. Unfortunately, dying people in institutional settings spend a great deal of time alone. With the advent of the electronic health record in most hospitals, nurses spend about one-quarter of their clinical day performing or reading computer documentation, and there are estimates that physicians can spend as much as half of their time on the computer, depending on unit acuity (Yates, 2020). Nurses and nursing assistants spent by far the greatest amount of time with the dying person, but most of this time is often broken into short, task-oriented visits. Despite the "busy-ness" of the environment and the many people present, an institution can be a lonely place in which to spend your final hours.

To establish rapport and maintain a therapeutic relationship with the recipients of care, the nurse needs to know as much as possible about the dying person and their loved ones, including personal and spiritual beliefs, cultural backgrounds, values, and personal experiences that might influence decision-making and the content of the advance directives for health care. Nurses must demonstrate verbally and nonverbally that they are approachable and are neither detached nor indifferent. A good way to start is by consistently addressing or referring to the dying person by name. This shows respect and helps the dying person to maintain a sense of self-worth and dignity. An empathetic word and gentle touch can demonstrate caring. Holding a hand, gentle repositioning, providing good basic hygiene, and maintaining an aesthetically pleasing environment free from odors, clutter, and unnecessary medical equipment communicate that the dying person is respected and valued.

Nurses must demonstrate willingness to listen to suggestions, requests, or criticisms made by the dying person or by the family. Near the end of life, emotions run high and people often feel powerless. The family members and friends of the dying person may deal with their feelings of powerlessness by voicing their frustrations with the quality of care. Nurses must listen to these criticisms without becoming defensive, whether the criticism is justified or not. Prompt response to requests and ongoing communication explaining the purpose and goals of care will communicate that the caregivers recognize the importance of the dying person's needs.

Answer all questions honestly and directly. If the information is not readily available or cannot be disclosed, make sure that the dying person and their loved ones receive the necessary information in a timely manner. Discussions regarding end-of-life experiences and care should be clear and truthful. The dying person and loved ones must receive as much information as possible about what to expect. Avoid using complicated technical terms and, whenever possible, provide explanations using plain language and simple statements. Even simple information or explanations can be confusing at stressful times and may need to be repeated. Try to prevent or correct any misunderstandings or mistaken perceptions by summarizing, clarifying, and restating what the patient has said. Allow time for responses and further clarification if necessary.

Within culturally acceptable parameters, actively involve the patient in discussions regarding the plan of care. Nothing is more demeaning or frustrating to a dying person than to have caregivers discuss and plan the care without their input. Nurses can help the patient work through fears and end-of-life decisions by taking the time to listen and doing so in a nonjudgmental manner. Sensitive communication cannot be hurried or scheduled, like a procedure. Therefore nurses need to manage the care in way that would allow them adequate time to engage with the dying person and loved ones. Nurses must make sure that the amount of care assigned to ancillary personnel does not limit the availability of professional nursing support to the ones who need it most.

Use reflective and open-ended statements such as, "There seem to be things that are worrying you," "If you want to talk, I'll listen," or "It must be hard. Do you want me to sit with you for a while?" as ways of encouraging a conversation. Start communication from where the patient is, then let the conversation go where they wish it to go. Ensure that the communication is focused on the patient rather than the caregiver. The dying person and loved ones should be free to discuss the things that concern them the most, not the topics concerning the caregivers.

Whenever possible, the dying person should have enough privacy to communicate freely and should be undisturbed by unnecessary noise and commotion. Reassurance that the nurse will keep information confidential may encourage the dying person to communicate feelings or concerns more freely. This may also encourage a dialogue that can help the dying person to begin a life review through which they can validate life experiences and develop a higher level of peace.

When death is near, family members or significant others may wish to remain with the dying person. Most facilities encourage this and provide some accommodations for their comfort. The nurse often needs to explain what to expect as death approaches; how to best communicate with the patient; and what, if anything, loved ones can do to help make the end of life as peaceful as possible.

After the person has died, the nurse need not be afraid to express emotion at the loss. Often, particularly in extended-care settings, the nurse and other caregivers have developed true affection for the person and will need to grieve the loss. Family members often report that seeing the nursing staff's grief actually helped them to cope with their loss because they knew that other people cared enough about their loved one.

PSYCHOSOCIAL PERSPECTIVES, ASSESSMENTS, AND INTERVENTIONS

CULTURAL PERSPECTIVES

Cultural beliefs influence the way one thinks, lives, and interacts with other people. Cultural beliefs also influence the way one views death and dying. Each person develops a unique set of beliefs and values over a lifetime, but as death approaches, those beliefs and values may be challenged. It would be much easier to understand people and their needs if there were predictable patterns and all people who shared a cultural heritage thought and acted identically. Of course that is not the case. Wide variations of belief and behavior exist within all cultures; therefore nurses need to assess each individual's unique preferences and viewpoints to develop a culturally sensitive plan of care. When nurses and patients come from different cultural and religious backgrounds, nurses must be careful not to impose their beliefs and should work to understand the perspectives of others. The four areas that need a particularly careful cultural assessment are (1) communication about death, (2) the decision-making process, (3) the amount and type of intervention that will be accepted, and (4) the significance of pain and suffering.

COMMUNICATION ABOUT DEATH

The way people communicate about death is to a great extent specific to their culture. For example, the Western cultural perspective is based on the person's "right to know" their diagnosis and prognosis in order to make informed decisions. In many other cultures, however, it may be considered insensitive or culturally inappropriate to discuss impending death (Givler, et al., 2021). Asking for the clarification of beliefs can enhance cultural awareness and ensure compliance with privacy issues. To accomplish this, use neutral and open statements such as, "Some people like to get information about their health directly; others prefer we speak to another family member instead. Which do you prefer?" Furthermore, make sure that the patient understands your questions and the information you provide. Follow "yes" or "no" responses with questions asking the patient if they understand. If there is a language barrier, use a professional translator rather than a friend or a family member who is emotionally involved.

DECISION-MAKING PROCESS

The dominant Western perspective tends to emphasize the right of the individual to make decisions regarding their care regardless of the views of the family or significant others. This is the basis of laws governing advance directives. However, members of many other cultures—including Asian Americans, African Americans, and Mexican Americans—may view life-and-death decisions as family issues that must be discussed and decided as a group. These groups are less likely to have initiated any form of advance directives (see the Cultural Considerations box). Don't automatically make assumptions based on ethnicity, however. It is important to get individual preferences. There are varying degrees of belief in and adherence to cultural norms.

Cultural Considerations

Religious Practices Regarding End of Life

- **Buddhism:** A person's state of mind at the time of death is of great importance. A peaceful state may be achieved by listening to friends, family, or monks; reading scriptures; and chanting mantras. Buddhists view death not as a continuation of the soul but as an awakening. Funeral rites last 49 days, ending in the rebirth of the individual. Cremation is common.
- **Christianity:** Christians believe in a union with Christ, necessary for the full enjoyment of God and the happiness of heaven. If possible, a special anointing (sacrament of the sick) is performed, and the dying person is given a chance to confess their sins. Depending on the branch of Christianity, cremation and organ donation may be prohibited.
- **Judaism:** Anything that may hasten death is forbidden. Death is viewed as a natural process in movement to a more rewarding afterlife. Extensive rituals are used to show respect for the dead and to comfort the living. After death, the body is not left alone before burial. Special washing and wrapping in a simple shroud with religious symbols are typically done by special religious volunteers. There is no viewing of the remains; a simple casket is used, and the body is always buried, never cremated. In general, autopsies are discouraged unless required by law.
- **American Indian (Lakota):** Death is a part of life and, after death, people enter a neutral spirit land. The spirit is believed to reside in the body and should not be disturbed, so burial is preferred over cremation. A religious celebration of the person's spirit is held a year after the death.
- **Islam:** Muslims believe that life on earth is a trial to prepare for the next realm of existence. When death is imminent, the patient must face Mecca, confess sins, and beg forgiveness in the presence of the family or a practicing Muslim. After death, the body is washed and wrapped in a clean white cloth and positioned facing Mecca. After a special prayer, burial is performed as soon as possible. Cremation is forbidden; autopsy is prohibited except for legal reasons.
- **Hinduism:** Hindus believe in the reincarnation and rebirth of the soul, leading to a higher state of completeness. Death is viewed as the temporary stopping of physical activity. The fate of one's soul after death is determined by the person's previous actions, their state of mind, the time and circumstances of the death, the activities of the person's children, and the grace of God. After death, the body is given a final bath and cremated, and the ashes are scattered in various places to allow the body to mingle with earth, air, and water and return to the elements.

AMOUNT AND TYPE OF INTERVENTION THAT WILL BE ACCEPTED

The Western perspective focuses on helping people to cope with death. Other cultures—such as African Americans, American Indians, Asians, Pacific Islanders, and Latinos—are more likely to focus on living and prolonging life. Members of these cultural groups may be inclined to choose aggressive interventions at the end of life. These cultures also appear to place greater responsibility and expectations on the family, church, or social network to provide end-of-life care. To some extent, this may explain why hospice care is becoming more accepted by some cultural groups but not by others.

SIGNIFICANCE OF PAIN AND SUFFERING

The Western perspective focuses on achieving freedom from pain and suffering. Some other cultures, however, may instead view pain as a test of faith or a preparation for the afterlife and something that is to be endured rather than avoided.

 QSEN Considerations: Patient-Centered Care

Spiritual Considerations

Religious and spiritual beliefs play an important part in the lives of many older adults and may grow even more important as they approach the end of life. Older people facing the reality of death and dying often lean on their spiritual beliefs to make sense of their lives and deal with the uncertainties of death. This may lead to greater spiritual or religious interest and concern, even among individuals who did not express any particular interest in religion for most of their lives.

Growing recognition of the importance of spiritual support to dying persons and their loved ones has enticed many health care agencies to develop specialized services that provide spiritual care. Often referred to as *pastoral care*, these may employ clergy, nurses, and other professionals trained to provide support to patients in need of spiritual support. To meet the spiritual needs of diverse populations, spiritual care services may use a variety of religious counselors including priests, pastors, rabbis, imams, mullahs, shamans, and other ministers. The counselors can be a valuable resource to nurses and other caregivers who are trying to tailor care to specific spiritual beliefs and practices.

 Critical Thinking

Spiritual Needs of the Dying

It has been said that there are no atheists in foxholes. What connection does this statement have to meeting patients' spiritual needs at the end of life?

Nurses play an important role in helping dying persons meet their spiritual needs. The following are some guidelines to remember when attempting to meet the spiritual needs of the dying person:

1. Determine whether or not any specific religious beliefs or practices are important to the patient or family members.
2. Assess whether or not the patient has a preferred spiritual counselor. When no particular individual is identified, ask the patient whether they wish to receive counsel from anyone else. Spiritual counseling is very personal, and the dying person should have the right to select whomever they wish.
3. Offer choices when available. Most hospitals or extended-care facilities maintain a list of ministers who will visit the dying regardless of denomination or church affiliation. Not all spiritual counselors are equally sensitive to the needs of the dying. If one spiritual counselor does not meet the patient's needs, make the patient aware that there are others available.
4. Determine whether or not the person wishes any spiritual counselor to be notified. Respect the wishes of people who do not want to have any spiritual counsel. Spiritual counseling can be very beneficial when it is desired. When it is not desired, intervention can cause more problems than it solves.
5. Demonstrate respect for the patient's religious and spiritual views. Provide the dying person time for private thought, prayer, or meditation when desired. Incorporate important activities and items into the care plan. The religious rituals related to dying can differ widely among cultures, and the nurse should help the family whenever possible to facilitate their practices even if this involves moving furniture to face a specific sacred direction, opening windows, or providing space for a large group of family members.
6. Do not impose your own beliefs on the patient. The nurse should keep the focus of spiritual discussions on the patient and their beliefs, not on the nurse's beliefs.
7. Be present, be available, and listen. The nurse cannot and should not attempt to solve the patient's problems, but empathy demonstrates acceptance and caring. This allows the patient to feel less alone and often mitigates spiritual distress.
8. Keep the patient's relevant religious symbols readily available, and treat them with respect.
9. Avoid moving beyond your role and level of expertise unless you have specific ministerial or pastoral training in death and dying.

DEPRESSION, ANXIETY, AND FEAR

An older man once said, "I think that waiting to die is worse than death itself." It is one thing to know that you will die eventually; it is another to realize that you have lived most of your life and that death is likely to be a reality soon. At that point, individuals must decide whether they will give up and let fear, anxiety, or depression overwhelm them or whether they will do something to remain in control of whatever time they have remaining.

Nurses can help dying people cope with emotional distress by listening to their concerns and helping them to find constructive ways of dealing with these concerns. Encourage the dying person and their loved ones to participate in creative and pleasurable activities. Art as well as poetry and other writings can provide a means for many dying patients to communicate their feelings and leave a tangible message for their family and loved ones. Physical activity can help reduce both physical and emotional tension. Relaxation classes or support groups designed to help people who are dealing with terminal conditions may lessen social isolation.

Everyone has good days and bad days. When there are more bad days, and these bad days seem to be getting worse, professional help may be necessary. A psychological evaluation may be needed to determine the nature and severity of the problem. Counseling and the use of antidepressant or antianxiety medications can help.

Anger is not uncommon, particularly soon after a terminal diagnosis is made. The nurse should accept this; allow patients the opportunity to verbalize their anger, and then help them find ways to move forward and cope with the future. More general approaches are discussed in Chapters 11 and 13.

PHYSIOLOGICAL CHANGES, ASSESSMENTS, AND INTERVENTIONS

No one can say exactly when a person will die, but a pattern of physiological changes can help to predict when the end is near. Typical physiological changes observed as death approaches include fatigue, dyspnea, gastrointestinal changes (dry mouth, anorexia, nausea and vomiting, constipation), anxiety, and delirium. Pain is not always present as death nears, but when it is, pain relief is a priority. As death approaches, the ultimate goal of care is to alleviate suffering and provide the dying person with the highest level of comfort possible. Effective end-of-life care requires commitment, creativity, and caring. This may involve use of a variety of traditional, complementary, and technologic approaches.

PAIN

Pain is often the most significant concern of the dying person and the loved ones. This is particularly true when the dying person suffers from a highly painful disease, such as cancer. Pain at the end of life can interfere with the dying person's ability to maintain control, to cope, and to complete end-of-life tasks. It increases the likelihood of fatigue, depression, and loss of appetite. Most importantly, pain interferes with the ability of the dying person to make thoughtful decisions and to communicate effectively with loved ones at a critical time.

Pain at the end of life is a form of suffering. Therefore treating pain is one of the most important priorities when caring for a dying person. The goal of pain management is to reduce pain to an acceptable level as defined by the dying person while maintaining a level of alertness that enables them to remain aware of daily activities and to interact with family and others. Although absolute pain relief may not be possible, the dying person should always be made comfortable.

Perform a thorough pain assessment as early as possible and as often as needed. The general rule that "pain is what the patient says it is" definitely applies to end-of-life care. However, older adults with multiple chronic conditions tend to underreport pain and often do not ask for pain relief until their pain reaches relatively high levels. Caregivers should review pain ratings with the patient and encourage them to report pain as soon as they experience it. Besides intensity, pain assessment should include evaluation of the frequency, location, quality, and duration of the pain as well as identification of the precipitating and relieving factors. Document all pain assessments carefully. Pain assessment flow sheets can be used to communicate changes in pain status. Teach the dying person and their loved ones how to keep a pain log that supplements nursing assessments. This log should be simple enough for a lay person to understand and should include all of the factors a nurse would assess. Self-reported logs are helpful because the patient and their significant others are more focused and attuned to subtle changes. Pain logs often reveal important information that would otherwise be missed (Fig. 15.3).

Meticulous pain assessment is particularly important when caring for dying persons who are unable to verbalize their distress. Changes in level of

Date	Time	Severity of Pain	Activity at Time of Pain	Medication Given	Comfort Measures	Severity of Pain in 1 Hour
6/2/16	0800	level 6 "mostly in my back"	walking in hallway	morphine sulfate 30 mg	encouraged to rest back massage given	level 2 "not entirely gone, but I can tolerate this"

Fig. 15.3 Sample pain management log.

consciousness do not affect the ability to feel pain—just the ability to express pain. Use alternative assessments with patients who cannot communicate verbally. Begin the assessment by reviewing whether the patient has an existing condition or has recently experienced some trauma that may cause pain. Perform a head-to-toe assessment to determine whether there are any objective data that might indicate the source of the pain, such as swelling, inflammation, or bruising. During the assessment, carefully observe the patient for any responses such as restlessness, moaning, guarding, grimacing, or striking out when body parts are touched or moved. The presence of any of these responses between assessments, especially during routine activities such as repositioning, can also indicate pain. Family members, friends, or staff members may be aware of behaviors the patient exhibits when in pain. This information should be indicated on the plan of care so that all care providers can respond appropriately.

Good pain management requires a thorough understanding of the patient's needs and wishes. This involves an in-depth evaluation of the dying person's physical needs, coping abilities, and support network as well as an evaluation of religious and sociocultural factors that may affect the pain experience. Recommendations for end-of-life pain management are constantly being updated as new evidence becomes available. Nurses and other health professionals must be aware of the new developments and continually update their pain management practices. The following is a list of evidence-based principles for end-of-life pain management:

1. **Do not give up trying to find an effective pain control regimen.** It may take several attempts to find the best combination of medication and nonpharmacologic approaches to reach a tolerable pain level.
2. **The likelihood of drug-drug and drug-disease interactions or adverse effects increases with the addition of new medication or higher doses.** Careful assessment is needed each time a medication change is made.
3. **Frequently evaluate the effectiveness of pain management.** Doses and frequencies of medications might need to be changed or adjusted based on the response. Thorough assessment reveals when the medication is no longer providing adequate pain relief.
4. **Consider using a variety of routes of administration.** Oral medication is the most common and accepted route for administration, but this may cause problems for the older adult who has difficulty swallowing pills. Never crush solid medications designed for sustained release, because this will result in rapid absorption. When the person has difficulty swallowing oral medication, consider switching to liquid, transdermal, or rectal formulations. Parenteral administration of medication may not be the first choice for an older adult unless they have an existing intravenous or central line, peripherally inserted central catheter, or implanted port.

5. **Pay attention to the timing of pain medication.** Pain medications are most effective when taken before the pain becomes severe. Long-acting or sustained-release opioids are commonly ordered because they are effective at maintaining pain control while also avoiding the need to disturb the patient to administer pain medication. Even with long-acting pain control, breakthrough pain may occur. Treat it promptly with a rapid-acting analgesic. Administer as-needed (prn) medications as soon as possible when requested.
6. **Never abruptly stop pain medications when they have been taken for an extended period.** Withdrawal symptoms including headache, shakiness, or diaphoresis can occur if medications are stopped suddenly.
7. **Use nonpharmacologic approaches to complement pharmacologic interventions when managing pain.** Discuss possible options and implement those that are most acceptable to the patient. Activities that may help provide relief include (1) hot or cold applications such as warm baths, showers, cool washcloths, or ice packs; (2) comfort devices such as cushions, pillows, and pads; (3) massage, foot rubs, or reflexology; (4) relaxation breathing or other relaxation exercises; (5) imagery or visualization; (6) distractions, such as socialization, listening to music, and watching television or movies; (7) biofeedback; (8) transcutaneous electrical nerve stimulation; (9) hypnosis; and (10) anything else that helps reduce stress. There are recent studies on the use of virtual reality that can distract the patient from pain and help lower the pain sensation (Stewart, 2019).
8. **Consider referral to a pain specialist.** If the dying patient does not experience adequate pain control, consult a pain specialist, such as clinical nurse specialist or a palliative care practitioner.

Sedation using atypical antipsychotics (neuroleptics), benzodiazepines, barbiturates, or high doses of opioids may be ordered when the pain is severe and not relieved by using standard narcotic medications. Use these with caution because they can induce dangerous side effects, especially when used together (NAMI, 2019). In general, sedation is not the ideal solution, but it may be used when it is the only way to alleviate extreme suffering and distress. It should be used only after the patient, family, or health care team has determined that it is in the person's best interest.

QSEN Considerations: Teamwork and Collaboration

Communication

The health care team must be aware of the need for ongoing communication with the family members regarding pain management. Some families have preconceived notions about medications, especially if there have been any addiction issues. Listen to their concerns while also advocating for effective pain control for the patient.

Once sedation begins, it may be reduced or terminated if the family or health care representative requests it. This, however, may result in the recurrence of physical and emotional distress for the dying patient. Therefore many health care agencies have policies guiding the use of sedation, including the types and amounts of medication that can be used. Careful documentation of all interventions is essential.

Some practitioners have expressed ethical concerns about the use of sedation in end-of-life care as a form of passive euthanasia. However, a majority of clinicians and legal experts do not support this view, because the purpose of sedation in end-of-life care is to reduce suffering, not to end life. This view has been supported by legal practice and the positions statements of the professional bodies representing nurses, physicians, and other health professionals.

⚖ Legal & Ethical Considerations

Physician Assisted Death

Physician assisted death (PAD), also known as physician assisted suicide, is a process whereby a physician provides a potentially fatal medication to a patient who is terminally ill, with the understanding that the patient may take it to end their own life. Federal law in the United States allows individual states to make their own laws on PAD. Nine states have laws allowing PAD as of 2021 (ProCon, 2021). Although it might be legal in one's state of practice, not everyone (medical professionals and nonprofessionals alike) agrees with it. The American Medical Association acknowledges the "moral tension at stake for physicians with respect to participating in assisted suicide" (AMA, 2021). The AMA has posted opinion pieces for both sides of the argument. The position of Stanford School of Medicine Palliative Care Department states that they are neither for it nor against it but are "anything but neutral on the issue of the profound suffering seriously ill patients experience" (Periyakoil, 2021). In the states where PAD is legal, hospice nurses may be asked to assist the patient, whether by opening up capsules or just providing support and comfort to the patient. Whatever the legality of this measure in your state, it is wise to examine your views on it as an ethical dilemma.

FATIGUE AND SLEEPINESS

Fatigue accompanies many conditions and is not specifically a sign of impending death. Fatigue can interfere with the dying person's ability to carry out necessary end-of-life tasks, including communicating with loved ones. Sometimes, stimulants, such as caffeine or prescription drugs, may help a person overcome fatigue and lethargy, but these should be used cautiously. Teach the patient to pace their physical activity and schedule frequent rest periods to reduce fatigue. Because of metabolic changes, the patient may begin to sleep more and may be difficult to arouse as the end of life nears.

CARDIOVASCULAR CHANGES

Diminished peripheral circulation, already common in older adults, is likely to worsen as death nears, resulting in dry, pale, or cyanotic extremities. Peripheral pulses are often weak and difficult to palpate. Blood pressure is typically decreased by 20 mm Hg or more from the normal range and may be difficult to auscultate. Body temperature may rise significantly as death nears.

Adjust room temperature and ventilation to promote comfort while avoiding chilling drafts. Use comfort measures such as bed socks, shoulder wraps, and warmed blankets (never electric blankets because of the risk for burns). Heavy or restrictive covers should not be used because they may increase discomfort.

RESPIRATORY CHANGES

Dyspnea is common as death nears. A dying person may experience shortness of breath, Cheyne-Stokes respirations, and other observable signs of respiratory difficulties. However, dyspnea is a subjective sensation of difficulty breathing and may not be easy to observe. Respiratory rate and oxygen saturation cannot predict the severity of dyspnea. A dying person may report feeling breathless even though oxygenation levels are satisfactory and typical signs of breathing difficulties are absent. Treatment should focus on symptom management and elimination of the underlying causes when possible.

Mild respiratory difficulty usually can be relieved by changing positioning, elevating the upper body, opening windows or using a fan to increase room ventilation, or administering oxygen by nasal cannula. Both physical and emotional stress can cause muscle tension, which exacerbates respiratory problems. Encourage the dying person and their visitors to minimize stressful experiences and to alternate episodes of activity with periods of rest. If they cause problems, excessive talking and visiting should be minimized. Visitors need to know that it is sometimes better to visit for shorter periods of time or to leave the room and allow the patient to have some quiet time if breathing difficulties occur. Resting in a reclining chair or elevating the head of the bed usually aids breathing. Listening to music and using relaxation exercises may help to reduce tension and improve breathing effort.

Severe breathing problems, such as those seen with chronic heart or lung disease, usually do not respond well to these simple measures and need treatment that is more aggressive. Acute distress, fear, and panic frequently accompany severe shortness of breath. When the dying person does not want aggressive medical treatment, the most common method used to manage shortness of breath is administration of morphine. The patient, family, and team of caregivers need to be aware of and be comfortable with the fact that morphine, when given in a dosage that is adequate to relieve the respiratory distress (via pulmonary vasodilation), can cause drowsiness, sleep, and even loss of consciousness.

GASTROINTESTINAL CHANGES

Loss of appetite (anorexia) and muscle wasting (cachexia) often accompany advanced terminal conditions, particularly some forms of cancer. Many factors contribute to poor appetite and weight loss in the terminal patient, including medications, mouth ulcerations, changes in taste, nausea and vomiting, metabolic changes, absorption problems, and emotional depression. The treatment of anorexia and cachexia is difficult because many of the underlying physiological actions are poorly understood.

The anorexic person should be encouraged but not forced to eat. Force-feeding will make the person more uncomfortable and can result in choking. Care should focus on the remaining pleasures attached to food. Inquire about food preferences and accommodate special requests when possible. The end of life is not a time for special or restricted diets. Encourage the person to eat anything that seems appealing. Present food in an appealing manner and in a quantity that is not overwhelming. Whenever possible, serve meals in an odor-free environment. Food is intimately attached to good times and social events. Watching a loved one waste away is very disturbing to family members. Enlisting the family to bring small amounts of special foods from home may bring back pleasant memories of happy times. Sharing a meal with family members can be a positive experience, even when the person consumes very little.

The issue of artificial feeding typically arises when a dying person is unable or unwilling to eat. Artificial nutrition and hydration can be delivered through a feeding tube or via the parenteral route. Artificial feeding bypasses normal mechanisms and response to thirst and hunger, thus increasing the risk for aspiration, nausea, vomiting, infection, and other complications. It also bypasses the usual processes associated with food ingestion, such as tasting, chewing, and swallowing food. Although it might provide energy, artificial feeding is generally uncomfortable and does not satisfy other needs normally met by eating. Therefore the need for artificial feeding and hydration has to be carefully considered because it might be more of a burden to a dying person than a benefit. Many health care consumers address this issue in their advance directives by specifying what forms of feeding, if any, they would permit.

The inability to take food and fluid by mouth is a part of the normal progression to death. The choice to stop eating is something different. People may stop eating as a method of hastening death. This may be a conscious decision or it may be a response to uncontrolled pain or severe depression. Be alert to these possibilities and find out the reasons. Adequate pain control and actions to reduce the depression may cause changes in the person's behavior. The idea of self-starvation is usually traumatic to family members and caregivers.

People can live for days without food. Prolonged fasting leads to ketosis, which depresses hunger and may even result in mood elevation or euphoria. There is no evidence that self-chosen food refusal causes suffering. Dehydration is more likely to cause death than is starvation. People can survive for only a few days without fluid. On the other hand, dehydration appears to have some benefits near the end of life. It is theorized that dehydration leads to the release of endorphins (i.e., natural chemicals that reduce pain). Dehydration also reduces fluid congestion in the lungs, making breathing easier, and it reduces respiratory secretions, decreasing the need for suctioning.

Dry mouth (xerostomia) and mouth ulcerations can be caused by many things, such as advanced age, medications, and decreased fluid intake. This problem increases distress and discomfort, which can and should be avoided as the end of life nears. A humidifier or pans of water (for evaporation) increase the amount of moisture in the air. Moist air helps to prevent drying of the skin and mucous membranes and may ease breathing. Common measures used to treat dry mouth include frequent swabbing with mouth sponges, spraying the mouth with water mist from an atomizer, and brushing the teeth. Avoid alcohol-based swabs because they tend to further dry mucous membranes. Commercial lip balms or liquid vitamin E may be helpful in easing the discomfort of dry lips. Petroleum-based products, such as Vaseline, may cause respiratory problems if they are inhaled and should not be used on the mouth.

Nausea and vomiting are not signs of impending death; rather, they are distressing symptoms of underlying problems such as adverse medication reactions, constipation, intestinal obstruction, or other physiological changes. Vomiting increases the risk for aspiration, so it is best to position the patient in a side-lying or sitting (Fowler) position rather than supine. Temporary relief from nausea and vomiting may be obtained by the rectal or parenteral administration of antiemetic medications, but the underlying cause must be identified and corrected before the symptoms will go away. If a medication reaction is suspected, contact the prescribing practitioner.

Constipation is a common and distressing problem for the terminal patient. Common causes of constipation near the end of life include disease factors such as tumor compression, calcium imbalance, adhesions, dehydration, inadequate fiber intake, pain, immobility, and medications (e.g., opioids, antidepressants, and antacids). Prevent constipation whenever possible. A high fiber diet, bulk-forming supplements such as psyllium, and adequate fluid intake might prevent problems while the patient is able and willing to eat. Stool softeners, laxatives, suppositories, or enemas are indicated when dietary intake inadequate, but they may cause an electrolyte imbalance. As the end of life approaches and muscle tone in the rectum decreases, manual disimpaction might be required to decrease rectal pressure and pain. Disimpaction should be done gently and carefully using adequate lubrication (K-Y Lubricating Jelly or petroleum jelly). When the person has thrombocytopenia, use extreme caution before performing a rectal examination or digital removal of feces.

Diarrhea is a less common problem at the end of life, but it may have a profound effect on the quality of life. Repeated episodes of diarrhea contribute to electrolyte imbalance, dehydration, skin breakdown, fatigue, and depression. Diarrhea can be caused by numerous factors, including disease processes, psychological factors, medications, herbal remedies, bacterial or parasitic infections, and antibiotic therapy. Treatment may include increasing the patient's intake of clear fluids to replace electrolytes and/or administering antibiotics to treat infectious diseases, steroids to decrease bowel inflammation, medications, or bulk-forming agents to slow intestinal peristalsis. To avoid an obstruction, use bulk-forming agents only when the person has an adequate fluid intake of approximately 2000 mL/d.

URINARY CHANGES

Oliguria is commonly observed because of decreases in fluid intake, blood pressure, and kidney perfusion. Urinary incontinence is also common. Absorbent pads or an indwelling catheter can be used to reduce the need for bed changes, which may disturb the dying person.

INTEGUMENTARY CHANGES

Skin breakdown is a problem with malnourished patients near the end of life. Interventions designed to prevent skin tears or pressure injuries include proper skin cleansing, careful handling of the skin, frequent turning and positioning, and measures to reduce pressure. Chapter 17 provides further information on the prevention of pressure injuries.

Soft, nonconstricting, nonirritating (free from harsh detergents and other chemicals) clothing promotes comfort and minimizes risk for skin dryness and rashes. Comfort should take precedence over style. Older, loose cotton clothing is often best, particularly when the person is diaphoretic. A major advantage of cotton is that it breathes, allowing perspiration to escape, which helps keep the skin dry.

SENSORY CHANGES

Vision diminishes, and the visual field narrows as death nears. To compensate for this change in vision, caregivers and loved ones must come close to the dying person to be seen. Indirect lighting with minimal shadows is most restful and least disturbing. Hearing remains acute until death, even if the dying person does not respond. All caregivers and visitors must remember this when they speak in the presence of a dying person. Calm, supportive, loving messages should be delivered to the person even when they do not respond. Avoid negative or disturbing conversations because they can cause the dying person to become distressed and agitated.

CHANGES IN COGNITION

Delirium, an acute change in mental status, affects the majority of older adults in the final days of life. As death nears, periods of delirium may be combined with periods of coherent thought. Common symptoms include a decreased ability to think and process information, perceptual changes, disorientation, loss of consciousness, insomnia with daytime sleepiness, nightmares, agitation, irritability, anxiety, hypersensitivity to light and sound, fleeting illusions, visual hallucinations, delusions, mood swings, attention deficits, and memory disturbances.

Many forms of delirium are treatable if they are recognized and reported promptly. Causes of delirium include hypotension, oxygen deprivation resulting from apnea or hypoventilation, fever, neurologic changes, metabolic abnormalities such as hyperglycemia and uremia, dehydration, and other physiological or emotional disturbances. Medications such as antibiotics and opioid analgesics can also contribute to delirium. Vital signs, oxygen saturation, and laboratory values may provide valuable information about underlying problems.

Delirium is disturbing to the dying person, their family and loved ones, and the caregivers. Some decrease in symptoms may occur with simple interventions, such as calm, reassuring support. Treatment is aimed at restoring the baseline cognitive level if possible. Individualize treatment to meet the needs of each person. Correction of underlying physiological or metabolic problems may bring some relief, as may discontinuation of some medications.

DEATH

The experience of death in an institutional setting is very different from that at home. Family members, significant others, and friends often wish to be present at the time of death. However, some families might be able to spend only a limited time with their dying loved one and wish to be called only when there is a significant change in the person's status. Others would rather be notified only after death has occurred. Family decisions are influenced by many factors including coping ability, access to resources, work situation, health of family members, and personal factors, such as individuals' age, health, and relation to the dying person. Everybody copes with the death of a loved one in a unique way and needs to be supported in a professional and nonjudgmental manner. The following strategies can help caregivers provide support to the family through this experience:

1. Discuss the family's wishes early, so that appropriate notification of family, clergy, and others can take place.
2. Record and communicate instructions on whom to call, how they can be reached, and whether there are any limitations regarding time of day.
3. Offer family members the opportunity to participate in the care of the dying person. Families often want to be helpful. Educate them and provide them with opportunities to participate in the care.
4. Allow family members to express their emotions and provide them with support. Some family members may be hesitant and may need permission to express their emotions, although others might be very demonstrative when it comes to grief. Ensure they feel comfortable and supported.
5. Provide frequent updates on the condition of the dying person and be available to answer questions. Families often need assurance that the dying person is comfortable. Provide comfort measures, and be sensitive to the needs of the family members.

RECOGNIZING IMMINENT DEATH

Some physiological changes may indicate approaching death, but there is no way to predict the exact moment or manner of death.

Indicators of imminent death may include the following:

1. Increased sleepiness
2. Decreased responsiveness
3. Confusion in a person who has been oriented
4. Hallucinations about people (sometimes deceased family members)
5. Increased withdrawal from visitors or other social interaction
6. Loss of interest in food and fluids
7. Loss of control of bowel and bladder in a person who has been continent
8. Altered breathing patterns, such as shallow breathing, Cheyne-Stokes respirations, and rattling or gurgling respirations
9. Involuntary muscle movements and diminished reflexes

Death may be sudden and quick, or it may be slow and gradual. Some individuals experience acute physiological changes leading to a relatively quick death. They are alert and talking one minute and gone the next. In other individuals, bodily functions shut down system by system, the heart rate slows, respiration fades, and the individual slowly slips away. Signs of death include absence of heartbeat and spontaneous respirations; open eyes without blink; nonreactive pupils; flaccid jaw with slightly open mouth; and lack of response to touch, speech, or painful stimuli. Legal pronouncement of death is made by the physician.

If family members are present when the patient dies, they should be allowed to sit at the bedside and say farewells or grieve as long as necessary. Discreetly remove oxygen, intravenous lines, and other visible medical devices and turn off monitors and other noise-creating equipment. Accommodate and show respect for cultural practices regarding grieving and preparation of the body whenever possible. Give the family adequate time and provide them with nursing care until they are ready to leave. This is not the time to avoid the family. A word of support, a simple hug, or any other demonstration of sympathy by the nurse is long remembered by family members.

Allow the deceased person to remain in the room if other friends or family members who were not present at the time of death wish to assemble. The deceased person may remain in the room until the funeral director arrives or may be transported to the morgue, depending on agency policy. When death occurs in a shared room, make arrangements to provide privacy without unduly disturbing the surviving resident. Some facilities provide a special room for these situations.

Perform postmortem care in accordance with cultural and spiritual preferences. Typically, this includes removing any soiling and applying a clean sheet or shroud according to agency policy. In most cases, the head is elevated slightly to prevent discoloration. Gently close the eyes, insert dentures, and position a small towel to close the mouth. This gives the face a more natural appearance if a funeral visitation is planned. Most health care facilities have policies and guidelines to guide the personnel through administrative and legal procedures related to death. The nurse in attendance needs to note and document the time of death if witnessed. When death is not witnessed, time of death needs to be approximated. Notify the physician and funeral director specified by the family according to agency policies. Identify, list, and bag personal belongings for return to the family.

Coordinated Care

Delegation and Supervision of End-of-Life Care

END-OF-LIFE CARE

- Nursing assistants who work with dying patients may have many concerns related to end-of-life care.
- Agency policies and licensed nursing personnel should provide guidance so that nursing assistants know what is expected of them.
- Some concerns that need to be addressed include (1) what information regarding changes in status they should report, (2) whether they should start cardiopulmonary resuscitation in light of the patient's code status, (3) how they should respond to questions from the family, and (4) how to respond to abusive or difficult family members.
- Supervising nurses can work to recognize and meet the needs of their staff.
- Many nursing assistants, particularly those in long-term care settings, become attached to older patients and grieve when they die. The nursing assistants may feel unprepared and have difficulty dealing with a death. They may need reassurance if they feel guilty of doing something wrong when a patient dies after an activity, such as bathing or ambulation. They may need guidance, and they may be concerned that they may have said something that upset the dying patient or the family. They may need support when they are criticized and demeaned by family members who rarely visited the patient during their life and who appeared only when death was near. Such staff may need empathy when they are obliged to prepare the body of the deceased at a time when they need an opportunity to grieve the loss.

FUNERAL ARRANGEMENTS

Many religious and cultural implications are related to the handling and burial of the deceased person. Older people have usually given some thought to their final resting place, and many have made specific plans, issued specific directions regarding their wishes, and even paid for their funeral. Activities following death are easier when advanced planning has taken place. Ideally, the family should not be forced to make difficult choices at a time of high emotion. It is common for grieving families to commit to expensive caskets or services that impose an unnecessary financial burden. Some patients do not want burial but prefer cremation.

Funeral services also are highly influenced by culture and religion. In most cultures, some type of service takes place after death to memorialize the life of the deceased and to allow the family to begin to work through their grief. Nurses and other caregivers sometimes want to attend services for long-term patients. This is appropriate when possible and is often greatly appreciated by the family.

BEREAVEMENT

Death typically elicits complex psychosocial and physical responses in everyone associated with the deceased person, be it as a significant other, a family member, a friend, or a caregiver. Entire books have been written on coping with death and dying. This chapter provides only general guidelines (Box 15.3). Nurses who deal with dying patients and their loved ones should plan to obtain additional resources from the library or online.

There is no single "good" or "right" way to feel after a person dies. Survivors often have ambivalent feelings regarding the death. On one hand, they feel a sense of relief that the struggle is over and that the

Box 15.3 Kübler-Ross's Stages of Grief

The following stages were identified by Dr. Elisabeth Kübler-Ross in her groundbreaking book, which was the first to address grief related to death and dying. Although listed in a sequence, these stages do not necessarily follow in this specific order. A person may move in and out of the stages unpredictably and erratically.

DENIAL
Numbness protects the survivor from the intensity of the loss. This typically decreases as the individual acknowledges the reality and permanence of the loss.

ANGER
Feelings of anger are often directed at the deceased or at a deity because the survivor feels abandoned. Anger is one method for dealing with the feelings of helplessness and powerlessness. Anger tends to decrease over time.

BARGAINING
Survivors try to identify whether they could have done something different to prevent the loss. Some may make resolutions to change their behavior or lifestyle based on these reflections. Remorse and guilt that they did not do enough are common and can slow the grief process.

DEPRESSION
Feelings of emptiness, loneliness, and isolation are common after the loss of a loved one. Frequent crying spells, inability to sleep, inability to concentrate or make decisions, and loss of appetite are typical. Some survivors describe their lives as colorless and meaningless. Many people try to hide their feelings and suffer needlessly. Support from family, friends, nurses, physicians, and bereavement groups can help the survivor work through feelings of depression. Antidepressant medications are sometimes used on a short-term basis.

ACCEPTANCE
There is no set time limit for grief over the loss of a loved one. Acceptance and healing occur slowly as the person works through their feelings and reestablishes a meaning and pattern to life.

Data from Kübler-Ross, E. (1970). *On death and dying*, New York: Macmillan.

loved one is at rest. On the other hand, they seriously grieve and miss the loved one's presence. Even when death is anticipated, the initial feelings of shock and numbness are unavoidable. For a few weeks after such a death, people describe their behavior as "being in a fog" or "going through the motions." After this initial time, the reality of the loss strikes and survivors are likely to experience signs of depression, such as loss of appetite, inability to sleep, avoidance of social interaction, and uncontrolled bouts of crying. They may also be angry with the person who died and voice statements, such as, "How could he do this to me?" Talking to the deceased loved one is not abnormal and may be useful for some individuals.

In normal grieving, the frequency and severity of these signs of grieving gradually decrease over time, but grief over loss of a loved one never dissipates completely. Life goes on, but it never seems to be the same without the loved one. Most people who lose a loved one require at least a year to work through the most severe emotional distress. Grief counselors often evaluate a person's responses at the first anniversary of the death as an indicator of their adjustment. It is common for grieving to last longer than a year, but severe adjustment problems at this point suggest the need for more aggressive help.

Nurses can help grieving individuals in several ways. They can encourage the grieving person to take time to cry and to express their feelings. They can listen to the grieving person talk about the loved one. Reviewing and reminiscing about good times may bring tears, but it gives the person opportunities to gain strength from having known the loved one. Avoid using phrases such as "it's time to move on," as that would minimize the important role that this person played in the lives of others. Realize that while there are assumed stages of grief (see Box 15.3), the process is rarely linear but tends to follow a messy, unpredictable path toward acceptance. People will move in and out of stages, sometimes returning to earlier stages, and many take a more circular route to healing.

When appropriate, recommend bereavement support groups, which use the sharing of mutual experiences to help individuals cope with their loss and grief. Collaborate with other health team members to provide support, and initiate a referral to a grief counselor for individuals who are experiencing severe or protracted grief.

Get Ready for the Next Generation NCLEX® Examination!

Key Points

- Most deaths in the United States occur in the older-than-65 population.
- Despite increased attention from professional organizations and groups, death and end-of-life care do not receive adequate attention in nursing education or society as a whole.
- Many older adults do not want aggressive medical intervention at the end of life, so caregivers need to be prepared to provide palliative and holistic interventions.
- Older patients and their families need to be included in planning for end-of-life care.
- Most older adults state that they wish to die at home, but most deaths occur in institutional settings.
- Culture and ethnicity play a role in beliefs and expectations related to the end of life.
- Most individuals fear that they will die in pain. Nurses must work to allay this fear and provide adequate pain control for dying patients.
- Although it is not possible to predict exactly when a person will die, several physiological changes occur as death approaches.
- The nurse needs to provide ongoing care to minimize preventable problems and discomfort.
- Family members need to be apprised of the significance of physiological and behavioral changes that occur as death nears.
- Nurses can play an important role in helping survivors deal with grief after the death of a loved one.

Additional Learning Resources

 SG Go to your Evolve website at http://evolve.elsevier.com/Williams/geriatric for the additional online resources.

Review Questions for the Next Generation NCLEX® Examination

1. **Which statement is incorrect?**
   a. If the patient complains of respiratory difficulties even though vital signs and oxygen saturation are normal, he is most likely developing delirium.
   b. A dying woman with end-stage kidney disease should be allowed to choose foods she enjoys even if they are not part of the meal plan.
   c. The primary goal of end-of-life care is to alleviate suffering and to give the dying person the best quality of life possible.
   d. Artificial nutrition and hydration may cause a greater burden than benefit to a dying person.

2. **A calorie-restricted, low-sodium meal plan was prescribed for Mr. Nguyen, a terminally ill patient. Mr. Nguyen has diabetes, is in kidney failure, and has a "do not resuscitate" order. Mr. Nguyen has been in the care of hospice for 4 months. He and his family have had many conversations with the medical team and are in agreement with the goals of end-of-life care. As death nears, Mr. Nguyen has very little appetite and picks at the food. Choose the appropriate nursing intervention.** *(Select all that apply.)*
   a. Continue meal plan as ordered.
   b. Encourage Mr. Nguyen's family to bring in small amounts of food from home.

c. Serve food in a place free from odors.

d. Encourage Mr. Nguyen to eat anything that appeals to him.

e. Require Mr. Nguyen to eat at least one bite of each food group.

f. Provide good oral hygiene.

g. Request an order for tube feeding.

h. Ask the family to delay visits until Mr. Nguyen has eaten.

i. Inquire about Mr. Nguyen's food preferences and accommodate requests.

j. Request an order for intravenous fluids.

3. **Dyspnea, shortness of breath, and irregular breathing patterns are common as death nears. Identify a simple measure taken by the nurse that would help alleviate mild respiratory difficulty. (Select all that apply.)**

a. Administer oxygen by nasal cannula

b. Administer atropine sulfate as needed

c. Institute measures to reduce anxiety or tension

d. Elevate the head of the bed

e. Remind visitors not to tire the patient

4. **List the 5 stages of death and dying identified by Kübler-Ross.**

a. _____

b. _____

c. _____

d. _____

e. _____

5. **Which is true about the presence of pain at the time of death? Pain is**

a. one of the greatest fears of the dying person.

b. usually of short duration and readily treated with analgesics.

c. normal, expected, and unavoidable.

d. likely to require high doses of narcotic analgesics.

6. **The nurse is interviewing a patient whose husband died 18 months ago. Which statement indicates that the patient is adjusting to the loss?**

a. "I miss my husband every day. Focusing on our children and going back to work help me focus on future."

b. "Seeing our children grow without a father is too hard for me. I often wonder if I can go on."

c. "I sent my children to my parents. I don't think I can be a good parent in my state."

d. "My career was important to me before my husband died, but it's been only 18 months and I don't feel capable of going back to work quite yet."

REFERENCES

American Medical Association: Physician-assisted suicide: 2021. https://www.ama-assn.org/delivering-care/ethics/physician-assisted-suicide

AGivler, A., Bhatt, H., & Maani-Fogelman, P. A. (2021). The importance of cultural competence in pain and palliative care. [Updated 2021 Jul 26]. In: StatPearls [Internet]. Treasure Island (FL): StatPearls Publishing; 2022. Available from: https://www.ncbi.nlm.nih.gov/books/NBK493154/

Cabarkapa, S., Nadjidai, S. E., Murgier, J., & Ng, C. H. (2020). The psychological impact of COVID-19 and other viral epidemics on frontline healthcare workers and ways to address it: A rapid systematic review. *Brain, Behavior, and Immunity – Health, 8,* Article 100144. doi:10.1016/j.bbih.2020.100144 Epub 2020 Sep 17. PMID: 32959031; PMCID: PMC7494453.

Kübler-Ross, E. (1970). *On death and dying.* Collier Books/Macmillan Publishing Co.

Maslow, A. H. (1943). A theory of human motivation. *Psychological Review, 50*(4): 370–396.

National Alliance on Mental Illness (NAMI) (2019). Benzodiazepine-associated risks. https://www.nami.org/Learn-More/Treatment/Mental-Health-Medications/Benzodiazepine-Associated-Risks

National Center for Health Statistics (2018). Older persons' health, https://www.cdc.gov/nchs/fastats/older-american-health.htm

National Hospice and Palliative Care Organization (NHPCO) (2020). Facts and figures: Hospice care in America. https://www.nhpco.org/wp-content/uploads/nhpco-facts-figures-2020-edition.pdf

Periyakoil, V. J. (2021). Physician assisted death. https://palliative.stanford.edu/physician-assisted-death/2021ProCon: States with legal phyisican-assisted suicide https://euthanasia.procon.org/states-with-legal-physician-assisted-suicide/.

Stanford School of Medicine (2021). Where do americans die? https://palliative.stanford.edu/home-hospice-home-care-of-the-dying-patient/where-do-americans-die/.

Stewart, D., Mete, M., & Groninger, H. (2019). Virtual reality for pain management in patients with heart failure: Study rationale and design. *Contemporary Clinical Trials Communications, 16,* Article 100470. doi:10.1016/j.conctc.2019.100470. Erratum in Contemporary Clinical Trials Communications, 20:100689. PMID: 31650079; PMCID: PMC6804617.

World Health Organization (WHO) (2020). WHO definition of palliative care. https://www.who.int/news-room/fact-sheets/detail/palliative-care

Yates, S. W. (2020). Physician stress and burnout. *American Journal of Medicine, 133*(2), 160–164. doi:10.1016/j.amjmed.2019.08.034. Epub 2019 Sep 11. PMID: 31520624.

Objectives

1. Develop an understanding of the impact of age on sexuality.
2. Discuss the effects of illness on sexual functioning.
3. Describe the assessment findings related to sexual functioning of an older adult.
4. Identify older adults at risk for experiencing problems related to sexuality.
5. Discuss the common concerns of aging lesbian, gay, bisexual, transgender, and queer/questioning persons.
6. Select appropriate problem statements related to sexuality.
7. Describe nursing interventions for older adults experiencing problems with sexuality.

Key Terms

altered sexual function (p. 279)

dyspareunia (dĭs pě-R-nē-ă, p. 279)

hysterectomy (hĭs-těr-ĔK-tō-mē, p. 280)

intercourse (ĬN-těr-kŏrs, p. 278)

masturbation (măs-tŭr-BĂ-shŭn, p. 283)

sexuality (sěk-shū-ĂL-ĭ-tē, p. 278)

Like food and water, sexuality is a basic human need that does not disappear with age. Although society may prefer to think of older adults as asexual, this is not the case. Individuals who have had an active sex life in younger years are likely to continue to do so as they age, and many adults continue to have sexually satisfying lives well into old age.

Women lose their childbearing capacity after menopause. However, with the assistance of reproductive technologies such as using a donor egg, women can sometimes have healthy children after their usual childbearing age. Unlike women, men are generally able to father children well into their 60s and 70s without medical assistance. Although uncommon, fathering children at 80 and 90 years of age does occur. Nevertheless, it is important to remember that the loss or decline of reproductive capacity does not mean a decline or loss of sexual desire. Even though the frequency and form of sexual activity tend to change, sexual needs do not disappear with age (Fig. 16.1).

Sexual touching, fondling, masturbation, intercourse, and other expressions of sexuality remain an important part of the lives of many older adults. Sexual thoughts and feelings are normal as people age. Studies indicate that the majority of older adults believe that sex is an important aspect of a romantic relationship regardless of age; 46% of adults over age 60 identify themselves as sexually active (Stein, 2020). The importance of sexuality goes beyond the biologic realm. It also includes psychological, social, and moral dimensions, all of which are essential components of sexual health. Sexuality is more than just a physical drive; it provides opportunities for the aging person to express and receive affection, connection, and emotional bonding. Therefore the preservation of sexual health should be an integral part of the care for older adults.

Nurses have a unique role in the promotion of sexual health in older people. The nurse has the responsibility to foster the sexual well-being of older adults by offering opportunities for discussion. Open the door to discussion of sexual concerns in a nonjudgmental manner by offering information and education to those who want to continue being sexually active, although making it clear that stopping sex is an acceptable option for those who choose to do so. Provide information and guidance to older people who desire it.

FACTORS THAT AFFECT SEXUALITY OF OLDER ADULTS

Age-related changes have a considerable impact on the sexual practices of older adults. Normal physiological changes in sexual function may raise concerns for older adults. In general, sexual response time slows with aging, but the ability to enjoy various expressions of sexuality remains throughout life. However, some changes may have a more significant

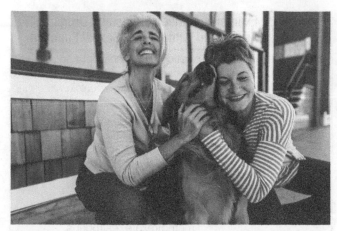

Fig. 16.1 Love and affection are important to older adults. (Copyright © istock.com/kate_sept2004.)

impact, leading to altered sexual function, which is a persistent impairment of a person's usual pattern of sexual functioning. Either way, older adults will benefit from holistic care with a focus on the promotion of sexual health.

AGE-RELATED CHANGES IN WOMEN

Older women experience normal changes in the reproductive system related to lower levels of progesterone and estrogen. Approximately one-third of women over the age of 65 experience discomfort during intercourse (dyspareunia) related to postmenopausal changes such as (1) irritation of the external genitalia (pruritus vulvae); (2) thinning and dryness of the vaginal walls (atrophic vaginitis); and (3) alteration in the levels of normal micro-organisms in the vagina, resulting in an increased risk for vaginal yeast infections. In many instances, dyspareunia can be treated with over-the-counter topical preparations (see Complementary Health Approaches box).

Menopausal hormone therapy (MHT), once widely prescribed to reduce perimenopausal hot flashes, is not commonly used because of serious safety risks including heart attack, stroke, some cancers, and dementia (National Cancer Institute, 2018). Women who are prescribed MHT should be closely monitored for blood clots and have regular health screenings, including annual mammogram and pap smear, as advised by their care provider.

Women may experience altered sexual function caused by other illnesses, stress, and medications. Medications such as anticholinergics, antidepressants, and chemotherapy may cause arousal disorders. Medications for depression may cause orgasmic disorders. Other conditions and treatments that may lead to female altered sexual function include uterine prolapse, rectoceles, cystoceles, and stress. In many instances, altered sexual function resolves when the primary disorder is treated.

Complementary Health Approaches

Remedies for Postmenopausal Discomfort

1. Over-the-counter (OTC) vaginal moisturizers or water-soluble lubricants may help decrease the symptoms of dryness. Vaseline or other petroleum-based products should be avoided. Very-low-dose estrogen preparations in the form of vaginal creams, gels, or rings that produce minimal systemic effects are sometimes prescribed to reduce localized symptoms.

2. Estrogen receptor agonist-antagonists (ERAAs), also known as *designer estrogens*, provide estrogen-like effects on some tissues while blocking the effect of estrogen (acting as an antiestrogen) on other tissues. Tamoxifen and raloxifene are two ERAAs currently in use.

3. Herbs and other "natural" remedies are sometimes used to reduce menopausal symptoms. Because the U.S. Food and Drug Administration does not regulate the quality or effectiveness of anything labeled as a dietary supplement, self-treatment with herbs may not be a safe practice. If a woman decides to try an herbal remedy, it is essential that she tell her primary care provider what she is taking so that the provider can monitor her for any untoward effects or possible interactions with other prescription and OTC drugs. Dong quai, ginseng, black cohosh, Vitex/chasteberry, dehydroeplandrosterone (DHEA), melatonin, and St. John's wort are commonly used herbal preparations.

Other natural products include phytoestrogens and wild yams (sweet potatoes). Phytoestrogens are chemicals that act as estrogens on some parts of the body and antiestrogens on others. Soybeans are a rich source of phytoestrogens. Research in this area is ongoing, and more scientific information is needed. Wild yams are thought to be helpful because they contain a chemical similar to one used for making the type of progesterone in birth control pills. Wild yam creams are considered nonhormonal and are currently being tested for effectiveness.

AGE-RELATED CHANGES IN MEN

Older men may experience a normal delayed reaction to sexual stimuli. They require a longer time to achieve an erection, and the erection is often less firm than it was at a younger age. Male orgasm takes longer to achieve and has a shorter duration than it did at a younger age. Ejaculation is less forceful, and a smaller volume of seminal fluid is released. Loss of erection occurs quickly after orgasm. In general, the time between orgasms increases, and orgasm may not occur with every episode of sexual intercourse.

The most common altered sexual function in older men is erectile dysfunction (ED). ED is the inability to achieve or maintain an erection sufficient for a satisfactory sexual intercourse in more than 50% of attempts. Diabetes, depression, and cardiovascular disease contribute to ED, even in younger men. Prostatectomy (removal of excess prostate tissue) does not always cause ED because newer surgical techniques may allow the surgeon to avoid cutting the nerves involved in achieving an erection. Medications such as sildenafil citrate or tadalafil are effective for many individuals suffering from ED.

IMPACT OF ILLNESS ON SEXUAL HEALTH

Illness of one or both partners is a common cause of changes in sexual well-being among older adults. For example, joint pain resulting from arthritis can interfere with sexual activity. Cardiac problems may interfere with normal sexual activity, although this is often more from fear than from actual danger. The risk for serious cardiac problems resulting from sexual *intercourse* is generally low, but older people with history of a heart attack should discuss their concerns with their primary care provider. Sexual activity does not need to be suspended because of stroke, as intercourse is unlikely to cause another stroke. However, a person with a history of stroke may require education about positioning and/or the use of assistive devices to compensate for any residual weakness or paralysis. Hysterectomy (removal of the uterus) and mastectomy (removal of a breast) do not change sexual functioning, although loss of these organs may make a woman feel less desirable or make her fear that she will be viewed as less desirable. Vaginal lubrication does diminish after hysterectomy, however, which may cause discomfort for the woman. Counseling may be helpful for women with these concerns. Chronic depression can decrease sexual interest and lead a woman to be less responsive to intimacy. Finally, it is important to recognize that incontinence itself does not interfere with the physical aspect of sexual function but may cause affected individuals to avoid sexual activity because of embarrassment. Incontinence treatment and education can alleviate this problem.

EFFECTS OF ALCOHOL AND MEDICATIONS ON SEXUAL HEALTH

Alcohol and medications can have a profound impact on sexual function in older adults. Excessive alcohol intake results in delayed orgasm in women and loss of the ability to achieve or maintain an erection in men. A wide range of medications and drugs (Table 16.1) can lead to sexual problems for both men and women. Changes in medication or dosage may help to resolve the problem. Interestingly, some antiparkinsonian medications actually enhance sexual desire but not necessarily the ability to perform sexually.

LOSS OF A SEX PARTNER

Loss of one's intimate partner is one of the most common causes of decreased sexual activity among older

Table 16.1	Examples of Medications and Drugs Associated With Altered Sexual Function
Antihypertensives	Diuretics; alpha and beta adrenergic blockers; angiotensin-converting enzyme inhibitors; calcium channel blockers
Central nervous system medications	Monoamine oxidase inhibitors (MAOIs); selective serotonin reuptake inhibitors (SSRIs); tricyclic antidepressants; anxiolytics; antipsychotics; lithium carbonate, opioids
Miscellaneous	Antiseizure medications; cimetidine, methotrexate, estrogens, amphetamines, cholesterol-lowering drugs
Over-the-counter medications	Some antihistamines, decongestants; antiinflammatories
Street drugs	Alcohol, cocaine, heroin, tobacco, marijuana

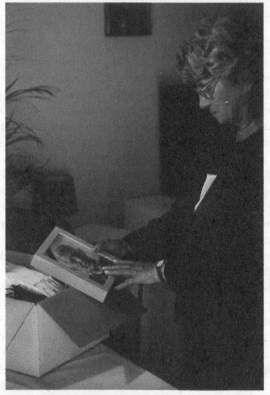

Fig. 16.2 Loss of an intimate partner has a huge impact on the sexual health and overall well-being of an older person. (Copyright © istock.com/KatarzynaBialasiewicz.)

adults (Fig. 16.2). This is especially true for older women. Some 32% of women over the age of 70 have partners, compared with 59% of men in the same age group—a situation termed the "partner gap" (Stein, 2020). Moreover, social norms may suggest to older women that their sexual interest in men is not socially acceptable. Older men more frequently voice an interest in sex, although older women are more likely to express a desire for companionship and love.

MARRIAGE AND OLDER ADULTS

Some older adults may view sex only within the context of marriage, while other older adults do not associate it with a linked partnership. It is important to be culturally sensitive regarding how individuals perceive sexuality.

Marriage or remarriage among older adults elicits many different responses, particularly from their families. Some are accepting and recognize the need for older adults to find affection and meaning in later life. Others believe that marriage at a late age is somehow unacceptable. Children may fear that the marriage discredits the memory of the deceased parent. They may fear that remarriage will displace them from their parent's affection or affect their inheritance. Regardless of the family's response, older adults have the right to determine what is best for them. Ideally, family and friends will be supportive of their decisions.

Marriage is not always an option for aging individuals. Some older adults, particularly widows, stand to lose a great deal if they remarry. Pensions, insurance benefits, and other financial concerns may be contingent on the person's remaining single. For this reason, some older people choose to live together without marrying. This may be a difficult decision for both older adults and their families because of their cultural and religious beliefs. Health care professionals must be able to recognize the value of these relationships and support older adults' choices.

CAREGIVERS AND THE SEXUALITY OF OLDER ADULTS

Sexuality is a difficult area to address at any age. Young people may not be comfortable with the thought of sexual activity among seniors, believing that it is somehow offensive or abnormal. Similarly, health professionals may harbor personal biases or may lack the necessary skills to address the sexual needs of older adults in a therapeutic manner. In addition, older adults are often reluctant to discuss their own sexuality. Discomfort or embarrassment over what younger persons may think leads many older people to hide their sexual interests and activity even from health professionals. Nurses and other health professionals who provide care to older adults must be nonjudgmental and sensitive to the values and attitudes of older individuals.

Caregivers should address issues of sexuality in private and ask open-ended questions, such as, "What have you noticed about how your sexuality has changed with age?" or "What concerns do you have about your sex life?" Open-ended questions allow the older person the opportunity to express a variety of concerns in their own words and in the manner acceptable to them. Caregivers must be aware and maintain control of their own personal and cultural beliefs in order to remain nonjudgmental and to preserve the therapeutic relationship. They need to indicate their willingness to listen and allow adequate time to discuss any concerns that may arise.

SEXUAL ORIENTATION OF OLDER ADULTS

The exact number of lesbian, gay, bisexual, transgender, and queer/questioning (LGBTQ) persons over age 65 is unknown. Studies estimate that about 2.4 million Americans over age 65 are LGBTQ—a figure that is expected to double by 2030 (Wardecker & Matsick, 2020). Female LGBTQ people are likely to be overrepresented in these numbers because of general population trends and the greater impact of human immunodeficiency virus (HIV)/acquired immunodeficiency syndrome (AIDS)–related deaths on the male population (Rosenfeld, 2018). LGBTQ older people face the "double stigma" related to their age and sexual orientation (Pereira & Silva, 2021). Health care providers must be sensitive to the sexual needs and concerns of LGBTQ older adults.

The LGBTQ population still faces considerable discrimination; LGBTQ older adults have faced it throughout their lives (Cahill, 2020). The regulatory protection of the rights of the LGBTQ population varies considerably from one jurisdiction to another. Consequently this population tends to be underserved because health care and social services are not always well equipped to provide adequate support to older LGBTQ people. Many older LGBTQ adults are reluctant to access a health care system focused on the heterosexual population—a system that often fails to address the concerns of the LGBTQ community (Cahill, 2020). Older LGBTQ persons may be uncomfortable about disclosing their sexual orientation because of confidentiality concerns or fears that resulting discrimination might lead to substandard care. For example, LGBTQ older adults may fear end-of-life care because of lack of recognition of their relationship or marriage and lack of mental health care as a widow or widower. Many aging LGBTQ people report becoming depressed and express concern about having to deny or conceal their life choices in order to gain acceptance (Cahill, 2020; Candrian & Cloyes, 2021). Nurses are expected to promote the sexual well-being of all older adults regardless of their sexual orientation. The development of services sensitive to the needs of the LGBTQ population is an important goal for health care.

SEXUALLY TRANSMITTED INFECTIONS

Older adults are often not considered when sexually transmitted infections (STI) are discussed, even though over half of all HIV/AIDS cases in the United States occur in people age 50 and older (CDC, 2020). HIV infection is commonly overlooked because older adults are not considered to be at high risk for it. The prevalence of HIV among older adults is likely to continue to increase as more individuals become infected later in life, and individuals infected in early adulthood live longer as a result of better disease treatment. Moreover, the decreasing responsiveness of the immune system that is associated with aging increases the older person's susceptibility to HIV and AIDS. AIDS in older adults is known as the "great imitator" because many of the associated symptoms are similar to those of other diseases and may be attributed to normal aging (HIVinfo.NIH.gov, 2021). Older adults with HIV are at higher risk of cognitive decline. Dementia associated with AIDS may be mistaken for Alzheimer disease. The threat of other STIs is equally important. Between 2015 and 2020, the rates of chlamydia, gonorrhea, and syphilis infections among the over-55 age group have doubled (Shaw, 2020). People are living longer and are in better health, and retirement communities, much like college campuses, provide ample opportunities for sexual activity. In addition, today's older adults were raised in an era before "safer sex" practices became the norm. Activities promoting sexually responsible behaviors should target older adults, as the risk of becoming infected clearly does not disappear with age.

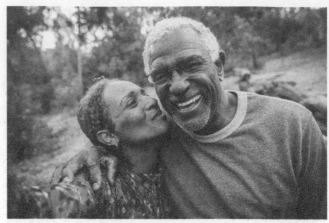

Fig. 16.3 Sexuality is an important need in late life and affects pleasure, adaptation, and a general feeling of well-being. (Copyright © istock.com/adamkaz.)

Health Promotion

Health Care Directives for Nonrelated Caregivers

LGBTQ people need to be aware of the laws regulating same-sex relationships in their respective states. In the states that do not provide protection to same-sex relationships, LGBTQ people may need to be made aware of the importance of completing advance directives if they wish to have their friends, partners, or other nonfamily members participate in their health care decision-making. Without these directives, even long-term partners may not have legal standing in decision-making and may even be prohibited from visiting in some situations.

PRIVACY AND PERSONAL RIGHTS OF OLDER ADULTS

Community-dwelling older adults generally have a right to manage their sex lives without interference. They are free to express affection and engage in sexual activities whenever they choose. However, institutional placement of one or both partners may interfere with their ability to maintain their usual sexual patterns. Finding privacy may be difficult, even for married couples who reside in the same institution, particularly if regular medical or nursing care is necessary (Fig. 16.3).

In the past, displays of sexual affection among older adults were discouraged. This perspective has changed as health care professionals gain better understanding

their understanding of the importance of sexual well-being across the lifespan. Many facilities and clinical agencies now have policies and programs that protect and promote the expression of sexuality among older adults. Touching, hand-holding, and cuddling are encouraged. Unmarried older adults are allowed to form whatever relationships they desire. A closed door must be respected when privacy for intimacy is desired. Of course, judgment is necessary when either person in a relationship suffers from cognitive impairment. When there is any sign of disinterest or resistance to sexual advances, the behavior cannot be permitted. It is important to protect vulnerable older adults from undesired physical contact, while mutually agreeable physical contact remains a right of older adults.

❖ NURSING PROCESS/CLINICAL JUDGMENT MODEL FOR ALTERED SEXUAL FUNCTION

◆ ASSESSMENT (DATA COLLECTION)

Recognize cues:
- Is the person sexually active?
- If they are sexually active, do they have any difficulties or discomfort during sexual activity?
- Does the person have any discharge or drainage from the genitals?
- Do they have any diseases or disabilities that interfere with sexual activity?
- Are there any emotional issues, such as depression, that interfere with sexual interest or activity?
- Does the person take any medications that may interfere with sexual activity?
- What level of sexual activity do they desire?
- Does the person have any real or perceived barriers to sexual activity?
- Do they have adequate privacy for sexual activity?
  Box 16.1 lists risk factors for altered sexual function in older adults.

Box 16.1	**Risk Factors Related to Altered Sexual Function in Older Adults**

- Loss of partner
- Problems with physical mobility
- Living in an institutional setting
- Physical illness or a reaction to therapeutic medications

◆ **DATA ANALYSIS/PROBLEM IDENTIFICATION**

Analyze Cues and Prioritize Hypotheses: Problem statement for older adults with an alteration in sexual functioning includes

Altered Sexual Function

◆ **PLANNING**

The patient goals for older adults with altered sexual function are to (1) verbalize feelings about sexual identity, (2) discuss concerns regarding sexuality, and (3) describe the effects of aging and illness on sexual functioning.

◆ **IMPLEMENTATION**

Take Action: The following nursing interventions should take place in hospitals, in extended-care facilities, and at home:

1. **Encourage verbalization of concerns.** Many older adults do not feel comfortable talking about sex to anyone, including nurses. Without undue prying into the older person's privacy, communicate a willingness to discuss any concerns older adults have, including those that deal with sexuality. Allow adequate time and provide a private place for these discussions.

2. **Provide privacy.** Older adults who wish to date or visit should have the opportunity to do so without interference. Private areas should be available for dating interactions. Older residents of extended-care facilities should have the opportunity for conjugal visits in the agency or at home if desired. Ensure that these visits meet all federal and state regulations that pertain to residents' rights. Carefully respect privacy during these visits.

3. **Protect the sexual dignity of confused older adults.** Confused individuals may display sexually inappropriate behaviors (e.g., exposing themselves in public, masturbating, and making inappropriate sexual advances to nursing staff). Implement interventions to protect their dignity. For example, undressing in public can be decreased by modifying clothing. For men, elastic waist pants can replace pants with zippers. For women, buttonless or back-opening tops and pants instead of skirts can help reduce exposure. Masturbation is common and is not abnormal. Distraction is often effective at reducing the incidence of public masturbation. If distraction is not effective, take the person to their room and provide privacy. Do not apply protective devices to prevent masturbation. If a confused older person makes inappropriate sexual advances, attempt to distract them and, if necessary, stop care temporarily. Confused individuals do not realize that their behavior is inappropriate. Do not overreact to the behavior, because this can precipitate violent or verbally abusive episodes (Nursing Care Plan 16.1).

⭐ **Nursing Care Plan 16.1   Altered Sexual Function**

Mr. Silver, age 89, has a history of hypertension and diabetes. Mrs. Silver, age 87, has severe osteoarthritis and heart failure. Both are residents of Pine Grove Care Center. They have been married for 67 years. Because of space constraints, they have been assigned to separate rooms. Mr. Silver spends a great deal of time at Mrs. Silver's bedside, where he holds her hand and talks to her. Both often verbalize the wish to hold and touch more intimately. They both state, "I wish we just had some privacy around here."

PROBLEM STATEMENT

Altered Sexual Function

SUPPORTING ASSESSMENT DATA

- Lack of privacy
- Separation from significant other
- Altered body function related to age and disease processes

PATIENT GOALS/OUTCOMES IDENTIFICATION

Mr. and Mrs. Silver will identify methods for satisfying their need for sexual expression.

NURSING INTERVENTIONS/IMPLEMENTATION

1. Allow opportunities for both parties to verbalize their feelings about continuing sexual contact.
2. Attempt to arrange for a shared room, if this is agreeable to both parties.
3. Develop a method such as hanging a "Do Not Disturb" sign for ensuring private time for the couple while recognizing the need for access in case of emergency.
4. Assist with hygiene needs so that both parties are physically clean and attractive.
5. Verbalize an understanding of the continued need for physical closeness throughout life.

⭐ **Nursing Care Plan 16.1** | **Altered Sexual Function—cont'd**

EVALUATION

Mr. and Mrs. Silver are observed spending time privately in Mrs. Silver's room with the door closed. After these visits, Mr. Silver states that "It feels good just to touch, share a kiss, and be together quietly for a while. It isn't how I thought we'd end up, but it's better than nothing." You will continue the plan of care.

APPLYING CLINICAL JUDGMENT

1. Some facilities permit or encourage married couples to share a room in long-term care facilities. Do you think that this is something that should be encouraged or discouraged? Why?
2. How can the nurse provide for privacy needs if a couple is still interested in sexual activity?
3. How can the nurse determine whether there is mutual consent to sexual activity?

Get Ready for the Next Generation NCLEX® Examination!

Key Points

- Sexuality is a concept that is often minimized or ignored in older adults.
- Older adults who are cognitively intact have the right to make decisions about their sexuality.
- Health problems, loss of a partner, and the normal physiological changes of aging all affect sexual practices.
- Age- and health-related changes affect the type and frequency of sexual activity, although many individuals maintain an active interest in sex into old age.
- Nurses must recognize that older adults are still sexual beings who continue to have sexual needs.
- Nurses must respect and protect older adults' right to enjoy sexual activities that meet their needs.
- Information about safer sex should be available to older adults, as the rates of sexually transmitted infections are on the rise in this age group.
- People over age 50 account for more than half of all HIV cases; the rates of chlamydia, gonorrhea, and syphilis infections among the over-55 age group have doubled in recent years.

Additional Learning Resources

SG Go to your Evolve website at http://evolve.elsevier.com/Williams/geriatric for the additional online resources.

⚡ Review Questions for the Next Generation NCLEX® Examination

1. A 70-year-old man confides to the nurse that he recently began to have difficulty achieving an erection. Which nursing response is appropriate?
   - a. "That's quite normal at your age."
   - b. "What do you think is wrong?"
   - c. "Are you having problems in your marriage?"
   - d. "Did you recently change any medications?"

2. A 69-year-old woman reports that she avoids intercourse because it is uncomfortable. Which nursing response is appropriate?
   - a. Suggest that she ask her primary care provider for an estrogen vaginal cream.
   - b. Describe herbal and natural products that have effects similar to estrogen.
   - c. Clarify what she means by "uncomfortable."
   - d. Explain that this is a normal and expected change of aging.

3. An older man with dementia often masturbates in the lounge area of a long-term care facility. Which nursing intervention is appropriate? *(Select all that apply.)*
   - a. Modify his clothing to make genital exposure more difficult.
   - b. Apply mitten protective devices to prevent self-stimulation.
   - c. Provide privacy by escorting him back to his room.
   - d. Explain repeatedly that this type of behavior is not acceptable.
   - e. Distract him with a different activity.
   - f. Administer an as-needed (prn) sedative medication.

4. Why might an older transgender person be reluctant to move into a long-term care facility?
   - a. Because they fear that they will receive substandard care.
   - b. Because they prefer not to associate with aging heterosexuals.
   - c. Because they fear that they will lose legal rights in the facility.
   - d. Because they believe that most caregivers will discriminate against them.

5. The nurse is precepting a new graduate licensed vocational nurse (LVN) at a nursing home. Which response by the LVN indicates that they have a good understanding of sexuality in aging population?
   - a. "Mr. Wang and Mrs. Levy would like some privacy while they are in Mrs. Levy's room. May I place a 'Do Not Disturb' sign on her room door?"
   - b. "Mr. Smith was masturbating in his bed yet again this morning. I asked him to refrain from doing it because it makes the staff uncomfortable."
   - c. "Mr. Nguyen told me that he does not feel comfortable discussing sexual issues with me. Should I ask his son to talk to him and relay the content of their conversation to me?"
   - d. "Mrs. Ball told me that she has been considering marrying her long-term companion. Should I warn her against it because it might upset her children?"

REFERENCES

Cahill, S. (2020). *LGBT aging 2025: Strategies for achieving a healthy and thriving LGBT older adult community in Massachusetts*. https://www.lgbtagingcenter.org/resources/pdfs/LGBT-Aging-2025-Report-December-2020.pdf

Candrian, C. & Cloyes, K.G. (2021). She's dying and I can't say we're married? End-of-life care for LGBT older adults. *The Gerontologist*, 61(8), 1197–1201. https://doi.org/10.1093/geront/gnaa186

Centers for Disease Control and Prevention [CDC] (2020). *HIV: People aged 50 and older*. https://www.cdc.gov/hiv/group/age/olderamericans/index.html#:~:text=HIV%20and%20Older%20Americans&text=In%202018%2C%20over%20half%20(51,2018%20were%20in%20this%20group/

HIVinfo.NIH.gov (2021). *HIV and older people*. https://hivinfo.nih.gov/understanding-hiv/fact-sheets/hiv-and-older-people

National Cancer Institute (2018). *Menopausal hormone therapy and cancer*. https://www.cancer.gov/about-cancer/causes-prevention/risk/hormones/mht-fact-sheet#r7

Pereira H., & Silva P. (2021). The importance of social support, positive identity, and resilience in the successful aging of older sexual minority men. *Geriatrics*, 6(4), 98. https://doi.org/10.3390/geriatrics6040098

Research & Evaluation Group at PHMC and Bradbury-Sullivan LGBT Community Center. (2020). 2020 *Pennsylvania LGBTQ Health Needs Assessment*. https://www.pacancercoalition.org/images/pdf/LGBTQ_resources/2020_pa_lgbtq_full_report_final_public_distribution.pdf

Rosenfeld, D. (2018). *The AIDS epidemic's lasting impact on gay men*. https://www.thebritishacademy.ac.uk/blog/aids-epidemic-lasting-impact-gay-men/

Shaw, G. (2020). STI rate has doubled among senior citizens. *Emergency Medicine News*, 42(11), 18–19. doi:10.1097/01.EEM.0000722388.18510.27

Stein, L. (2020). Sex and seniors: The 70-year itch. https://consumer.healthday.com/encyclopedia/aging-1/misc-aging-news-10/sex-and-seniors-the-70-year-itch-647575.html

Wardecker, B.M., & Matsick, J.L. (2020). Families of choice and community connectedness: A brief guide to the social strengths of LGBTQ older adults. *Journal of Gerontological Nursing*, 46(2). https://doi.org/10.3928/00989134-20200113-01

17 Care of Aging Skin and Mucous Membranes

Objectives

1. Discuss changes related to aging that have an effect on skin and mucous membranes.
2. Identify the older adults who are most at risk for problems related to the skin and mucous membranes.
3. Describe interventions that assist older adults in maintaining intact skin and mucous membranes.

Key Terms

alopecia (ăl-ō-PĒ-shē-ă, p. 290)
aseptic technique (ā-SĔP-tĭk, p. 296)
caries (KĂR-ēz, p. 301)
dysgeusia (dĭs-goózhah, p. 304)
edentulous (ē-dĕn-chū-lŭs, p. 302)
exudate (ĔKS-ū-dāt, p. 294)
gingivitis (jĭn-jĭ-VĪ-tĭs, p. 301)
halitosis (hăl-ĭ-TŌ-sĭs, p. 301)

hyperkeratosis (hī-pĕr-kĕr-ă-TŌ-sĭs, p. 290)
leukoplakia (lū-kō-PLĂ-kē-ă, p. 302)
pigmentation (pĭg-mĕn-TĂ-shŭn, p. 288)
pressure injuries (p. 286)
pruritus (prū-RĪ-tŭs, p. 286)
scabies (SKĂ-bēz, p. 288)
shearing forces (p. 289)
xerostomia (zēr-ō-STŌ-mē-ă, p. 302)

With aging, the skin undergoes changes that make it more susceptible to damage. Over time, the epidermal layer becomes thinner and the subcutaneous padding diminishes, increasing the risk for traumatic injuries such as skin tears or pressure injuries. Bruises are more common because capillary walls are more fragile. Skin tears can turn into chronic wounds if not treated properly. Medications used to treat various health issues can cause problems. Corticosteroids make the skin more fragile, and anticoagulants increase the risk for bleeding with even minor trauma. Decreased sebaceous secretions and circulatory changes contribute to the dry skin and scaliness of the lower extremities commonly seen with aging. Older skin is also more susceptible to inflammation, infection, and rashes. Pruritus (itching), which is a common complaint among older adults, may be caused by dryness, irritation, or infection, but it can also be related to diseases such as diabetes mellitus, kidney disease, malignancy, or anemia. Changes in the function of dermal receptor cells result in the decreased ability of older persons to perceive sensations such as touch and pressure, thus increasing the risk for pressure-related disorders. Although skin problems are not usually life-threatening, they are significant because they can distress the older person and lead to a decreased quality of life. Skin problems should be prevented whenever possible. In situations where the problems are not preventable, they should be recognized, treated, and resolved in a timely manner.

AGE-RELATED CHANGES IN SKIN, HAIR, AND NAILS

Changes in the skin, hair, and nails may indicate a variety of problems related to poor nutrition and circulation. Because these structures are the ones most easily observed, they can provide a great deal of information about the metabolic health of the entire body. See Table 17.1 for a complete list of these changes.

Complete assessment of skin, hair, and nails is best done when the person is undressed so that all skin surfaces can be inspected. Skin assessment can be performed during a bath, during daily personal hygiene, at bedtime, or at any other convenient time for the older person. Independent older adults should be aware of what is normal for themselves, and they should bring any changes to the attention of the primary care provider. Privacy must be maintained and modesty protected during the skin inspection. Assessment of the skin and related structures is an important responsibility of nurses. Instruct nursing assistants and attendant health care workers who assist with bathing or other care to promptly report any unusual or

Table 17.1	Age-Related Changes in Skin, Hair, and Nails	
	AGE-RELATED CHANGE	**RELATED ASSESSMENT FINDINGS**
Hair		
Color	Decreased production of melanin	Graying of hair
Texture	Many hair follicles stop producing; as hair falls out, less is replaced	Thinner hair
Distribution	Hormonal changes	Decreased axillary, pubic, and extremity hair; increased facial hair in women
Nails		
Growth	Nail plate growth rate decreases	Slower growing nails
Texture, color	Nail plate morphology changes	Thick or thin nails; brittle, discolored nails
Skin		
Appearance	Thinning of the epidermis	Thinner, more translucent skin
	Fewer melanocytes; remaining melanocytes tend to be larger	Paler looking skin; large pigmented spots ("age spots") More frequent bruising, cherry angiomas
	Fragile blood vessels in the dermis	Dry skin
	Decreased oil production by sebaceous glands	
Sensation/Safety	Decreased subcutaneous fat	Feeling "cold"; risk of developing hypothermia
	Decreased production of sweat by sweat glands	Harder to keep cool in hot weather; risk of hyperthermia

Data from Martin, L. J. (2016). Aging changes in hair and nails. https://medlineplus.gov/ency/article/004005.htm. Martin, L. J. (2018). Aging changes in skin. https://medlineplus.gov/ency/article/004014.htm; Touhy, T. A., & Jett, K. (2018). *Ebersole and Hess' toward healthy aging: human needs and nursing response*. St. Louis, MO: Elsevier Mosby.

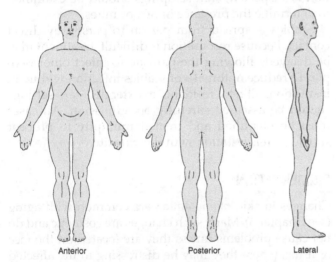

Fig. 17.1 Example of a body diagram that can be used in assessing older adults for skin impairment. (From Mosby [2010]. *Mosby's field guide to physical therapy*, St. Louis, MO: Mosby.)

questionable observations to a nurse for further investigation. Inspection should follow a logical order so that no pertinent observations are missed. Most nurses find that a head-to-toe progression is the most helpful, as is a body diagram on which observations are indicated (Fig. 17.1).

SKIN COLOR

Changes in skin color can indicate a variety of disorders. When assessing skin for color, it is important to be aware of the differences in skin pigments among ethnic groups. Examine the skin in good, preferably natural, light and compare one side of the body with

the other. Use touch to determine skin temperature or the presence of rashes or irritation. Stretching the skin slightly may help in determining the underlying tones. Color changes—including pallor, cyanosis, jaundice, or erythema—can indicate a variety of problems. Record and report the extent and location of any color changes promptly.

🌐 Cultural Considerations

Pressure Injuries

When assessing people with dark skin tones, changes in tissue color that indicate stage 1 pressure injuries can be better distinguished using a halogen light, which may reveal a purple hue. Be sure to use touch to determine changes in tissue temperature or sensation and palpate for signs of localized edema over pressure points.

DRY SKIN

Dry skin is one of the most common problems of aging. Studies have shown that 75% of people older than 65 years of age experience dry skin. Physiological changes, excessive bathing, the use of harsh soaps, and a dry environment all contribute to problems with dry skin.

Dry skin can result in pruritus, burning, and cracking of the skin (Fig. 17.2). Older people may develop a habit of scratching or picking at dry or cracked skin, increasing their risk for further tissue damage and infection. Skin irritation can be severe and can cause intense discomfort to older adults. In fact, it may be so distracting that affected individuals stop participating in social activities.

Fig. 17.2 Dry scaly skin as commonly seen in older adults. (From White, G. M., & Cox, N. H. [2006]. *Diseases of the skin: A color atlas and text* [2nd ed.]. St. Louis, MO: Mosby.)

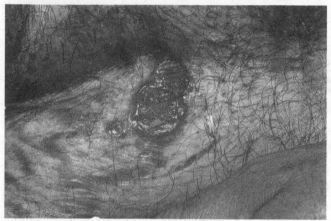

Fig. 17.3 Drug-induced skin reactions are seen more commonly in older patients than younger ones. Here the use of a potent topical corticosteroid has caused in severe striae. The atrophy was so severe that the skin tore, forming an ulceration. (From White, G. M., & Cox, N. H. [2006]. *Diseases of the skin: A color atlas and text* [2nd ed.]. St. Louis, MO: Mosby.)

RASHES AND IRRITATION

Rashes and skin irritation can be caused by factors other than dryness. Medications, communicable diseases, and contact with chemical substances are common causes of skin rashes and pruritus (Fig. 17.3).

Allergic response to medications can manifest as diffuse rashes over the body. Whenever a rash develops soon after administration of new medication, a drug allergy should be suspected. It would then be appropriate to withhold that particular medication and contact the primary care provider to report the symptom.

One communicable source of skin irritation and severe pruritus is scabies, a superficial infection caused by a parasitic mite (*Sarcoptes scabiei* var. *hominis*) that burrows under the skin (Fig. 17.4). Older adults—especially individuals who suffer from chronic illness, dementia, or a depressed immune system—are particularly vulnerable to scabies infections. Signs of scabies include intense itching and fine dark wavy lines at the flexor surface of the wrist or elbow, the webbed area of

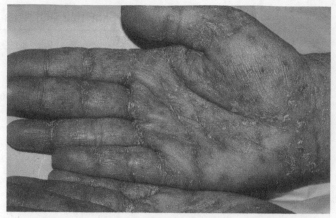

Fig. 17.4 Scabies lesions at three different stages are evident on this patient's hand. The lesion at the far left features a well-demarcated round border surrounding a blister, whereas the lesion nearest the thumb fold has already erupted and appears to be healing. (From White, G. M., & Cox, N. H. [2006]. *Diseases of the skin: A color atlas and text* [2nd ed.]. St. Louis, MO: Mosby.)

the fingers, the axillae, and the genitals. Recognition of scabies may be difficult in older adults because it has an asymptomatic incubation period of 4 to 6 weeks and atypical presentations are common. When infestation is suspected, skin scrapings should be examined to determine the presence of ova or mites.

Scabies is spread from person to person by direct contact. Because recognition is difficult, treatment may be delayed, allowing the parasite to infect other people. To reduce outbreaks of scabies infection within an institution, all new residents in extended-care settings should be assessed carefully on admission. All cases must be identified and treated promptly to prevent spread or reinfestation with the parasite.

PIGMENTATION

Changes in skin pigmentation are common with aging (see Chapter 3). Many such changes are cosmetic and do not cause problems unless they are located on the face or arms, where they may be distressing to the affected person. Common conditions such as acne rosacea can be treated with topical medications, which help heal the skin and reduce redness, whereas others can be concealed by appropriate use of cosmetics. Changes in the size or pigmentation of moles are of greater significance and must be reported because these changes may indicate the presence of a precancerous or cancerous condition that needs immediate medical attention.

TISSUE INTEGRITY

Breaks in tissue integrity increase the older person's risk for infection and often result in the need for costly, time-consuming treatments. These breaks can cause disfigurement and are frightening to older adults. Skin tears, abrasions, lacerations, and ulcers most often result from pressure or pressure combined with

Table 17.2	Quick Guide to Prevention of Pressure Injuries
RISK FACTOR	**NURSING INTERVENTIONS**
Immobility	Establish individualized turning schedule; reduce shear and friction by using trapeze and/or turning sheet; elevate head of bed lower than 30 degrees; provide pressure relief surface.
Inactivity	Provide assistive devices to increase activity.
Incontinence	Assess the need for incontinence. management; clean and dry skin after soiling.
Malnutrition	Provide adequate nutritional and fluid intake; assist with snacks and meals, monitor intake and output (I&O); consult the dietitian for nutritional evaluation.
Diminished sensation, decreased mental status	Assess the patient's and family's ability to provide care; educate caregivers regarding pressure injury prevention.
Altered skin integrity	Avoid pressure; do not use donut-shaped cushions or sheepskin; lubricate skin; apply barrier ointments to protect skin from moisture; do not massage red areas; do not use heat lamps, heating pads, or hot water.

Modified from Catania, K., Huang, C., James, P., Madison, M., Moran, M., & Ohr, M. (2007). PUPPI—The pressure ulcer prevention protocol interventions. *American Journal of Nursing, 107*(4), 44-52.

shearing forces. Even simple incidents—such as bumping a leg into an open dishwasher door, sliding across bed linens, or the removal of tape—can result in significant skin trauma to the older person.

PRESSURE INJURIES

Pressure injuries are a particular risk to older adults who suffer from compromised circulation, restricted mobility, altered level of consciousness, fecal or urinary incontinence, or nutritional problems (Table 17.2). Studies estimating the occurrence of pressure injuries vary widely, but one consistent point is that they occur in all settings. Although most studies show that the incidence of pressure injuries has declined, there is still much work to do regarding prevention. Pressure injuries have negative effects on the overall health of an older adult. They can lead to infection, pain, loss of function, and even death.

⚖️ Legal Considerations

The occurrence of pressure injuries can leave care facilities and nurses vulnerable to lawsuits for negligence. A single pressure injury can cost up to $40,000 to treat, which does not include the human cost of pain and suffering. New Medicare rules specify that a hospital will not be reimbursed for the care of a patient who develops a "reasonably preventable" pressure injury after being admitted. In some states, it is mandatory to report the development of a stage 3 or 4 pressure injury to the Department of Health. It is important to carefully assess and document any pressure injuries that are present upon admission.

Excessive pressure on tissues, particularly over bony prominences, can quickly lead to skin breakdown (Fig. 17.5). The development of pressure injuries depends on the amount of pressure, the length of time the pressure is exerted, and the underlying status of the tissues involved. Tissue that is subjected to excessive pressure does not receive adequate oxygen or nutrients. This can result in ischemia and increases the skin's susceptibility to breakdown. When tissue is deprived of necessary nutrients for a longer period, necrosis and tissue destruction can result. Tissue that is fragile because of poor nutrition or circulation is most susceptible to breakdown. Early danger signs indicating a risk for breakdown include pale or reddened tissue. Pressure injuries are categorized or staged based on their appearance and the depth of tissue penetration (Fig. 17.6).

Individuals who have had one pressure injury are at greater risk for future development of more injuries. Additional factors that contribute to the development of pressure injuries include:

- Obesity
- Malnutrition
- History of alcohol and tobacco use
- Edema
- Moisture: bladder and/or bowel incontinence, use of incontinence briefs
- Immobility
- Shearing forces
- Cognitive impairment

It is recommended that a formal risk assessment be performed at the time of admission, upon discharge, upon any change in patient condition, and then at regular intervals. Guidelines recommend that this assessment should include a complete history and physical examination, skin inspection, and use of a pressure injury risk assessment tool. The tools most commonly used for this are the Braden and Norton scales (Tables 17.3 and 17.4). A nutritional assessment is also needed to determine whether the patient is ingesting the nutrients needed to promote wound healing (Boyko et al., 2018). Nurses use the information from this assessment

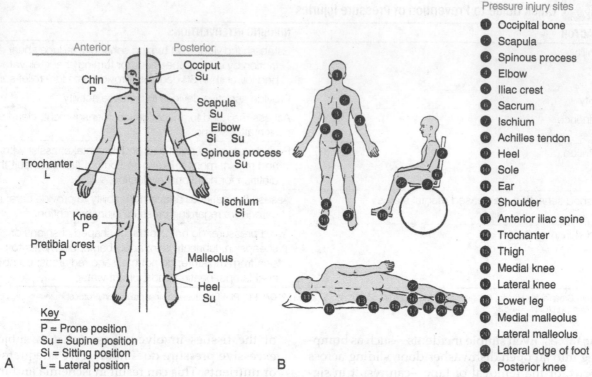

Fig. 17.5 **A,** Bony prominences most often underlying pressure injuries. **B,** Pressure injury sites. (From Trelease, C. C. [1988]. Developing standards for wound care. *Ostomy Wound Management, 26,* 50.)

to develop a plan of care that minimizes risk factors and promotes skin integrity.

AMOUNT, DISTRIBUTION, APPEARANCE, AND CONSISTENCY OF HAIR

The amount, distribution, appearance, and consistency of the hair change with aging. Hair typically becomes thinner and has a finer consistency with advanced age. Heredity and gender play a role in hair loss patterns. Men tend to lose more hair than do women, although some men retain a full head of hair throughout life. Male pattern baldness typically results in progressive loss of hair at the temples and back of the head. Sudden and excessive hair loss (alopecia) or breakage is likely to indicate a systemic problem. Abnormal hair loss can be related to high fevers, medications, nutrition problems, fungal or bacterial infections, endocrine disorders, or stress. Sudden or unusual hair loss should be reported so that the primary care provider can determine the cause.

The amount and distribution of body hair also change with aging. Diminished or absent hair on the lower legs or feet—particularly when combined with excessively dry, scaly, or flaky skin and weak or absent pedal pulses—indicates decreased blood supply to the lower extremities.

TISSUE OF THE FEET

Inspection of the tissue on the feet warrants special attention in older adults. Because many aging individuals are unable to bend adequately to view their feet, a family member or friend can perform this inspection for independent older adults (Fig. 17.7). In an institutional setting, nursing staff should perform foot inspection. Many older adults neglect their feet simply because they cannot see or reach them. Unless foot inspection is done on a regular schedule, severe problems can occur before anyone is aware of them.

NAILS

Aging results in hyperkeratosis of the nails, particularly the toenails. Thick, hard nails are difficult to cut using normal foot care equipment. The strength and effort required to cut these nails may exceed the older person's abilities, resulting in overgrowth. Soaking the feet in warm water before attempting to cut the nails may soften them and make them easier to cut. Assistance from a family member or health care provider is appropriate when there is no history of circulatory problems or diabetes. When diabetes or circulatory problems are present, care should be provided by a foot care specialist, because nails can be thick and the underlying tissue is easily injured, which can lead to infection. Special heavy duty equipment may be needed to accomplish proper nail care.

> **QSEN Considerations: Safety**
>
> During nail care, the use of safety glasses is recommended to prevent eye injuries resulting from flying nail particles.

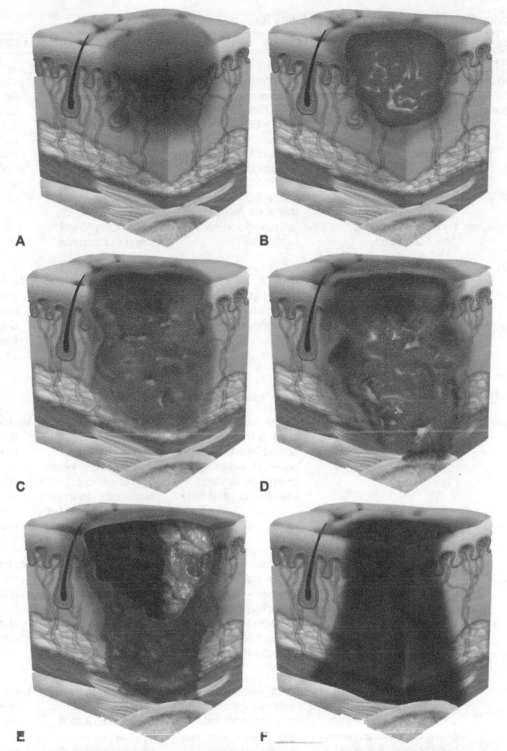

Fig. 17.6 Stages of pressure injuries. **A** = stage 1; **B** = stage 2; **C** = stage 3; **D** = stage 4; **E** = unstageable; **F** = suspected deep tissue injury. (Used with permission from the National Pressure Injury Advisory Panel, September 2016.)

If proper nail care is neglected, uncut nails confined in shoes often begin to curl under the toes, resulting in a condition called *ram's horn nails*. In this condition, the nail curls over the top of the toe and grows into the flesh on the bottom, causing pain. When the discomfort becomes severe, the older person may stop wearing shoes and decrease ambulation in an attempt to reduce the discomfort. In such severe cases, care from a podiatrist is needed. Nail fungus is increasingly common with aging. Fungi cause the nails to become thick, brittle, misshapened, and discolored. Fungal infections are more likely to affect the feet because the environment in shoes (dark, moist, and warm) supports growth of these micro-organisms. Fungal infections are more common in older adults with diabetes or other conditions of diminished peripheral circulation. These infections need to be recognized and treated so that they do not cause more widespread problems.

Table 17.3   **Braden Scale for Predicting Pressure Injury Risk**

ASSESSMENT TOOL	1 POINT	2 POINTS	3 POINTS	4 POINTS
Sensory Perception				
Ability to respond meaningfully to pressure-related discomfort	Completely limited: Unresponsive (does not moan, flinch, or grasp) to painful stimuli because of diminished level of consciousness or sedation *or* Limited ability to feel pain over most of body surface or discomfort over half of body	Very limited: Responds only to painful stimuli; cannot communicate discomfort except by moaning or restlessness *or* Has a sensory impairment that limits the ability to feel pain on one or two extremities	Slightly limited: Responds to verbal commands but cannot always communicate discomfort or the need to be turned *or* Has some sensory impairment, which limits ability to feel pain or discomfort	No impairment: Responds to verbal commands; has no sensory deficit that could limit ability to feel or voice pain or discomfort
Moisture				
Degree to which skin is exposed to moisture	Constantly moist: Skin is kept moist almost constantly by perspiration, urine, and the like; dampness is detected every time patient is moved or turned	Very moist: Skin is often, but not always, moist; linens must be changed at least once a shift	Occasionally moist: Skin is occasionally moist, requiring an extra linen change approximately once a day	Rarely moist: Skin is usually dry; linen requires changing only at routine intervals
Activity				
Degree of physical activity	Bedridden: Confined to bed	Chairfast: Ability to walk severely limited or nonexistent; cannot bear own weight and/or must be assisted into chair or wheelchair	Walks occasionally: Walks occasionally during day, but for very short distances, with or without assistance; spends majority of each shift on bed or chair	Walks frequently: Walks outside room at least twice a day and inside room at least once every 2 hours during waking hours
Mobility				
Ability to change and control body position	Completely immobile: Does not make even slight light changes in body or extremity position without assistance	Very limited: Makes occasional slight changes in body or extremity position but is unable to make frequent or significant changes independently	Slightly limited: Makes frequent although slight changes in body or extremity position independently	No limitations: Makes major and frequent body position changes without assistance
Nutrition				
Usual food intake pattern	Very poor: Never eats complete meal; rarely eats more than one-third of any food offered; eats two servings or less of protein (meat or dairy products) per day; takes fluids poorly; does not take a liquid dietary supplement *or* Receives nothing by mouth and/or is maintained on clear liquids or intravenous fluids	Probably inadequate: Rarely eats a complete meal; generally eats only approximately half of any food offered; protein intake includes only three servings of meat or dairy products per day; occasionally takes a dietary supplement *or* Receives less than optimal amount of liquid diet or tube feeding solutions for more than 5 days	Adequate: Eats more than half of most meals; eats a total of 4 servings of protein (meat or dairy products) each day; occasionally refuses a meal, but usually takes a supplement if offered *or* Is on a tube feeding or total parenteral nutrition regimen that probably meets most of nutritional needs	Excellent: Eats most of every meal; never refuses meal; usually eats total of 4 or more servings of meat and dairy products per day; occasionally eats between meals, does not require supplements

Table 17.3	Braden Scale for Predicting Pressure Injury Risk—cont'd			
ASSESSMENT TOOL	**1 POINT**	**2 POINTS**	**3 POINTS**	**4 POINTS**
Friction and Shear				
	Problem: Requires moderate to maximal assistance in moving; complete lifting without sliding against sheets is impossible; frequently slides down in bed or chair, requiring frequent repositioning with maximal assistance; spasticity, contractions, or agitation leads to almost constant friction	Potential problem: Moves feebly or requires minimal assistance; during a move, skin probably slides to some extent against sheets, chair, protective or other devices; maintains relatively good position in chair or bed most of the time but occasionally slides down	No apparent problem: Moves in bed and in chair independently and has sufficient muscle strength to sit up completely during move; maintains good position in bed or chair at all times	

Instructions: Score patient in each of the 6 subscales. The maximum score of 23 has the best prognosis and the minimum score of 6 has the worst prognosis. A patient is at risk for pressure injury if the score is equal to or greater than 16.

From Bergstrom, N., Braden, B.J., Laguzza, A., & Holman, V. (1987). The Braden scale for predicting pressure sore risk. *Nursing Research, 36*(4), 205-210.

Table 17.4	Norton Risk Assessment Scale									
PHYSICAL CONDITION		**MENTAL CONDITION**		**ACTIVITY**		**MOBILITY**		**INCONTINENT**		**TOTAL SCORE**
Good	4	Alert	4	Ambulant	4	Full	4	Not	4	4
Fair	3	Apathetic	3	Walk/help	3	Slightly limited	3	Occasional	3	3
Poor	2	Confused	2	Chairbound	2	Very limited	2	Usually/Urine	2	2
Very bad	1	Stupor	1	Bed	1	Immobile	1	Doubly	1	1
Name										
Date										

From Norton, D., McLaren, R. & Exton-Smith, A. N. (1962). *An investigation of geriatric nursing problems in the hospital*. Published by the National Corporation for the Care of Old People. Reproduced with permission from the Centre for Policy on Ageing, London (formerly NCCOP).

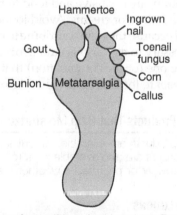

Fig. 17.7 Common foot problems in older adults. (From Ebersole, P., & Hess, P. [2008]. *Toward healthy aging: Human needs and nursing experience* [7th ed.]. St. Louis, MO: Mosby.)

OTHER COMMON FOOT PROBLEMS

Other common foot problems include corns, calluses, blisters, and bunions, which usually result from years of wearing poorly fitted footwear, including high heels. These conditions often cause discomfort for older adults and lead to some degree of activity restriction.

QSEN Considerations: Safety

Foot Care

Many independent older adults use commercially available foot remedies or attempt to remove corns or calluses with a knife or scissors. This practice is dangerous and significantly increases the risk for serious foot infections, which may necessitate amputation of a toe, toes, or the entire foot. Older people with diabetes or impaired peripheral circulation are particularly prone to develop foot ulcers or infections and are at greatest risk for amputation.

❖ NURSING PROCESS/CLINICAL JUDGMENT MODEL FOR ALTERED SKIN INTEGRITY

◆ ASSESSMENT (DATA COLLECTION)

Recognize cues:
- What is the general appearance of the person's skin?
- Are any lesions evident on the scalp?
- What is the skin color? Are there any signs of pallor, jaundice, cyanosis, or erythema? If so, where?
- Are there any areas of dry skin? If so, where?
- Does the person complain of itching?
- Is there any evidence of scratching?

Box 17.1	Risk Factors for Alterations in Skin, Hair, or Nails in Older Adults

- Circulatory problems
- Restricted mobility
- Nutritional or fluid imbalances
- Cognitive impairments
- Exposure to irritating chemicals, including body secretions or waste products
- Exposure to communicable diseases
- Lack of adequate hygiene facilities or assistance in the home

- Are there any signs of scabies (fine wavy dark lines, or spots at the webs of the fingers or folds of the skin)?
- Are there any rashes? If so, where are they located? What is their appearance (e.g., macular, papular, or vesicular)?
- Is there any sign of pallor or erythema over bony prominences?
- Are there any breaks in the skin? If so, where? What do they look like?
- Are any abrasions or skin tears evident?
- Is there any change in the amount, distribution, or appearance of the hair?
- What is the appearance of the toenails? Are they thickened? Difficult to cut? Discolored?
- Are any lesions evident on the feet or ankles?
- What is the person's nutritional status? Are they overweight or underweight?
- Is the person alert and able to move freely? If not, what is the person's level of immobility?
- Is the person incontinent of bladder or bowel?
- Are there pedal pulses? Are they easy or difficult to palpate?

Box 17.1 lists risk factors for skin, hair, or nail alterations in older adults.

◆ DATA ANALYSIS/PROBLEM IDENTIFICATION

Analyze Cues and Prioritize Hypotheses: Problem statements for older adults with skin integrity issues include

Altered Skin Integrity
Potential for Altered Skin Integrity
Altered Tissue Integrity
Potential for Altered Tissue Integrity

◆ PLANNING

Generate Solutions: The patient goals for older individuals with or at risk for altered skin or tissue integrity are to (1) remain free from excessive skin dryness or skin breakdown; (2) display timely healing of wounds, lesions, and ulcerations; and (3) maintain optimal nutritional status to promote tissue integrity and healing.

◆ IMPLEMENTATION

Take Action: The following nursing interventions should take place in hospitals or extended-care facilities:

1. **Assess the level of alteration and the contributing factors.** Perform a daily skin inspection; measure the location, size, and depth of the affected area or areas; and identify any conditions or changes that may have caused the problem. Changes in skin condition can occur rapidly in older adults. Measure and document all areas of concern so that improvement or further breakdown can be evaluated. Explore any possible causes for the problem and institute nursing measures to prevent or reduce further tissue damage.

2. **Institute measures to reduce the potential for skin and tissue breakdown.**
   - *Reduce the frequency of complete bathing.* The type and frequency of baths or showers depend greatly on the individual. The condition of the skin and the presence of perspiration or other body wastes must be considered.

> **Nursing Tip**
> Some individuals require a complete bath or shower daily; others benefit more from a complete bath on a biweekly or weekly basis. On days when total baths are not taken, partial or sponge baths of the face, axillae, and perineum can provide adequate cleanliness and prevent body odors.

   - *Keep the skin free from wastes and exudate by using mild nondetergent soaps.* If dryness is a problem, reducing the frequency of bathing is suggested. Use of mild, nondetergent, nonperfumed, superfatted soaps (e.g., Basis Sensitive Skin, Neutrogena Transparent [fragrance free]) for cleansing decreases excessive skin dryness.
   - *Use emollients, lotions, creams, and oils to maintain skin moisture.* Emollients help keep moisture in the skin and reduce dryness. This can reduce the risk of skin tears. Because most preparations are effective for only a short period of time, apply them frequently. A variety of preparations are available at a wide range of costs. Ointments, particularly those containing petrolatum, are occlusive and tend to be longer lasting than lotions or creams. Avoid lotions containing alcohol because they can contribute to drying. It may be necessary to try various emollients and lotions to find the one (or the combination) that provides the most relief to the older individual (Box 17.2).

Box 17.2	Products That Help Moisturize the Skin

All of these products are available without a prescription. Other moisturizers are also available in stores. Ask the primary care provider or pharmacist whether these moisturizers would work well.

CREAMS AND LOTIONS
- Aveeno Daily Moist Lotion
- Aveeno Intense Relief Hand Cream
- Eucerin smoothing repair dry skin lotion
- Kiss My Face Foot Cream
- Moisturel therapeutic lotion
- Planet Botanicals Ugandan Shea Butter Hand Cream
- St. Ives Intensive Healing Hand Cream, Fragrance Free

OINTMENTS
- Africare 100% Glycerine
- Aquaphor natural healing ointment
- Burt's Bees Miracle Salve
- Crisco vegetable shortening
- Vaseline pure petroleum jelly
- Walgreen's Advanced Therapy Dry Skin Treatment Ointment

This Lotion May be Hazardous to Your Health!

Many untested chemicals are allowed into our personal care products. A common misconception is that if a product is available for sale in the United States, it must be safe; but in fact, companies are allowed to use any ingredient or raw material without government review or approval except for a very few prohibited substances and colors. For example, over 1000 additives in sunscreens are banned from use in the European Union; only about 10 are prohibited in the United States. SkinDeep, a database maintained by the Environmental Working Group (EWG), lists over 73,000 commonly used products. EWG ranks these products on the basis of scientific data, assigning them a hazard score of low (0-2), moderate (3-6), or high (7-10). [Author's note: I became extremely interested in this topic after having too many friends diagnosed with cancer and having had a cancer scare of my own. After going on the SkinDeep website, I was shocked at the scores of some of my favorite products and makeup. Because of this, only products with a hazard score of "low" are included in this chapter.] Check your own products and learn more at http://www.ewg.org/skindeep

- *Rinse skin carefully.* Soaps tend to dry the skin and should always be rinsed off completely before drying. If a basin is being used, complete rinsing may require frequent water changes.
- *Dry skin tissue gently and thoroughly.* To decrease skin irritation, dry the skin by patting rather than rubbing. If the skin is severely irritated, use soft towels that have been rinsed carefully to remove all detergents.
- *Turn and position the person frequently and reduce sources of pressure by keeping bed linen tight and clear of foreign objects.* Pressure over bony prominences restricts blood flow to the tissues that are being compressed (Fig. 17.8). These areas are most likely to become ischemic or necrotic. Redistributing pressure is an important component of pressure injury prevention. Frequent position changes allow reestablishment of blood flow and reduce the risk for skin breakdown.

Position Changes

The maximum time a person should be in one position must not exceed 2 hours. More frequent turning is necessary for individuals at high risk for skin problems. Base the frequency of position changes on your assessment of pressure points after the person is turned. A turning schedule will help ensure that repositioning is done at appropriate times.

A 30-degree lateral position (Fig. 17.9) is preferred to a full lateral position. Pressure points over bony prominences are most susceptible to breakdown, but anything that exerts resistance against the skin can become a pressure point. Foreign objects such as large wrinkles, personal belongings (rosary or prayer beads), or needle caps trapped under the body can also contribute to skin breakdown. Each time the person is repositioned, inspect the skin for signs of circulatory reduction such as blanching or hyperemia. If these signs are present, establish a more frequent turning

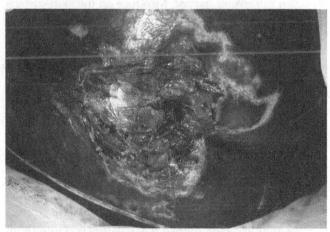

Fig. 17.8 A stage 4 pressure injury in the sacral area of an 85-year-old man. Note the sacrum (*white area*) and necrotic surrounding muscles. (From Swartz, M. H. [2006]. *Textbook of physical diagnosis: History and examination* [5th ed.]. Philadelphia, PA: Elsevier.)

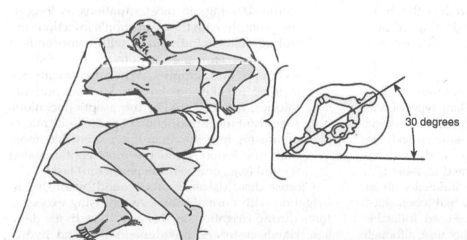

Fig. 17.9 To avoid pressure points, a 30-degree lateral position is best. (Modified from Bryant, R. A., & Nix, D. P., Eds. [2012]. *Acute and chronic wounds: Current management concepts* [4th ed.]. St. Louis, MO: Mosby.)

30 degrees

schedule. Treat reddened areas with caution, and do not massage them because massage can increase the risk for pressure injury formation.

- *Wash the skin and supply clean, dry linens after episodes of incontinence.* Urine and stool contain waste products that are highly irritating to the skin and must be cleansed promptly with gentle washing and rinsing. Apply barrier ointments to clean skin to reduce contact with body wastes. Check people who are known to be incontinent of stool or urine frequently to reduce the chance of prolonged exposure to moisture and body wastes. Special absorbent pads or garments that wick moisture away from the skin may be appropriate. Problems of incontinence are addressed in greater depth in Chapter 18. Once the skin has been thoroughly washed and dried, moisture barriers (e.g., Desitin) can be applied to protect the skin. These types of preparations must be removed from the skin at regular intervals to prevent bacterial overgrowth.
- *Keep the skin dry after episodes of diaphoresis; check skin surfaces where moisture caused by normal perspiration can become trapped.* Moisture on the skin surface can cause maceration (whitening and softening) and tissue breakdown. Moisture caused by perspiration usually evaporates and causes few problems unless perspiration is excessive or is trapped between skin surfaces (e.g., under pendulous breasts). Frequent sponging with clear water and thorough drying, exposure to air, or use of a drying substance such as cornstarch helps reduce the amount of moisture and friction between skin surfaces.
- *Move and transfer the person carefully.* The skin of older individuals is thinner, less elastic, and has less subcutaneous padding than that of younger people. This makes it particularly vulnerable to shearing forces during movement. When the head of the bed is elevated, it is recommended that the elevation be kept at or below 30 degrees to reduce the shearing force that may occur when a person slides down in bed. To reduce the shearing forces that occur when tissue is dragged over bed linens, use transfer sheets or other assistive devices when turning, repositioning, or transferring a frail older person.
- *Provide appropriate pads, cushions, mattresses, or beds that are designed to reduce pressure.* Many types of beds and mattresses that are designed to distribute weight over a larger area and reduce pressure on body tissues are available. The advantages and disadvantages of some of these are presented in Table 17.5. Wheelchair pads made of gel or inflated with air help to reduce pressure on the ischial tuberosities. Only full chair cushions should be used. Inflatable "donuts" are not recommended because, although they reduce pressure on one area, they increase pressure on surrounding tissues. This can lead to more ischemia and result in extending the area of tissue damage.

- *Encourage older adults at high risk for skin tears to wear long sleeves, long trousers, or knee-high socks.* Shin guards and leg protectors have also been found to help those who experience repeated tears on their shins (see Fig. 3.1).

3. Institute measures to promote tissue healing.
- *Encourage adequate rest.* Tissue healing uses energy and places additional physiological stress on the aging body. Older adults may require additional rest periods during the day.

Nutritional Considerations

Promote Adequate Nutritional Intake

Tissue regeneration occurs more slowly in older adults than in younger individuals. It is particularly important to increase the intake of calories, with emphasis on protein and vitamin C, because these nutrients are necessary for tissue repair.

- *Check wounds daily for signs of inflammation or infection, and obtain cultures of wound drainage if appropriate.* The typical signs of inflammation or infection may be absent or diminished in older adults; therefore pay special attention to any open areas. Wound cultures are indicated if any purulent or foul smelling drainage is observed. Infection delays healing and imposes additional stress on older adults.
- *Avoid using adhesive strips for skin tears.* If possible, hold the dressing in place with a stocking-like or tubular bandage, but make sure that it is not excessively tight.
- *Follow aseptic technique (sterile technique) when cleansing wounds, changing dressings, or applying medications.* A variety of preparations are available for wound care; the particular type selected by the primary care provider or wound care specialist depends on the location and stage of the lesion (Table 17.6). Use clean rather than sterile dressings in most situations as long as they comply with the institution's infection control guidelines. Individuals with compromised immune systems may require the use of sterile technique and supplies. When treatments are ordered for skin breakdown, such as pressure injuries, it is essential to use aseptic technique to prevent the introduction of pathogenic microorganisms into the area. If a patient has more than one lesion, clean the most contaminated wound (e.g., one near the perineum) last.

Cleanse dead tissue from a wound by rinsing or irrigating with normal saline. Avoid using excessive force during irrigation, as this can cause tissue damage. Harsh cleansers, povidone-iodine, and hydrogen peroxide should be avoided because they can

Table 17.5 Mattress Surface Types

SUPPORT SURFACES			
CATEGORY AND MECHANISM OF ACTION	**INDICATIONS FOR USE**	**ADVANTAGES**	**DISADVANTAGES**
Support Surfaces and Overlays			
Foam Overlay (Available as an Overlay or in a Full Mattress)			
Reduces pressure; the cover (top) can reduce friction and shear. Base height of 7.5-10 cm (3-4 in); see manufacturer guidelines regarding amount of body weight supported.	Use for patients with moderate to high risk.	• One-time charge • No setup fee • Cannot be punctured • Available in various sizes (e.g., bed, chair, operating room table) • Little maintenance • Does not need electricity	• Elevated body temperature • Hot and may trap moisture • Limited life span • Plastic protective sheet needed for incontinent patients or patients with draining wounds • Not indicated for patients with existing stage 3 or stage 4 pressure injuries
Water Overlay (Available as an Overlay or in a Full Mattress)			
Reduces pressure and pressure points because surface provides flotation with pressure reduction by redistributing patient's weight evenly over entire support surface.	Use for patients with high risk.	• Readily available • Some control over motion sensations • Easy to clean	• Easily punctured • Heavy • Fluid motion may make procedures (e.g., dressing changes, CPR) difficult • Maintenance needed to prevent micro-organism growth • Patient transfers out of bed are difficult • Difficult to raise and lower head of bed
Gel Overlay			
Reduces pressure and pressure points because surface provides flotation by redistributing patient's weight evenly over entire support surface.	• Use for patients with moderate to high risk. • Use for patients who are wheelchair dependent.	• Low maintenance • Easy to clean • Multiple-patient use • Impermeable to needle punctures	• Heavy • Expensive • Lacks airflow for moisture control • Variable friction control
Nonpowered Support Surface			
Reduces pressure by lowering mean interface pressure between patient's tissue and mattress.	• Use for patients with moderate to high risk. • Use for patients who can reposition themselves.	• Easy to clean • Multiple-patient use • Low maintenance • Potential repair of some air-filled products • Durable	• Damaged by punctures from needles and sharps • Requires routine monitoring to determine adequate inflation pressure • Patient transfers out of bed are difficult
Low-Air-Loss Overlay (Available as an Overlay or in a Full Mattress)			
Maintains constant and slight air movement against patient's skin, also assists in managing heat and humidity (microclimate) of the skin.	Use for patients with moderate to high risk.	• Easy to clean • Maintains constant inflation • Deflates to facilitate transfer and CPR • Moisture control • Fabric covering overlay is air permeable, bacteria impermeable, and waterproof • Reduces shear and friction • Setup provided by manufacturer	• Damaged by needles and sharps • Noisy • Requires electricity, but some are available with short backup battery • In home may need to purchase backup generator in case of loss of electrical power

Continued

Table 17.5   **Mattress Surface Types—cont'd**

SUPPORT SURFACES			
CATEGORY AND MECHANISM OF ACTION	**INDICATIONS FOR USE**	**ADVANTAGES**	**DISADVANTAGES**
Specialty Beds			
Air-Fluidized Bed			
Bed frame contains silicone-coated beads and provides pressure redistribution by the fluidlike medium that is created by forcing air through beads resulting in immersion and envelopment of patient.	• Use for patients at high risk. • Use for patients with stage 3 or 4 pressure injuries or burns.	• Less frequent turning or repositioning • Improved patient comfort • Quickly becomes firm for CPR or other treatments when device is turned off. • Reduces shear, friction, and edema to site • May facilitate management of copious wound drainage or incontinence • Setup provided by manufacturer	• Continuous circulation of warm, dry air may increase patient risk for dehydration • Possible increase in room temperature • Patient may experience disorientation • Patient transfer difficult • Heavy • Expensive • May not be wide enough for use with obese patients or patients with contractures • Patient cannot lie prone because of risk of suffocation
Low-Air-Loss Bed			
Bed frame with series of connected air-filled pillows. Flow of air controls the amount of pressure in each pillow and assists in managing heat and humidity (microclimate) of the patient's skin.	• Use for patients who need pressure relief, who cannot be repositioned frequently, or who have skin breakdown on more than one surface. • Contraindicated in patients with unstable spinal column.	• Can raise and lower head and foot of bed • Easy transfer in and out of bed • Less frequent turning schedule • Pillows can be transferred to stretcher with patient • Setup provided by manufacturer	• Portable motor is noisy • Bed surface material is slippery; patients can easily slide down mattress or out of bed when being transferred
Kinetic Therapy			
Provides continuous passive motion to promote mobilization of pulmonary secretions and low air loss, which provides pressure relief.	• Use primarily for patients needing spinal stabilization. • Should not be used when the patient is hemodynamically unstable.	• Reduces pulmonary complications associated with restricted mobility • Reduces risk for urinary stasis and urinary tract infections • Reduces venous stasis	• Does not reduce shear or moisture • Cannot be used with cervical or skeletal traction • Possible motion sickness initially • Possible sensations of claustrophobia

CPR, Cardiopulmonary resuscitation.

Data from Doughty, D., & McNichol, L. (2016). *Wound, ostomy, and continence nurses society core curriculum: Wound management.* Philadelphia, PA: Wolters Kluwer. Wound Ostomy and Continence Nurses (WOCN) Society (2016). *Guideline for prevention and management of pressure ulcers.* WOCN Clinical Practice Guidelines Series, Mount Laurel, NJ: 2016, The Society.

cause damage to underlying healthy tissues. It is important to keep dressings clean to prevent cross-contamination between lesions.

 QSEN Considerations: Evidence-Based Practice

Thorough handwashing between patient contacts and strict adherence to body substance precautions is essential. Each older adult should have their own supply of dressing materials that are kept apart from others' supplies; multipatient treatment carts should be avoided. All supplies used for wound care should be protected from environmental contamination by dust, water, or other such substances.

4. **Provide thorough foot care.** The feet of older adults are particularly susceptible to problems. Poor circulation leads to a greater number of problems—such as bunions, excessively thick toenails, and the results of years of wearing poorly fitted shoes—contribute to foot issues in older adults. The feet should be soaked regularly to remove old dry skin. After a good soaking, dry the feet by patting rather than rough rubbing. Thoroughly dry the feet, paying careful attention to the areas between the toes. If permitted, cut the toenails straight across and file the sharp edges off. The toenails of people with diabetes and other older adults with circulatory

Table 17.6 Dressings by Injury Stage

PRESSURE INJURY STAGE	PRESSURE INJURY STATUS	DRESSING	COMMENTS[a]	EXPECTED CHANGE	ADJUVANTS
1	Intact	None	Allows visual assessment	Resolves slowly without epidermal loss over 7–14 days	Turning schedule Support hydration Nutritional support
		Transparent dressing	Protects from shear Not to be used in presence of excessive moisture		
		Hydrocolloid	Does not always allow visual assessment		Pressure-redistribution surface or chair cushion
2	Clean	Composite film	Limits shear	Heals through reepithelialization	Turning schedule Support hydration Nutritional support
		Hydrocolloid	Change when seal of dressing breaks; maximal wear time 7 days		Manage incontinence
		Hydrogel	Provides a moist environment		
3	Clean	Hydrocolloid	Must change when seal of dressing breaks; maximal wear time 7 days	Heals through granulation and reepithelialization	See previous stages; evaluate pressure-redistribution needs
		Hydrogel covered with foam dressing	Applied over wound to protect and absorb moisture		
		Calcium alginate	Used with significant exudate; must cover with secondary dressing		
		Gauze	Used with normal saline or other prescribed solution; must unfold to make contact with wound		
		Growth factors	Used with gauze per manufacturer instructions		
4	Clean	Hydrogel covered with foam dressing	Applied over wound to protect and absorb moisture	Heals through granulation and reepithelialization	Surgical consultation often necessary for closure (see stages 1, 2, and 3)
		Calcium alginate	Used with significant exudate; must cover with secondary dressing		
		Gauze	Used with normal saline or other prescribed solution; must unfold to make contact with wound; fill all dead space with gauze		
		Growth factors	Used with gauze		
	Unstageable: wound covered with eschar	Adherent film	Facilitates softening of eschar	Eschar lifts at edges as debridement progresses	See previous stages, surgical consultation sometimes considered for debridement
		Gauze plus ordered solution	Delivers solution and wick wound drainage and softens eschar	Eschar softens	
		Enzymes	Facilitate debridement	Eschar softens	
		None	If eschar is dry and intact, no dressing used, allowing eschar to act as physiological cover; may be indicated for treatment of heel eschar		

[a]As with all occlusive dressings, wound should not be clinically infected.
From Potter, P.A., Perry, A.G., Stockert, P.A., & Hall, A.M. (2013). *Fundamentals of nursing* (8th ed.). St. Louis, MO: Mosby.

problems should be cared for by a foot specialist. Use emollients if the skin on the feet is very dry. When emollients are used on the feet, teach older adults to be aware of the importance of wearing socks to prevent slipping. Encourage a daily change into clean socks or stockings, because clean footwear reduces the risk for infection. Encourage older persons with diabetes or circulatory impairment of the lower extremities to wear clean white cotton socks to promote cleanliness and provide early recognition of injury or drainage. Use caution to ensure that the socks fit properly and do not cause excessive constriction around the ankles or calves. Document and report promptly signs of foot irritation, color or temperature change, skin break-down, or changes in the appearance of the nails.

The following interventions should take place in the home:

1. **Encourage adequate fluid intake and good nutrition.** When inadequate intake is suspected, a more complete assessment (including a food and fluid diary) is appropriate. This helps nurses determine the cause or causes (e.g., depression and illness) and plan suitable interventions.

Nutritional Considerations

Nutritious foods and adequate fluid intake are needed to maintain healthy tissue. Inadequate intake of nutrients such as protein, vitamin A, and vitamin C can result in fragile tissue that is more susceptible to bruising, shearing force injuries, and breakdown.

---

2. **Maintain adequate humidity in the environment.** Exposure to hot, dry air, whether in the desert or in overly warm living quarters, results in excessively dry skin. Such an environment intensifies the tendency toward dryness, which is already a problem in older adults. The result is skin that is rough, dry, cracked, irritated, and more susceptible to breakdown and infection. Dry mucous membranes usually accompany dry skin, increasing the risk for epistaxis (nosebleeds). Living spaces should be maintained at a temperature of approximately 70 to 72 degrees F. A relative humidity between 40% and 60% is most comfortable and beneficial for the skin and mucous membranes. Commercial humidifiers or even open pans of water set around the home will help to increase the amount of moisture in the room.

3. **Avoid excessive exposure to the sun.** Older adults have fewer melanocytes, which are unevenly distributed over exposed body areas. Excessive exposure to sunlight can cause irregular, blotchy, and cosmetically unacceptable tanning. Use of a safe sunblock is recommended when sun exposure is expected. Encourage older adults to wear loose, lightweight, light-colored clothing and wide-brimmed hats to prevent exposure to the ultraviolet rays in sunlight, which increase the risk for skin cancer.

⚠ Safety Alert

Sunscreens Can Be Dangerous Too!

Many sunscreens contain harmful chemicals. For example, vitamin A, useful in many night creams, can cause skin damage and potentially skin cancer when the skin is exposed to sunlight (EWG, 2018b). Higher–sun protection factor (SPF) formulas contain higher concentrations of chemicals. The safety rating of various sunscreens by EWG is surprising; however, not all high-SPF formulations are high risk, and a surprising number of pink-bottled "baby" sunscreens rank terribly. The following are some sun safety tips:

- The best sunscreens are protective clothing, shade, avoidance of both midday sun (highest radiation) and long periods of sun exposure.
- Avoid getting sunburned: each sunburn increases your risk for skin cancer.
- Wear sunglasses to avoid cataracts.
- Do not fall for a high-SPF rating. SPF 15 to 50 is the safest zone for sunscreens.
- Avoid sunscreens and lip balms containing vitamin A (also called *retinol palmitate* or *retinol*).
- Avoid sunscreens containing oxybenzone (a synthetic estrogen and potential hormone disruptor).
- Avoid using insect repellant/sunscreen combination products. If you need insect repellant, apply it first.
- Use cream, not spray: spray contains tiny particles that are potentially unsafe to breathe in. Choose a safer sunscreen (according to the SkinDeep website) and reapply it often.

Data from Environmental Working Group (2018a). Make sunscreen part of your outdoors routine. https://www.ewg.org/sunscreen/top-sun-safety-tips/#.WuiddYgvw2w

4. **Obtain regular professional foot care.** Older people, particularly those living alone, often find that foot care is difficult because of the loss of flexibility. Regular appointments with a foot care specialist reduce the risk for trauma or infection. Professional foot care is essential for individuals with diabetes or impaired peripheral circulation.

5. Use any appropriate interventions that are used in the institutional setting.

AGE-RELATED CHANGES IN ORAL MUCOUS MEMBRANES

Problems in the oral cavity may render an older adult unable to chew certain foods. Inspection of the oral cavity is an important part of the head-to-toe assessment and is needed to determine the status of the individual's teeth, tongue, and oral mucous membranes. Changes in the condition of the gums and oral mucous membranes may be related to several factors.

Studies show that poor oral hygiene is a major problem for the older population. Reasons for this include (1) failure of older adults to see dental care as a priority; (2) the cost of dental care; (3) restricted access caused by transportation problems or inadequate availability of dental services, which is particularly a problem in rural areas; and (4) physical or cognitive limitations.

Many older adults are unable or unwilling to maintain good oral hygiene practices.

Unfortunately, nursing staff members too often place oral hygiene at a lower priority than other more visible aspects of care. In recent years, oral hygiene has been proven to be a high priority; however, cases of pneumonia have been linked to inadequate oral care in intensive care unit patients (Modi & Kovacs, 2020). Some nursing experts tell others that if you are able to perform only one assessment to determine a person's overall quality of care, inspect the person's oral cavity. When oral care is good, there is a high probability that all of the care is good. Nurses need to recognize the importance of this aspect of care and give it the attention it deserves.

❓ Did You Know?

Dental care was not readily available to many of today's older adults during their youth because of the cost and the associated discomfort. Therefore older individuals who neglected their teeth now suffer tooth loss. Even those who maintained good dental practices are likely to experience tooth decay and loss because preventive dental techniques were not as advanced as they are today. Water fluoridation, which started in the 1940s, has helped to prevent some dental problems, resulting in a larger percentage of today's older adult population who have retained at least some of their teeth.

❓ Did You Know?

Oral Hygiene Care Plan

Development of an oral hygiene care plan (OHCP) has been recommended by experts as the best framework for preventive oral care in dependent older adults. The American Dental Association (2010) recommends that older adults brush their teeth 2 or more times per day, preferably with a rotating or oscillating toothbrush, a topical fluoride, and attention to dietary recommendations. For older adults with limitations—physical, sensory, or cognitive—additional care and assistance will be necessary to meet these recommendations.

DENTAL CARIES

Tooth decay, loose teeth, and lost teeth are ongoing problems in the older adult population. Poor nutrition and decreased appetite in older adults can often be attributed to dental problems. Decay, or caries, is caused by the action of bacteria that penetrate through the enamel shield of the tooth and cause destruction (Fig. 17.10). If caries is not recognized early, a significant amount of the tooth structure may be destroyed. If the caries extends deep into the tooth, a nerve may be exposed, and painful neuritis (toothache) may result. Replacement of the lost tooth material with amalgam restorations (fillings) can help rebuild the tooth, but this leaves a weakened structure that remains susceptible to problems. Lost restorations leave rough edges that cause irritation of the oral mucous membranes, particularly the cheek and tongue.

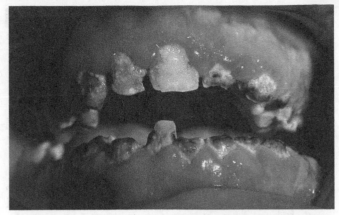

Fig. 17.10 Extensive dental caries in an older adult. (From Fillit, H., Rockwood, K., & Woodhouse, K. [2010]. Brocklehurst's textbook of geriatric medicine and gerontology [7th ed.]. Philadelphia, PA: Saunders. [Reprinted with the permission of Mirriam Robbins, DDS, New York University College of Dentistry].)

PERIODONTAL DISEASE

Food debris and plaque accumulate in the mouth and on the teeth when oral hygiene is inadequate. The activity of bacteria on this debris, especially on the tongue, causes halitosis, or bad breath, which is often disturbing to older persons and to anyone who has close contact with them. Periodontal disease is a less obvious but potentially more serious complication of poor oral care. One form of periodontal disease is gingivitis, or inflammation of the gums. Gingivitis causes gum swelling, tenderness, and bleeding and eventually leads to recession of the gum tissue away from the tooth. As the gums recede, the teeth lose support, become loose in the sockets, and eventually fall out. When a tooth is lost, a gap is created. Healthy teeth shift position or move into the space, resulting in an uneven bite. Chewing becomes increasingly difficult when significant numbers of teeth, particularly the molars needed for chewing and grinding food, become loose or lost. Periodontal disease is suspected to play a role in thromboembolitic disorders, bacterial endocarditis, and myocardial infarction. Individuals with a cardiac history are typically given prophylactic antibiotics before or following any dental work.

PAIN

Dental caries and periodontal disease are the most common reasons for oral pain, but oral lesions, such as stomatitis or altered sensations in the mouth, are frequently reported. Pain may be limited to the oral cavity or may affect the face and jaw. Oral pain can cause loss of appetite and decreased food intake and can have a negative effect on the overall quality of an older person's life. Pain leads to impaired ability to perform physical activities and can even lead to physical, psychological, and social disability when the pain originates from the teeth (Petersen & Ogawa, 2018).

Carefully Assess Jaw Pain

Jaw pain can be an "atypical presentation" of a myocardial infarction, a medical emergency! Take into consideration the patient's medical and dental history, carefully assess the entire patient, and report the jaw pain to the registered nurse or primary care provider for follow-up.

DENTURES

If only a few teeth are missing, the dentist may attempt to bridge the gaps by attaching artificial teeth to the good teeth. If too many teeth are missing, a partial plate may be required. When all of the upper or lower teeth are removed, a complete set of dentures is needed. Both partial plates and dentures can cause problems for the wearer. Partial plates tend to catch particles of food and may weaken the healthy teeth to which they are attached. Complete dentures are expensive and difficult to fit.

Dentures that fit properly at one time may not fit properly if the older person loses or gains a significant amount of weight. Fit is also a problem when dentures are left out of the mouth for a prolonged period. Many older adults refuse to wear their dentures because of the discomfort caused by an improper fit. This is because the arch of the jaw changes to compensate for the edentulous state. Professional dental attention is needed to repair or rebuild the dentures in these cases.

Dentures can cause irritation, inflammation, and ulceration of the gums and oral mucous membranes. Older adults should inspect their mouths regularly and promptly report any problems to the dentist. Sometimes a minor adjustment of the denture or use of a fixative agent or cushion is all that is required to prevent painful problems.

DRY MOUTH

Xerostomia, or dry mouth, is common with aging. Dryness may result from the normal age-related reduction in saliva secretion, inadequate hydration, or disorders such as diabetes. In turn, xerostomia makes chewing and swallowing more difficult, promotes tooth decay, and alters the sense of taste.

 Medication Therapy

Medications such as diuretic agents, antidepressants, sedatives, hypnotic agents, antihistamines, and anticholinergic medications also contribute to xerostomia.

LEUKOPLAKIA

Inspection of the mouth can reveal a number of abnormalities. White patches in the mouth, called leukoplakia, are often precancerous and require prompt medical attention (Fig. 17.11). Lesions on the posterior third or the sides of the tongue are often abnormal and should be brought to the attention of the primary care provider.

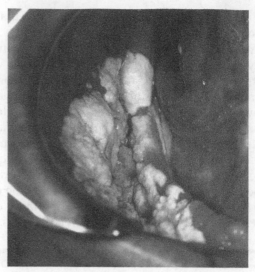

Fig. 17.11 Leukoplakia. Note the formation of white spots, which may become malignant. (From White, G. M., & Cox, N. H. [2000]. *Diseases of the skin: A color atlas and text.* St. Louis, MO: Mosby.)

| Box 17.3 | **Symptoms of Oral Cancer** |

- A mouth lesion that does not heal within 2 weeks
- A lump or thickening in the cheek
- Red or white patches on the gums, tongue, tonsil, or oral mucosa
- Sore throat or sensation of something being caught in the throat
- Difficulty chewing or swallowing
- Difficulty moving the tongue or jaw
- Numbness in the mouth
- Swelling of the jaw; uncomfortable fit of dentures
- Chronic hoarseness

Data from Oral Cancer Foundation. Diagnosis. n.d. https://oralcancerfoundation.org/discovery-diagnosis/diagnosis/

CANCER

According to the Oral Cancer Foundation, as many as 45,750 people are diagnosed with oral or pharyngeal cancer each year (Oral Cancer Foundation, n.d.). The incidence of this cancer increases with age. These forms of cancer have a poor prognosis, primarily because they are often discovered late. Early recognition and treatment before the cancer has metastasized to other tissues offer the best hope. Symptoms of oral cancer are listed in Box 17.3.

 Nutritional Considerations

Disorders Caused by Vitamin Deficiencies

Vitamin deficiencies—particularly deficiencies of riboflavin, niacin, and vitamin C—can affect the oral mucous membranes. A smooth, purplish, sore tongue may be related to riboflavin deficiency. Complaints of a burning sensation or soreness of the mouth may be related to niacin deficiency. Multiple painful ulcers of the oral mucous membranes with enlargement of the cervical lymph glands, difficulty swallowing, and foul odor may indicate Vincent angina. This is a condition caused by opportunistic micro-organisms that normally live in the mouth but cause infection only when the individual becomes malnourished.

Medication Therapy

Suprainfections

Suprainfections of the mouth are relatively common in older individuals who receive broad-spectrum antibiotic therapy for some other infection. Antibiotics destroy the normal mouth flora and allow opportunists or yeast colonies to become established and grow. Candidiasis, a yeast infection (also known as *thrush*), appears as white patches that adhere to the tongue, lips, and gums. Attempts to remove these patches may result in sore, bleeding tissue. A hairy tongue is the result of enlargement of the papillae on the tongue; this often follows antibiotic therapy. These conditions are more commonly observed in malnourished older adults and those with poor oral hygiene practices. Yeast infections are usually treated by direct oral application or swishes of prescription medication. Hairy tongue usually resolves without medical treatment.

ALCOHOL AND TOBACCO-RELATED PROBLEMS

Alcohol and tobacco, even in small amounts, can harm mucous membranes. Alcohol is chemically irritating and drying to the mucous membranes. Tobacco, whether smoked, chewed, or taken as snuff, increases the risk for oral cancer. Black or brown discoloration on the tongue may be caused by tobacco use or by a chromogenic (color-producing) bacterium.

 Did You Know?

The main risk factors for oral cancer are a history of alcohol and tobacco use or the presence of human papillomavirus version 16 (HPV-16), the same virus responsible for most cervical cancers.

PROBLEMS CAUSED BY NEUROLOGIC CONDITIONS

Good oral hygiene practices are part of routine health maintenance; however, it may be difficult for older individuals who have lost strength, coordination, or cognitive processes to meet their oral hygiene needs. Neurologic conditions such as stroke, multiple sclerosis, or Parkinson disease decrease coordination and strength, making it difficult for the person to manipulate the equipment needed for oral hygiene. Individuals with severe arthritis may not only find the equipment hard to manage, but they may also find it difficult to open their mouths adequately for thorough cleaning. Older people who take medication for epilepsy or other seizure disorders need to use special precautions because these medications often cause hyperplasia of the gingiva. Oral hygiene with soft toothbrushes or swabs is recommended to prevent excessive trauma and bleeding from the tender, swollen tissues. Providing oral hygiene to persons with Alzheimer disease can be a challenge because affected people do not understand the need for oral hygiene and may resist care.

❖ NURSING PROCESS/CLINICAL JUDGMENT MODEL FOR ALTERED ORAL MUCOUS MEMBRANES

◆ ASSESSMENT (DATA COLLECTION)

Recognize cues:
- Does the person have their own teeth? If so, how many?
- What is the condition of the teeth? Are any teeth loose or decayed?
- Does the person have halitosis?
- Do they wear dentures? If so, are they uppers, lowers, or both? Partial plates or bridges?
- Are the dentures worn during meals or removed? How do they fit?
- Are there any signs of irritation in the mouth? Any bleeding?
- Are food particles trapped under the dentures at meals?
- Is any residual food or debris evident in the mouth?
- How good is the person's appetite? What types and consistencies of food do they prefer to eat?
- What is the condition of the oral mucous membranes? Are they moist or dry?
- What is the condition of the tongue? Is it coated, pale, red, or irritated?
- Does the person use tobacco or have a history of tobacco use?
- What medications are they receiving?
- Does the person have any physical conditions that would interfere with performing oral hygiene?

Box 17.4 lists risk factors for problems with oral mucous membranes in older adults.

◆ DATA ANALYSIS/PROBLEM IDENTIFICATION

Analyze Cues and Prioritize Hypotheses: Problem statement for older adults with oral mucous membrane issues includes

Altered Oral Mucous Membranes

◆ PLANNING

Generate Solutions: The patient goals for older individuals diagnosed with altered oral mucous membranes are to (1) obtain regular professional dental care; (2) demonstrate techniques for maintaining or restoring the integrity of the mucous membranes; (3) inspect the oral cavity regularly and seek care promptly if any symptoms arise; (4) experience no unusual signs or

---

Box 17.4	**Risk Factors for Problems With Oral Mucous Membranes in Older Adults**

- Impaired cognitive, neurologic, or musculoskeletal function
- Inadequate fluid intake
- Medication that affects the oral mucous membranes
- Complete or partial artificial teeth
- Tobacco use (smoking or chewing)
- Poor health maintenance practices

symptoms, such as irritation, inflammation, or ulceration; (5) ingest foods and fluids without discomfort; and (6) verbalize specific actions to promote healthy oral mucous membranes.

◆ IMPLEMENTATION

Take Action: The following nursing interventions should take place in hospitals or extended-care facilities. Individuals who are able to provide their own oral hygiene should be encouraged to do so. When individuals are not capable of meeting their own oral hygiene needs, nurses or nursing assistants must provide the care. When you are providing oral hygiene, wear gloves and other appropriate protective devices to maintain universal precautions.

1. **Complete a thorough assessment of the oral mucous membranes.** Individuals who require intermediate or skilled nursing care are likely to have more oral hygiene problems and greater oral hygiene needs. If one wishes to judge the quality of nursing care provided in an extended-care facility, the first place to look is in the mouths of the patients or residents. For whatever reason, oral hygiene seems to be the area of hygiene that is most often neglected. This is troubling, because oral care is a very important component of nursing care. Good oral hygiene promotes comfort, enhances appetite, and fosters a sense of well-being.

2. **Initiate referral to a dentist or dental hygienist.** If any problems with the teeth or oral mucous membranes are observed, the individual should be seen by a dentist. Hospitals may have outpatient dental clinics that will see in-house patients if necessary. If the problem is not urgent, encourage the individual to make an appointment with their own dentist after discharge. Extended-care facilities should have a clinic or dentist on staff that sees residents on a scheduled or referral basis. If there is no dentist on the premises, arrange transportation with the family or a transport service.

 Health Promotion

It is important to refer individuals to a dentist as soon as a problem is detected in order to prevent the development of more serious conditions. Patients with problems related to ill-fitting dentures should also be referred. Nurses must send the improperly fitting dentures along on the visit. Dental hygienists can perform more detailed oral assessment, provide cleanings and other preventive treatments, and assist the nurse in developing strategies for providing effective oral hygiene.

---

3. **Provide oral hygiene.** Provide thorough oral hygiene a minimum of twice a day. Brushing after each meal and at bedtime is more desirable for individuals suffering from halitosis, xerostomia, or gingivitis. Individuals who have poor nutritional intake because of dysgeusia (funny tastes in the mouth) should have additional oral hygiene before meals. Frequent oral hygiene is also necessary for individuals with upper respiratory infections. Excessive respiratory secretions coat the mouth and tongue, leaving a bad taste; in addition, the infectious agent can easily be aspirated. The frequency of oral hygiene should be determined by the nurse and stated specifically in the care plan (e.g., "oral hygiene every 2 hours and as needed [prn]"). Use toothbrushes, not foam swabs, to clean the teeth, as swabs are ineffective in removing plaque. Swabs should be used only to clean oral mucosa in someone who is edentulous.

Dentures should be cleansed using warm water and a nonabrasive cleanser. Brush dentures over a basin of water or over a towel to prevent breakage. Ultrasonic cleaning devices are available in some facilities and are very effective at removing particles of debris, particularly from the wire clasps on partial plates. Clean the oral cavity thoroughly and inspect before reinserting dentures.

Patient Education

Patients should be discouraged from removing and wrapping their dentures in paper napkins or tissue. Many dentures wrapped this way have been accidentally thrown away. It is also wise for anyone who wears dentures to have their name etched into each plate. This can prevent permanent loss of these costly items if, for some reason, the owner is separated from them. Dentures should be removed from the mouth before sleep to prevent slippage, which could result in trauma to the mouth or problems with breathing.

Nursing Tip

When providing oral hygiene for an unconscious patient, take special care to prevent aspiration. Place unconscious individuals in a side-lying position, and use enough towels to protect the bedding and clothes. Prop the mouth open with gauze or padded tongue blades. Cleanse all surfaces of the teeth, tongue, and oral mucous membranes with a soft brush, damp gauze, sponge-tip swab, or clean moistened washcloth. Special toothbrushes that attach to suction machines are available in some facilities.

Use lemon and glycerin swabs with caution because they may be irritating to open areas on the mucous membranes and may ultimately cause drying (glycerin tends to draw moisture away from tissues).

Dry lips may require the application of Vaseline, mineral oil, or a lip balm, such as Burt's Bees. Petroleum-based products should be used with extreme caution because of the potential for aspiration and resulting pneumonia.

4. **Promote adequate intake of nutrients and fluids.** If the individual is avoiding certain foods or fluids because of dental problems, contact the primary care

provider or dietary department to obtain a change in food consistency. Soft, chopped, or puréed foods may be necessary for persons who are unable to chew because of loose teeth or improperly fitting dentures. If food tends to become trapped under the dentures, remove and cleanse them promptly after each meal. Excessively hot or cold foods may irritate the mucous membranes or teeth and should be avoided if they cause problems. Document any temperature modification in the care plan so that consistent approaches can be used. For example, if the individual tolerates beverages at room temperature, all fluids, including the water at the bedside, should be provided this way. Keep fluids at the bedside, and offer them to the individual at planned intervals throughout the day.

5. **Provide lozenges or topical analgesics as prescribed.** If severe or painful lesions are present in the mouth, the primary care provider may order the use of topical analgesics in lozenge or viscous form (viscous lidocaine). Drinking and eating should be avoided for 1 hour after administration of these preparations.

6. **Communicate suspected oral side effects of medication therapy to the primary care provider and dentist.** If a drug is suspected of causing untoward side effects on the oral mucous membranes, promptly communicate this information to the provider so that any necessary adjustments in dosage or drugs can be made.

The following interventions should take place in the home:

1. **Complete a thorough assessment of the oral mucous membranes.** A thorough assessment is necessary to detect the presence and severity of any problems. Specific interventions are based on the information gathered.

2. **Stress the importance of regular dental visits.** Dental hygiene is essential for older adults. Periodic dental visits should be part of ongoing health maintenance practice, even for edentulous individuals.

Home Care Considerations

Encourage and remind those living at home to make and keep regular dental appointments. If cost is prohibitive, dental clinics and schools of dentistry and dental hygiene may offer care at reduced rates. Some dentists also give price reductions to older people if requested.

3. **Review the person's oral hygiene practices.** Teach older adults who have their own teeth to brush, floss, and irrigate the mouth at least once daily. If problems of halitosis, plaque formation, bad taste, or gingivitis are present, more frequent brushing may be required. Brushing is best done with a soft to moderate bristle brush. Too firm a bristle may scratch or irritate the oral cavity. Commercial fluoridated toothpastes are available at a reasonable cost.

Special toothpastes are available for individuals with sensitive teeth and gums.

Patient Education

Older adults who have been in the habit of using salt or baking soda as a dentifrice should be counseled to avoid ingesting these products because they are high in sodium.

Flossing between the teeth helps remove trapped food and maintain healthy gums. If the older adult has difficulty holding the floss, a loop tied at each end of the string can help provide a better grip, or prethreaded flossers may be a better choice. A handheld water flosser is also a good choice for someone with limited hand strength.

Irrigation of the mouth is best accomplished with a commercial irrigator. If a commercial irrigator is too costly, a bulb syringe can be used. Even the swish-and-swallow technique of rinsing the mouth with water is better than doing nothing. Teach the person to gently brush the tongue to prevent halitosis and to inspect the entire oral cavity for signs of irritation.

Individuals who wear dentures should also be instructed in proper oral hygiene. Dentures should be cleansed thoroughly every day. In some people, food debris tends to become trapped under the dentures. If this is a problem, instruct the person to remove the denture and rinse it after each meal to prevent irritation. Thorough cleansing can be done by brushing with a commercial dentifrice or by using a soaking cleanser. Some people choose to use both. Many individuals use a powder or pad to help the dentures adhere to the gums. It is important that all of the fixative be removed at each cleansing. If it is not removed, an uneven surface may result and irritate the gums. Cleanse and store dentures in tepid water, because hot water may cause them to warp. When the dentures are out of the mouth, cleanse the entire oral cavity with a soft to moderate-bristle brush and inspect the entire oral cavity for signs of irritation. If signs of irritation from the dentures are present, the individual should see the dentist. Dentures can be reworked until they fit comfortably.

4. **Provide assistive devices as needed.** If the individual has difficulty holding the toothbrush because of arthritis or a weakened grip, modifications may be needed. Wrapping tape, aluminum foil, a small sponge, a polystyrene ball, or other padding around the handle of the brush may make it easier to grasp. Handle extenders made of a ruler or dowel rod may help those who are unable to reach the mouth easily (Fig. 17.12).

5. **Obtain the assistance of family members, friends, or community agencies.** Some older adults may require the assistance of family members, friends, or transportation services in order to keep dental

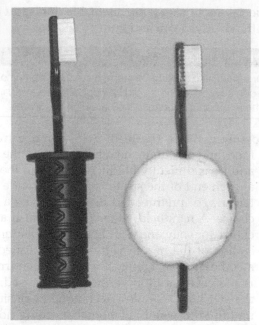

Fig. 17.12 Adaptive aids for brushing. (From Daniel, S. J., Harfst, S. A., & Wilder, R. [2008]. *Mosby's dental hygiene* [2nd ed.]. St. Louis, MO: Mosby.)

appointments. Family and friends can also help by purchasing and setting up oral hygiene equipment. A family member or friend can be shown how to modify a toothbrush or prepare floss for use by the older person.

6. **Explain the need to avoid alcohol and tobacco.** Because alcohol and tobacco are likely to irritate the mucous membranes and cause significant health problems, it is important to stress the importance of eliminating or at least restricting their use.

7. **Promote adequate intake of nutrients and fluids.** Nurses should explain how nutrients, particularly vitamins, can contribute to healthy mucous membranes. Instruction about diet may be necessary if inadequacies are detected. Stress the importance

of fluid intake for saliva formation and for use as a rinse for the mucous membranes. Encourage older adults to keep a glass of water by the chair or bedside as a reminder to drink enough fluids. Highly sugared beverages should be avoided because they encourage tooth decay. Many older adults with altered oral mucous membranes prefer to avoid ice in beverages, which can stimulate toothache. If the individual has difficulty chewing food because of loose or missing teeth, a food processor, grinder, or blender can be used to change the food's consistency.

8. **Discuss the benefits of adequate moisture in the environment.** If the environment is dry or if the individual is a mouth breather, an additional source of moisture may be needed. A freestanding humidifier or one attached to the furnace increases the moisture present in the air so that less is drawn away from the mucous membranes.

9. **Suggest use of hard candy, chewing gum, or artificial saliva to increase moisture in the mouth.** Sucking on hard candy or chewing gum stimulates the production of saliva. If a sugar-based candy or gum is used, the teeth must be brushed more frequently to prevent tooth decay. Individuals on sugar-restricted meal plans should use only sugar-free candy or gum. Artificial saliva preparations may be used according to package directions if there is no medical contraindication.

10. **Discuss the relationship between medications and oral hygiene.** If the individual is receiving any medications that could affect the oral mucous membranes, teach the person any necessary observations or precautions. For example, people who are taking phenytoin or those who are on antibiotic therapy should know the possible side effects indicating the need to contact the primary care provider.

11. **Use any appropriate interventions that are used in the institutional setting.**

Get Ready for the Next Generation NCLEX® Examination!

Key Points

- Under normal conditions, the aging skin and mucous membranes are more susceptible to damage than are the comparable tissues of younger individuals. When disease factors are present, the risk for damage is even greater.
- Careful assessment allows nurses to recognize normal changes and identify any abnormalities that may indicate more serious problems.
- Nursing interventions are designed to reduce the risk for damage or trauma to fragile tissues.

Additional Learning Resources

SG Go to your Evolve website at http://evolve.elsevier.com/Williams/geriatric for the additional online resources.

Review Questions for the Next Generation NCLEX® Examination

1. A nurse is caring for a 71-year-old immobile patient who has been in a wheelchair for 2 hours. While repositioning the patient, the nurse observes a reddened area at the base of the buttocks. How would this observation be best documented?

   a. Stage 2 pressure injury at greater trochanter
   b. Stage 1 pressure injury at ischial tuberosity
   c. Stage 1 pressure injury on iliac crest
   d. Stage 0 pressure injury on posterior superior iliac spine

2. A nurse is caring for an older adult who is bedridden because of advanced Parkinson disease. What is the most appropriate problem statement for this patient?

   a. Potential for altered skin integrity related to immobility
   b. Immobility related to Parkinson disease

   c. Altered skin integrity related to incontinence

   d. Ischemia related to disuse syndrome

3. A nurse is caring for an older patient who complains of dry itchy skin. What advice should the nurse offer?

   a. Advise the patient not to scratch and to trim the nails so that they will be less likely to break the skin and acquire an infection.

   b. Advise the patient to drink more fluids, use cool water when bathing, and only wear cotton clothing.

   c. Advise the patient to ask the primary care provider for an antihistamine prescription to decrease the itching.

   d. Advise the patient to bathe less often, use soap sparingly, and apply a skin emollient after each bath.

4. The nurse notices that an older adult is using a large amount of denture fixative paste. The patient states that this is because the denture hurts otherwise. What is the most important nursing action?

   a. Make a note about this practice in the patient's care plan and another note to tell the dentist.

   b. Check that the denture does not have rough spots and that all of the old fixative has been removed.

   c. Assess the patient's oral cavity to make sure that there is no irritation or breakdown.

   d. Assist the patient with oral hygiene and request an order for a topical anesthetic to reduce the patient's oral discomfort.

5. Family members are caring for their aging mother at home. Which statement by the daughter indicates the need for further teaching? (Select all that apply.)

   a. "I change Mom's brief whenever it is really wet."

   b. "I make sure Mom eats good meals and gets extra snacks."

   c. "We try to change Mom's position at least every 2 hours."

   d. "I try to use lotion on Mom's skin every morning and evening."

   e. "I'm glad we don't have to see the dentist anymore now that Mom has dentures."

6. In helping the registered nurse perform an admission and assessment of a new patient, you mutually recognize that this patient is at risk for skin tears. Which would be appropriate to include in the care plan? (Select all that apply.)

   a. Apply lotion after the daily bath to moisten the skin.

   b. Dress the patient in short sleeves to allow for better visualization of skin.

   c. Apply Steri-Strips if a skin tear appears.

   d. Move and position the patient gently and carefully.

   e. Use a safe sunblock when sun exposure is expected.

7. An 87-year-old female patient was discharged to home 3 days a following an open reduction and internal fixation of the left hip. Since she's returned home, she has developed a stage 2 pressure injury to her left ischium. **Place an "X" for the nursing actions listed below that are Indicated (appropriate or necessary), Contraindicated (could be harmful), or Nonessential (makes no difference or is not necessary) for the patient's care at this time.**

NURSING ACTION	INDICATED	CONTRAINDICATED	NON-ESSENTIAL
Recommend a hydrocolloid or hydrogel dressing for the site of injury.			
Bathe the patient daily using a mild soap and warm water.			
Gently massage reddened areas to help increase circulation to the skin.			
Make sure that 3 nutritious meals and adequate fluids are provided throughout the day.			
Offer a relaxing massage at bedtime to encourage restful sleep.			

REFERENCES

American Dental Association: *Aging and dental health*, 2019, https://www.ada.org/en/member-center/oral-health-topics/aging-and-dental-health

Boyko, T. V., Longaker, M. T., & Yang, G. P. (2018). Review of the Current Management of Pressure Ulcers. *Advances in wound care*, 7(2), 57–67. https://doi.org/10.1089/wound.2016.0697

Environmental Working Group (EWG) (2018a). *Make sunscreen part of your outdoors routine*. https://www.ewg.org/sunscreen/top-sun-safety-tips/#.WuiddYgvw2w2018a

Environmental Working Group (EWG) (2018b). *The problem with vitamin A*, https://www.ewg.org/sunscreen/report/the-problem-with-vitamin-a/?gclid=CjwKCAjwoKDXBRAAEiw A4xnqvwVH9GSymlUOFqBCG74_mcDPliVZUHI9K9nO6zG-dU3Oq3elPa3kq3xoCW7gQAvD_BwE#.WuicP4gvw2w2018b

Modi, A. R., & Kovacs, C. (2020). Hospital-acquired and ventilator-associated pneumonia: Diagnosis, management, and prevention. *Cleveland Clinic Journal of Medicine*, 87(10), 633–639. https://doi.org/10.3949/ccjm.87a.19117

Oral Cancer Foundation (2018). *Diagnosis*. https://oralcancerfoundation.org/discovery-diagnosis/diagnosis/

Petersen, P. E., & Ogawa, H. (2018). The global burden of periodontal disease: Towards integration with chronic disease prevention and control. *Oral Health and Preventive Dentistry*, 16(2), 113–124. http://www.quintpub.com/userhome/ohpd/ohpd_16_2_petersen_p113.pdf

18 Elimination

Objectives

1. Describe the normal elimination processes.
2. Examine age-related changes in bladder and bowel elimination.
3. Identify the older adults who are most at risk for problems with elimination.
4. Discuss methods for assessing elimination practices.
5. Choose common problem statements related to elimination.
6. Describe interventions used to prevent or reduce patient problems related to elimination.

Key Terms

catheterization (kă-thĕ-tĕr-ĭ-ZĀ-shŭn, p. 316)
constipation (kŏn-stĭ-PĀ-shŭn, p. 308)
defecation (dĕf-ĕ-KĀ-shŭn, p. 308)
diarrhea (dī-ă-RĒ-ă, p. 308)
diuretics (dī-ŭ-RĔ-tĭks, p. 311)
enemas (ĔN-ĕ-măs, p. 309)

fecal impaction (FĒ-kăl ĭm-PĀK-shŭn, p. 310)
incontinence (ĭn-KŎN-tĭ-nĕns, p. 308)
laxatives (LĂK-să-tĭvs, p. 309)
parasitic (păr-ă-SĬ-tĭk, p. 315)
retention (rē-TĔN-shŭn, p. 316)
sphincter (SFĬNGK-tĕr, p. 308)

To function properly, the body must be able to rid itself of waste products effectively. The two major systems involved in waste elimination are the urinary system and the gastrointestinal (GI) system. Small amounts of urea (a by-product of protein metabolism) and sodium chloride can be eliminated through the skin, but the skin is not considered a major site of elimination.

NORMAL ELIMINATION PATTERNS

Every adult develops unique patterns for bowel and bladder elimination. As long as the pattern is within normal limits and is effective for the individual, no special intervention is required. Diet, fluid intake, activity, and lifestyle influence these patterns. Even in young adults, elimination patterns can be disrupted by illness, medications, or changes in daily routine.

The typical adult bowel movement consists of a moderate amount of formed brown stool that is passed without difficulty. The normal frequency of bowel elimination varies from several stools per day to only two or three per week. Most adults experience bowel elimination every 1 to 2 days. The urge to defecate most commonly occurs 30 to 45 minutes after a meal, when the gastrocolic and defecation reflexes stimulate peristalsis. Another common time for defecation is first thing in the morning after consumption of a warm beverage. Many people develop a daily routine or establish rituals

over their lifetimes to promote normal elimination. Attempts to change these habits late in life can create problems.

Urine elimination in adults also follows patterns. The typical adult experiences the urge to urinate when the bladder contains approximately 300 mL of urine. Voluntary control of the external sphincter muscles enables healthy adults to hold larger amounts within the bladder until urination is convenient. Most adults void between 6 and 10 times per day, but this may vary greatly depending on fluid consumption, personal habits, and emotional state. For example, urinary frequency can be a physical response to emotional stress.

ELIMINATION AND AGING

A large percentage of the older adult population suffer from problems with elimination. The most common elimination problems experienced by older adults are constipation, diarrhea, and incontinence of bladder and/or bowel. These problems may result from changes in the function of the GI system or the urinary system, or they may be related to changes in other body systems, such as the musculoskeletal and nervous systems.

Incontinence of bladder and/or bowel is one of the most common reasons that older adults are institutionalized. Many families who can cope with other problems are often unable to deal with incontinence.

Box 18.1	Rome IV Criteria for Constipation

A diagnosis of constipation must include two or more of the following symptoms for the previous 3 months. Symptoms must have an onset at least 6 months before the diagnosis and be present at least 25% of the time.
- Straining
- Hard or lumpy stools
- Sensation of incomplete evacuation
- Fewer than three spontaneous bowel movements per week
- Sensation of obstruction or blockage
- Use of manual maneuvers, such as digital stimulation, to facilitate defecation

Modified from Basson, M. (2020). What are the Rome IV Criteria for Constipation? Medscape. https://www.medscape.com/answers/184704-23237/what-are-the-rome-iv-criteria-for-constipation

CONSTIPATION

Constipation is not a disease but rather a symptom of some other problem. Constipation is defined as hard, dry stools that are difficult to pass. Because bowel elimination patterns can differ widely from person to person, the frequency of elimination is not a good measure. For some people, regularity means more than 1 bowel movement a day; for others, it means 3 bowel movements a week. Other people who were reared with the idea that a daily bowel movement is essential to health may spend undue amounts of time worrying about their bowels. The Rome Criteria have been developed as an objective way to classify functional GI disorders. The most recent Rome Criteria for constipation can be found in Box 18.1. Constipation, both real and perceived, is a common complaint of older adults. Studies show that up to 27% of older adults experience constipation and that it is more commonly a problem for women. The following changes related to aging or chronic illness increase the risk for constipation: decreased abdominal muscle tone, inactivity, immobility, inadequate fluid intake, inadequate dietary bulk, disease conditions, medications, dependence on laxatives or enemas, and various environmental conditions.

Peristalsis normally slows somewhat with aging. Loss of abdominal muscle tone and inadequate physical activity contribute to even slower peristalsis. About half of those with chronic constipation have delayed intestinal transit time. Older individuals with weak abdominal muscles and those who are inactive or immobile are highly likely to become constipated.

Water is absorbed as waste products pass through the large intestine. Inadequate fluid intake or excessive fluid loss through perspiration, emesis, or wounds increases the body's need to recover as much fluid as possible. Because many older adults suffer from some degree of fluid volume deficit, their bodies attempt to reabsorb as much fluid from the stool as possible. The physiological need to absorb water combined with a slower rate of peristalsis results in stools that are drier, harder, and more difficult to pass. Fluid volume deficit also leads to a decrease in urine production.

Dietary fiber plays an important role in promoting normal bowel elimination because this indigestible substance is effective at trapping moisture and providing bulk to the wastes. Foods such as whole grains, fruits, vegetables, and lean meats are high in fiber. Fiber-rich foods are often lacking in the older person's diet because these foods are more difficult to chew, particularly when teeth are loose or missing. Foods such as dairy products, eggs, refined breads, desserts, and many convenience foods consumed by older adults contain very little fiber. When the diet lacks adequate fiber, a smaller amount of stool is produced. This stool then moves more slowly through the intestine, further contributing to excessive dryness. The small mass of stool produced without fiber is inadequate to stimulate the normal defecation reflex, resulting in infrequent elimination with as many as 4 or more days between bowel movements.

The potential for constipation is increased with a number of disease processes, including stroke, diabetes, hypothyroidism, uremia, lupus, scleroderma, multiple sclerosis, Parkinson disease, dementia, and depression. Cancerous tumors located in the GI tract can result in a partial or total obstruction that can be mistaken for constipation or impaction. Medications often contribute to constipation in older adults. The more medications an older person takes, the greater the risk of medication-induced constipation. Medications that increase the potential for constipation include
- Narcotic analgesics, particularly those containing codeine
- Anticholinergics, including many tricyclic antidepressants and antipsychotics
- Diuretics
- Iron supplements
- Calcium channel blockers
- Antacids containing calcium or aluminum
- Anticonvulsants
- Antidepressants
- Antiparkinson medications
- Nonsteroidal anti-inflammatory agents
- Antihypertensives, such as angiotensin-converting enzyme inhibitors

Repeatedly ignoring the urge to defecate can lead to suppression or even extinction of the defecation reflex. Changes in neurologic sensitivity or fear of pain may cause older adults to ignore or delay defecation. Those with neurologic disorders may not be aware of the need to defecate because the strength of nerve impulses transmitted to and from the sphincter muscles is decreased.

With no urge to defecate, individuals may go for many days unaware of the fact that their bowels have not emptied. Older individuals who encounter pain with defecation are more likely to avoid or deliberately delay what they know will be a painful experience. Pain can originate from the decreased production of mucus in the intestine, which is typical with aging. Without the lubrication provided by mucus, the stool becomes

Safety Alert

Risks Associated With Chronic Laxative Use

Many older individuals who have had problems with constipation over the years may have developed a habit of taking laxatives or enemas. In fact, laxatives are one of the most frequently purchased over-the-counter products sold in the United States. Some older adults started taking laxatives when they were quite young because absolute regularity (having a daily bowel movement) was at one time considered important for good health. Thus some people have been taking laxatives or enemas daily for as long as 50 to 60 years. We now recognize that this is dangerous because the body can become dependent on laxatives and require this assistance to stimulate elimination. Chronic laxative use has other risks as well: it has even been associated with an increased risk for falls (Sharif et al., 2018). Reestablishing normal bowel elimination in a laxative-dependent older person is almost impossible because the body has forgotten how to work on its own.

excessively dry and irritating to the rectal tissues. The presence of hemorrhoids or anal fissures further contributes to the likelihood of pain. Delaying defecation creates a vicious circle. When defecation is delayed, the stool becomes harder, drier, and more difficult to pass. This, in turn, leads to more painful defecation, which results in further avoidance of defecation. Active interventions are needed to break this cycle. Untreated constipation can result in fecal impaction.

 Nursing Tip

Timely Assistance for the Older Person

Delays in defecation are not always chosen by the older person. An older adult who requires assistance may need to suppress the defecation reflex while waiting for help getting to the bathroom. If this occurs repeatedly, the individual may lose sensitivity to the urge to defecate and become constipated. If unable to suppress the urge, the person runs the risk of being considered incontinent.

Environmental factors can play a role in constipation, particularly with institutionalized older adults. The older adult may be embarrassed by the sounds or odors involved with bowel elimination. Lack of privacy may cause anxiety or may result in the person's ignoring or suppressing the urge to defecate.

Difficulty assuming an anatomically suitable or comfortable position can also interfere with effective bowel elimination. Sitting upright or squatting are the preferred positions for defecation because it is easier to bear down in these positions (bearing down straightens out the anorectal angle, which is necessary for bowel elimination), and gravity assists elimination when the entire body is upright. People confined to bed find that bedpans are uncomfortable and difficult to use. Although sometimes necessary, bedpans should be avoided whenever the use of a toilet or commode chair is possible.

FECAL IMPACTION

Fecal impaction, the presence of a mass of hardened feces that is trapped in the rectum and cannot be expelled, is a result of unrelieved constipation. In severe cases, the fecal mass may extend up into the sigmoid colon. Individuals who have a history of chronic constipation are most at risk for impaction.

Symptoms of impaction include a delay in defecation that is longer than usual. More than 3 days without a bowel movement warrants close attention. Passage of small amounts of liquid stool without any formed fecal material can also indicate impaction. This liquid stool is fecal material from higher in the colon that is able to pass around the hardened mass. It typically oozes from the rectum and differs from a diarrheal stool, which passes with normal force.

Older adults suffering from fecal impaction are likely to complain of cramping or rectal pain, abdominal distention, and loss of appetite. Digital examination of the rectum typically reveals the presence of a hardened mass of feces. Sometimes the impacted mass is higher in the intestinal tract and cannot be detected by digital examination. In these cases, abdominal x-rays may be necessary. Before deciding that an older adult has a problem with bowel elimination, nurses should thoroughly assess the total situation, including the frequency, amount, and consistency of stools. Assessment should also include identification of factors that contribute to the development of bowel elimination problems. This enables the development of a plan that promotes sound elimination patterns.

 Safety Alert

Digital Examination for Fecal Impaction

Perform digital examination with extreme caution because it is uncomfortable and traumatic to the rectal tissues. Use particular caution when examining older persons with a history of cardiac problems, because rectal examination can stimulate the vagus nerve, resulting in a sudden decrease in heart rate accompanied by syncope and loss of consciousness. Some facilities require written orders before a digital rectal examination can be performed.

 Patient Education

When It May Be More Than Constipation

Older adults should be taught to contact their primary care provider when

- There is severe vomiting or abdominal pain.
- The frequency of bowel movements slows dramatically.
- Blood is present with bowel movements.
- There is a continuous sensation of pressure, fullness, or pain in the rectal area but they are unable to pass stool.
- Only small amounts of loose stool are passed or there is leaking of stool.

❖ NURSING PROCESS/CRITICAL THINKING MODEL FOR CONSTIPATION

◆ ASSESSMENT (DATA COLLECTION)

Recognize cues
- How often does the person have a bowel movement?
- Is there any pattern to when bowel elimination occurs?
- Is the person continent or incontinent of stool?
- What is the amount, consistency, and color of the stool?
- Is there evidence of blood, mucus, undigested food, or other unusual substances in the stool?
- Has the stool been checked for occult blood?
- Does the person have to strain to have a bowel movement?
- Is the stool expelled with excessive force, or does it ooze from the body?
- Does the person report or has the nurse observed any particular foods that affect bowel movements?
- Do these foods cause diarrhea or constipation?
- Does the diet have adequate bulk?
- Does the person rely on any aids for bowel elimination (e.g., suppositories, laxatives, and enemas) or bulk enhancers?
- How long have they been using this aid?
- Is the abdomen distended?
- If the person cannot speak, do they rub their abdomen?
- Has their appetite decreased?
- If the person cannot sense rectal fullness, what does a digital examination of the rectum reveal?
- What do they say about their bowel habits? Have these habits changed recently?
- Does the person report any concerns related to bowel elimination?

Box 18.2 lists risk factors for constipation in older adults.

◆ DATA ANALYSIS/PROBLEM IDENTIFICATION

Analyze Cues and Prioritize Hypotheses: Common problem statement for older adults with difficulties in bowel elimination includes

Constipation.

Box 18.2	**Risk Factors Related to Constipation in Older Adults**

- Neurologic problems that decrease the ability to sense the need for elimination or to control the sphincter muscles
- Reduced mobility
- Inadequate intake of dietary bulk
- Tube feedings
- Gastrointestinal obstructions or disease (e.g., Crohn disease and diverticulosis)
- Inadequate fluid intake
- Cognitive impairment (e.g., Alzheimer disease and dementia)

◆ PLANNING

Generate Solutions: The patient goals for older individuals with constipation are to (1) exhibit regular patterns of bowel elimination, (2) identify behaviors that promote normal bowel functioning, and (3) modify behaviors to enhance regular bowel elimination.

◆ IMPLEMENTATION

Take Action: The following nursing interventions should take place in hospitals or extended-care facilities:

1. **Assess bowel elimination patterns and contributing factors.** It is important to determine whether the older adult actually has a problem with constipation or only perceives a problem. Because many older people cling to the idea that daily bowel elimination is necessary, they may consider themselves constipated when no real problem exists. If this is the case, explain the normal range of variation. If the person is truly experiencing constipation, determine the causes and direct the plan of care toward eliminating or reducing the causative factors. Regularly assess older adults with a history of constipation or risk factors for constipation to avoid fecal impaction.

2. **Increase physical activity.** Physical mobility, even as little as twisting the body, turning from side to side, flexing the trunk, or lifting the legs to the abdomen, can help stimulate peristalsis. If possible, encourage older adults to participate in activities that are more vigorous, such as walking, bending, and stretching.

3. **Increase intake of dietary fiber and fluids.** Fluid and dietary bulk enhance the normal process of defecation. The recommended daily allowance for women over the age of 50 is 21 g/d of fiber; for men, the recommendation is 30 g/d (Carter, 2020). Cereal fiber is more effective at preventing constipation than other types, and older adults typically find it palatable. Some foods, such as bran or prunes, have bulk and a natural laxative effect. Many older adults accept these foods if they are offered as part of the breakfast meal. Some people find that other foods, such as cabbage or licorice, are helpful in stimulating bowel elimination. Adequate fluid intake (2 L/d is recommended) reduces the risk for constipation from excessive fluid absorption in the large intestine. Additional fluid is necessary during hot summer months or when illness results in excessive fluid loss.

 Safety Alert

Medication Safety

Older people who take **diuretics** should be encouraged to consume adequate fluids as long as their cardiovascular status is stable.

4. Schedule or encourage toileting at times when the person's defecation urge is strongest. If the urge to defecate is suppressed, the individual will be at greater risk for constipation. Encouraging older adults to use the toilet (or taking them there) at a time when defecation is likely may enable a healthy pattern to develop. The most likely times are early in the morning, after drinking the first warm beverage of the day, and shortly after a meal.

QSEN Considerations: Patient-Centered Care

There is value in seeing health care situations "through patients' eyes." According to QSEN, in providing compassionate and coordinated care based on respect for patients' needs, it is important to recognize the patient as the source of control. Some older people go through established rituals that support normal elimination. Determine the existence and nature of these rituals by talking with the person and use this information in care planning.

5. **Position the person to facilitate ease of elimination.** Use of a toilet is best for normal elimination. If this is not possible, a bedside commode is the next best option. Position a small footstool under the feet of the older person to increase intra-abdominal pressure and facilitate defecation. A bedpan is the least desirable option. Bedpans are uncomfortable, and their use makes it difficult for the person to achieve the normal bearing-down force needed for defecation.

6. **Provide privacy for elimination.** Privacy reduces the risk for constipation that results from suppressing elimination to prevent embarrassment. To prevent unpleasant odors, promptly remove soiled bedpans and use an air freshener.

Coordinated Care
Supervision

Patient Privacy

- The supervisory nurse should ensure that all older patients are given adequate privacy for elimination and that cultural modesty standards are observed.
- This is particularly important when the nurse is assisting an incontinent patient.

7. **Administer stool softeners or bulk-forming laxatives as prescribed.** Stool softeners keep fecal material moist and reduce the chance of anal irritation when stool is passed. Bulk-forming substances, such as psyllium, expand and trap moisture in the feces. Take care to administer these bulk-forming laxatives with adequate amounts of fluid. If adequate fluid is not ingested, these substances can cause constipation or bowel obstructions (Table 18.1).

8. **Administer prescribed osmotic agents, stimulant laxatives, or enemas if other methods have not been effective, as ordered.** If other methods of stimulating defecation have not been effective, it may be necessary to administer osmotic agents, which draw fluid into the colon through osmosis, either orally (e.g., magnesium hydroxide) or via suppository (glycerin suppositories). Stimulant laxatives, such as bisacodyl, stimulate peristalsis but may produce cramping. Bisacodyl can be given orally or via suppository. Older adults are more apt to accept suppositories because they are generally less traumatic and less invasive than are enemas.

9. **Perform digital rectal examination and impaction removal as ordered or according to agency policies.** Provide privacy and emotional support.

Table 18.1   Considerations Related to Certain Laxatives

TYPE	CONSIDERATIONS
Stimulant Laxatives	
Castor oil Bisacodyl Sennosides	Use with caution in older adults; can cause cramping or vomiting; may lead to electrolyte imbalance (loss of potassium), altered fat absorption, fat-soluble vitamin deficiency, and dependency; less expensive than some other forms.
Bulk Laxatives	
Psyllium Calcium polycarbophil Methylcellulose Wheat dextrin	Work effectively; safe for long-term use in older adults; can cause flatulence; resistance or nonadherence is common because of taste; risk for worsened constipation or impaction if fluid intake is inadequate.
Osmotic Agents	
Polyethylene glycol Lactulose Sorbitol Magnesium hydroxide Glycerin suppositories	Most are safe and effective even in frail older adults; magnesium salts should only be administered after consulting with patient's primary care provider, because they interact with numerous medications and are contraindicated for certain medical conditions (e.g., kidney disease, seizure disorder).
Fecal Softeners	
Docusate sodium	Do not have a laxative action so are not effective for chronic constipation; result in softer stool, allowing easier passage when straining is dangerous.

Safety Alert

Medication Safety

Enemas should be used with caution because they can lead to damage of the rectal mucosa and contribute to electrolyte imbalance. If performed incorrectly, enemas increase the risk for rectal perforation.

 Did You Know?

New Medications for Chronic Constipation

Two newer categories of constipation medications have shown promising results:

- Prokinetic drugs increase intestinal peristalsis. The main one, prucalopride, is being used in Europe, Canada, and Israel and was approved by the U.S. Food and Drug Administration (FDA) for use in the United States in 2019.
- Intestinal secretagogues increase intestinal chloride, thereby moving fluid into the bowel. Lubiprostone has been approved by the FDA for narcotic-related constipation in patients with chronic, noncancerous pain as well as those with cystic fibrosis and diabetes.

Verify that there are no preexisting conditions that contraindicate digital manipulation. Perform digital examination with a well-lubricated gloved hand. Some agencies use a lubricant containing a topical anesthetic to reduce discomfort. When an impaction is detected, oil-retention enemas may be ordered to soften the mass, followed by large-volume enemas to evacuate the mass. If this is not successful, digital removal may be necessary. With the patient positioned in a side-lying position, manually break the fecal mass into smaller pieces and remove.

 Safety Alert

The nurse must use caution during digital removal of fecal impaction to prevent trauma to the rectal tissues. This process may need to be done in increments to reduce the risk for damage.

The following interventions should take place in the home:

1. **Provide information regarding high fiber foods, and encourage increased consumption of these.** Many older individuals prefer processed foods that are easy to prepare and chew. Provide information about the value of foods that are easily obtained—such as cereals, whole wheat breads, bran muffins, and prunes—to help older adults select foods that may reduce the incidence of constipation. If family members prepare the meals, discuss the importance of fiber in preventing constipation.
2. **Encourage adequate fluid intake.** Approximately 2000 mL of fluid should be taken each day. This should include approximately 6 glasses of water, juice, and other beverages. Some individuals drink senna tea, which has laxative properties.
3. **Encourage adequate activity and exercise.** Activity enhances peristalsis and, along with good dietary practices, is most important in preventing constipation. Walking after meals may effectively stimulate the urge to defecate. Older adults should stay near toilet facilities so that they can act immediately when the urge arises. Suppressing the urge to defecate increases the risk for constipation.
4. **Discuss the risks involved with the use of laxatives without medical supervision.** Many older adults are unaware of the side effects and problems related to laxative use. Discuss these concerns, and encourage older adults to discuss any bowel elimination problems with the primary care provider before using laxatives.
5. **Use any appropriate interventions that are used in the institutional setting** (Nursing Care Plan 18.1).

DIARRHEA

Diarrhea is defined as the frequent passage of liquid, unformed stools. The stools are liquid because they pass through the large intestine too rapidly and are expelled before sufficient water has been absorbed in the large intestine. Diarrhea is a symptom and can have many causes, such as malabsorption syndromes, tumors of the GI tract, lactose intolerance, diverticulosis, and pathogenic organisms. Older adults who receive large amounts of concentrated tube feedings often experience diarrhea.

Many older people with diarrhea complain of nausea, vomiting, and abdominal cramps in addition to frequent stools. Rectal pain and skin irritation of the anus and buttocks are common because fecal material is very irritating.

Diarrhea can easily result in excessive fluid loss. This is a major concern in older adults, who are already at risk for fluid volume deficit. Because diarrhea can quickly result in dehydration, notify the primary care provider promptly so that the cause can be isolated and treatment begun.

❖ NURSING PROCESS/CRITICAL THINKING MODEL FOR DIARRHEA

◆ ASSESSMENT (DATA COLLECTION)

Recognize cues

See the assessment for constipation on page 312.

◆ DATA ANALYSIS/PROBLEM IDENTIFICATION

Analyze Cues and Prioritize Hypotheses: Common problem statement for older adults with excessive bowel elimination includes

   Diarrhea

Nursing Care Plan 18.1   Constipation

Mrs. Port, who is 85 years old, resides at Shady Grove Nursing Home. She has mild osteoarthritis, and she prefers to sit and visit or do crafts. She can move about using a walker. When her osteoarthritis pain is severe, she takes acetaminophen combined with 30 mg of codeine.

She eats with friends in the dining room and prefers to eat meat, white bread, and desserts. She eats very little of the fruits or vegetables served, and she consumes about 1200 mL of fluid per day.

Mrs. Port reports that she has bowel movements about every 2 or 3 days. "I used to have a bowel movement every other day. Now I really have to push, and it hurts." The nursing assistant reports that the stool is hard and dry.

PROBLEM STATEMENT
Constipation

SUPPORTING ASSESSMENT DATA
- 2 to 3 days between bowel movements
- Complaints of straining at stool
- Hard, dry stools
- Less than normal frequency of bowel movements

PATIENT GOALS/OUTCOMES IDENTIFICATION
Mrs. Port will have regular bowel movements at 1- to 2-day intervals, experience no difficulty passing stool, and describe dietary changes that promote regular elimination.

NURSING INTERVENTIONS/IMPLEMENTATION
1. Assess bowel elimination pattern for the frequency, amount, consistency, and effort required.
2. Explain the importance and effect of adequate fluid intake on bowel elimination.
3. Design a plan for increasing fluid intake to 2000 mL/d, including beverages favored by Mrs. Port.
4. Encourage consumption of fruits, vegetables, and whole grain breads or cereals.
5. Discuss alternative measures for pain control to decrease reliance on codeine-based medication.
6. Encourage increased frequency of physical activity.

EVALUATION
Mrs. Port has increased her fluid intake to 1800 mL/d. She reports eating bran cereal, whole wheat toast, and prune juice for breakfast and a fruit or vegetable with lunch and dinner. Formed, soft bowel movements have been reported every other day and documented in Mrs. Port's health record She states, "It feels so much better when I don't have to strain." You will continue the plan of care.

APPLYING CLINICAL JUDGMENT
Mrs. Port has decided that the high fiber foods and prune juice are upsetting her stomach and has stopped eating them. She reports that problems with elimination have returned.
1. What else could she do to help stimulate regular elimination?
2. What teaching does Mrs. Port require if she chooses to use a bulk-forming preparation such as psyllium?

◆ PLANNING

Generate Solutions: The patient goals for older individuals experiencing diarrhea are to (1) exhibit regular patterns of bowel elimination, (2) identify behaviors that promote normal bowel function, and (3) modify behaviors to enhance regular bowel elimination.

◆ IMPLEMENTATION

Take Action: The following nursing interventions should take place in hospitals or extended-care facilities:
1. **Assess the elimination pattern and suspected causative factors.** Diarrhea in older adults can result from many factors. Pay close attention to the frequency and nature of stools. Assess the time of day when diarrhea occurs and any factors that appear related to the onset of loose stools.

For example, a loose stool that follows a meal, a tube feeding, or administration of a medication is significant and should be reported. Assess for additional complaints, such as pain, cramping, fever, and force of expulsion. If the liquid stool seeps from the rectum, fecal impaction must be suspected. Removal of the impaction corrects this problem.

2. **Maintain adequate fluid intake.** Diarrheal stools lead to an excessive loss of body fluid. Fluid replacement to prevent dehydration is essential. In addition to simple fluid balance, electrolyte levels may be disturbed if the episodes of diarrhea are severe or prolonged. Provide oral fluids within dietary restrictions. Offer fluids that are rich in electrolytes (e.g., juices, Gatorade, and broth) instead of plain water. Avoid offering fluids high in fiber, caffeine,

and milk because they tend to induce diarrhea. If the individual is unable to take fluids orally, intravenous infusions may be necessary. Monitor older adults carefully for signs of dehydration, such as decreased skin turgor, orthostatic hypotension, tachycardia, and altered laboratory values.

3. **Institute measures to maintain skin integrity.** Cleanse the skin immediately after each episode of diarrhea. Diarrheal stool is very irritating to the skin and can rapidly lead to skin breakdown. Wash the anal area after each stool, and apply a protective ointment or lotion to provide a barrier against the caustic body wastes. If the skin becomes excessively irritated and tender to touch, sitz baths followed by air drying may help promote healing. Take care to prevent further trauma to the tissue. Keep bed linens clean and dry at all times.

4. **Promptly report observations to the primary care provider, and follow up on care provider's orders regarding medications that decrease intestinal motility.** Diarrhea in older adults is a serious concern. Because it can have many causes, report diarrhea to the primary care provider promptly so that its origin can be determined. The provider will probably prescribe fluid maintenance and medications to decrease the rate of intestinal motility and increase water absorption. The timing for administering these medications is usually related to the frequency of diarrheal stools. It is important to administer the medications as prescribed. If diarrhea persists, diagnostic tests on stool specimens may be ordered to determine whether the diarrhea is parasitic or bacterial in origin. Standard precautions and proper handwashing must be followed when obtaining or handling stool specimens.

The following interventions should take place in the home:

1. **Explain the importance of seeking medical attention if the person is experiencing diarrhea.** Many older people become severely dehydrated from diarrhea before they seek medical attention. Teach the importance of calling the primary care provider if diarrhea is severe or lasts more than 1 day. Any additional complaints, such as abdominal pain, cramping, or fever, also indicate the need to call a provider immediately. Many prescription and nonprescription medications can cause diarrhea. Because many older adults have prescriptions from multiple providers, it is important that they tell each provider every medication they are taking, including over-the-counter preparations and supplements.

2. **Explain the importance of proper food preparation and storage in preventing bacterial diarrhea.** Many cases of diarrhea are related to improper food preparation or storage. Some older adults allow food to sit out longer than it should. If unrefrigerated, food becomes a good medium for the growth of bacteria, many of which can cause diarrhea. Teach the importance of refrigerating all dairy products, meats, and other prepared foods immediately after purchase or after the meal and to not allow food to warm up on the counter before preparation.

3. **Use any appropriate interventions that are used in the institutional setting.**

FECAL INCONTINENCE

Incontinence of the bowel is most common among older adults who are unable to recognize and respond to normal sensations because of mental impairment or problems with mobility. Less frequently, colon or rectal disorders—such as cancer, inflammatory bowel disease, diverticulitis, or weak rectal muscles—cause or contribute to incontinence. Fecal incontinence is more common than suspected and is the second leading cause for nursing home admission. The exact incidence of incontinence is unknown because of varying definitions and underreporting, but studies reveal numbers varying from 2% to 18%. In some cases, incontinence is slight, consisting of just a small leakage of stool. In other cases, incontinence is a daily occurrence. Frequent incontinence of the bowel is a significant problem because fecal wastes are very irritating to tissues and can contribute to skin breakdown. Inability to control bowel elimination is also psychologically disturbing and embarrassing for older adults. Many community-dwelling older adults are unwilling to bring up concerns regarding this problem with health caregivers. They attempt to manage the problem themselves by using incontinence pads or briefs. In severe cases, they may stop participating in social activities for fear of embarrassment. Identification of underlying health problems and planning additional preventive strategies can help affected older adults maintain a more comfortable lifestyle.

❖ NURSING PROCESS/CRITICAL THINKING MODEL FOR FECAL INCONTINENCE

◆ ASSESSMENT (DATA COLLECTION)

Recognize cues
See assessment for constipation on page 312.

◆ DATA ANALYSIS/PROBLEM IDENTIFICATION

Analyze Cues and Prioritize Hypotheses: Common problem statement for older adults experiencing unpredictable expulsion of feces includes
Fecal Incontinence

◆ PLANNING

Generate Solutions: The patient goals for older individuals with fecal incontinence are to (1) exhibit regular patterns of bowel elimination, (2) identify behaviors that promote normal bowel functioning, and (3) modify behaviors to enhance regular bowel elimination.

◆ IMPLEMENTATION

Take Action: The following nursing interventions should take place in hospitals or extended-care facilities:

1. **Assess patterns of elimination and causative factors.** It is important to know how often and when the individual is incontinent. If these episodes have a regular pattern, use this information to plan nursing care. For example, many individuals have a pattern of defecating 30 to 45 minutes after a meal. If the person is taken to the bathroom at that time, an episode of incontinence will be prevented. Unfortunately, not all individuals have such a regular pattern of defecation.

2. **Establish a toileting schedule.** If a defecation pattern is detected, take the person to the bathroom at the time they are most likely to defecate. If no detectable pattern is present, the care provider may order the use of digital stimulation or glycerin suppositories. When repeated daily or every other day, these measures may establish a regular pattern of defecation. When planning a toileting schedule, consider the older adult's daily routines and scheduled appointments (e.g., physical therapy).

> 💡 **QSEN Considerations: Teamwork and Collaboration**
>
> To be effective, all individuals and departments that have contact with the individual should be aware of the patient's toileting plan and follow through with it.

3. **Take measures to prevent or reduce episodes of constipation.** It is difficult to prevent incontinence when an individual is constipated. Measures used to prevent constipation increase the likelihood of regular elimination.

4. **Use appropriate aids or garments.** It is best if episodes of incontinence are prevented by regular toileting or other methods discussed previously. If these measures are not completely successful, use special pads or garments to reduce the embarrassment of soiling the bed or clothing. However, do not use these aids in place of other nursing measures that promote bowel control.

5. **Clean the person promptly after each episode of incontinence.** Incontinence can easily lead to skin breakdown. It is essential to remove any soiled linens or garments as soon as possible to reduce skin irritation. Provide this care tactfully to reduce damage to the self-esteem of older adults, most of whom are acutely embarrassed by their incontinence and are sensitive to any negative verbal or nonverbal communication from the nursing staff. Remove all soiled materials from the room and put into appropriate containers to reduce environmental odors.

6. **Use any appropriate interventions that are used in the institutional setting.**

URINARY RETENTION

Urinary **retention** is an abnormal accumulation of urine in the bladder because the bladder is unable to empty completely. Normally, no more than 50 mL of urine remains in the bladder after voiding. The person experiencing urinary retention often has several hundred milliliters remaining after voiding. Urinary retention in older adults can result from decreased muscle tone in the bladder wall, decreased fluid intake, prostate gland enlargement, trauma to the muscles of the perineum, neurologic damage, medications, or anxiety.

Symptoms of retention include a feeling of fullness, discomfort or tenderness in the bladder, restlessness, and diaphoresis. People experiencing urinary retention may complain of a total inability to void or of passing small amounts (between 25 and 50 mL) of urine at frequent intervals. This pattern is called *retention with overflow*. Severe retention results in bladder distention that can be detected by inspecting or palpating the area over the symphysis pubis. Treatment of urinary retention depends on the cause. If retention is caused by perineal trauma or anxiety, noninvasive measures, such as medications or a sitz bath, may be enough to stimulate effective voiding. If severe retention is caused by an obstruction, such as an enlarged prostate, **catheterization** or surgery may be necessary to prevent serious bladder damage that may result from persistent or excessive bladder distention.

URINARY TRACT INFECTION

Urinary tract infections (UTIs) are a common problem, particularly for older women (see Chapter 3).

URINARY INCONTINENCE

Urinary incontinence (UI) is the involuntary loss of urine in sufficient amount or frequency to be a social or hygiene problem. UI is not a normal part of aging, but it is a major problem in the aging population. More than 17 million adults in the United States are affected by UI, women twice as often as men. Up to 46% of community-living older adults experience UI, and institutionalized older adults have even higher rates of UI. Prevalence of UI in persons with dementia is as great as 90% (Box 18.3). The national cost of UI currently exceeds 16 billion dollars a year in the United States. UI is among the leading causes of long-term institutional placement.

UI has medical, emotional, social, and economic consequences for older adults. It can result in skin irritation or breakdown and can contribute to pressure

Box 18.3	**Risk Factors Associated With Urinary Incontinence in Older Adults**

- Advanced age
- Caffeine intake
- Immobility/functional limitations
- Diuretics/other medications
- Obesity
- Smoking
- Fecal impaction/fecal incontinence
- Malnutrition
- Depression/delirium
- Enlarged prostate and treatment for prostate cancer
- Hearing or visual impairment
- Low fluid intake
- Environmental barriers
- Disorders: Diabetes, Parkinson disease, stroke, chronic obstructive pulmonary disease, arthritis/back problems
- Estrogen depletion
- Pelvic organ prolapse
- Institutionalization

Modified from National Institute on Aging. (2017). Urinary incontinence in older adults. https://www.nia.nih.gov/health/urinary-incontinence-older-adults

injuries; it can lead to guilt, frustration, and psychological distress; it can lead to social isolation; and it can be costly because of the need to purchase expensive undergarments and replace or launder clothing more frequently. Ultimately, it can lead to the emotional, social, and economic costs of institutional care.

Home Health Considerations

Community Education Programs

Community education programs can be helpful in reducing the extent and severity of urinary incontinence (UI) among community-dwelling older adults, particularly women. These programs should stress that UI is not a part of normal aging and emphasize behavioral management of UI, including the use of incontinence diaries, identification of dietary triggers, recognition of signs and symptoms of urinary tract infections, and performing pelvic muscle strengthening exercises.

Older adults may hesitate to discuss UI problems with care providers because they are embarrassed or because they think that incontinence is simply a problem of aging that they must endure. Therefore the topic must be introduced in a sensitive manner by caregivers. In some cases, UI is curable using surgery, medications, or other treatments. In other cases, it can be better managed, thus allowing the older person to lead a more normal life.

A number of normal age-related physiological changes or common diseases seen with aging can cause or contribute to UI. Different forms of incontinence (e.g., stress, urge, reflex, overflow, functional, and mixed UI) are recognized as problems in older adults.

QSEN Considerations: Teamwork and Collaboration

Prevention of Urinary Incontinence

Urinary incontinence (UI) can be reduced if there is a commitment to success rather than a defeatist attitude. Stressing the benefits to the patient and identifying the benefits to caregivers can help motivate the process. All members of the health care team are essential to reduce UI. The physician, nurses, nursing assistants, physical therapists, occupational therapists, and facility management need to be actively involved in the development, communication, and implementation of the plan. A staffing system designating specially trained certified nursing assistants to implement restorative interventions to prevent incontinence has been shown to be effective. However, no staff members should consider themselves "too important" to respond to the needs of patients. A successful plan can improve the self-esteem of residents and enhance the perceptions of the level of care held by family members and the community.

STRESS URINARY INCONTINENCE

Stress UI is leakage of urine during conditions that increase intraabdominal pressure, such as exercise, lifting heavy objects, laughing, coughing, or sneezing. When a full bladder is compressed against weakened urinary sphincters, incontinence occurs. This problem is most commonly observed in women, particularly those who have weakened perineal muscles resulting from aging and childbearing. In general, the amount of urine lost is small.

URGE URINARY INCONTINENCE

Urge UI is caused by involuntary contraction of the detrusor muscle of the bladder. It is characterized by a sudden strong urge to void. Individuals suffering from urge incontinence are often unable to hold back the urine long enough to reach a commode or toilet. Urge UI is often seen in older individuals who suffer from diseases that affect nerve transmission to the bladder (e.g., Parkinson disease, multiple sclerosis, stroke, and dementia). Urge UI is also observed when there is increased bladder stimulation caused by lower UTIs, concentrated urine, and irritating chemicals, such as caffeine or alcohol. Atrophic urethritis, uterine prolapse, fecal impaction, or prostate enlargement also increases the likelihood of urge UI. Even healthy older adults with no known medical problems may experience occasional episodes of urge UI.

The basis of urge UI is in the physiological changes seen with aging. With aging, the bladder decreases

QSEN Considerations: Safety

Fall Risk

People who experience urge UI once or more per week are at greater risk for falls and fractures, most likely caused by the individual rushing to the restroom to avoid an incontinent episode.

in size; it can hold less volume (often 200 mL or less) and needs to be emptied more often. This results in the increased urinary frequency seen with aging. When larger volumes of urine are produced in response to excessive fluid intake or increased use of diuretics, the problem of urinary frequency is magnified. In addition, many older adults experience involuntary spasms of the muscles of the bladder wall, called *detrusor spasms*. These spasms can occur even when the bladder contains small volumes, resulting in a sense of urgency to empty the bladder. When the need to void is frequent and urgent, the result is urge UI.

Urge UI is likely to occur after the removal of an indwelling catheter. When an indwelling catheter is placed, the result is diminished bladder capacity. Frequency, urgency, and incontinence are likely to occur when a catheter is removed suddenly without incremental clamping, which allows the bladder muscles to stretch gradually to accommodate larger volumes.

REFLEX URINARY INCONTINENCE

Reflex UI is the involuntary loss of urine at a fairly predictable interval after a certain bladder volume has been reached. When this level is reached, the bladder empties, like a reflex. This type of UI occurs when there is an exaggerated reflex of a bladder muscle in patients with neurologic disorders, such as spinal cord injury. The patient may or may not feel the urge to void or have any sensation of bladder fullness.

OVERFLOW URINARY INCONTINENCE

Overflow UI is defined as leakage of small amounts of urine from an overly full bladder. The bladder cannot hold the amount of urine being produced, so it overflows. Overflow UI is a common problem for people with diabetes suffering from loss of bladder muscle tone because of neuropathy or those experiencing polyuria related to hyperglycemia. Overflow UI is also common in older men with benign prostatic hyperplasia. Enlargement of the prostate restricts the flow of urine, so the bladder never empties completely. This contributes to overflow problems (see the earlier section on urinary retention). Women who have an obstruction at the outlet of the bladder resulting from a prolapsed uterus, cystocele, or rectocele may experience similar problems. Those with neurologic disorders, such as multiple sclerosis or spinal cord injuries above the sacral area, are also prone to have overflow UI. Anticholinergic medications may also cause excessive relaxation of smooth muscle.

FUNCTIONAL URINARY INCONTINENCE

Functional UI is seen in older adults who have normal urethral and bladder function. It is caused by a

| Table 18.2 | Medications That Affect Continence |
MEDICATION	POTENTIAL EFFECT
Diuretics	Cause rapid filling of the bladder resulting from the rapid increase in urine production
Anticholinergics	Interfere with normal contraction of the muscles of the bladder wall
Sedatives and hypnotics	Interfere with alertness and recognition of the need to urinate
Narcotics	Interfere with normal contraction of the muscles of the bladder wall; decrease awareness of sensations from the bladder
α-Adrenergic agonists	Increase tone of the internal sphincter muscle
α-Adrenergic antagonists	Decrease tone of the internal sphincter muscle
Calcium channel blockers	Decrease tone of the bladder wall muscles

poor relationship between the aging person's abilities and their environment. Changes in functional ability may be cognitive or physical in nature. The inability to recognize a toilet and perform simple tasks—such as using a zipper or pulling down underwear, walk to the bathroom, transfer to the toilet, or ask for assistance—can result in functional UI. Environmental factors contribute to the problem of functional UI and increase its likelihood. Functional UI is likely to occur when there are not enough toilets, when toilets are difficult to access because of their location or height, when there are not enough caregivers to provide needed assistance, and when protective devices prevent free movement. Weakness, changes in dexterity, and decreased ability to manipulate clothing contribute to problems. Medications that interfere with cognition or mobility, alter bladder tone, and increase urine production often contribute to functional UI (Table 18.2).

MIXED URINARY INCONTINENCE

Some older adults with incontinence appear to have more than one form of UI. This problem is sometimes called *mixed UI*. For example, many older adults report that when they have the urgent need to urinate, they cannot respond quickly enough because of decreased functional ability and environmental limitations. UI can be a continuous and ongoing problem or may occur only occasionally. Careful history taking and medical examination are needed to determine the specific type of UI and the underlying causes so that appropriate medical treatment and nursing interventions can be initiated.

❖ NURSING PROCESS/CRITICAL THINKING MODEL FOR ALTERED URINARY FUNCTION

◆ ASSESSMENT (DATA COLLECTION)

Recognize cues
- Is the person continent or incontinent?
- Does the incontinence occur at a specific time of day or under special conditions?
- Does the person have a history of any medical conditions that would interfere with urine elimination (neurogenic bladder)?
- Do they have a history of any medical condition that would decrease awareness of the need to void?
- What is the volume of a typical voiding?
- How much urine is produced each day?
- What is the odor, color, and consistency of urine?
- Are there any signs of a UTI (burning, pain with urination, frequency)?
- Has a urinalysis been done recently? What are the results?
- What is the person's normal pattern of voiding?
- Do they experience any difficulty in starting to urinate?
- Is there any involuntary loss of urine when they cough, laugh, or sneeze?
- What is the pattern of fluid intake?

Box 18.4 lists the risk factors for altered urinary function in older adults.

◆ DATA ANALYSIS/PROBLEMS IDENTIFICATION

Analyze Cues and Prioritize Hypotheses: Common problem statements for involuntary expulsion of urine include

Urinary Incontinence
Altered Urinary Function

◆ PLANNING

Generate Solutions: The patient goals for older individuals diagnosed with altered urinary function are to (1) exhibit a reduction in episodes of UI or retention, (2) urinate at acceptable times in acceptable places, (3) identify measures that reduce episodes of UI or retention, and (4) establish a routine to reduce or prevent the occurrence of bladder elimination problems.

Box 18.4	Risk Factors Related to Altered Urinary Function in Older Adults

- Neurologic problems that decrease the ability to sense the need for elimination or to control the sphincter muscles
- Endocrine disorders
- Altered structures that interfere with elimination (prostate enlargement or tumors)
- Decreased mobility (especially people on bed rest)
- Inadequate or excessive fluid intake
- Cognitive impairment (Alzheimer disease, dementia)

◆ IMPLEMENTATION

Take Action: The following nursing interventions should take place in hospitals or extended-care facilities:

1. **Assess elimination patterns.** Older adults may experience a variety of urinary problems. Careful assessment of elimination patterns and problems enables nurses to develop a plan of care that addresses the unique needs of a specific person. Determine how often the person voids and how much is voided each time. If the older person is incontinent, investigate how often and when incontinence occurs. Consider whether the person is receiving medications that affect continence. For example, if incontinence occurs only at night when the older person is receiving diuretic medications, the timing of administration should be considered.

2. **Assess fluid intake patterns.** Fluid intake has a direct effect on urine elimination. Many older individuals with urination problems attempt to correct the problem by drinking less. This is likely to increase problems with incontinence because the highly concentrated urine produced is more likely to irritate the bladder, increasing the risk for an episode of incontinence. Fluid restriction also increases the risk for problems with fluid balance and bowel elimination. Encourage older adults to consume most of the day's fluids early in the day and to reduce fluid intake after 7 P.M. to reduce the incidence of incontinence during sleep. Fluids that irritate the bladder, such as alcohol or caffeine, should be avoided.

3. **Explain measures that help improve tone of the sphincter muscles.** Kegel exercises are helpful in improving the tone of the sphincter muscles (Box 18.5). These exercises include starting and stopping the stream of urine when voiding. Improved muscle tone can help the person hold the urine until they can reach a toilet or obtain assistance. Biofeedback has also shown promise as a method of reducing stress and urge incontinence.

4. **Modify clothing to make toileting easier.** The time that is spent manipulating buttons or zippers may be long enough to cause incontinence. Use of Velcro closures and elastic waists with loops may speed undressing and reduce functional problems related to toileting.

5. **Reduce environmental barriers by providing grab bars in the bathroom, installing toilet risers, keeping the urinal or bedpan readily available, and providing a call light for assistance.** Minimizing environmental barriers to safe elimination can help older adults function more effectively and will reduce the incidence of incontinence caused by mobility problems.

6. **Answer call lights promptly.** Decreased muscle tone and neurologic changes hinder the ability of

Box 18.5	Modified Kegel Exercises

The purpose of Kegal exercises is to strengthen the pelvic floor muscles and the squeezing action that helps hold back the flow of urine. It is important that these exercises be done faithfully for 3 to 4 months to see improvement. If no improvement is seen in this time, consultation with a urologist is suggested.

A. Follow these instructions to identify the muscles you will be exercising.

  1. Sit or stand. Without tensing the muscles of your legs, buttocks, or abdomen, imagine that you are trying to hold back a bowel movement by tightening the ring of muscle around the anus. Do this exercise only until you identify the back part of the pelvic floor.

  2. When you are passing urine, try to stop the flow, then restart it. This helps you identify the front part of the pelvic floor. Now you are ready to do the complete exercise.

B. Do this exercise for 2 minutes at least 3 times daily (at least 100 repetitions).

  Working from back to front, tighten the muscles while counting to 4 slowly, and then release them. You can do this exercise anywhere; sitting or standing, while watching television, or while waiting for a bus. There is no need to interrupt your normal daily activity. To feel only the pelvic muscles, do not tighten the abdominal, thigh, or buttock muscles or cross your legs. Their movement is distinct and separate from that of the other muscles and can be checked by women while they are in the bath or shower by placing one finger inside the vagina and contracting the muscles. Men can check success only through improved urine control.

C. Do this exercise every time you urinate.

  Start and stop your stream 5 times each time you urinate (i.e., start the flow of urine, squeeze to hold back, then let go to resume the flow). Repeat this sequence several times. Remember, do this every time you urinate. You will probably notice that you have much more control of the flow of urine in the morning than you do in the afternoon. That is because your muscles are not so tired earlier in the day.

From National Association for Continence (NAFC), PO Box 1019, Charleston, SC 29402.

many older adults to delay urination. An older adult cannot wait as long as a younger person for assistance to the bathroom. Respond promptly to call lights or other requests for assistance with toileting, or an episode of incontinence will be likely. An occurrence of incontinence caused by lack of staff response is embarrassing for the older adult and frustrating to all involved because it need not happen. Routine scheduling of trips to the bathroom at regular intervals throughout the day can help to reduce the need for the person to call for assistance (Table 18.3).

7. **Develop a toileting schedule.** Planning a regular toileting schedule encourages emptying of the bladder at regular intervals. This reduces the likelihood of urgency and incontinence. The schedule should be based on the individual's urinary elimination patterns; there is no absolute best time. If the person is frequently incontinent, begin by scheduling toileting at 2-hour intervals. Because urine is produced at a rate of approximately 50 to 75 mL/h and the older person's bladder capacity is approximately 150 to 200 mL, this frequency will reduce episodes of incontinence. Toileting too frequently can actually decrease the ability of the bladder to hold an adequate amount of urine, increasing the risk for incontinence. When a 2-hour schedule is successful, the time should be increased gradually to retrain the bladder to accommodate larger volumes of urine. A regular schedule of every 3 to 4 hours is desirable. Monitor the patient's response to scheduled toileting and praise successes.

8. **Familiarize older adults with the locations of bathrooms throughout the facility.** Many older adults who experience urgency or incontinence are afraid to leave their rooms because they fear being unable to reach a bathroom when necessary. This may result in isolation and withdrawal from others. Even a short distance may be too far for an older person with an urgent need to urinate. Reassurance that toilets are available nearby can reduce these fears.

9. **Provide support and encouragement.** Incontinence is disturbing to alert older adults. Episodes of incontinence are embarrassing and can lead to frustration and loss of self-esteem. Even those involved in bladder training programs are likely to have accidents. It is essential to focus on successes and minimize failures.

10. **Initiate actions to maintain skin integrity.** Aging skin is particularly susceptible to damage from moisture and the waste products in urine. Remove wet clothing and linens immediately to prevent maceration and irritation. Thoroughly wash and dry the skin after each episode of incontinence.

11. **Provide incontinence pads or garments when appropriate.** Incontinence pads or garments reduce the need to completely change the bed linens or clothing after an episode of incontinence (Figs. 18.1 and 18.2). Use these items with caution, however, because they tend to trap moisture next to the skin. Some of the newer incontinence garments are constructed with a barrier that keeps moisture away from the skin. Because newer incontinence garments are also smaller and less conspicuous, they are more acceptable to older people than are the bulkier diaper-type garments. The newer garments allow wearers more freedom to move about without fear of embarrassing themselves. These pads and garments should not be used as a replacement for toileting, however. The cost of incontinence supplies can be significant for people with limited financial resources. When incontinence pads or garments are soiled, change and

Table 18.3   **Promoting a Continence-Friendly Environment**

ASSESSMENTS	MODIFICATIONS OR INTERVENTIONS
Accessibility	
Are restrooms close to bedrooms and activity centers?	Schedule activities in locations with convenient restrooms.
Are restrooms clearly identified?	Use signs that contrast with walls and have large, bold, dark lettering.
Can the resident recognize restrooms?	Show residents where restrooms are located.
Can the resident read signs regarding restroom locations?	Use universal picture symbols for restrooms in addition to words.
Is the resident able to ask for assistance to the restroom?	Watch for nonverbal signs of discomfort. Assist resident to toilet on a 2-hour schedule.
Does the resident ask for assistance to the restroom?	Assist resident to restroom before start of activities. Answer call lights promptly.
Are adequate staff assistants available?	Plan to have adequate staff available based on number of residents with continence issues.
Are there any physical barriers or protective devices that restrict mobility?	Minimize use of restrictive devices or other barriers to movement.
Safety	
Are the restrooms equipped with call lights and grip bars?	Verify presence of safety devices. Develop plan for acquisition if not in place.
Are floors level, dry, and nonskid?	Check condition of floors regularly. Post safety signs during cleaning sessions.
Are restrooms free from clutter?	Remove all clutter from restroom floors promptly.
Is there adequate lighting in restrooms?	Use adequate wattage in restroom. Leave lights on in restroom at night.
Does the resident have and wear appropriate footwear?	Remind resident to wear shoes or slippers when going to restroom.
Does the resident require assistive devices, such as a walker or wheelchair?	Consult with physical therapist regarding need for assistive devices. Encourage resident to use recommended devices.
Does the resident need help transferring from wheelchair to toilet?	Verify that resident and staff are both aware of proper transfer techniques between wheelchair and toilet.
Privacy	
Does the resident share a restroom with other people?	Be aware that more than one person may need to use the restroom at the same time. Have an alternative restroom identified.
Do restrooms have doors and locks?	Doors with safety locks that can be released by staff promote a sense of privacy.
Are toileting requests handled tactfully?	Ask resident tactfully if he or she needs to use the toilet. Do not shout.
Is modesty protected during toileting?	Close curtains and doors. Make sure resident is adequately dressed when moving in room or public spaces.
Comfort	
Are toilets and toilet seats in good condition, clean, and secure?	Check regularly for chips or cracks, and check cleanliness on a regular basis. Report any need for cleaning or repairs promptly.
Are special needs addressed?	Consult with a physical therapist and/or occupational therapist regarding the need for seat riser or padded seat based on resident needs.
Are residents assisted off of the toilet promptly?	Assist resident off of toilet when finished. Excessive waiting time is uncomfortable and can result in unsafe actions.
Does the resident have the opportunity to wash hands after toileting?	Assist to sink, or provide washcloths or hand sanitizer after toilet use.

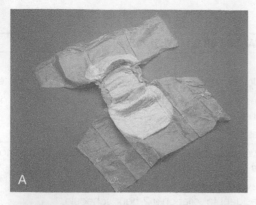

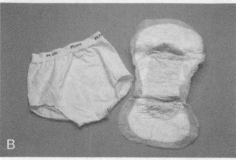

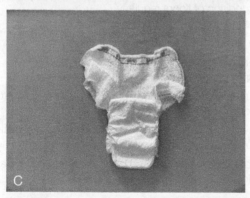

Fig. 18.1 Disposable garment protectors. **A,** Complete incontinence brief. **B,** Pant liner and undergarment. **C,** Pull-on brief. (A and B: From Kostelnick, C. [2020]. Mosby's textbook for long-term care nursing assistants [8th ed.]. St. Louis, MO: Mosby.)

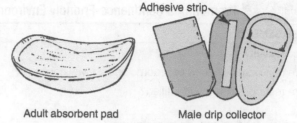

Adult absorbent pad   Male drip collector

Fig. 18.2 Disposable incontinence pads. (From Gray, M. [1992]. Genitourinary disorders. St. Louis, MO: Mosby.)

dispose of them promptly to reduce environmental odors.

12. **Administer medications as prescribed by the primary care provider.** Uroseptic medications, such as sulfonamides, are often used to treat UTIs. Always check for allergies to sulfa before administering these medications. Medications such as oxybutynin or imipramine may be prescribed to reduce bladder spasms that cause incontinence. Nurses must administer these medications as prescribed and assess the patient for signs of medication effectiveness. Many of the medications prescribed to treat incontinence cause side effects such as dry mouth, dry eyes, confusion, constipation, orthostatic hypotension, and tachycardia. Comfort measures and safety precautions are necessary if these side effects occur.

13. **Insert a straight catheter as prescribed by primary care provider.** Straight catheterization requires an order by a physician or care provider with prescriptive authority (Fig. 18.3). The insertion of an indwelling catheter is not recommended for treating incontinence. The risk for UTIs increases dramatically with this invasive procedure. Catheters should be used only when the benefits to the patient outweigh the risks involved. Sterile technique must be used when inserting an indwelling catheter. When the catheter is in place, thorough perineal care is essential to reduce the possibility of ascending UTI. Many older adults who have had an indwelling catheter even for a limited time are at increased risk for incontinence once it is removed. When the catheter is in place, the bladder is decompressed. Once the catheter is removed, the bladder is unable to adapt to holding a significant volume of urine. Before removing the catheter, this problem can be reduced by following a procedure whereby the catheter is clamped intermittently to increase bladder capacity.

The following interventions should take place in the home:

1. **Encourage the individual to establish a pattern of urine elimination.** A pattern of voiding on awakening, after meals, before leaving home, before becoming interested in a lengthy activity, before exercise, and before bed can reduce the risk for incontinence.

2. **Stress the importance of good skin care and hygiene after episodes of incontinence.** Poor hygiene increases the risk for skin irritation or breakdown and increases the risk for UTIs. Teach the importance of changing soiled clothing promptly, careful handwashing after toileting, and (for women) proper wiping from front to back.

3. **Encourage discussion of concerns with the primary care provider.** Nurses working in a home setting may be aware of urinary problems that have not been shared with the medical team. Older adults should be encouraged to reveal their problems and concerns with their care provider so that an appropriate diagnosis can be made and treatment initiated. Document all observations regarding urine elimination in the person's record, and notify the primary care provider.

4. **Provide encouragement during treatment for urinary problems.** Problems with urinary retention or incontinence do not usually respond quickly to

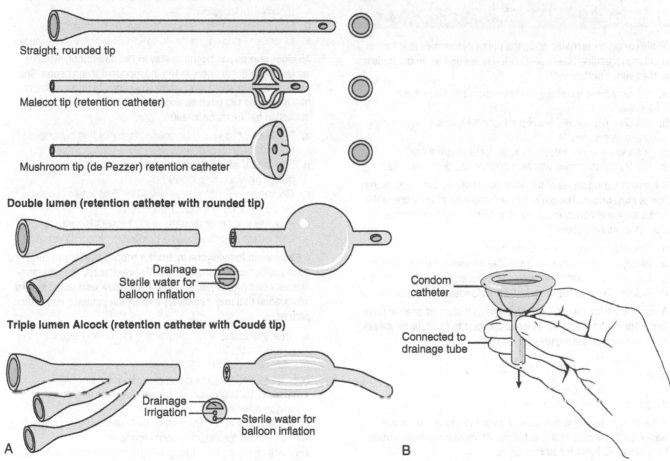

Single lumen

Straight, rounded tip

Malecot tip (retention catheter)

Mushroom tip (de Pezzer) retention catheter

Double lumen (retention catheter with rounded tip)

Drainage

Sterile water for balloon inflation

Triple lumen Alcock (retention catheter with Coudé tip)

Drainage

Irrigation

Sterile water for balloon inflation

A

Condom catheter

Connected to drainage tube

B

Fig. 18.3 Examples of catheters. **A,** Single-, double-, and triple-lumen catheters. **B,** Condom catheter. (From Williams, P. A. [2022]. deWit's fundamental concepts and skills for nursing [6th ed.]. St. Louis, MO: Elsevier.)

treatment. Weeks or months of treatment may be required before any improvement is noticed. This can easily result in nonadherence with the treatment plan. Encourage older adults to take medications, practice exercises, or follow through with other medical recommendations.

5. **Discuss methods for coping with incontinence.** Older adults are more likely to become socially isolated rather than embarrass themselves in public. Developing strategies for coping (e.g., use of incontinence garments and learning the location of toilets in stores or theaters) can help to prevent this.

6. **Use any appropriate interventions that are used in the institutional setting.**

Get Ready for the Next Generation NCLEX® Examination!

Key Points

- Bladder and bowel elimination is essential for normal body functioning.
- Unless waste products are removed effectively from the body, serious consequences will result.
- Aging results in less effective removal of waste products, but a problem more significant to older adults is any alteration in the ability to control the elimination process.

- Urinary incontinence is not a normal part of aging, but it is a major problem in the aging population.
- Problems related to elimination are serious concerns for older adults, and a great deal of physical and mental energy is devoted to dealing with changes in elimination function.

Additional Learning Resources

SG Go to your Evolve website at http://evolve.elsevier. com/Williams/geriatric for the additional online resources.

Review Questions for the Next Generation NCLEX® Examination

1. While caring for an older adult, the nurse determines that further teaching regarding bowel elimination is needed when the patient makes which statement?

   a. "I'll do some exercise and increase my daily fluid intake."
   b. "I'll give myself an enema if I don't have a bowel movement every day."
   c. "I'll increase my intake of fruits and vegetables."
   d. "I'll try to eat more whole grain foods, like bran, daily."

2. A nurse is caring for an older adult who recently had small watery bowel movements. The patient now complains of pressure in the rectal area and abdominal cramping. Which is the most appropriate initial nursing action?

   a. Administer an oil-retention enema.
   b. Notify the primary care provider of these observations.
   c. Digitally stimulate the rectal sphincter.
   d. Administer the "as needed" (prn) laxative medication.

3. A nurse is caring for an older adult with a history of cardiac problems. The nurse knows it is most important to institute measures to prevent which outcome?

   a. Constipation
   b. Diarrhea
   c. Urinary tract infection
   d. Bladder incontinence

4. A nurse is caring for a patient with urge urinary incontinence. Based on the nature of this problem, which nursing intervention is appropriate? *(Select all that apply.)*

   a. Avoid placing throw rugs in their room.
   b. Offer the patient a cup of tea to reduce detrusor muscle spasms.
   c. Place the patient close to the restroom, and remind them of its location.
   d. Use safety pins to secure the patient's pants.
   e. Orient the patient to the location of nearby restrooms.

5. An older woman has begun to stay in her apartment, avoiding socializing with her peers in the independent living center. She states that she cannot wait when she needs to urinate. She is afraid that she will have an accident. What is the most appropriate action for the nurse to take?

   a. Tell her not to worry because many of the other ladies have the same problem.
   b. Suggest that she begin to wear an adult incontinence garment when she goes out.
   c. Recommend that she restrict her fluid intake so the problem does not occur as often.
   d. Provide encouragement, and discuss Kegel exercises and other approaches to cope with incontinence.

6. A 69-year-old female yoga instructor tripped over a yoga mat and fractured her pelvis. She is currently hospitalized for pain management and evaluation. Place a check mark next to the patient information that may negatively impact the patient's elimination pattern.

   i. Temperature: 97.8 degrees F (36.6 degrees C)
   ii. Heart rate: 92
   iii. Blood pressure: 139/87
   iv. Takes oxycodone 5 mg po q4h for pain
   v. Takes furosemide 10 mg po daily for treatment of hypertension
   vi. Has eggs and drinks milk for breakfast every morning
   vii. Must call for assistance to the toilet
   viii. Will get out of bed to chair only for breakfast. Refuses all other activity.
   ix. Has trouble sleeping at night

REFERENCES

Carter, C. (2020). What should your diet be like after 50? AARP. https://www.aarp.org/health/healthy-living/info-2020/nutrition-after-age-50.html

Sharif, S. I, Al-Harbi, A. B., Al-Shihabi, A. M., Al-Daour, D. S., & Sharif, R. S. (2018). Falls in the elderly: assessment of prevalence and risk factors. Pharmacy Practice (Granada), 16(3), 1206. Epub 14 de octubre de 2019. https://dx.doi.org/10.18549/pharmpract.2018.03.1206

Objectives

1. Describe normal activity and exercise patterns.
2. Examine how activity and exercise patterns change with aging.
3. Discuss the effects of disease processes on the ability to participate in exercise and activity.
4. Describe methods of assessing changes in the ability to participate in activity or exercise.
5. Identify older adults most at risk for experiencing problems related to activity and exercise.
6. Select appropriate problem statements related to activity and exercise problems.
7. Select nursing interventions appropriate for older individuals experiencing problems related to activity and exercise.
8. Differentiate between a custodial focus and a rehabilitative focus in nursing care.
9. Discuss the impact of nurses' attitudes on care planning.
10. Identify the benefits of a rehabilitative focus on older adults.
11. Identify the goals of rehabilitation nursing.

Key Terms

agility (ă-JĬL-ĭ-tē, p. 326)
alignment (ă-LĬN-měnt, p. 330)
arthritis (ăhr-THRĬ-tĭs, p. 328)
coordination (kō-ŏr-dĭ-NĂ-shŭn, p. 326)
custodial (kŭ-STŌ-dē-ăl, p. 348)
dexterity (děk-STĚR-ĭ-tē, p. 326)
diversional activities (dĭ-VŬR-zhăn-ăl, p. 345)
dyspnea (DĬSP-nē-ă, p. 338)

hemiparesis (hěm-ē-pă-RĒ-sĭs, p. 330)
hemiplegla (hěm-ē-PLĒ-jă, p. 330)
isometric (ī-sō-MĚT-rĭk, p. 330)
isotonic (ī-sō-TŌN-ĭk, p. 330)
rehabilitation (rē-hă-bĭl-ĭ-TĂ-shŭn, p. 328)
rehabilitative (rē-hă-bĭl-ĭ-TĂ-tĭv, p. 342)
tachycardia (tăk-ē-KĂR-dē-ă, p. 337)

NORMAL ACTIVITY PATTERNS

The activity-exercise health pattern deals with behaviors related to exercise, activity, leisure, and recreation. Nurses must consider the wide range of behaviors within this pattern that fall under the general term *activity*. Activity is anything that requires the expenditure of energy. Some activities require only a small expenditure of energy, whereas others require a great deal of energy.

Basic body functions—such as breathing, temperature control, and metabolism—expend the least amount of energy. Sitting, resting, watching television, reading, and playing cards or bingo are sedentary activities that require little energy. Activities of daily living (ADLs)—such as dressing, grooming, eating, bathing, and toileting—require a greater expenditure of energy. Cooking, cleaning, driving, and shopping require still more effort and expend more energy. Walking can be a mild or vigorous activity, depending on the pace. Running, swimming, dancing, aerobics, and other forms of active exercise require the greatest energy expenditure. Although the amount and type of exercise one performs changes over the life span, exercise and activity remain an essential part of life. People who were not physically active as young adults can become more physically active as they age, but the activity must be increased gradually to avoid injury. A healthy pattern of activity and exercise is best established early in life, however, to ensure that these behaviors become habitual and are carried into old age.

Exercise helps people look and feel better. Physical activity is necessary to maintain joint mobility and muscle tone. When people do not participate in regular activity, all body systems suffer. Preventing mobility problems is easier than trying to overcome the problems once they develop. Older adults should be encouraged to be as active and independent as possible. Because existing medical conditions may restrict activity, nurses should be aware of any problems that may affect someone's ability to participate in activities and assist them to do as much as is permitted.

Many older adults remain physically active. It is common to see individuals in their 60s, 70s, and older leading active, self-sufficient lives. Aging does not imply that a person must sit in a recliner and vegetate. Visit a park or shopping mall early in the morning, and you will see many older adults walking for their health. Golf courses are filled with older adults teeing up. Activity is good for people of all ages. Aging may change the type and amount of participation, but active participation in a variety of activities is the best way to maintain high level function.

Physical activity requires a complex interaction of physiological processes, primarily those of the neurologic, musculoskeletal, cardiovascular, and respiratory systems. Anything that interferes with the coordination of these systems can alter the ability to participate in physical activity.

Of major importance is the function of the nervous system, which is the primary coordinating system of the body. The brain controls the involuntary activities of the body, including metabolism, respiration, and temperature control. Areas of the brain control the high level processes of perception and cognition. Before any voluntary activity occurs, individuals must be able to recognize that a need for action exists. Once the need is recognized, the individual must have the desire and the ability to perform that action. The brain is also the motor control center of the body, and it communicates with the somatic peripheral nervous system. Any physiological age- or disease-related change that alters the function of the brain's motor centers or interferes with the transmission of impulses from the brain to the musculoskeletal system can interfere with activity.

The musculoskeletal system must then be able to respond to these messages from the brain. Normal and pathologic changes in muscles or bones can interfere with normal activity. Even if the nervous and the musculoskeletal systems are intact, problems in the cardiovascular and respiratory systems can lead to alterations in activity. Muscles, including the heart muscle, require an adequate supply of oxygen and nutrients to function properly. Anything that interferes with the oxygen supply to tissues affects a person's ability to perform activity.

ACTIVITY AND AGING

With advancing age, most people experience some changes in their ability to perform or tolerate activity; such changes vary widely from one person to another. In general, the more active a life a person has lived, the more active they are likely to remain with aging.

The first change noticed by most aging people is a decrease in the rate or speed of activity. Things that could be done quickly in the past now take longer. Many older individuals complain that it now takes them much longer to dress, shop, or do other simple activities. Normal aging does not interfere with the

transmission of nerve impulses, but it does slow the speed of nerve transmission.

A loss of muscle mass can interfere with activities that require muscular strength. Activities such as moving furniture, lifting bags of groceries, shoveling snow, and vacuuming may become increasingly difficult.

Loss of cushioning cartilage can result in arthritic joint pain, which inhibits motion and makes a person less inclined to exercise. Ligaments and tendons become stiff, contributing to decreased joint flexibility. This can result in problems with performing ADLs. Reaching for objects on shelves, dressing, bending to put on shoes, and even washing one's feet or back may become more difficult.

Agility, the ability to move quickly and smoothly, decreases with age. This may cause difficulty when older adults try to climb ladders or avoid hazards while walking. Dexterity, the ability to perform fine manipulative skills, is also likely to decrease with age. Gross motor skills remain intact longer than do fine motor skills. However, skills that were perfected when one was younger, such as playing a musical instrument or sewing, may be maintained at a high level if used regularly.

Decreased stamina is typically seen with aging. This is most often a result of decreased oxygen supply to body tissues. Impairment of oxygen exchange may be caused by decreased elasticity in the lungs and a smaller chest cavity. The decreased availability of oxygen may lead to the need for frequent pauses during activity or a slower pace while activities are being performed.

! Safety Alert

The ability to coordinate multiple activities is likely to decrease with aging. Activities that require simultaneous perception of many stimuli and quick physical responses (as in driving) are often affected. Older adults with impaired vision and hearing, decreased strength, slow reaction time, and decreased coordination may not be able to perform these types of complex activity safely.

 Elder Care Points

Because these changes appear gradually, older individuals generally learn to compensate for or cope with them. Many strategies—such as pacing activities, finding alternative methods of performing activities, and simplifying activities—demonstrate older adults' capacity to adapt and adjust.

EXERCISE RECOMMENDATION FOR OLDER ADULTS

Regular planned exercise is of benefit to all ages, and it is of particular benefit as we age. Scientific evidence indicates that regular physical activity can extend one's years of active independent life, reduce disability, and improve the quality of life. Exercise promotes muscle mass, strength, balance, coordination, and joint flexibility. It helps to decrease stress and promotes normal sleep. Exercise does not have to be demanding to be beneficial. Moderate exercise done for 30 minutes a day is more beneficial than strenuous exercise done infrequently. It is recommended for older adults that they participate in moderate-intensity exercises for 150 to 300 minutes each week. For those who are able to perform vigorous-intensity aerobic activity, 70 to 150 minutes each week is recommended. Muscle-strengthening exercise should be included on at least 2 days each week (Administration for Community Living, 2020).

Because there may be medical reasons for contraindicating certain activities, older people should check with their primary care provider before starting an exercise program. Care providers often refer older patients to a physical therapist, who can develop a plan specific to their needs. Older adults with physical limitations will need an individualized plan developed to meet their unique needs. The proper exercise plan for a frail older adult will be quite different from one best suited to a high-functioning 65-year-old individual. Physical therapists can recommend exercise programs designed for use by wheelchair-bound individuals or anyone with special needs. Before starting an exercise program, the older person should know the importance of acquiring good supportive footwear and clothing appropriate for the environment and type of exercise. Because older adults are more at risk for thermal imbalance, they should be aware that it is wise to avoid excessive exercise during extreme weather conditions.

> A 94-year-old man was interviewed at a private health club where he spends 1 hour a day, 6 days a week. He said that he started coming to the club when he was in his late 70s in order to give his wife, who had Alzheimer disease, some privacy while she received personal care at home. He said he thought it would help him decrease his stress and increase his physical strength so that he could help her. She has since died, but he keeps coming to the club to use the treadmill and flexibility machines. When asked why he likes to come to the club to exercise, the man replied, "It keeps me young." He also mentioned that he likes the social atmosphere and "watching the youngsters sweat."

Specific types of exercise provide unique benefits. Aerobic exercise promotes cardiovascular and respiratory function. Aerobic exercise includes activities that increase the heart rate, such as walking, jogging, or bicycling. Many residential facilities, the Young Men's Christian Associations (YMCAs), and senior centers provide additional opportunities for aerobic exercise, providing equipment such as treadmills, elliptical trainers, and rowing machines. The individual must know how to use the equipment properly to avoid injury. Swimming is a pleasurable aerobic exercise for many seniors, and

water exercises can help individuals with sore joints because the water provides support and eases movement. Even doing routine household chores and yard work can be considered aerobic if done for a long enough time. Strength training will help maintain muscle mass and can be performed at home or at the gym using exercise balls, inexpensive elastic stretch bands, or weights. Weight-bearing exercise, such as walking, helps maintain bone strength. Stretching exercises are important to promote range of motion and joint flexibility. Most aerobic or strength-training exercises cause muscles to tighten, so stretching major muscle groups after exercising will help maintain flexibility. Little equipment is needed for these exercises; but if someone has balance problems, caution should be used when doing standing exercises. Balance training is particularly important for older adults. Technologic innovations, such as the Nintendo Wii and other interactive games appear to have the potential of stimulating interest in activity within the aging population. They have the added benefit of being able to be performed at home.

QSEN Considerations: Evidence-Based Practice

Physical Fitness

The plan of care for older adults should include activities that improve physical fitness. Studies have demonstrated that strength and balance training not only improves physical fitness but also reduces fall risk in community-dwelling older adults (World Health Organization, n.d.).

Clinical Situation

Keeping motivated to exercise is a major problem at any age, perhaps more so as a person gets older. Nurses should educate older persons about the importance of exercise and emphasize the benefits, such as weight loss, improved mobility, improved blood glucose control, lower blood pressure, decreased fall risk, and living a longer and healthier life. Here are some guidelines for nurses that can help older adults make a regular exercise program a reality:

- Keep it simple. Simple exercise programs are more likely to be successful than complicated ones that are hard to remember or difficult to perform.
- Have a plan. Set up a weekly calendar with a planned time for exercise to keep on track.
- Do it with a friend. Encourage the older adult to enlist the company of a friend or group of friends who can provide mutual encouragement and support as a way of staying motivated. Even a pet can be a great exercise companion.
- Keep it interesting. Encourage the older adult to join an exercise or dance class as a way of trying some new form of exercise that is more interesting and motivating (see Complementary Health Approaches box, further on).
- Try music. Upbeat rhythms or waltzes can help coordinate your movements. Music designed specifically for exercise is available online for download. Exercise videos are also available, but choose one that is appropriate for your needs and abilities.

- Get a coach. A physical therapist can provide additional teaching and motivation and can design a safe workout routine that can be done at home.
- Set a goal. Goals should be realistic but challenging. Focus on small but measurable gains in the areas of strength and flexibility, such as increasing strength to walk an additional block or being able to put on shoes more easily. Remember, anything that you can do now but had trouble with before is a gain. In fact, not losing function as you age is a significant gain in itself.

Complementary Health Approaches

Qi Gong and Tai Chi

Qi gong and tai chi are forms of exercise from Asia that are gaining popularity because they are less stressful to the body and yet require more focus and concentration. This makes these exercises beneficial for both body and mind. The major components include body posture adjustments, gentle motion, regulated breathing, meditation, and other purposeful relaxation. Some forms also include massage or hand resistance. These exercises can be done vigorously or gently, making them suitable for a variety of individuals. They are typically performed while standing but can also be adapted for walking, sitting, or lying. They are inexpensive to perform because they require no special equipment or facilities. Research conducted abroad and in the United States has shown many benefits from these exercises, including increased oxygen consumption, decreased blood pressure, improved flexibility, increased lower extremity strength, increased bone density, improved posture and balance, and improved immune system function. Additional reported benefits include decreases in stress, anxiety, and depression.

These exercise practices have gained some support in the United States, but many health care providers and potential older participants are unaware of them or remain skeptical of their benefits. This may be because of lack of familiarity with the techniques and a perception of difficulty. In addition, there are not enough teachers who are prepared to explain the principles and skills of these exercises appropriately. Further research and dissemination of information are being funded by the Robert Wood Johnson Foundation and others. Many articles and video training materials are now available.

Focusing on the positive outcomes of exercise is key to maintaining a regular program. See the Nursing Process/Clinical Judgment Model for Altered Mobility on pages 330–336 for additional benefits that can increase an older adult's motivation to continue exercising.

EFFECTS OF DISEASE PROCESSES ON ACTIVITY

In addition to normal changes, if the older adult has health problems that affect critical body systems, their ability to participate in activity will be further impaired. Cognitive disorders such as delirium, Alzheimer disease, and stroke can affect both the high-level thinking functions and motor functions of the brain. Severely affected persons may not recognize the need for the most basic activities, such as moving, eating, dressing, bathing, or toileting. Even if they do recognize these needs, their altered motor function may prevent them from meeting such basic needs.

Neurologic damage resulting from head injury, infection, degenerative disease, Parkinson disease, or toxic drug reactions can interfere with the transmission of normal nerve impulses. People suffering from these conditions may recognize a need and have the desire to perform an activity yet are unable to carry it out. The nervous system does not transmit appropriate messages to the muscles to enable them to perform the activity. Abnormal nerve transmission can result in difficulty getting started with movement or in uncoordinated muscle activity (e.g., a staggering gait), which further limits the ability to participate in normal activities.

Diseases or injury to the musculoskeletal system can interfere with the ability to perform some activities. Fractures can lead to limited or extensive mobility restriction depending on the body part affected. Fracture of a small bone, such as a finger, results in limited loss of mobility. Fracture of a large bone, such as the femur, results in a severe loss of mobility. The fracture itself restrict mobility, and the treatment limits it further. Even after surgical repair, the person with a fractured hip is not permitted to participate in certain activities (e.g., weight bearing on the extremity) until healing has occurred. Preventive nursing interventions are important to preserve strength and mobility of joints.

Diseases such as gout and arthritis cause joint pain, which leads to restricted activity. A person with severe gout or arthritis may avoid using the painful joints to reduce discomfort. Unfortunately, this inactivity can lead to further loss of joint mobility and muscle strength, thus even more reducing the person's ability to perform activities. Joint degeneration with aging severely restricts mobility, particularly in the weight-bearing joints in the knees and hips. Joint replacement surgery is an increasingly common option for older adults. After a period of rehabilitation, older adults generally achieve a greatly improved activity level.

Elder Care Points

Foot conditions commonly seen in older adults (e.g., bunions, hammertoes, and calluses) may interfere with ambulation, particularly if footwear does not fit properly. Painful feet are a common reason for decreased activity in older adults.

Any disease or condition that interferes with the intake or distribution of oxygen to body tissue significantly interferes with a person's ability to participate in activity and exercise. These conditions include diseases of the respiratory system that prevent adequate gas exchange in the lungs (e.g., asthma, emphysema, bronchitis, and pneumonia) and diseases of the cardiovascular system that prevent adequate distribution of oxygen to body tissues and heart muscles (e.g., myocardial infarction, heart failure, heart block, arteriosclerosis, and hypertension).

Inadequate oxygenation places additional stress on the cardiovascular and respiratory systems. Pulse and respiratory rates increase to compensate for the decreased amount of oxygen. If additional demands for oxygen occur, as they do with even moderate activity, older adults may experience yet more symptoms. With oxygen deprivation, fatigue with minimal activity is common. Pain may be reported with activity. Most common are angina (chest pain that may radiate down the left arm or present as vague gastrointestinal discomfort) and intermittent claudication (a cramping pain in the legs during or after walking), both of which are caused by inadequate tissue oxygenation. Initially, this pain occurs with activity only; in severe cases of oxygen deprivation, it also occurs at rest. Severe oxygen deprivation can result in cardiac or respiratory distress.

To compensate for these symptoms, older adults spontaneously restrict their activities. Individuals may become homebound because the effort of dressing is too much for them. Some are unable to eat or perform basic hygiene because it is too exhausting. Sometimes the activity limitation is so severe that such individuals are able to maneuver around the home only by placing chairs at 10-foot intervals. They move that short distance and then sit and rest until they are able to move to the next chair.

🍎 Nutritional Considerations

Malnourishment can also contribute to the reduced ability to perform activities. Inadequate intake of nutrients can result in muscle atrophy. Malnourished individuals lack adequate protein to build muscle tissue, an adequate supply of glucose to fuel the muscles, and adequate iron to form hemoglobin. Inadequate iron intake can result in anemia, which leads to a decrease in the oxygen available to tissues and further reduces the ability to perform activities.

Although not physiological in origin, emotional disorders such as severe grief, anxiety, or depression can lead to decreased participation in normal activity. Individuals who are emotionally disturbed may be directing all of their energy inward and may not be willing or able to summon the energy required for physical activity. It is important to remember that these people need to continue to use their bodies to prevent loss of physical function.

❖ NURSING PROCESS/CLINICAL JUDGMENT MODEL FOR ALTERED MOBILITY

Older adults typically experience some changes in their ability to perform physical activities. These changes may result from the normal changes of aging or from pathologic changes.

◆ ASSESSMENT (DATA COLLECTION)

Recognize cues:

- Does the person have full range of motion in the joints?
- Do they have any contractures or deformities?
- Does the person experience any pain or tenderness in the joints?
- Is there any particular motion that aggravates joint pain?
- What relieves pain?
- Describe the muscle tone of the arms and legs.
- Is muscle strength equal on both sides of the body?
- Is there any muscle tenderness?
- Is the person bedridden, wheelchair bound, or ambulatory?
- If ambulatory, what is the pattern of the gait? Steady? Shuffling? Ataxic? Slow? Rapid?
- Is the person able to lift their feet when walking or do they shuffle?
- Does the person maintain an upright posture when walking?
- Do both sides of the body move evenly?
- How well can the person maintain balance?
- What kind of footwear do they wear for walking?
- Does the person have any foot problems (e.g., bunions and calluses) that interfere with walking?
- How far can they ambulate without discomfort?
- Does the person require any assistive devices (walkers or canes) for ambulation? Are they used properly?
- Does the person feel comfortable and confident using these aids?
- Do they require the assistance of another person to ambulate?
- If the person is not ambulatory, what is their activity level?
- Does the person use a wheelchair?
- Can they operate the wheelchair independently?
- Does the person receive passive range-of-motion exercises?
- Is the environment safe for the person?

Box 19.1 lists risk factors for altered mobility in older adults.

◆ DATA ANALYSIS/PROBLEM IDENTIFICATION

Analyze Cues and Prioritize Hypotheses: Common problem statements for older adults with mobility difficulties include

Altered Mobility

◆ PLANNING

Generate Solutions: The patient goals for individuals with altered mobility are to (1) increase participation in physical activities that maintain strength and mobility, (2) maintain normal anatomic position and function in all joints, (3) remain free from joint contractures and foot

Box 19.1 **Risk Factors Related to Altered Mobility in Older Adults**

- Altered activity tolerance because of medical conditions that decrease endurance or strength
- Pain
- Neuromuscular or musculoskeletal conditions
- Cognitive impairment (Alzheimer disease or dementia)
- Severe anxiety or depression
- Prescribed bed rest
- Restrictive devices (protective devices, casts, splints, and immobilizers)

drop, and (4) maintain or increase strength and mobility using assistive devices.

◆ **IMPLEMENTATION**

Take Action: The following nursing interventions should take place in hospitals or extended-care facilities:

1. **Identify the prescribed activity level.** The activity level is established by the primary care provider based on the older adult's overall health status. The patient should be as active as possible yet not exceed the prescribed activity level.

⚠ Safety Alert

It is particularly important to be aware of any weight-bearing restrictions related to fractures or joint replacements. Failure to take proper precautions can lead to serious and permanent harm.

2. **Continue to assess strength and joint mobility.** Strength and joint mobility are not always consistent in older adults. Changes may be caused by something as simple as a change in the weather, or they may be an early indication of a change in the older person's health status. Carefully assess mobility if the older adult has experienced weakness or falls. Promptly report any acute changes in the assessment, such as one-sided weakness or severe pain, to the primary care provider.

3. **Perform physical mobility activities in conjunction with daily care.** Provide passive range-of-motion exercise in conjunction with the bath. Incorporate active exercise as part of dressing, meals, grooming, toileting, and other ADLs. Even minimal participation in ADLs can increase physical mobility. Any exercise performed by the older individual during bathing, hair combing, and oral hygiene that uses the joints and muscles can be beneficial.

4. **Provide good body alignment and frequent position changes.** Bedridden older adults are at high risk for loss of joint mobility. Poor alignment can result in muscle fatigue, which enhances the likelihood of contractures. Flexion contractures of the hip, knee, and foot occur when the stronger flexor

muscles dominate. These contractures can result in permanent loss of the ability to stand or ambulate. To prevent this, always provide good alignment and positioning. Use positioning devices (pillows, trochanter rolls, and foot supports) when needed to maintain proper alignment.

5. **Avoid unnecessary protective devices that limit physical mobility.** Protective devices limit mobility. Any device that restricts mobility is a considered to be a restraint, including vests, wheelchair tables, foot pedals, and even safety bars. Many of these devices that historically have been used to protect older adults from falls have actually increased the likelihood of injury. An older adult who is prevented by these devices from using joints and muscles loses strength and function and becomes increasingly susceptible to injury. Ensure that splints or other devices do not unnecessarily restrict joint movement.

6. **Create a suitable activity/exercise plan that maintains muscle strength and joint mobility.** Passive range-of-motion exercises help keep the joints flexible, but they do little to maintain muscle strength. Passive range of motion should be provided a minimum of twice a day for immobile older individuals. Active range of motion helps with both joint flexibility and muscle toning. Teach older people with hemiplegia or hemiparesis to use the stronger side of the body to exercise the weaker extremities.

💡 QSEN Considerations: Teamwork and Collaboration

Physical Therapy

The physical therapist may be able to suggest exercises that will benefit a specific individual. These exercises should become part of the nursing care plan and be included in the day's activities (Fig. 19.1).

Many facilities provide exercise programs adapted to meet the ability levels of the residents. Exercise is often done to music because the rhythm encourages motion. Isometric exercises—such as alternately tightening and relaxing the muscles of the arms, abdomen, or buttocks— may benefit some older adults by helping them maintain the strength of their abdominal and gluteal muscles and quadriceps. Isometric exercise does not affect the joints. Isotonic exercise—which helps to improve muscle strength, muscle tone, and joint mobility—includes such movements as lifting the body off of the bed with a trapeze (Fig. 19.2), pressing against a footboard, or pushing against the bed to lift the buttocks off the mattress. Isometric and isotonic exercises should be used with caution by persons with cardiac problems because these exercises increase stress on the cardiovascular system.

LYING DOWN

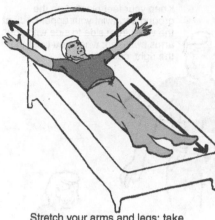

Stretch your arms and legs; take a deep breath.

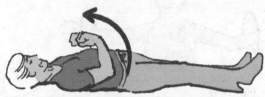

With your arms at your sides, bend at the elbow and curl your arms as if making a muscle.

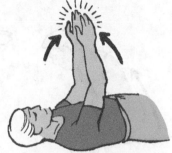

Clap your hands directly above your head.

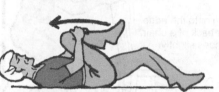

Grab each leg with both hands below the knee and pull toward your chest slowly.

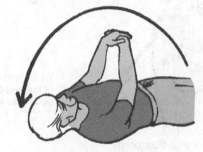

Fold your hands on your stomach; raise your arms over your head toward the headboard.

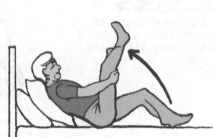

Lift each leg off the bed, but try not to bend your knee. Use an arm to help.

SITTING

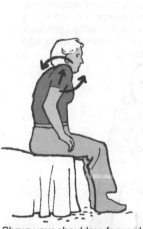

Shrug your shoulders forward, then move them in a circle, raising them high enough to reach your ears.

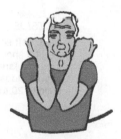

Touch your elbows together in front of you.

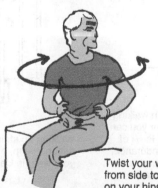

Twist your whole upper body from side to side with your hands on your hips.

Bend forward and let your arms dangle; try to touch the floor with your hands.

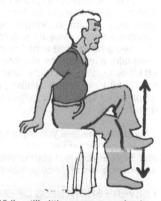

While still sitting, move each of your knees up and down as if you are walking; each time your right foot hits the ground, count it as one. Lift your knee high.

Fig. 19.1 Various exercises that can be done while lying down, sitting, standing up, and walking. (From Johnson-Paulson, J. E., & Koshes, R. [1985]. Exercise is for everyone. *Geriatric Nursing, 6*[6], 322.)

STANDING UP

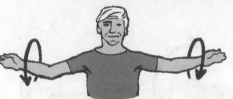

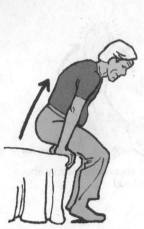

Using your arms, push off from the bed and stand up; if you get dizzy, sit down and try again.

Hold your arms out and turn them in big circles.

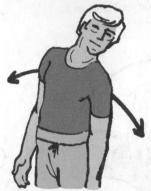

With hands at your side, bend at the waist as far as you can to the right side, then to the left.

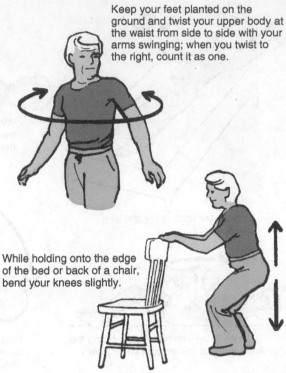

Keep your feet planted on the ground and twist your upper body at the waist from side to side with your arms swinging; when you twist to the right, count it as one.

While holding onto the edge of the bed or back of a chair, bend your knees slightly.

WALKING PLACES

Walking is good exercise. It helps in toning muscles and maintaining flexibility of joints. It also is good exercise for the heart and circulatory system. Walking briskly for 20 minutes a day, 3 times a week can be as effective a heart conditioner as jogging, but it does take a longer time to achieve the same effect as jogging. For those who cannot walk rapidly for long periods, walking to the point of muscular fatigue also helps maintain good muscle tone.

Your body may give you signs to indicate you are overdoing exercise. Stop, rest, and if necessary, call your physician if you experience any of these symptoms:

• SEVERE SHORTNESS OF BREATH
• CHEST PAIN
• SEVERE JOINT PAIN
• DIZZINESS OR FAINT FEELING
• HEART FLUTTERS

In all walking exercises, go only as fast as you are able to walk and still carry on a conversation. If you cannot, slow down.

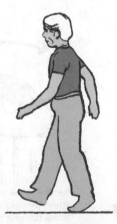

INSIDE

It is important to maintain walking ability. Determine how far you can walk and each day walk to 3/4 of that distance, building endurance. Wear supportive shoes and use whatever aids are necessary.

OUTSIDE

Wear soft-soled shoes with good support, (i.e., jogging shoes). When walking, push off from your toes and land on your heels. Swing arms loosely at your sides. Begin with 10-minute walks and build to 20 to 30 minutes.

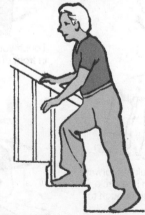

Walking up stairs requires effort. Place one foot flat on a step, push off with the other and shift your weight. Use a railing for balance if necessary.

Fig. 19.1, Cont'd

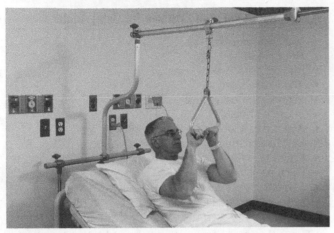

Fig. 19.2 Patient using a trapeze bar. (From Kostelnick, C. [2020]. *Mosby's textbook for long-term care nursing assistants* [8th ed.]. St. Louis, MO: Mosby.)

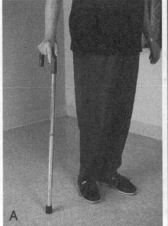

Fig. 19.3 Types of canes. **A,** Single-tip cane. **B,** Four-point (quad) cane. Note that proper footwear is being worn. (From Kostelnick, C. [2020]. *Mosby's textbook for long-term care nursing assistants* [8th ed.]. St. Louis, MO: Mosby.)

? Did You Know?

These exercises may result in elevation of the blood pressure and use of the Valsalva maneuver, which can slow the heart rate dangerously, even to the point of cardiac arrest in someone with cardiac disease. To prevent this problem, older adults should be instructed to breathe through the mouth while exercising.

7. **Verify that the older adult is appropriately dressed for activity and has the proper footwear.** Proper clothing and footwear should be selected for exercise. Clothing should not be constricting (to allow for freedom of movement) and should be suitable to the environment. Many older adults choose comfortable footwear instead of footwear that provides proper support. Most slippers do not provide adequate support and are intended for rest, not ambulation.

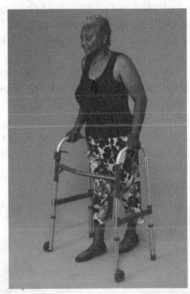

Fig. 19.4 Patient using a wheeled walker. (From Kostelnick, C. [2020]. *Mosby's textbook for long-term care nursing assistants* [8th ed.]. St. Louis, MO: Mosby.)

💡 QSEN Considerations: Safety

Reduce Fall Risk

Encourage the wearing of shoes whenever possible. Shoes should fit well and support the foot in order to to decrease the likelihood of falls. If the individual has foot problems, special footwear may be necessary. Gait changes, particularly the inability to lift the feet freely, increase the risk for falls. If footwear is too loose or is not supportive, the fall risk increases. Shoes should fit snugly enough that they do not slip off the heel when walking. Older women, particularly those with kyphosis, should be encouraged to wear low heels when walking so as to provide better balance.

8. Provide pain medication in a timely manner so that maximal benefits from the medication occur when greatest physical effort is expected. Pain is a common reason for decreased physical mobility. Be aware of particular activities that intensify or relieve an individual's pain. Pain increases with fatigue; therefore pace activities so that they do not overly fatigue the individual. Administer

anti-inflammatory medications or analgesics so that the older adult will be as comfortable as possible when physical activity is scheduled.

9. Verify that the individual knows the correct method for using assistive devices and that they do, in fact, use them for activity. Explain proper use if needed. If assistive devices such as wheelchairs, walkers, or canes are needed, verify that the older adult knows how to use them properly (Figs. 19.3 and 19.4). Assess the older adult's ability to use the walker, particularly when climbing stairs. Check that the person holds the cane in the correct hand when they are is walking. To prevent falls, remind older adults to lock the wheels of their wheelchair before sitting down. In addition, ensure that assistive devices are kept nearby so that they will be readily available to the older person. If the individual suffers from one-sided

weakness, place the device on the stronger side. Many older adults do not like to use these devices because they are cumbersome and also constant reminders of failing health. Stress the importance of using the devices if they are needed for safety.

10. Encourage wheelchair-bound patients to move by using their arms or feet whenever possible. If they are unable to walk, older adults may still be able to move about in a wheelchair, which involves using either the arms to turn the wheels or the legs and feet to propel the chair.

11. Provide adequate assistance during ambulation. Gait belts and the assistance of 1 or 2 helpers may be needed to provide safety and a sense of security. The loss of balance seen in some older people increases the risk for falls. Use a gait belt when assisting an unsteady person. A gait belt is not a lifting device. Gait belts that are properly secured around the person's waist allow the caregiver to prevent injury to both the individual and the caregiver. The belt is near the person's center of gravity; thus the caregiver can sense subtle changes in balance and anticipate problems (Fig. 19.5). If the belt is too loose, it may slide up under the rib cage and cause injury. Regular belts on trousers or dresses should be used only as a last resort because they are usually narrower and may not fasten as securely as a proper gait belt. Holding the arm of the older adult to provide support should be avoided, as it can lead to shoulder dislocation in a fall.

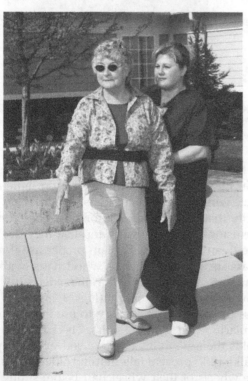

Fig. 19.5 Assist with ambulation by walking behind and slightly to the side of the person. Use a gait belt for the person's safety. (From Kostelnick, C. [2020]. *Mosby's textbook for long-term care nursing assistants* [8th ed.]. St. Louis, MO: Mosby.)

Box 19.2 Benefits of Exercise for Older Adults

- Maintain independence
- Retain mobility
- Prevent or reduce depression
- Encourage sleep
- Improve self-esteem
- Improve appetite
- Improve cardiovascular status
- Maintain or improve musculoskeletal function
- Prevent obesity
- Decrease stress level
- Expand social network
- Enhance appreciation for life

The following interventions should take place in the home:

1. **Teach or reinforce the benefits of regular activity and exercise.** Remind and encourage older adults about the benefits of exercise (Box 19.2). Important information to communicate to older adults includes the fact that moderate or higher levels of physical activity are associated with lower mortality rates. Physical activity has been associated with many beneficial physiological effects, including improved cardiovascular status, decreased risk for colon cancer, beneficial effects on type 2 diabetes, maintenance of normal muscle strength and joint function, reduced risk for falling, and decreased incidence of obesity. Activity also has psychological benefits, including a decreased incidence of depression, improved mood, and an enhanced sense of well-being.

2. **Assess the home for safety hazards or conditions that may interfere with mobility.** The home may present conditions that interfere with mobility or increase the risk for falls. Modifications of the environment may be required to prevent accidents or injury. Chapter 9 addresses the assessment of home safety in detail.

3. **Help older adults develop a schedule for regular physical activity that is appropriate for their prescribed activity level.** The primary care provider

---

🏠 **Home Health Considerations**

Older adults who do not have limiting health conditions should participate in 150 minutes of aerobic physical activity each week as well as muscle strengthening activities that work every major muscle group twice a week (Centers for Disease Control and Prevention, 2020). The physical activity can be broken down into small, even 10-minute sessions. Midmorning is a good time for exercise, but afternoon and early evening are also good. Much of the timing depends on the individual's peak energy time. Blood supply may be diverted to digestion for up to 2 hours after large meals; therefore intense physical activity should not be scheduled immediately after meals. Walking is an excellent exercise for older adults. Swimming and cycling are also recommended (Fig. 19.6).

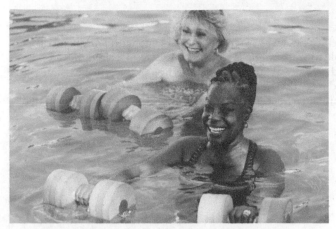
Fig. 19.6 Healthy aging. (Copyright © istock.com/kali9.)

should be consulted before an older person who has a chronic disease or has lived a sedentary lifestyle starts an exercise program. Once an appropriate target level is established, teach the older adult to start slowly and build up to the optimal level over time. Encourage active older adults to participate in regular physical activity. Incorporate exercise into the daily activity plan. If exercise is not viewed as important enough to plan for, it will not be done.

 Community Considerations

Exercise programs, including aerobics classes, are sponsored by many senior citizen centers. Before joining an exercise program, older adults should see their primary care providers to ensure that the program is appropriate and safe for them. In addition to providing exercise, these programs offer an opportunity for socialization. Exercising with others provides motivation and makes the effort more worthwhile and pleasant.

4. **Explain the importance of warm-up and cool-down exercise.** Before starting an exercise session, the individual should warm up for approximately 5 minutes. Simple exercises that make the joints limber and slowly stretch the muscles are recommended. Older adults better tolerate exercises that do not put undue stress on bones and joints.

Patient Education

Explain to older adults the importance of a cool-down period after exercise. Five minutes of slower activities (similar to the warm-up) help blood return from the muscles to the central circulation. If someone stops exercise abruptly, they may experience fainting (syncope) because of inadequate blood flow to brain tissue.

5. **Explain the importance of proper dress for environmental conditions and proper footwear for safety.** Consider environmental conditions—including heat, cold, high humidity, and air pollution—when planning activity. Older persons should try to minimize exercise on excessively hot or cold days. On very hot days, activity is best planned for early in the day or later in the evening, when the temperature is cooler. Some large cities experience ozone alerts because of excessive air pollution. On ozone alert days, it is wise for all individuals, particularly older adults, to minimize their activity. On warm days, lightweight, loose clothing should be worn to allow the body to cool by evaporation. On extremely cold days, it is wise for older adults to exercise indoors. Cold weather can be extremely stressful for individuals with cardiac or respiratory conditions. If older adults must go outside in cold weather, clothing should be layered to trap heat. A mask or scarf worn over the face and mouth helps to warm the air before it enters the respiratory tract.

6. **Review signs and symptoms that necessitate contacting the primary care provider.** Older adults should be aware that any new or unusual pain, weakness, or other untoward symptoms experienced during activity should be reported promptly to the care provider.

7. **Use any appropriate interventions that are used in the institutional setting** (Nursing Care Plan 19.1).

❖ NURSING PROCESS/CLINICAL JUDGMENT MODEL FOR ALTERED ACTIVITY TOLERANCE

When an older adult has altered activity tolerance, that individual has insufficient physiological or psychological energy to accomplish necessary or desired daily activities. Altered activity tolerance is a common problem among older adults who live sedentary lifestyles.

◆ ASSESSMENT (DATA COLLECTION)

Recognize cues:
- Does the person complain of shortness of breath, fatigue, or weakness?
- How much exertion can they tolerate before shortness of breath or fatigue sets in?
- Has participation in normal or routine activities decreased?
- Does the person complain of decreased interest in activities?
- What are their vital signs? Do vital signs remain within normal limits with activity?
- Does the person experience orthostatic hypotension?
- Is their nutritional intake adequate?

See Box 19.3 for a list of risk factors for altered activity tolerance in older adults.

◆ DATA ANALYSIS/PROBLEM IDENTIFICATION

Analyze Cues and Prioritize Hypotheses: Problem statement for older adults with decreased tolerance for activities includes

Altered Activity Tolerance

Nursing Care Plan 19.1 | **Altered Mobility**

Mrs. King, 73 years old, lives at Poplar Bluff Long-Term Care Facility. She, was diagnosed 3 years ago with Parkinson disease. She has bilateral tremors in the upper extremities. She is able to walk but does so very slowly with a rigid, flexed posture. Her coordination and balance are poor. She has experienced occasional falls when ambulating in the hall. She states, "I get tired so easily. My bones and muscles ache all the time, and recently I've noticed that my fingers and toes tingle." The care provider has ordered physical therapy 3 times a week to maintain Mrs. King's strength and flexibility. She participated in a pottery class until recently. She states that these activities are "just too hard for me now."

PROBLEM STATEMENT
Altered Mobility

SUPPORTING ASSESSMENT DATA
- Impaired coordination and balance
- Muscle rigidity
- Altered posture
- Slowed movements
- Tremors

PATIENT GOALS/OUTCOMES IDENTIFICATION
Mrs. King will participate in mobility activities and exercises and maintain mobility at the highest level possible.

NURSING INTERVENTIONS/IMPLEMENTATION
1. Provide passive range-of-motion exercises twice daily.
2. Encourage active range-of-motion exercises whenever possible.
3. Encourage participation in ADLs.
4. Consult with occupational therapy regarding assistive devices for feeding and dressing.
5. Discuss the exercise program with the physical therapist so that exercises can be incorporated into daily routine.
6. Assist with ambulation, using a gait belt.
7. Provide massage for tight muscles.
8. Schedule daily or every-other-day tub baths for muscle relaxation.
9. Encourage continued participation in activities such as music therapy or other relaxing pastimes.
10. Provide positive encouragement for successes.

EVALUATION
Slight tremors are still noted in both arms, and Mrs. King moves slowly but with slightly less rigidity than noted previously. No falls have been reported in the past 2 weeks. She states, "I feel stronger since I've been getting the therapy and doing exercises. I even helped get myself dressed today." You will continue the current plan of care.

APPLYING CLINICAL JUDGMENT
1. What other activities that are appropriate for Mrs. King can you identify?
2. What modifications in the plan of care are likely to be necessary as the disease process progresses?

Box 19.3	**Risk Factors Related to Altered Activity Tolerance in Older Adults**

- Sedentary lifestyle
- Decreased sense of self-worth, self-esteem, or independence
- Generalized weakness, immobility; restriction to bed rest
- Problems related to oxygenation
- Cognitive impairment (Alzheimer disease or dementia)
- Malnourishment

◆ **PLANNING**

Generate Solutions: The patient goals for older adults with altered activity tolerance are to (1) demonstrate an increased ability to tolerate activity and (2) identify factors that contribute to altered activity tolerance.

◆ **IMPLEMENTATION**

Take Action: The following nursing interventions should take place in hospitals or extended-care facilities:

1. **Identify factors that contribute to altered activity tolerance.** People stop participating in physical activity for a variety of reasons. Plan nursing interventions specific to the reason why the participation stopped. For example, an older person who stops participating in activities because of depression after the death of a spouse has a very different problem from that of the person who has altered activity tolerance because of cardiac problems. Some older adults have no real reason for their declining activity levels other than a belief that it is expected and accepted with old age. As they age, older adults become increasingly sedentary and consequently lose functional abilities.

Active Participation in the Plan of Care

Before creating the plan of care for the older adult, the nurse must determine the specific concerns and problems experienced by the individual so that an effective plan of care can be developed.

2. **Identify the activities that older adults view as essential or desirable.** The activities that nurses think are important are often different from those that older adults value. Consult with and include older adults in the planning and structuring of activities. It is easier to motivate people to work toward goals or activities that they consider important.

3. **Plan activities so that older adults can progress from easier activities to those that are more demanding.** Activities should build from least strenuous to most strenuous. Those unable to tolerate low levels of activity must progress slowly, because rapid progression leads to exhaustion, a feeling of failure, loss of motivation, and possible injury. Once mild activities are tolerated, activities that are more physically demanding can be attempted. The pace at which activities are introduced depends on the specific needs and abilities of the individual. Some older adults are able to resume near-normal levels of activity; others always experience some degree of altered activity tolerance.

4. **Encourage older adults to pace their activities throughout the day, alternating periods of activity with periods of rest.** Attempting to do too much in too short a period of time is a common cause of altered activity tolerance in older adults. Older adults often benefit from a planned approach to activity that includes periods of activity and periods of rest. By pacing activities, individuals usually find that they can accomplish more and feel better.

5. **Monitor vital signs to assess the physiological response to activity.** Vital signs are good indicators of the older person's tolerance of activity. Individuals who have been immobile or sedentary may experience significant changes in vital signs with increased activity. Tachycardia is a common occurrence when an activity program is started. An elevated pulse in an older adult takes longer to return to its normal rate than it would in a younger person.

Changes in blood pressure, particularly orthostatic hypotension, may pose safety risks to older adults. Those who are sedentary or have been on bed rest often experience dizziness or light-headedness when changing position, which may result in falls. Changing position more slowly and waiting after each positional change can help to prevent injuries or falls.

6. **Teach methods of conserving energy. Simple modifications in activity can help the older adult conserve energy.** Putting on clothing while sitting requires less energy than doing so while standing. Dressing in clothing with Velcro grips and zippers is less exhausting than dressing in clothing with small buttons or other difficult fasteners. Slip-on shoes require less energy than do laced shoes. Occupational therapists can provide assistance in modifying the environment so that a maximal amount of activity can be performed with a minimal amount of exertion.

7. **Teach older adults and their families methods of reducing stress.** Both psychological and physiological stress place extra demands on the body and decrease the older person's activity tolerance. Methods for reducing stress are discussed in Chapter 13.

The following interventions should take place in the home:

1. **Modify the environment to reduce energy expenditure and promote safety.** All frequently used objects should be readily accessible. Remote controls for the television, stereo, or lights are desirable. Arrange furniture to provide easy access to resting places. Take care to ensure that the environment is safe. Remove hazards such as throw rugs and other clutter on the floor.

2. **Identify family or community resources to assist with energy-intensive activities.** The family should be encouraged to assist the aging person with energy-intensive activities, such as cleaning, cooking, and laundry. If this is not possible, service agencies such as Meals on Wheels may be available.

3. **Use any appropriate interventions that are used in the institutional setting** (see Nursing Care Plan 19.1).

❖ NURSING PROCESS/CLINICAL JUDGMENT MODEL FOR PROBLEMS OF OXYGENATION

To survive, body tissues and organs must have an adequate supply of oxygen. The respiratory and cardiovascular systems work together to meet the oxygen needs of the body. If either system functions inadequately, a variety of physiological changes will be observed.

In general, the aging heart and lungs are able to meet the demands of a normal activity level. However, under conditions of emotional or physical stress, they may not be able to supply the body's physiological needs fully.

◆ ASSESSMENT (DATA COLLECTION)

Recognize cues:
- Does the person experience excessive fatigue?
- What level of activity causes this fatigue?
- Does the person have any complaints of nausea, vomiting, or anorexia?
- Do they complain of dyspnea? Is this worse at any specific time of day, such as during the night?
- Does the person complain of chest pain?

- What is the heart rate? Respiratory rate?
- Is the breathing silent and effortless? If not, describe.
- Does the chest expand evenly with respiration?
- Is the breathing deep or shallow?
- Does the person adopt a posture that is more comfortable for breathing?
- Do they have a cough? Is it productive? Describe the sputum.
- Is there an order for supplemental oxygen?
- Does (or did) the person smoke?
- Is there a history of exposure to air pollution? Secondhand smoke?
- Are any signs of cyanosis present? Is the skin cold, clammy, or diaphoretic?
- Are the jugular veins distended? At what angle (30 degrees, 45 degrees)?
- Are peripheral pulses palpable? Are they equal bilaterally?
- What color are the nail beds and fingers?
- What is the capillary refill time?
- Is there a normal amount of body hair present over the feet and lower legs?
- Does the person experience any leg pain with ambulation? If so, how severe is it? Is it relieved by rest?
- Does the person complain of cold hands and feet?
- Are signs of peripheral edema present?
- Is the urinary output low despite normal fluid intake?
- Has there been a rapid weight gain of more than 10 pounds? Over what period of time?
- Has the person shown signs of confusion?
- Do they complain of anxiety, loss of ability to concentrate, or insomnia?
- Are there any changes in relevant laboratory values (e.g., hemoglobin, hematocrit, cardiac enzymes, and electrolytes)?
- If an electrocardiogram (ECG) was done, what were the findings? Are these different from the baseline ECG?
- If chest radiography was done, are there any signs of heart enlargement or congestion?

Box 19.4 lists risk factors related to altered cardiac output in older adults.

◆ DATA ANALYSIS/PROBLEM IDENTIFICATION

Analyze Cues and Prioritize Hypotheses: Common problem statements for older adults with difficulty with oxygenation may include:

Altered Cardiac Output
Altered Gas Exchange
Alteration in Airway Clearance
Altered Breathing Pattern

◆ PLANNING

Generate Solutions: The patient goals for older individuals with oxygenation problems are to (1) maintain

---

Box 19.4	Risk Factors Related to Altered Cardiac Output in Older Adults

- Arteriosclerotic changes in the blood vessels
- Heart failure
- Myocardial infarction
- Obstructive pulmonary disease
- Increased physiological or psychological stress, including anxiety and pain
- Severe anemia

---

an open, patent airway; (2) exhibit an effective respiratory pattern; (3) experience fewer episodes of dyspnea, angina, and cyanosis; (4) demonstrate an increased activity tolerance; (5) identify methods to reduce physical and psychological stress; and (6) manifest signs of improved cardiac function (e.g., stable vital signs, adequate urinary output, and adequate tissue perfusion).

◆ IMPLEMENTATION

Take Action: The following nursing interventions should take place in hospitals or extended-care facilities:

1. **Assess pulse and respiration before, during, and after activity.** Vital signs are good indicators of activity tolerance. These should be assessed while the individual participates in various levels of activity to determine which specific activities cause the greatest problems. Tachycardia may be a sign of altered cardiac output, although it is an expected sign of increased oxygen demand during vigorous physical activity. To provide more oxygen and blood to the body, the heart beats more rapidly. Once the heart rate is elevated, it takes longer for the heartbeat of older adults to return to a normal resting rate. Consistent tachycardia or an excessive delay in return to a normal rate indicates serious cardiac problems. The respiratory rate should also increase with the heart rate in the body's attempt to meet oxygen needs. With severe cardiac problems, fluid may back up into the pulmonary circulation, interfere with oxygenation, and further stress the heart.

2. **Monitor laboratory values, radiographic reports, and other diagnostic studies.** Laboratory tests, including hematocrit and arterial blood gases, provide information regarding the blood's oxygen carrying capacity. Results of cardiac enzyme studies (e.g., elevated levels of creatinine kinase and troponin) can indicate cardiac damage from a myocardial infarction. Electrolyte levels should be evaluated, particularly if the person is receiving diuretics. Chest radiographs can reveal the presence of pulmonary congestion, which could indicate respiratory tract infection or pulmonary edema. Other diagnostic tests (e.g., ECGs) may reveal pathologic conditions of the heart before other symptoms are obvious. Any abnormal test results

should be reported immediately to the primary care provider.

3. **Observe respiratory effort, including the use of accessory muscles.** An individual who has difficulty breathing appears to labor when breathing. Use of the accessory muscles of the abdomen and shoulders is an indication that the individual is working harder than normal to breathe.

4. **Evaluate oxygenation by observing for signs of cyanosis and checking capillary refill time.** To meet the life-sustaining needs of the body, blood flow to the extremities may be reduced. This results in cold, clammy skin, slow capillary refill time (more than 3 seconds), pallor, and cyanosis. These changes are most often observed in the lips and fingertips. Delayed capillary refill time indicates that blood supply to the extremities is restricted.

5. **Assess the peripheral pulses, particularly in the lower extremities.** Assessment of the peripheral pulses reveals any areas of the body that are not receiving adequate oxygen. The lower extremities are most at risk because of the arteriosclerotic changes of aging. Inadequate oxygen can result in ischemia and necrosis. Mild ischemia can result in hair loss from the lower extremities. Severe ischemia may result in stasis ulcers and in necrosis of the toes, which may necessitate amputation.

6. **Position the person to maximize chest expansion, and encourage frequent changes of position.** Age-related changes tend to reduce the size of the chest cavity. To maximize oxygen exchange, the person should be encouraged to stand or sit in a position that is as upright as possible. Bedridden individuals should change position frequently to prevent stasis and the pooling of respiratory secretions within the lungs.

7. **Clear secretions, and teach effective coughing.** Older adults may find it difficult to cough effectively because of loss of muscle strength and tone. The inability to remove secretions from the respiratory tract can increase the risk for respiratory tract infections. If the older person is very weak and unable to remove secretions, suction may be necessary. When suctioning is performed, care should be taken to avoid excessive stimulation of the respiratory tract, which increases the production of secretions.

8. **Administer medication as ordered to promote cardiovascular and respiratory function.** Medications such as cardiotonics may be ordered to strengthen the pumping ability of the heart. Mucolytics, bronchodilators, and expectorants may be ordered to enhance the person's ability to remove respiratory secretions. Observe all precautions regarding these medications and monitor vital signs closely.

9. **Administer supplemental oxygen as ordered.** Increasing the amount of available oxygen by using supplemental oxygen may make breathing easier.

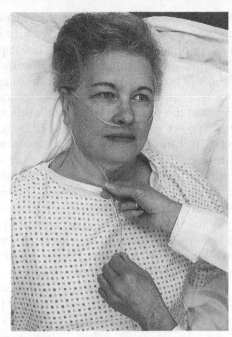

Fig. 19.7 Nasal cannula. (From Potter, P. A., Perry, A. G., Stockert, P. A., & Hall, A. M. [2015]. *Essentials for nursing practice* [8th ed.], St. Louis, MO: Mosby.)

Oxygen should be prescribed by the primary care provider and administered at the prescribed rate. Low doses are normally used because high oxygen concentrations can decrease respiratory effort in some people. Supplemental oxygen is most commonly administered through a nasal cannula (Fig. 19.7). When oxygen is being administered, good care of the nasal passages is essential. Keep the nares free of secretions, and inspect the skin regularly for breakdown where the plastic tubing presses at the nares and over the ears. Post "No Smoking" signs when oxygen is in use.

10. **Use incentive spirometers to improve ventilation.** Incentive spirometers are often ordered to improve respiratory effort. Many older people are unfamiliar with these devices and need clear explanations regarding their use. An older adult who is confused or cognitively impaired may have difficulty performing the correct action with the incentive spirometer. Some older adults find these devices unpleasant and may avoid using them. Reinforce the importance of these devices and encourage the patient to use them at regular intervals.

11. **Assess for the presence, location, and duration of pain.** Pain that occurs during activity should be assessed and reported. Determine the location and severity of the pain as well as whether it radiates or stays in one area. Ask if the pain occurs during an activity or afterward. Anginal pain originates in the heart and occurs when the heart muscle is deprived of oxygen because of coronary artery narrowing or increased oxygen demand. This pain classically starts in the upper left chest

and radiates down the left arm. In some individuals, the pain is referred to the jaw; jaw pain of a cardiac origin can exist without the chest pain in some people, such as women, people with diabetes, and older adults. Coronary vasodilators, such as nitroglycerin, are used to improve blood flow and decrease the pain. Intermittent claudication is a specific type of pain that is described by some as cramping, tightness, or aching. This pain is most commonly in the foot or calf, but it may extend to the thigh or buttock. It typically occurs during activity and disappears with rest. Intermittent claudication is an indication of inadequate oxygen supply to the tissues of the leg, and the pain is a result of ischemia. Most care providers recommend daily walking for 60 minutes, pausing when pain occurs. Any activity that causes vasoconstriction (e.g., smoking) must be stopped. Cold environments should also be avoided because cold further aggravates the condition.

QSEN Considerations: Patient-Centered Care

Pain Relief

Nurses can improve a patient's participation in activities by providing adequate pain relief beforehand. It is important for the nurse to understand that each patient has different expectations when it comes to pain relief.

12. **Administer sedatives and analgesic medications with caution.** Many sedatives and analgesics affect the rate or depth of respiration. Assess and document respiratory rate and depth before administering these medications to verify that the initial rate is adequate for safety. Assess and document respirations again after administration.

13. **Maintain a calm, restful environment, and provide emotional support.** Stress places additional demands for oxygen on the body. A calm, restful environment decreases the effects of stress. Decreasing the number of interruptions, closing doors, playing soft music, or making other environmental changes may benefit an individual who is experiencing stress. If the stress is severe or if it is made worse by interaction with unpleasant roommates, a private room may be medically indicated. Take time to listen to the concerns of older adults so as to reduce their stress.

14. **Explain stress reduction techniques.** Stress can be controlled by means of nonmedical interventions, including meditation, guided imagery, biofeedback, and relaxation techniques. These techniques are particularly helpful to older adults because they enable individuals to control their own behavior and lack the side effects of antianxiety medications.

15. **Promote good fluid and nutritional intake within medical restrictions.** Adequate fluid intake keeps respiratory secretions liquefied, making them easier to expectorate. If the older person has heart failure or other disease processes that lead to fluid retention, it is important to give fluids with caution and assess for signs of fluid overload.

Nutritional Considerations

Adequate nutrition, particularly adequate iron intake, is essential for the production of adequate hemoglobin, which is necessary for oxygen transport.

The following interventions should take place in the home:

1. **Explain how to use oxygen equipment safely.** If oxygen is required, teach the older adult and family safety precautions related to its use. Also teach them how to operate the equipment. Patient education should include the reasons that smoking and open flames are dangerous. All people having contact with the oxygen should be familiar with the various modalities of home oxygen use and should know the proper precautions to take when handling oxygen tanks and equipment (Fig. 19.8). They should know how to verify that adequate oxygen is available and who to call if any equipment problems arise (Box 19.5). A power outage may present a problem to individuals who use an oxygen concentrator. The older adult must keep a backup tank

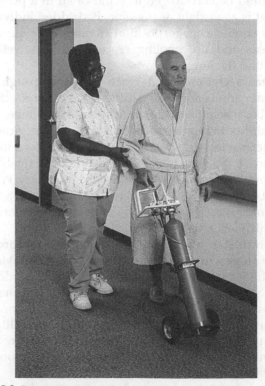

Fig. 19.8 Portable oxygen cylinder used during ambulation. (From Kostelnick, C. [2020]. *Mosby's textbook for long-term care nursing assistants* [8th ed.]. St. Louis, MO: Mosby.)

| Box 19.5 | **Home Oxygen Systems** |

LIQUID OXYGEN

Portable[a] unit can be refilled by patient from reservoir. A portable unit holds 6 to 8 hours of supply at 2 L/min; reservoir will last approximately 7 to 10 days at 2 L/min when used continuously. Patients normally do not use the reservoir continuously because of the expense. Instead, patients use the oxygen (O_2) concentrator because the cost is much lower. Liquid systems are strictly for portable and emergency use. They are not available everywhere but generally limited to urban areas.

COMPRESSED O_2 CYLINDERS

Cylinders or tanks come in various sizes (e.g., D, M, E, H, and J). Their duration varies with tank size and liter flow (e.g., a J tank at 2 L/min flow lasts about 50 hours). Portability is possible with a cart, and some of the smaller tanks may be refilled from large cylinders. Smaller tanks weighing about 10 pounds can be carried on a shoulder strap, in a backpack, or in a fanny pack, or they may be carried or placed in a portable cart.

CONCENTRATOR OR EXTRACTOR

Because the O_2 supply is produced from room air, these devices never need to be "filled." They are typically on wheels and are movable from room to room, but they are usually kept centrally located in the dwelling with extension tubing reaching to the furthest area. Patients need to be very cautious to prevent falling over the tubing. This is a compact, excellent system for rural or homebound patients. It is convenient, safe, and reliable. The patient will need a backup O_2 tank in case the electricity fails. The concentrator noise may be bothersome; therefore it should be kept in a room other than the bedroom.

PORTABLE OXYGEN CONCENTRATOR

These are lighter-weight devices (8.5 to 17 pounds) that are portable via carts or shoulder straps. They may provide pulsed or continuous O_2 flow of 5 to 6 L/min depending on the particular device. Batteries provide up to 8 hours of operation with recharging via AC or DC (e.g., in a car), and they are approved by most airlines. This combined with another stationary system in the patient's dwelling provides the patient with exceptional freedom and mobility, as the system continuously provides a renewable source of O_2 outside the home. Commercial brands include EverGo, Inogen One, and Eclipse Oxygen Generator.

O_2-CONSERVING OR PULSED DEVICES

These deliver a pulse of O_2 only during inhalation, which conserves O_2. They give the patient better mobility as the devices are relatively light in weight, varying from approximately 3 to 6 pounds with a supply of O_2 up to 20 hours. Such a system may clip onto a belt or be contained in a backpack or shoulder bag. The audible pulses may be annoying, and some devices may require batteries. They becomes less efficient at higher O_2 flow rates and are usually best for low activity levels. The patient's O_2 saturation should be monitored during rest and exercise to determine whether the level of oxygenation is acceptable.

[a]*Portable* usually refers to units weighing more than 10 pounds (4.5 kilograms) and *ambulatory* units weighing less than 10 pounds.
Modified from Lewis, S.L., Dirkson, S.R., Heitkemper, M.M., Bucher, L., & Camera, I.M. (2011). *Medical-surgical nursing* (8th ed.). St. Louis, MO: Mosby.

of oxygen for use in such an emergency as well as a portable oxygen concentrator with several charged batteries. It is also wise to notify the power company in advance that the resident needs to have power returned quickly. Persons needing oxygen or other medical equipment are usually a priority for power companies.

2. **Explain the signs and symptoms of possible complications and the measures to take if these occur.** Teach older adults and their families the signs and symptoms of a change in condition that may indicate complications. The telephone number of the care provider and emergency services should be prominently displayed next to the telephone or stored in their smartphones so that help can be summoned rapidly if needed.

3. **Use any appropriate interventions that are used in the institutional setting.**

❖ NURSING PROCESS/CLINICAL JUDGMENT MODEL FOR ALTERED SELF-CARE ABILITY

When a person is partially or totally restricted in the ability to perform the most basic ADLs (i.e., bathing, dressing, grooming, eating, and toileting), their ability to manage self-care is altered. With advancing age or the onset of disease, many individuals experience some degree of difficulty with self-care. Problems related to self-care can be devastating to older adults because of their effect on self-esteem. People who cannot meet these needs become dependent on others and lose much control over the most basic elements of their lives. Older adults who cannot feed themselves must eat what they are fed. Those who cannot dress themselves must wear what another person chooses. Those who cannot bathe or groom themselves are only as clean and well-groomed as another person makes possible. Those who cannot go to the bathroom alone are likely to become incontinent. Nurses must be able to recognize the individual's specific difficulties and degree of limitation with self-care so that appropriate nursing interventions can be planned. These interventions should be directed toward maintaining the individual's functioning at the highest possible level. The previously discussed concepts of rehabilitation form the basis for working with older individuals with altered self-care ability.

◆ ASSESSMENT (DATA COLLECTION)

Recognize cues:
* Can the person feed themself? If not, what level of assistance is required (0–4)?
  0 = Completely independent
  1 = Requires devices or equipment
  2 = Requires help, supervision, or teaching from another person
  3 = Requires devices and help from another person
  4 = Is totally dependent

Box 19.6	Risk Factors Related to Altered Self-Care Ability in Older Adults

- Decreased strength or endurance resulting from respiratory or cardiovascular changes
- Altered neuromuscular or musculoskeletal function related to disease or aging
- Pain
- Cognitive or perceptual problems (Alzheimer disease or dementia)
- Severe anxiety or depression
- Mobility limitations

- Can the person toilet themself? If not, what level of assistance is required (0–4)?
- Can the person bathe themself? If not, what level of assistance is required (0–4)?
- Can the person dress themself? If not, what level of assistance is required (0–4)?

Box 19.6 lists risk factors for altered self-care ability in older adults.

◆ DATA ANALYSIS/PROBLEM IDENTIFICATION

Analyze Cues and Prioritize Hypotheses: Problem statements for older adults with altered self-care abilities include

Altered Self-Care Ability: Feeding
Altered Self-Care Ability: Bathing
Altered Self-Care Ability: Dressing
Altered Self-Care Ability: Toileting

◆ PLANNING

Generate Solutions: The patient goals for older individuals with altered self-care ability are to (1) perform self-care at the highest possible level within limitations, (2) demonstrate the use of modified techniques and assistive devices to accomplish self-care, (3) verbalize improved self-esteem related to self-care ability, and (4) identify the resources available to provide assistance.

◆ IMPLEMENTATION

Take Action: The following nursing interventions should take place in hospitals or extended-care facilities:

1. Assess the individual to determine the factors that cause or contribute to the altered self-care ability, such as age-related changes, disease processes, medications, and cognitive or perceptual changes. Each aging individual presents a unique set of problems to which nurses must respond when planning care. Unless the specific needs of each person are identified, the plan of care is meaningless. Some individuals are able to regain many skills and become less dependent; others remain at lower levels of function. A thorough assessment covers the person's strengths and limitations so that the most appropriate care plan can be developed.
2. Include older adults in problem identification and care planning. A plan that does not include the individual is likely to fail. Overcoming an altered self-care ability requires the person's total commitment and cooperation. The only way nurses can hope to ensure this level of commitment is by including the older person in the entire process.

💬 Communication

If the older adult is unable to communicate verbally, nurses should observe nonverbal communication. Many individuals who cannot express their needs verbally will respond to simple directions and positive encouragement.

3. **Allow adequate time for the completion of activities.** With aging, even healthy, active persons require more time than younger individuals to accomplish a task. Those experiencing altered self-care ability require even more time than older adults who are well. Most facilities and nurses are geared toward getting things done as quickly as possible. In many facilities, older individuals who are perfectly capable of completing self-care activities are not allowed to do so because it would take too long. This practice is in direct opposition to those of the rehabilitative focus. Encouraging and allowing older adults to perform self-care does take more time than having the care provided by the nursing staff. This fact must be taken into consideration when decisions regarding staffing and assignments are made so that adequate time will be available. If these adjustments are not made, any chance of success will be undermined.
4. **Develop a plan that moves in stages toward the highest possible level of function, and give positive feedback to reinforce positive changes.** The plan to increase self-care ability should be structured in stages so that the individual will be able to achieve some successes. If too much is expected, the individual may become frustrated and give up. It is better to work toward and build on small successes. For example, if the person has not been performing any personal hygiene, successfully washing the face would be a major accomplishment. Successes of this nature should not be ignored but should be reinforced by a comment, such as, "You did a good job of washing your face." Use a simple checklist to enable the person to see that they are making progress. Reinforcing the positives while minimizing the negatives is the best way to achieve the desired goals and increase motivation.
5. **Consult with occupational and physical therapists to identify alternative methods and equipment that would most benefit the individual.** Occupational and physical therapists are specialists in rehabilitation. They have extensive knowledge of the techniques and equipment available to improve self-care ability. Modification of an activity (such as sitting instead of standing) may enable an

individual to perform self-care activities (Fig. 19.9). Modified clothing or eating utensils may mean the difference between complete dependence and independence.

6. **Modify the environment with assistive devices designed to meet the specific needs of the individual.** Once the need for special assistive devices has been identified, make certain that these devices are available (Figs. 19.10 and 19.11). Identifying the need for a toilet riser, grip rail, or special spoon does no good if the item is not available. The staff may have to wash special eating utensils so that they don't get lost. Residents sharing a bathroom may have to adjust to the presence of a toilet riser.

They must either use the riser or be willing and able to remove and replace it when they use the toilet. In some situations, modification of the environment with assistive devices may necessitate room changes so that individuals with common needs are grouped together.

The following interventions should take place in the home:

1. **Assess the ability of the family or significant others to provide safe care.** Today, many totally dependent older adults are being cared for in the home setting. Nurses may make regular visits, but much of the responsibility for care falls on spouses or other family members. These caregivers may have little

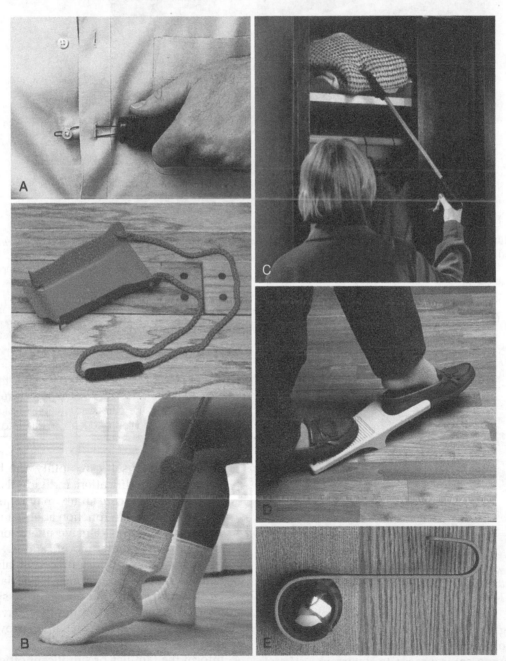

Fig. 19.9 **A,** A button hook is used to button and zip clothing. **B,** A sock assist is used to pull on socks and stockings. **C,** "Reachers" are helpful to remove items from high shelves. **D,** A shoe remover is used to take off shoes. **E,** A doorknob turner increases leverage to help turn the knob.
(A–C, E, Courtesy Northcoast Medical Inc., Morgan Hill, CA. D, Courtesy AbilityOne Corporation, Germantown, WI.)

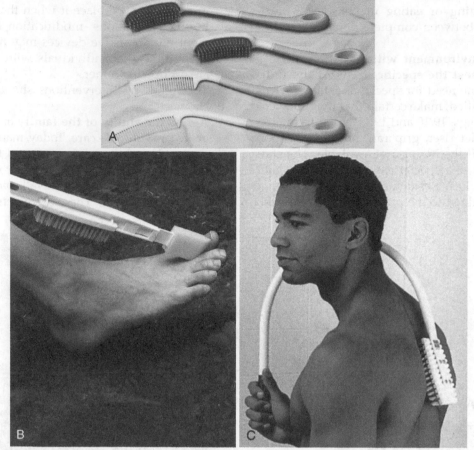

Fig. 19.10 A, Long-handled combs and brushes for hair care. **B,** Long-handled brushes for bathing. **C,** Brush with a curved handle.
(A–B, Courtesy Northcoast Medical Inc., Morgan Hill, CA. C, Courtesy Sammons Preston: An AbilityOne Company, Bolingbrook,)

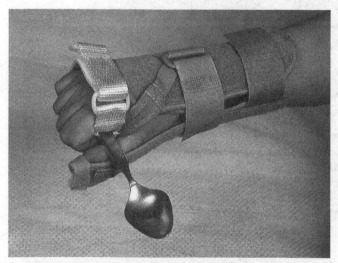

Fig. 19.11 Eating device attached to a splint. (From Kostelnick, C. [2020]. *Mosby's textbook for long-term care nursing assistants* [8th ed.]. St. Louis, MO: Mosby.)

or no training for the tasks involved. Often, the caregiver is also older or debilitated.

2. Assess the home environment to determine safety and the need for modifications such as grip rails, bath chairs, or toilet risers. Depending on the level

> **Family Teaching**
>
> Nurses are responsible for ensuring that no harm comes from the home care situation. If the care needs exceed the ability of the caregivers, nurses may have to contact other family members or social services to ensure the older individual's safety. If the caregiver is capable of providing care, they may need additional education related to providing care.

of alteration of self-care ability, the home may require major modification. Individuals with minimal alteration in self-care ability may require only a few assistive devices to function adequately (Fig. 19.12). Those with more extensive alterations in self-care ability require greater modifications.

3. Identify community resources available to help obtain the necessary equipment. Special assistive devices can be costly and may require special skill for installation. Many communities have agencies or volunteer groups that can help to provide the necessary assistance.

4. Inform the families or significant others of the need to allow older adults to do as much as possible for themselves. Family members are often too helpful

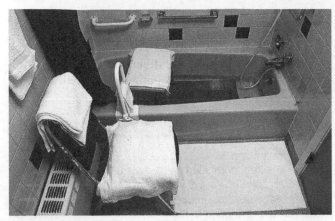

Fig. 19.12 Bathtub with grab bars. (From Sorrentino, S. A., & Gorek, B. [2003]. *Mosby's textbook for long-term care assistants* [4th ed.]. St. Louis, MO: Mosby.)

and do not expect older individuals to do anything for themselves, which can lead to a loss of functional ability. Teach the family the importance of allowing and encouraging aging individuals to do as much as possible on their own. Stress that this is the best thing caregivers can do for their loved ones and that they are not being thoughtless or neglectful in enabling it.

5. Discuss respite care and other options with caregivers. People who provide long-term care in the home place themselves at risk for both physical injury and psychological distress. Home care is often exhausting for the caregivers. Discuss the possibility of some form of respite care so that caregivers will be able to maintain their own health and mental well-being.

6. Assist the family with arrangements for hospitalization or extended-care placement. When the aging individual becomes completely dependent, the spouse or family may have to consider alternative methods of providing care. This is a very difficult topic, both financially and emotionally. Nurses may be able to provide some guidance or to contact other social service agencies that can help the family through this difficult process.

7. Use any appropriate interventions that are used in the institutional setting (see Nursing Care Plan 19.1).

❖ NURSING PROCESS/CLINICAL JUDGMENT MODEL FOR DEFICIENT DIVERSIONAL ACTIVITY

Diversional activities play an important role in the lives of older adults. Diversional activities can help to pass the time and to provide creative outlets, particularly when they are meaningful to the older person. Older adults are especially at risk for loneliness and depression from the lack of social interaction due to the COVID-19 pandemic. The role of the nurse may include teaching the older adult how to use video conferencing apps such as Zoom and Skype in order to remain connected with friends and family while also protecting themselves from exposure to the virus.

◆ ASSESSMENT (DATA COLLECTION)

Recognize cues:
- What activities does the person enjoy?
- How often do they participate in these activities?
- Does the person prefer solitary or social activities?
- How much time do they spend alone? With others?
- Does the person interact with other individuals? With whom? How often?
- Can the person interact with others through Zoom, Skype, or other conferencing apps?
- Can the person undertake the usual hobbies/activities in the present setting?
- Can the person afford, financially, to participate in the activities they enjoy?
- Is the person able to get to the desired activities? Is transportation required?
- Do sensory or cognitive changes interfere with pursuing their interests?
- Do physical changes interfere with pursuing their interests?
- Is the person napping because of boredom? If so, how often?
- What is their psychological state of mind (e.g., are they depressed)?

Box 19.7 lists risk factors for deficient diversional activity in older adults.

◆ DATA ANALYSIS/PROBLEM IDENTIFICATION

Analyze Cues and Prioritize Hypotheses: Problem statements for older adults experiencing a deficit of diversional activities include

Deficient Diversional Activity

◆ PLANNING

Generate Solutions: The patient goals for older individuals with deficient diversional activity are to (1) identify activities that might be of interest, (2) express interest in participating in diversional activities, (3) participate in selected diversional activities, and (4) demonstrate socially acceptable behaviors while participating in activities.

Box 19.7	Risk Factors Related to Deficient Diversional Activities in Older Adults

- Restricted mobility
- An environment with limited activities
- Anxiety, depression, or grief
- Limited financial or transportation resources
- Cognitive or perceptual problems

◆ IMPLEMENTATION

Take Action: The following nursing interventions should take place in hospitals and extended-care facilities:

1. **Assess current and past hobbies, activities, and interests.** The best way to prepare for a good old age is to have as many interests as possible when one is young. Young adults are so busy raising families and working that they often neglect to develop and nurture hobbies or interests outside of family and work. Individuals who have developed a wide range of interests seem to adjust to aging better than those with few interests. After their families have grown and they have retired from work, many men and women finally get the opportunity to participate in favorite hobbies and activities. Some older adults have a steady stream of activities that keep their days full. Others complain of boredom. Lack of interests and diversions makes time seem to pass slowly and may lead to depression and social isolation.

2. **Include the individual in selecting and planning diversional activities.** Older adults should have the right to choose the activities they find most meaningful. Purposeful activity is good for maintaining self-esteem; busywork is not. Older adults who reside in extended-care facilities because of illness or infirmity may have fewer opportunities and diversions available. Nurses can help these individuals maintain active interests by exploring those activities that they had enjoyed at an earlier age. The nurse's interest and a little creativity can go a long way toward meeting the social and diversional needs of older adults.

3. **Provide suitable reading materials, such as large-print books or audiobooks.** Many older persons enjoy books but are not able to read because of visual changes. Books with large print may be usable and are available through most libraries. If visual impairments are severe, audiobooks can be downloaded to book readers and smartphones.

4. **Focus on what the individual can do rather than on what they cannot do.** Successes, even small ones, are likely to lead to more successes. It is often depressing to older adults to focus on activities in which they can no longer engage. Directing their attention to accomplishments can help them to maintain a more positive attitude.

5. **Suggest activities that are occurring in the facility, such as music or discussion groups, occupational therapy, activity therapy, or religious activities.** Many older adults are not able to leave the care setting to participate in offered activities. Physical or economic changes may interfere with normal diversional activities. Hospitalization or a change in living accommodations can lead to a variety of restrictions and inconveniences. Nurses can help individuals maintain social contacts and interests by exploring other activities. Occupational and activity therapists may suggest activities and provide assistance in learning new skills. Activity and occupational therapy are provided in most residential care settings. Therapists can help individuals learn new activities or ways to modify existing interests. For example, if physical changes make knitting too difficult, lap weaving may be possible. Music therapy provides another form of diversion and allows individuals to express their feelings nonverbally.

QSEN Considerations: Evidence-Based Practice

Music Therapy

Music is often combined with exercise because rhythm seems to enhance activity. Interestingly, people unable to speak because of a stroke can sometimes sing beautifully because different parts of the brain are involved. This author once developed a routine of singing with a stroke patient during morning care. The smile on the resident's face once he realized that he could sing words was priceless!

6. **Work with the activities department to plan new or different activities based on patient input.** Many facilities tend to fall into habits or patterns of repeating the same activities. Many older adults are very creative and should have input into decision making. Some facilities are progressive and offer a variety of activities; others do not. Nurses play a more important role in this department of extended-care facilities and home care than in acute care settings.

7. **Encourage social interaction among residents with similar interests.** People of all ages find shared activities enjoyable. Those who share common interests are more likely to want to spend time together (Fig. 19.13).

8. **Spend time with individuals to demonstrate interest in their personal pursuits.** We all need to know that we are special. Even a few minutes spent with an older person will help nurses know that person better and will elicit responses that are more personal. Commenting on older adults' latest craft projects or asking how they are enjoying a television show demonstrates interest and caring.

9. **Change the physical environment to increase stimulation and interest (e.g., use of bulletin boards of currently scheduled activities, seasonal themes, and flyers about topics of interest).** Lack of stimulation can lead to loss of interest and disengagement from others. Any device that helps to maintain interest and contact with the rest of society will help the aging person remain alert and interested.

10. **Enlist the help of volunteers to read, play games, or just talk with residents.** There is not enough time for nursing staff to meet the needs of all the patients in an institution. Many groups—such as Scouts, social clubs, and school groups—are interested in providing community service. Volunteering to work with older adults is a very rewarding activity. The resulting intergenerational mix can be a learning experience for both old and young.

11. **Display the results of residents' activities in a prominent place, and give recognition to all**

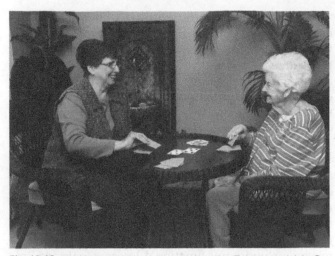

Fig. 19.13 Residents enjoying a game of cards. (From Kostelnick, C. [2020]. *Mosby's textbook for long-term care nursing assistants* [8th ed.]. St. Louis, MO: Mosby.)

participants. Displaying what residents have created (e.g., craft work, creative writing, and other achievements) recognizes their accomplishments and enables the staff and visitors to realize that creativity and productivity do not end with old age.

12. **Explore the possibility of new activities, such as pet therapy, to stimulate interest of withdrawn individuals.** Pet therapy is becoming increasingly common. The benefits of association with animals have been documented in many studies. Older individuals who have pets are healthier and able to live longer than do those without pets. Institutionalized individuals, even those who have isolated themselves from most human contact, seem to respond to the unquestioning affection given by animals. Some residential care centers have pets that live in the home (Fig. 19.14).

13. **Ensure that an individual's physical needs are met before and during diversional activities.** Make sure assistance is available for toileting, snacks, and transfers. Many older adults with

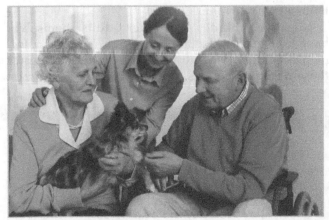

Fig. 19.14 Pets can be a great comfort to older adults. (From Webb, M., Kostelnick, C., & Scott, K. [2018]. *Long-term caring* [4th ed.]. St. Louis, MO: Elsevier.)

physical deficits are reluctant to leave their rooms or care units because of fear. Many are afraid that they will not get to a bathroom in time and will embarrass themselves. Others are afraid that no one will be available to help them move from place to place or meet other physical challenges. Make certain there is adequate help to meet physical care needs before and during activities. Provide older adults the opportunity to use the toilet before leaving the care unit and at regular intervals during the activities. Even diversional activities require increased energy expenditure, so snacks should be made available that are in keeping with the prescribed meal plans.

The following interventions should take place in the home:

1. Provide information regarding community resources for older adults, including senior citizen centers, libraries, museums, and volunteer activities. Many senior citizen centers offer a variety of craft programs, including painting, weaving, woodworking, and pottery. Participation in these activities may provide exposure to crafts that the individual never had the opportunity to try before. Some individuals discover real talents that they never suspected they had. Travelogs, movies, or speakers on topics of current interest help older adults maintain an interest in world events. Activity centers can provide an opportunity for social interaction and a chance to meet new friends and reduce the sense of isolation. Some senior citizen centers also offer classes in subject, such as foreign languages, history, and computer skills. Some colleges have special programs that offer free, noncredit courses to older adults as long as they are not already full. The older adult benefits from the stimulation of the course, and the younger students benefit from the different perspective of the older individual. Road Scholar (Elder Hostel) is a program through which older adults can travel around the world by staying in hostels and expanding their knowledge. There are many volunteer opportunities for older adults, including being a foster grandparent, working as a docent/tour guide, volunteering in one's former profession, or helping with literacy programs, the work of a humane society, or disaster relief.

2. Identify community resources that provide transportation to desired activities. Lack of transportation is a common cause for social isolation and failure to participate in activities. Many communities have special programs that provide buses or vans to transport older adults to shopping centers or activities for a nominal fee. Research these services, and assist the older adult with making contact if they are hesitant to call for help. Once you guide someone the first time, it will be easier for them to use the service for future occasions.

3. Encourage participation in new and meaningful activities and interests. Many older adults need encouragement to explore new interests and seek new possible diversional activities. Many are interested in participating in new activities but are afraid to try them because of their age. They often fear that others will not accept them or will laugh at their inexperience. Provide information that will familiarize the person with the activity beforehand. Knowledge about the activity can reduce fear of the unknown. Exploration of past successes in facing new or different challenges may provide the necessary encouragement to try something new.

4. Assist with setting up conferencing apps or other tools for online interactions. In order to protect older adults during a pandemic or local infectious disease outbreak, it may be necessary to avoid face-to-face interactions with friends and family. Teaching the older adult how to connect with loved ones in an online platform may help decrease the feelings of social isolation and loneliness.

5. Use any appropriate interventions that are used in the institutional setting.

REHABILITATION

Our attitudes affect our expectations, and our expectations affect our plans. If caregivers do not expect much from older adults, they will not get much; if caregivers keep their expectations high, much is possible.

The attitudes held by nurses regarding aging and older adults have a significant impact on their planning of nursing care. Attitudes about the value of older persons and their potential for leading active, meaningful lives influence the priorities, goals, and interventions that nurses select during the planning process. Attitudes also influence the extent to which nurses include and involve older adults in the planning process.

Low expectations for older adults lead to a low level, or custodial, focus in care planning. High expectations of older adults lead to a high level, or rehabilitative, focus.

NEGATIVE ATTITUDES: THE CONTROLLING OR CUSTODIAL FOCUS

Nurses who take a negative view of aging see aging as a process of deterioration and loss. With this negative perspective, older adults are viewed as helpless, passive, dependent, and incapable of making decisions regarding their own care. Nurses who have these negative attitudes generally see little potential for improvement in older adults. Although this may be true for a small percentage of older adults, it is not the norm.

If nurses have predetermined that older adults are incapable of making their wishes known or that they are not interested in what happens, then the nurses will not consider older adults' input important or necessary for care planning. Preferences or desires often go unnoticed merely because the nurse chose not to listen to verbal or nonverbal communication.

Once nurses predict or anticipate little potential for improvement, their expectations are kept low. With a negative attitude toward aging and older adults, priority is given to slowing the process of physical deterioration. Maintenance of function is supported, but no improvement or higher level of functioning is expected or encouraged. Little if any attempt is made to reverse or undo any functional losses. Goals are limited to maintaining the existing level of function, or the status quo.

With maintenance as the goal, the care plan is often limited to physiological and safety concerns. In general, according to Maslow (1943), interventions address the lowest level of needs. Older adults are kept clean, groomed, clothed, and fed. Basic elimination needs are met. Accommodations are clean and reasonably comfortable. Medications are administered and treatments performed. However, higher level needs—such as security, love, and a sense of belonging—are minimized or ignored.

Nurses then control all aspects of the planning process and take total responsibility for determining what is best for the older person. The care plan requires the nurse to be active and the older adult to be passive. By its very nature, this type of care plan promotes helplessness, loss of function, and dependence. Little is expected; even less is achieved. A few older adults are severely impaired and have experienced a profound loss of mental and physical capabilities because of aging and disease. Some are so severely affected that they are truly unable to communicate their wishes or do anything for themselves. However, it is amazing how much even severely impaired persons can and will communicate about their care, often nonverbally, if nurses pay attention.

Negative attitudes that older adults themselves have may lead to declining function. They may feel helpless, hopeless, or afraid to try. If nurses reinforce these negative feelings, nothing positive will occur.

Clinical Situation

If functional losses are so severe that the person is unaware of reality or is absolutely unable to function, then and only then should all needs be anticipated and provided by nurses or other caregivers. However, this determination should not be made quickly. Many seemingly hopeless and helpless older adults have more ability and potential than we give them credit for. Often, the potential remains hidden because we do not expect to find it.

Older adults who have potential for improvement but are given only custodial care are likely to lose hope. Loss of the will to fight and of the ability to strive for something better is the most destructive attitude.

POSITIVE ATTITUDES: THE REHABILITATIVE FOCUS

When nurses have a positive attitude toward aging and believe that older adults are able and willing to participate in their care, the outcome is very different. These nurses recognize that, as older adults experience the normal physiological changes of aging or the impact of disease, they are more likely to require nursing care. This care may be given in the home, in the hospital, or in an extended-care facility. Nurses who have a positive attitude toward aging recognize that older adults often have a great deal of unused and unrecognized potential. Consider the following anecdote:

Clinical Situation

Diana, a nursing instructor at a long-term care facility, was checking on her students' assignments when she met a resident who had had several strokes. His health record read "dementia; cannot speak or understand." Diana began reading the greeting cards above the resident's bed. He had been a highly decorated colonel in the military. There were letters from soldiers formerly under his command and cards from world dignitaries. When the resident noticed Diana reading his memorabilia, he stared at her. Diana decided to assume that he could understand and chose to speak to the man he had been before the strokes, saying, "on behalf of the families of your soldiers ... thank you for putting yourself in danger to keep their sons safe. They have no idea what it cost you when you couldn't." To Diana's astonishment, he clearly and quietly replied, "thank you." The following week, Diana dropped off a book about the war in which Col. X. had served; he later returned it to her without saying anything. When she placed it in her bookshelf, however, the flap of the dust jacket was positioned halfway through the book; not how she had left it. Had he placed it there intentionally? The following week, she brought a different book written by a soldier who had made several mistakes during his time in the war. When Col. X. returned it to Diana at the end of the day, he said, "They promoted him too quickly and he never learned from his mistakes." This man, previously "written off" by caregivers, could read, think, understand, critique, and speak quite clearly, and had evaluated the young soldier through the eyes of a commanding officer.

Why did the nurses underestimate Col. X.'s cognitive abilities? Is it possible that when we expect very little from someone, they deliver very little? Did Diana's "breakthrough" occur because she had spoken to him on the assumption that he could understand her whereas others perhaps had not?

Nurses with a positive attitude toward aging recognize that most older adults want to retain control of their lives. A rehabilitative care focus addresses both true and potential problems older adults are likely to experience. A nurse with a rehabilitative focus does not wait until problems occur. It is a proactive approach to planning that deals with the prevention of problems, not just reactions to them. Always speak to someone as if they were able to understand you, even if you believe they may not.

QSEN Considerations: Patient-Centered Care

Active Involvement of the Older Adult

All older adults benefit from a rehabilitative focus in care planning. To plan care with a rehabilitative focus, nurses must (1) acknowledge that older adults have intrinsic worth greater than their limitations; (2) accept that older adults have the right to make informed decisions regarding their care; (3) recognize that loss of function or disability has a serious impact on older adults, their families, and significant others; and (4) recognize that older adults, their families, and significant others are important members of the health care team and should play a role in decision making.

The long-term goal of rehabilitative nursing care is to help older adults achieve and maintain maximal physical, psychosocial, and spiritual health. When planning care with a focus on rehabilitation, nurses must (1) attempt to prevent complications of physical disability, restore optimal functioning, and help the individual adjust to alterations in lifestyle; (2) attempt to minimize the impact of physical changes or disease processes that interrupt or alter functioning and life satisfaction; (3) focus on maintaining the highest achievable level of independent function; (4) provide for comfort needs and adjustments in lifestyle that are conducive to health; (5) support the ability of older adults to adapt to change; (6) help older adults reestablish and maintain control over their lives; and (7) work to reduce the impact of societal factors that restrict the older adult's ability to maintain independence.

Under these guiding principles, nurses work with older adults and establish priorities based not on the nurse's values but on the older adult's values. It is vital for nurses in acute care settings to avoid neglecting the rehabilitative focus while focusing on more urgent medical problems. If the older adult is discharged from acute care in a less independent state than they were admitted, unless it is directly related to the reason for hospitalization (e.g., hip fracture), a disservice has been done to that person. Establish goals with the older adult that are challenging yet realistic. In the plan of care, select and communicate those nursing interventions that are most likely to help these persons achieve their goals.

When a formal meeting is held in a hospital or extended-care facility, it is commonly referred to as a *staffing*. Regular reviews of the care plan are scheduled in order to determine whether modifications are necessary. Information should be shared by all concerned

QSEN Considerations: Teamwork and Collaboration

When planning care with a rehabilitative focus, look beyond the nursing interventions and act as coordinator for all of the various disciplines that enable the older adult to achieve the highest level of physical, mental, psychosocial, and spiritual functioning. Seek input from a wide range of specialists, including physicians, pharmacists, dietitians, physical therapists, occupational therapists, speech therapists, activity therapists, dentists, podiatrists, chaplains, and social workers. For older individuals residing in their own homes, consider the environmental impact of the surroundings and the community services available.

All of these specialists, along with the older adult and the family, should have input into the development of the care plan.

parties and communicated clearly. Clearly document interventions in enough detail so all parties will be aware of their roles. Remind older adults of their right to change or modify the plan of care.

A rehabilitation focus is not limited to the care provided in institutional settings. Rehabilitation is also directed toward improving or maintaining the ability of disabled older adults to function in society. Like other healthy, capable adults, nurses are often unaware of environmental barriers that prevent the disabled from accessing goods and services. Box 19.8 provides a

good way of assessing the world through the eyes of a disabled person. Nurses who believe that older adults have the desire and ability to maintain high-level function at home and in the community must become social activists and work to make others aware of the needs of the disabled. Much work is needed to make the everyday world accessible to them.

I have traveled extensively with my 89-year-old mother-in-law, along with her wheelchair and oxygen; I can attest to an enormous range in accessibility throughout the world. We found a shortage of elevators in restaurants in France, and at an American ski resort, we followed the signage for "wheelchair route" to the outdoor café, only to hear the door close and lock behind us, leaving us on an actual ski run! Other cities, such as London, do incredibly well. We cut the queue and were escorted onto the London Eye in record time. We were immediately seated at a popular new restaurant while others were turning back because of the long wait time (we felt guilty about that). We toured Buckingham Palace and were directed to have our taxi driver deliver us to a private entrance; at the end of our tour, we were taken to a special gift shop, with items placed at a lower level where someone in a wheelchair could properly view them! Touring with my mother-in-law certainly made me look at the accessibility of the world very differently.

Patricia Williams

Box 19.8 Accessibility of Public Places

The term *accessible* means that public transportation and public places (as well as objects therein) are approachable and usable by someone with a physical disability. The following questions can be used as a guideline to help determine accessibility:

- Does public transportation allow entry and appropriate space for people who use wheelchairs?
- Do streets have crosswalk signals for people with vision loss?
- Does the facility have access to someone who can use sign language?
- Are there parking spaces reserved for the disabled? If so, are these parking spaces clearly marked with the access symbol on a raised sign?
- Is there an unobstructed path from the parking area to the curb cut to the building entrance or event area?
- If the front door is not at ground level, are there alternative entrances (e.g., ramp, side door at ground level)? Are there alternate methods of entry (e.g., personnel willing and able to assist)? Are doorways to public areas at least 32 inches wide?
- Is the doorway threshold no higher than half an inch?
- How many doors are at the entrance? The restroom entrance? If there are consecutive sets of doors, how much space is between them?
- Are entrance doors easily opened (automated, opened with a button or levered handles and a minimum of force)?

- Are reception areas well marked and lit with desk space available at a suitable height for wheelchair users?
- Are steps leading to the restrooms? Are restroom doors at least 32 inches wide? Do they swing outward with 32 inches of clearance? Is there a wider stall (56 inches wide × 60 inches deep)? Are grab bars installed?
- Are walkways and hallways at least 36 inches wide and free of obstacles?
- Do directional signs and menus use large print and/or Braille?
- Are any ramped or steep areas sloped 1:10 to 1:12 with handrails on either side?
- Are drinking fountains no higher than 48 inches from the floor? If not, are drinking cups provided?
- Do elevator doors open at least 32 inches wide? What are the internal dimensions of the elevator? Are elevator buttons set lower? Are there Braille elevator buttons?
- Are public telephones set no higher than 48 inches from the ground? Do they have sound amplifiers?
- Are there clear routes to emergency exits?
- Are alarm and alert systems both audible and visible?
- Are telephones no higher than 48 inches from the floor and equipped with sound amplifiers?
- Is there a TDD (telephone device for the deaf)?
- Are guide dogs allowed? Is there an outside area where they can relieve themselves?

Modified from Centers for Disease Control and Prevention, *Disability Inclusion*, 2020. https://www.cdc.gov/ncbddd/disabilityandhealth/disability-inclusion.html
Work Group for Community Health and Development at University of Kansas, *Tool 3: Accessibility checklist*, 2018. https://ctb.ku.edu/en/table-of-contents/implement/access-barriers-opportunities/increase-access-disabilities/tools

Get Ready for the Next Generation NCLEX® Examination!

Key Points

- The ability to perform activity and exercise requires that the musculoskeletal, respiratory, cardiovascular, and nervous systems work together effectively.
- Age- and disease-related changes in these systems contribute to the decreased level of activity common with aging.
- Difficulty with activity and exercise can result in lifestyle changes for older adults.
- Assessment and prompt initiation of appropriate nursing interventions help older adults achieve and maintain the highest level of function possible.

Additional Learning Resources

SG Go to your Evolve website at http://evolve.elsevier.com/Williams/geriatric for the additional online resources.

Review Questions for the Next Generation NCLEX® Examination

1. A home health nurse is visiting her patients and evaluating their exercise routines. Which patient(s) meet the current recommendations for physical activity? *(Select all that apply.)*
   - a. Tom, a former marathon runner, power walks 30 minutes every weekday.
   - b. Marge, a retired nurse, swims 25 minutes every day except Sundays and does strength training with weights on Tuesdays and Fridays.
   - c. Jose lifts weights in his home gym every day and walks to the grocery store twice a week.
   - d. Yi-Lin plays video fitness 3 times each day, 10 minutes each time, and performs weight lifting 3 times a week.

2. A nurse is asked to speak to a group of older adults about exercise, activity, and aging. What are 5 benefits of exercise and activity for older adults that the nurse can discuss?
   - a. _____
   - b. _____
   - c. _____
   - d. _____
   - e. _____

3. The nurse is teaching an older adult with a history of severe cardiac problems that the goal is to use exercise to maintain the highest level of function possible. Which directions should be included in the patient education to prevent hypertension or use of the Valsalva maneuver?
   - a. Breathe through your mouth while exercising.
   - b. Start slowly and work up until you feel short of breath.
   - c. Limit exercises to range of motion and stretching.
   - d. Perform isotonic and isometric exercise frequently.

4. A patient with altered activity tolerance was found to have oxygenation problems. Which statement made by the patient would indicate to the nurse the need for further teaching?
   - a. "I'll need to rest if my pulse rate gets too fast."
   - b. "I need to do my activities quickly to get everything done."
   - c. "I need to work on strategies that reduce my stress."
   - d. "I'll use my oxygen so I can breathe easier."

5. The nurse is caring for an older man residing in a community-based residential facility. The patient states, "I just don't know what to do except sleep. I worked hard all my life; I never had the time or money to do lots of things." Which nursing intervention is the most appropriate to meet this patient's diversional activity needs?
   - a. Schedule the patient to join a museum trip sponsored by the local senior center.
   - b. Select books and videos from the library to occupy his time.
   - c. Refer him to occupational therapy for evaluation.
   - d. Explore the variety of activities that are now available to him.

6. A 72-year-old female patient sustained a left hip fracture after a mechanical fall. She underwent an open reduction and internal fixation (ORIF) of the left hip and is now being discharged to a rehab facility. Her anticipated length of stay is 1 month to increase strengthening and her self-care abilities. Mark with "X" to indicate nursing actions listed below that are indicated, contraindicated, or nonessential for the patient's care.

NURSING ACTION	INDICATED	CONTRAINDICATED	NON-ESSENTIAL
The only focus while in rehab should be on keeping the patient fed, groomed, and clean.			
Encourage exploration of new interests and activities offered while in rehab.			
Pace activities throughout the day, allowing for periods of exercise and periods of rest.			
Include the patient's security, love, and sense of belonging in the plan of care.			

NURSING ACTION	INDICATED	CONTRAINDICATED	NON-ESSENTIAL
On admission, create a long-term exercise schedule for the patient to follow after being discharged home.			

NURSING ACTION	INDICATED	CONTRAINDICATED	NON-ESSENTIAL
Avoid weight-bearing activities that put weight on the patient's hips and knees.			

REFERENCES

Administration for Community Living. (2020). 2019 Profile of older Americans. Special section: Aerobic activity and muscle-strengthening activities. https://acl.gov/aging-and-disability-in-america/data-and-research/profile-older-americans

Centers for Disease Control and Prevention (CDC) (2020). *Physical activity: How much physical activity do older adults need?* https://www.cdc.gov/physicalactivity/basics/older_adults/index.htm2020

Maslow, A.H. (1943). A theory of human motivation. *Psychological Review, 50*(4): 370–396.

Sleep and Rest

Objectives

1. Describe normal sleep and rest patterns.
2. Discuss how sleep and rest patterns change with aging.
3. Examine the effects of disease processes on sleep.
4. Explain methods of assessing changes in sleep and rest patterns.
5. Identify older adults who are most at risk for experiencing disrupted sleep patterns.
6. Choose problem statements related to sleep or rest problems.
7. Describe appropriate nursing interventions for older individuals experiencing problems related to disrupted sleep patterns.

Key Terms

apnea (ĂP-nē-ă, p. 355)
boredom (p. 360)
circadian (sĭr-KĂ-dē-ăn, p. 353)
cognitive behavioral therapy for insomnia (CBTI) (p. 357)
diurnal (dī-ŬR-năl, p. 353)
fatigue (p. 353)

hypnotic (hĭp-NŎT-ĭk, p. 357)
insomnia (ĭn-SŎM-nē-ă, p. 355)
nocturnal (nŏ-TŬR-năl, p. 355)
orthopnea (or-THŎP-nē-ă, p. 358)
phase advance (p. 354)
sedative (SĔD-ă-tĭv, p. 357)

SLEEP-REST HEALTH PATTERN

The sleep-rest health pattern describes the patterns of sleep, rest, and relaxation exhibited throughout the 24-hour day. Individual perceptions, rituals, and aids used to promote sleep and rest are included in the sleep-rest health pattern.

No one knows exactly why we sleep, but we all require sleep to function normally. Sleep apparently allows the body time to rejuvenate and to respond to life's daily stresses. Lack of adequate sleep can affect one's health and behavior. Studies have connected sleep deprivation and insomnia to altered appetite, fatigue, decreased ability to perform tasks that require high-level coordination, increased traffic accidents, home accidents, falls, irritability, emotional instability, weakened immunity, difficulty with short- and long-term memory and concentration, pain, impaired judgment, low sex drive, and heart disease (Watson & Cherney, 2020).

Many older people experience problems related to sleep. It is estimated that more than half of older adults have sleep disturbances, and the figure is likely higher among institutionalized older adults. Sleep-related problems can be troubling to the aging individual and are often the basis of visits to the primary care provider and complaints to the nurse. Some of these problems result from changes that normally occur with aging, but they are more likely a result of changes that accompany aging, such as illnesses, medications, and changes in the circadian rhythm. Nurses must understand normal sleep patterns and be able to identify common age-related changes in sleep patterns and common sleep disorders to assess, plan, and intervene appropriately and effectively.

NORMAL SLEEP AND REST

Periods of sleep and wakefulness occur in regular and somewhat predictable cycles. Most humans develop a pattern that repeats approximately every 24 hours. This cycle occurs in response to the day-night cycle of the sun and is referred to as circadian (from the Latin word meaning "about a day") or diurnal (from the Latin word meaning "daily") rhythm. Within this cycle, individuals develop their own unique patterns for waking and sleeping.

The usual times for going to bed and rising differ widely among individuals. Some go to sleep at 10 PM and rise at 6 AM; others go to sleep at midnight and rise at 8 AM. These sleep-wake patterns can be disrupted by shift work, time zone changes, illness, emotional stress, medications, and numerous other factors. The amount of sleep needed also varies among individuals. Some individuals function normally with less than 6 hours of sleep, whereas others require 9 hours of sleep or more to feel rested. The average amount of sleep required for people ages 20 to 60 is 7.5 hours per day.

Sleep is under the control of the central nervous system. Current research indicates that wakefulness is regulated by the neurotransmitter norepinephrine. Sleep appears to be controlled by the release of serotonin within the brainstem. Melatonin, which is produced by the pineal gland, is released when the level of light decreases. Because of medical conditions and living situations such as institutionalization, older adults are less likely to receive adequate bright light to promote the sleep-wake cycle. Levels of cortisol and growth hormone also affect sleep. Sleep is not a uniform state of unconsciousness; rather, it is divided into a series of cycles of lighter and deeper stages of sleep. Immediately before falling asleep, most adults experience a stage of increased relaxation and drowsiness lasting from 10 to 30 minutes. This is followed by 4 to 6 complete sleep cycles lasting between 1 and 2 hours each. Each cycle consists of 4 non–rapid eye movement (NREM) stages and one rapid eye movement (REM) stage (Box 20.1 and Fig. 20.1). As the night's sleep progresses, REM periods increase in length and NREM periods decrease in length. If sleep is interrupted at any time, the individual goes back to stage 1 of NREM sleep and begins a new cycle.

SLEEP AND AGING

As a person ages, the levels of hormones associated with sleep change. Decreases in melatonin (which regulates the sleep-wake cycle) and growth hormone (which promotes sleep) lead to a shift in the circadian rhythm, causing many older adults to feel sleepy earlier in the evening and to wake up earlier in the morning, a phenomenon known as **phase advance**.

Because sleep efficiency decreases as age increases, many older adults complain that they do not feel refreshed after sleep. Although the amount of time spent in bed may increase with age, the amount of time actually spent sleeping may decrease. The average 70-year-old individual sleeps for 7 hours per night, about the same as reported by younger adults; however, the nature of the sleep changes. Older individuals experience more stage 1 and fewer stages 3 and 4 (deeper) NREM sleep and somewhat less REM sleep. REM sleep occurs earlier in the sleep cycle than is seen in younger adults. These changes result in less deep restorative and refreshing sleep. The phase advance in circadian rhythm also appears to change with age, resulting in earlier bedtime and earlier rising. (Not surprisingly, this is the opposite of the "phase delay" observed in teenagers, who easily sleep until noon.) It is suspected that this alteration in circadian rhythm in the older adult results from an earlier drop in core body temperature, decreased light exposure, or genetic factors. In addition, sleep interruption and nocturnal awakening are common because older adults are more easily aroused by environmental noise or other stimuli.

Box 20.1   Stages of Sleep Cycle

STAGE 1: NREM
Stage includes the lightest level of sleep.
Stage lasts a few minutes.
Decreased physiological activity begins with gradual fall in vital signs and metabolism.
Person is easily aroused by sensory stimuli, such as noise.
Awakened, person feels as though daydreaming had occurred.

STAGE 2: NREM
Stage is a period of sound sleep.
Relaxation progresses.
Arousal is still relatively easy.
Stage lasts 10 to 20 minutes.
Body functions continue to slow.

STAGE 3: NREM
Stage involves initial phases of deep sleep.
Sleeper is difficult to arouse and rarely moves.
Muscles are completely relaxed.
Vital signs decline but remain regular.
Stage lasts 15 to 30 minutes.

STAGE 4: NREM
This is deepest stage of sleep.
It is very difficult to arouse sleeper.
If sleep loss has occurred, sleeper will spend a considerable portion of the night in this stage.
Vital signs are significantly lower than during waking hours.
Stage lasts approximately 15 to 30 minutes.
Sleepwalking and enuresis may occur.

REM SLEEP
Vivid, full-color dreaming may occur. Less vivid dreaming may occur in other stages.
Stage usually begins about 90 minutes after sleep has begun.
It is typified by autonomic response of rapidly moving eyes, fluctuating heart and respiratory rates, and increased or fluctuating blood pressure.
Loss of skeletal muscle tone occurs.
Gastric secretions increase.
It is very difficult to arouse the sleeper.
The duration of REM sleep increases with each cycle and lasts an average of 20 minutes.

NREM, non–rapid eye movement; REM, rapid eye movement.

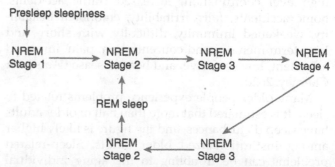

Fig. 20.1 The adult sleep cycle. *NREM*, Nonrapid eye movement; *REM*, rapid eye movement. (From Potter, P. A., Perry, A. G., Stockert, P. A., & Hall, A. M. [2017]. *Fundamentals of nursing* [9th ed.]. St. Louis, MO: Mosby.)

SLEEP DISORDERS

INSOMNIA

The risk for sleep disorders increases with age. The most common sleep disorder is insomnia, which is defined as difficulty falling asleep or remaining asleep or the belief that one is not getting enough sleep. Insomnia is frequently associated with an underlying medical problem. It can be acute (occurring on one or several nights) or chronic (lasting longer than one month). Different types of insomnia are identified based on the phase of sleep affected: (1) sleep onset problems: those related to falling asleep; (2) sleep maintenance problems: those related to staying asleep; or (3) terminal insomnia problems: those related to abnormally early awakening. Identification of the type of insomnia can help nurses determine the underlying cause or causes and implement the best interventions.

> **? Did You Know?**
>
> Baby boomers have been found to be chronically sleep deprived, with more than half of adults over age 50 reporting that they get fewer than 7 hours of sleep per night. According to the American Sleep Association (2021), 50 to 70 million Americans suffer from sleep disorders, which have been associated with a wide range of adverse health conditions including increased risk for hypertension, diabetes, obesity, depression, heart attack, stroke, and likely Alzheimer disease. Sleep deprivation and insomnia have been shown to be associated with the development of Alzheimer disease by mechanisms such as inflammation, beta-amyloid accumulation, and aggregation of tau protein, the protein in the brain associated with Alzheimer disease (Sadeghmousavi et al., 2020).

Older adults with existing health problems are more likely to experience sleep problems than are those who report themselves to be in good health. Insomnia can be related to a variety of medical conditions, medications, and psychological, behavioral, or environmental factors. Medical conditions that cause pain, interfere with breathing, or cause frequent bladder or bowel elimination contribute to frequent awakening. Common medical problems that may lead to insomnia include arthritis, bursitis, chronic pain, diabetes, gastroesophageal reflux, chronic obstructive pulmonary disease (COPD), heart failure, sleep apnea, prostatic problems, cystitis, and others. Nocturnal movement disorders—including restless leg syndrome, which is an irresistible urge to move the lower extremities, or nocturnal myoclonus, which causes sudden repetitive jerking or kicking movements of the lower extremities—also contribute to insomnia in older adults.

Anxiety is likely to be related to difficulty falling asleep and interrupted sleep. Depression is most likely to be associated with early awakening, but may also be related to hypersomnia (excessive sleepiness at a time of normal wakefulness). People with dementia often experience abnormal sleep cycles and are prone to waking and wandering during the night. Many prescription and over-the-counter (OTC) medications affect sleep in older adults. Commonly prescribed insomnia medications are listed in Table 20.1. Many medications prescribed for various disorders interfere with sleeping (Table 20.2). There are also other medications that can result in hypersomnolent responses.

Behaviors that contribute to sleep problems include physical inactivity, poor sleep routines, late night eating

Table 20.1 Medications to Treat Insomnia[a]

CLASSIFICATION	EXAMPLES	NOTES	PRECAUTIONS
Benzodiazepines (FDA approved for insomnia)	• Estazolam • Flurazepam • Quazepam • Temazepam • Triazolam	Older medications, high potential for dependence	Short-term use only; cautious use in respiratory or liver problems
Benzodiazepines (FDA approved for anxiety)	• Lorazepam • Clonazepam • Alprazolam	Same as above	Same as above
"Nonbenzodiazepines" (FDA approved for insomnia)	• Eszopiclone • Zaleplon • Zolpidem tartrate (extended release)	Newer medications; safe for older adults; fewer side effects	Cautious use in respiratory or liver problems; depression or psychiatric disorders
Melatonin receptor agonist (FDA approved for insomnia)	• Ramelteon	Newer medication; can cause paradoxical (opposite) reactions including anxiety and excitement; unusual activities (e.g., cooking, driving) not remembered the next day have been reported by patients taking this medication	Caution advised in patients with COPD, sleep apnea, liver disease; should not be used in anyone at risk for suicide

COPD, chronic obstructive pulmonary disease; FDA, U.S. Food and Drug Administration.

[a]Observe anyone taking medications for grogginess or "medication hangover" the following day; report any patient mention of suicidal thoughts immediately.

Data from Stanford Hospital and Clinics (2021). *Treating insomnia with medications*. https://stanfordhealthcare.org/medical-conditions/sleep/insomnia/treatments/treating-insomnia-with-medications.html.

Medscape (2021). *Drugs and diseases: Ramelteon*. https://reference.medscape.com/drug/rozerem-ramelteon-342928#5

Table 20.2   **Common Medication Categories That Cause Insomnia**

DRUG CATEGORY	EXAMPLES	REASON TAKEN	HOW THEY INTERRUPT SLEEP
Beta blockers	Atenolol, carvedilol, metoprolol, acebutolol	Treatment of angina; tremors; migraine headaches	Inhibits melatonin; leads to nighttime awakening and nightmares
Corticosteroids	Cortisone, methylprednisolone, prednisone	To reduce inflammation; treatment of arthritis; gout; allergic reactions	Stimulates the adrenal gland to release cortisol
SSRI antidepressants	Citalopram, escitalopram, fluoxetine, paroxetine, sertraline	To improve mood and sense of well-being	Decreases REM sleep; can make it difficult to fall asleep and stay asleep
ACE inhibitors	Benazepril, captopril, enalapril, fosinopril, lisinopril, moexipril	Treatment of hypertension and heart failure	May interrupt sleep due to the common side effects of hacking, dry cough; potassium overload in the body leading to aching bones and muscles
ARBs	Candesartan, irbesartan, losartan, telmisartan, valsartan	Treatment of hypertension and heart failure	May cause potassium overload in the body leading to aching muscles and bones
Cholinesterase inhibitors	Donepezil, galantamine	Treatment of Alzheimer disease and other memory loss conditions	Disrupts sleep by increasing your body's level of acetylcholine; can cause nightmares
Statins	Atorvastatin, lovastatin, rosuvastatin, simvastatin	To lower cholesterol and risk of heart disease	Insomnia caused by the common side effect of muscle pain

ACE, angiotensin-converting enzyme; *ARBs*, angiotensin II-receptor blockers; *FDA*, U.S. Food and Drug Administration; *SSRI*, selective serotonin reuptake inhibitor; *REM*, rapid eye movement.

Data from Freeland, M. N. (2020). 11 medications that can cause insomnia and what you can do about it. https://www.goodrx.com/blog/could-your-medication-be-causing-insomnia/.

Lewis, S. (2020). 10 drugs that affect your sleep. https://www.healthgrades.com/right-care/symptoms-and-conditions/10-drugs-that-affect-your-sleep.

Mayo Clinic (2021). Insomnia. https://www.mayoclinic.org/diseases-conditions/insomnia/symptoms-causes/syc-20355167.

or exercise, the use of tobacco, and consumption of alcohol or caffeine. Environmental factors—such as excessive noise, light, activity, or other distracting stimuli—can also contribute to the problem. Afternoon sleepiness is common with aging. Naps may adversely affect nighttime sleeping, particularly if the nap is taken late in the afternoon or lasts too long. Occasional naps of less than 30 minutes are usually not a problem. Box 20.2 lists risk factors for problems related to sleep or rest in older adults.

Occasional problems with insomnia are experienced by individuals of all ages, but if not properly addressed, these random, acute episodes are likely to result in chronic insomnia. Chronic insomnia can result in daytime sleepiness, irritability, decreased ability to concentrate, and other problems related to sleep deprivation. Daytime sleepiness is often ignored or excused as a normal change of aging rather than viewed as a symptom of sleep deprivation.

Health Promotion

Sleep Hygiene Practices

- Establish a regular bedtime and wake-up time, and follow this schedule as closely as possible.
- Develop a daily exercise program, preferably outdoors.
- Increase overall light exposure.
- Avoid naps, or limit them to no more than 30 minutes and no later than the early afternoon.
- Avoid caffeine, alcohol, and tobacco after lunchtime.
- Eat a light snack before bed, but avoid large meals.
- Take a warm bath or shower before going to bed.
- Use relaxation breathing or meditation techniques.
- Listen to relaxing music.
- Establish a restful sleep environment with a comfortable bed, good pillow and covers, shades or curtain to block out light, and a slightly cool temperature.
- If you cannot fall asleep after 30 minutes, do not get upset. Get up. Read, watch TV, or do something relaxing until you feel tired. Then go back to bed.

Box 20.2	**Risk Factors Related to Sleep or Rest Problems in Older Adults**

- Pain
- Chronic respiratory or cardiovascular problems
- Frequent elimination
- Nocturnal movement disorders
- Anxiety, depression, or delirium
- Drugs likely to interfere with sleep
- Excessive environmental stimuli
- Excessive caffeine, alcohol, or tobacco use
- Sedentary lifestyle

Treatment of insomnia includes both nonpharmacologic and pharmacologic approaches. Nonpharmacologic approaches include sleep hygiene education, relaxation therapies, **cognitive behavioral therapy for insomnia (CBTI)**, and other behavioral interventions. Industry has taken notice; helping people sleep has become a $30 billion to $40 billion industry, selling an extensive array of products touted to promote sleep, including napping pods, weighted blankets, and a special "sleep spray."

QSEN Considerations: Evidence-Based Practice

Based on numerous randomized controlled trials, cognitive behavioral therapy for insomnia (CBTI) has been shown to be the preferred nonpharmacologic therapy for insomnia. It has been found to be effective in decreasing insomnia symptoms, improving sleep efficiency, and decreasing sleep fragmentation. Nurse-guided internet-delivered CBTI has been shown to be an accepted, accessible option for patients (Van der Zweerde et al., 2020).

The cognitive part of CBTI deals with retraining one's expectations about sleep, such as the absolute number of hours of sleep needed. The behavioral part of CBTI includes teaching behaviors promoting sleep, such as sleep hygiene practices: for example, breaking the mental association between the bedroom and being awake, using the bed only for sleep, and getting rid of thoughts that hinder sleep, such as, "It's no use!" and "I'll never get to sleep." There is a mobile CBTI app that people who suffer from insomnia can download and use. Pharmacologic approaches include the use of drugs, such as antidepressant agents (most often benzodiazepines) and **hypnotic** agents. These medications are usually prescribed temporarily while the person is learning CBTI techniques. The common rule, as with all medications for the older adult, is to "start low (dosage) and go slow." Sleep-inducing medications are likely to have adverse effects on older adults, such as urinary retention, drowsiness, fatigue, confusion, and disturbed coordination, which increases fall risk.

Complementary Health Approaches

Alternative Treatments for Insomnia

- Valerian root: May help with sleep onset and sleep maintenance, although effectiveness is not proven, and it may interact with other medications.
- Chamomile: Shown to be an effective and safe sleep aid in animals. There is an increased risk of bleeding if the patient is on blood thinners, and people with allergies to ragweed and certain other plants may experience allergic reactions.
- Melatonin: A hormone produced by the pineal gland, melatonin helps to regulate the sleep-wake cycle. It may produce coronary vasoconstriction and paradoxical reactions (increased alertness). The Mayo Clinic lists it as "generally safe" but notes that it can interact with numerous medications (Mayo Clinic, 2021).
- Acupuncture: Has been shown to improve sleep quality in people with insomnia.
- Relaxation, meditation, yoga: Can be very effective but it can take several weeks to master the technique. May increase blood levels of melatonin.
- Exercise, tai chi: Helpful in enhancing sleep quality as long as not done late in the day.

SLEEP APNEA

Sleep apnea, also called *sleep disordered breathing*, is a common problem with aging. Sleep apnea is more common in older adults, in part because of changes in how the brain controls breathing during sleep (L'Heureux et al., 2021). Obstructive sleep apnea caused by airway blockage or collapse is the most common problem experienced. Men are more likely to experience sleep apnea, and about half of sleep apnea sufferers are overweight. Other things correlated with sleep apnea are hypertension, metabolic syndrome, smoking, and diabetes.

Cultural Considerations

A recent study has revealed that sleep apnea is very likely underdiagnosed in African American patients (Johnson et al., 2020).

Signs of sleep apnea include excessively loud snoring interspersed with periods of apnea lasting 10 to 30 seconds. Lack of oxygen causes the person to awaken frequently throughout the night, although they may not be aware of it. This cycle repeats hundreds of times each night. Recurrent disruptions of sleep results in daytime sleepiness. Individuals experiencing obstructive sleep apnea are also at increased risk for developing cardiovascular complications, including hypertension, arrhythmias, myocardial infarction, and stroke. People experiencing sleep apnea should try to lose weight and avoid alcohol, **sedatives**, and muscle relaxants, which can worsen the condition. Sleeping in the supine position may also make the condition worse; therefore a side-lying position is recommended. Mechanical oral or dental devices that prevent the relaxation of tissues may help some individuals. Continuous positive airway pressure devices are another common treatment. Occasionally, surgery is recommended. Many individuals need a combination of interventions to control the problem.

CIRCADIAN RHYTHM SLEEP DISORDERS

Changes in the circadian rhythm can cause unusual sleep disorders. This can occur for many reasons, such as working the night shift, jet lag, and certain medications. It has been long documented that blind people often experience a change in circadian rhythm known as non–24-hour sleep-wake disorder, or "non-24," because light does not stimulate their brains and they cannot synchronize their body clocks to the 24-hour light-dark cycle. In 2014, the U.S. Food and Drug Administration approved a medication called tasimelteon, which stimulates melatonin receptors and theoretically improves sleep disorders caused by changes in circadian rhythm. Because of the exorbitant cost of this medication, however ($700 per tablet), you are unlikely to see it on your clinical unit anytime soon.

REM SLEEP-BEHAVIOR DISORDER

REM sleep-behavior disorder is another less common problem; it is seen most often in men in their 60s and 70s. Muscle activity is normally inhibited during REM, so little or no gross muscle movement occurs during dreams. However, when a person experiences the disorder, this protective mechanism does not operate effectively. Thus the older individual may thrash around in bed, jump or fall out of bed, or sustain an injury (or injury to the partner) as they attempt to escape from vivid or violent dreams. Manifestation of this disorder may be a predecessor to the development of Parkinson disease or dementia. Long-acting benzodiazepines are frequently effective in treating this disorder; studies have also shown melatonin to have promising results.

❖ NURSING PROCESS/CLINICAL JUDGMENT MODEL FOR DISRUPTED SLEEP PATTERN

To assess sleep patterns in older adults, use a combination of objective and subjective data. Simply because an older individual's eyes are closed during nighttime checks does not mean that the person is asleep. Watch closely for signs of fatigue and decreased participation in activities and ask older adults how they feel about the adequacy of their sleep and rest.

◆ ASSESSMENT (DATA COLLECTION)

Recognize cues:
- Does the person feel rested after a night's sleep?
- At what times does the person normally go to bed and get up?
- Are they allowed to choose their bedtime, or is it chosen by someone else?
- Does the person sleep continuously through the night, or is their sleep interrupted?
- Does the caregiver or bed partner report any abnormal breathing pattern, excessive snoring, or unusual movement during sleep?
- What causes the person to wake up? Pain? Noise? Other factors?
- Does the person have difficulty falling asleep?
- Do they wake up early?
- Does the person nap or sleep during the day?
- Do they ever fall asleep during daytime activities?
- Has the person's behavior changed? Are they increasingly irritable, disoriented, or lethargic?
- Does the person appear tired? Do they complain of tiredness? When?
- Have any signs such as yawning or dark circles under the eyes been observed?

◆ DATA ANALYSIS/PROBLEM IDENTIFICATION

Analyze Cues and Prioritize Hypotheses: Common problem statements for older adults with a disruption in their sleep pattern include
Disrupted Sleep Pattern.

◆ PLANNING

Generate Solutions: The patient goals for older individuals experiencing a disrupted sleep pattern are to (1) verbalize an understanding of sleep changes associated with aging, (2) verbalize appropriate interventions to promote sleep, and (3) report feeling rested and refreshed on rising.

◆ IMPLEMENTATION

Take Action: The following interventions should take place in hospitals and extended-care facilities:
1. **Identify the factors that contribute to sleep disruption.** Identify the cause of sleep disruption so that the most appropriate interventions can be selected. Various internal and external factors can interfere with sleep. Pain, whether chronic or acute, interrupts or prevents sleep. Identify the causes of pain and take measures to make the older person as comfortable as possible. Medical conditions and the medications taken to treat them can affect sleep. Older people with cardiovascular disease may experience anginal pain during REM sleep that causes them to awaken. Patients with ulcers secrete excessive amounts of acid during REM sleep, causing pain and awakening. Individuals with COPD may experience dyspnea related to lying flat, also known as orthopnea. This can result in oxygen hunger and anxiety and may interfere with sleep. Anxiety and depression often result in early morning rising and an inability to return to sleep once awakened. Medications for hypertension commonly cause altered sleep patterns. Environmental

factors—including brighter lighting, noise, and temperature change—should also be considered.

2. **Schedule nursing interventions to allow for adequate uninterrupted sleep.** Nursing and medical interventions can interfere with sleep. Medication administration, dressing changes, or toileting can interrupt sleep. Although you may not have total control over the scheduling of medication and treatments, attempt to formulate a plan that causes the least interference with sleep. For example, if diuretic medications are given close to bedtime, urinary frequency may prevent the individual from getting continuous sleep. By scheduling the diuretic agent early in the morning, this problem can be minimized. If a procedure is not essential for the well-being of an individual, it should not be scheduled during the night. Many treatments and medications are now specifically ordered to be given to the patient "while awake" to eliminate any confusion or concern regarding interpretation of the order. The benefits to the patient must be weighed against the risks of sleep deprivation.

 Clinical Pitfall

Sleep and Rest

Mrs. Nguyen, age 79, had some problems with incontinence but no difficulty participating in her activities of daily living until she was placed on a toileting schedule. At that point she was reminded to use the bathroom every 3 hours, day and night. After being awakened 5 nights in a row, she began to become unable to dress and feed herself. Staff members began to search for symptoms of illness or disease to account for this change, but they found none. Nursing notes indicated that Mrs. Nguyen was attending fewer activities, and she was observed napping in her room on several occasions. On the sixth night of toileting, Mrs. Nguyen remarked, "If you would just let me sleep, I'd feel better."

The nurse put these pieces of information together and realized that, although the toileting schedule reduced problems with incontinence, it caused other problems related to sleep. After a discussion with Mrs. Nguyen, her primary care provider, and her family, it was determined that using incontinence briefs during the night would be a better alternative. After three nights of uninterrupted sleep, Mrs. Nguyen began to dress and feed herself again and to participate in social activities instead of napping.

3. **Plan bedtimes and wake-up times to meet the individual's needs and desires rather than those of the institution.** Although a regular bedtime schedule is advisable, set the schedule with input from the older adult. The fact that an older person resides in an institutional setting does not mean that sleep patterns established over a lifetime should change to fit the institution's convenience. The institution should allow for individual preferences. Many older adults find that they cannot sleep once they have gone to bed. They often lie awake and become increasingly anxious. This anxiety further interferes with their ability to fall asleep. If a person is unable to sleep after 20 to 30 minutes, encourage them to get up and quietly watch television, read, or listen to music. A lounge should be available so that this activity will not disrupt the sleep of others. When the person is tired, they should then return to bed. This supports the mental connection that bed is a place for sleep.

4. **Allow the individual to maintain rituals that help to induce sleep.** Many older adults have rituals that help them sleep. These presleep rituals are highly individual and include hygiene, the use of special pillows, praying, and a variety of other activities. Discuss individual preferences and incorporate these into the plan of care.

5. **Assist in providing an environment that is conducive to sleep.** To prevent awakening roommates, use the minimal amount of light necessary and make as little noise as possible when checking patients or performing required treatments. Ideally, individuals sharing a room should have similar sleep schedules. Establish a schedule for routine rounds so that even if nightly sleep is interrupted, it occurs at the same time each night. If possible, place individuals who have sleep difficulties in rooms away from noisy work areas. Noise that goes unnoticed during the day, particularly conversation near the nurses' station and unanswered call systems, can disrupt sleep at night. Because of circulatory changes, many older individuals need an extra blanket for comfort at night. A warm light blanket that does not feel heavy is preferred by many older adults.

QSEN Considerations: Teamwork and Collaboration

Minimizing Nighttime Disruptions

Schedule activities such as treatments and medications to minimize the number of times a patient will be disturbed during the night. In addition, communicate to other staff members that excessive noise from conversations or equipment use should be minimized because it can easily disrupt the sleep of older patients who already may have difficulty sleeping.

6. **Modify lighting through the day to imitate normal daily patterns.** Most institutions do not provide adequate light during the day to allow the body to maintain its normal circadian rhythm. Bright lighting should be provided during the daytime, particularly during the winter months. Dark rooms are best for sleep, but this may not be feasible in institutional settings. Provide lighting that allows for

safety but does not interfere with sleep. Ensure that curtains and doors are positioned to block light. Some individuals can sleep only if there is a night light; others are easily awakened by any light.

7. **Provide comfort measures to promote sleep.** A comfortable environment promotes sleep. Provide clean, dry, wrinkle-free bed linens. Tighten or loosen top linens to provide the greatest comfort. Sleepwear should be nonrestricting and of the type preferred by the individual (Fig. 20.2). Encourage or provide oral hygiene. Remind the older adult to empty their bladder before going to bed to avoid the need to get up once they become sleepy. Nocturia occurs most commonly within a few hours of going to sleep. In addition, if an older adult is left wet, their sleep will be disrupted for several hours. Waking the person and changing the wet clothes usually result in a return to normal sleep.

8. **Administer sleep medications (sedatives and hypnotics) as a nursing intervention of last resort, and watch carefully for side effects.** Assess patients or residents for desired effects and untoward effects of sleep medications. Because many medications that are used to promote sleep can cause orthostatic hypotension, observe the individuals for dizziness, make positional changes slowly, and assist with ambulation to reduce the risk for falls or other injuries. Offer medications to promote sleep only as a last resort, because many sedative and hypnotic drugs can leave older adults with lingering or hangover effects and can contribute to insomnia. These drugs can disrupt sleep because they alter the nature and quality of sleep. Long-acting drugs can be retained in the body for an excessive period of time, potentially leading to confusion, disorientation, and daytime sleepiness. Use medications that affect respiration with extreme caution in older adults. Low doses of drugs with short half-lives are best tolerated by older adults.

9. **Provide nutritional supplements that aid sleep.** A light snack or beverage before bed is commonly requested. Discourage caffeinated beverages, such as coffee, because caffeine can interfere with sleep. Decaffeinated coffee, herbal tea, and milk are good choices. Milk is often suggested because it contains tryptophan, which has sleep-inducing properties. Heavy meals put extra stress on the body and should be avoided near bedtime. Discourage alcoholic beverages because they may interfere with normal sleep cycles and may lead to awakening because of diuresis.

10. **Promote emotional comfort by spending time listening to patients' concerns.** Anxiety and depression interfere with sleep. A back rub or a few minutes of quiet conversation at bedtime may help relieve the concerns of the day and promote sleep in older adults. Relaxation training or other stress management techniques may be appropriate for some individuals.

11. **Observe patients for patterns of fatigue or napping throughout the day.** Excessive napping or fatigue during the day can interfere with nighttime sleep. Assess for daytime behaviors that affect sleep. If individuals spend too much time napping, determine the reason. If boredom is the cause, encourage diversional activities. If the individual is too fatigued or stimulated by the day's activities, encourage more frequent rest periods.

The following interventions should take place in the home:

1. **Use a journal to assess sleep and rest patterns.** Many older individuals who complain of sleep problems are unaware of their daily routines. Keeping a journal to record naps, bedtimes, periods of being awake, and time of rising in the morning often yields important information. If the individual cannot do this alone, a spouse or relative may assist. Any information that may be relevant (e.g., pain and nocturia) should be noted. Loud snoring and apnea are more likely to be noticed by a close family member than by the affected party. Refer any reports of these behaviors to the primary care provider for follow-up.

2. **Explain the importance of adequate activity and exercise throughout the day.** Adequate exercise and activity help promote good sleep. Excessive activity should be avoided within 2 hours of bedtime because such activity may raise body temperature and interfere with sleep.

3. **Assist older adults to establish an environment that promotes rest and sleep.** Verify that the conditions in the home promote rest and sleep and that the older adult has an adequate bed and suitable covers. Make sure that the heating is adequate. If noise from neighbors or traffic is a problem, discuss possible ways of dealing with this.

4. **Discuss limiting fluid intake at night if nocturia is a problem.** If nocturia is interrupting sleep, encourage older adults to decrease their fluid intake for 1 to 2 hours before bedtime. However, it is important

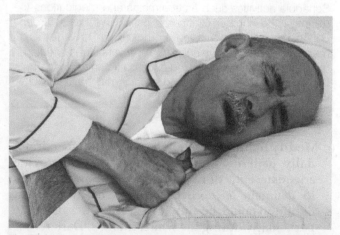

Fig. 20.2 Nonrestricting sleepwear. (© 2010 Photos.com, a division of Getty Images. All rights reserved.)

that adequate fluid be consumed earlier in the day to prevent fluid balance problems.

5. **Encourage the use of relaxation exercises, creative visualization, self-hypnosis, or other relaxation techniques.** Many techniques that promote relaxation can be used to help induce sleep. Numerous DVDs, downloads, podcasts, and books are available to describe these techniques, many of which could benefit older adults and are unlikely to cause the problems that are caused by medications.

6. **Use any appropriate interventions that are used in the institutional setting** (Nursing Care Plan 20.1).

★ Nursing Care Plan 20.1 | Disrupted Sleep Pattern

Mrs. Star, age 83, lives at Larkspur Court Residence Center. Her room is near the nurses' station and is frequently observed to be awake during the night. She often does not want to get up for breakfast, stating, "I'm too tired." She yawns often during the day and takes frequent naps in her room. She complains, "I can't get comfortable. There is just too much noise around here."

PROBLEM STATEMENT
Disrupted Sleep Pattern

SUPPORTING ASSESSMENT DATA
- Change from normal sleep pattern
- Observed periods of wakefulness at night
- Complaints of feeling tired
- Alteration in daytime functioning

PATIENT GOALS/OUTCOMES IDENTIFICATION
Mrs. Star will report feeling adequately rested.

NURSING INTERVENTIONS/IMPLEMENTATION
1. Identify specific factors that make sleep difficult for Mrs. Star.
2. Ask Mrs. Star whether she can identify any changes that would help her sleep.
3. Consider a room change if possible.
4. Close her door to reduce extraneous noise.
5. Place a "QUIET" sign on her door at night.
6. Discourage daytime napping.
7. Encourage daytime physical activities, outdoors if possible.
8. Recommend that she avoid caffeine after dinner.
9. Teach relaxation techniques.
10. Provide comfort measures at bedtime.
11. Assess the need for further therapies.

EVALUATION
Mrs. Star now states, "I really like my new room. It's much quieter, so I don't have trouble sleeping at night. In fact, I've even started going to more activities now that I'm feeling more rested during the day. The lawn bowling club is really fun!" She is observed to be sleeping soundly when checked at night. Fewer daytime naps are documented in her health record. You will continue the plan of care.

APPLYING CLINICAL JUDGMENT
A new resident who calls out loudly day and night was admitted to the room next door. Mrs. Star states to another resident, "I just started getting a good night's sleep, and now he's keeping me awake again."
1. What would your most appropriate response be to Mrs. Star's concerns?
2. How could you resolve this problem for her and other residents who may be disturbed?

Get Ready for the Next Generation NCLEX® Examination!

Key Points

- Changes related to sleep are a major concern for many older adults.
- Because sleep problems can result from normal age-related changes or other problems, concerns about sleep should not be taken lightly.
- A thorough assessment of sleep behaviors and appropriate interventions help older adults achieve the rest and sleep they require to function at the highest possible level.
- Sleep medications should be implemented only as an intervention of last resort and for as short a time as possible.

Additional Learning Resources

SG Go to your Evolve website at http://evolve.elsevier.com/Williams/geriatric for the additional online resources.

Review Questions for the Next Generation NCLEX® Examination

1. In promoting sleep hygiene practices for her older adult patient, what should the nurse suggest? *(Select all that apply.)*

   a. Implement a routine of bedtime cocoa.
   b. Make the bedroom warm for a comfortable sleep.
   c. Eat a light snack before bedtime.
   d. Develop a daily exercise program, preferably outdoors.
   e. If the older adult cannot fall asleep, tell her to lie there until it eventually happens.

2. List four factors that are likely to cause sleep problems in older adults.

   a. _____
   b. _____
   c. _____
   d. _____

3. The wife of an overweight older adult reports that her husband snores very loudly, then stops breathing several times each night. In addition to recommending a visit to the primary care provider, what should the nurse suggest?

   a. The husband should have a glass of wine at bedtime to promote relaxation.
   b. The husband should use an OTC decongestant to open his respiratory passages.
   c. The husband should sleep in the supine position with two pillows.
   d. The husband should try to lose weight and sleep in a side-lying position.

4. An older patient requests an evening snack. Which food is most appropriate to facilitate sleep?

   a. Graham crackers with banana and milk
   b. Cheese, toast, and hot chocolate
   c. Slice of cake and hot tea
   d. Fruit, cheese, and a glass of wine

5. A patient who lost his wife 6 months ago has been diagnosed with clinical depression. He plans to ask his primary care provider for a prescription for sleep medication. He asks for advice about what else he can do. The lack of sleep is interfering with his daytime activities, making him feel like he's "in a fog," and he states that his COPD is getting worse. What should the nurse keep in mind when providing an answer?

   a. Most of the newer sleep medications are safe choices for people with depression.
   b. Benzodiazepines carry a low risk of dependence.
   c. CBTI is more effective than medications in treating insomnia.
   d. Ramelteon, a newer medication, is the best choice for someone with COPD.

6. Which of the following are true statements regarding insomnia and its treatment? *(Select all that apply.)*

   a. Sleep medications can be useful in the short-term management of insomnia.
   b. CBTI may be indicated when sleep medications fail.
   c. Valerian root is the most effective herb for the treatment of insomnia.
   d. Tai chi at bedtime has been shown to be effective in preventing insomnia.
   e. Taking the medication cortisone, especially late in the day, can contribute to insomnia.

REFERENCES

American Sleep Association (2021). Sleep and sleep disorders statistics. https://www.sleepassociation.org/about-sleep/sleep-statistics/

Johnson, D. A., Sofer, T., Guo, N., Wilson, J., & Redline, S. (2020). A sleep apnea prediction model developed for African Americans: The Jackson Heart Sleep Study. *Journal of Clinical Sleep Medicine.* https://doi.org/10.5664/jcsm.8452

L'Heureux, F., Baril, A., Gagnon, K., Soucy, J.P., Lafond, C., Montplaisir, J., & Gosselin, N. (2021). Longitudinal changes in regional cerebral blood flow in late middle-aged and older adults with treated and untreated obstructive sleep apnea. *Human Brain Mapping,* 42(11), 3429–3439.

Mayo Clinic (2021). Melatonin. https://www.mayoclinic.org/drugs-supplements-melatonin/art-20363071

Sadeghmousavi, S., Eskian, M., Rahmani, F., & Rezaei, N. (2020). The effect of insomnia on development of Alzheimer's disease. *Journal of Neuroinflammation,* 17, 289. https://doi.org/10.1186/s12974-020-01960-9

Van der Zweerde, T., Lancee, J., Slottje, P., Bosmans, J.E., Van Someren, E.J.W., & van Staten, A. (2020). Nurse-guided internet-delivered cognitive behavioral therapy for insomnia in general practice: results from a pragmatic randomized clinical trial. *Psychother Psychosom,* 89, 174–184. https://doi.org/10.1159/000505600

Watson, S., & Cherney, K. (2020). The effects of sleep deprivation on your body. https://www.healthline.com/health/sleep-deprivation/effects-on-body

Laboratory Values for Older Adults

TEST NAME	ADULT NORMALS	OLDER ADULT NORMALS	SIGNIFICANCE OF DEVIATIONS
Hematology			
Red blood cells (RBCs)	M 4.7–6.1 million/unit F 4.2–5.4 million/unit	Unchanged with aging	Low: hemorrhage, anemia, chronic illness, kidney disease, pernicious anemia High: high altitude, polycythemia, dehydration
Hemoglobin	M 14–18 g/dL F 12–16 g/dL	Values may be slightly decreased	Low: anemia, cancer, nutritional deficiency, kidney disease High: polycythemia, heart failure (HF), chronic obstructive pulmonary disease (COPD), high altitude, dehydration
Hematocrit	M 42%–52% F 37%–47%	Values may be slightly decreased	Low: anemia, cirrhosis, hemorrhage, malnutrition, rheumatoid arthritis High: polycythemia, severe dehydration, severe diarrhea, COPD
White blood cells (WBCs) (total)	5,000–10,000/mm³	Unchanged with aging	Low: drug toxicity, infections, autoimmune disease, dietary deficiency High: infection, trauma, stress, inflammation
Neutrophils	55%–70%	Unchanged with aging	Low: dietary deficiency, overwhelming bacterial infection, viral infections, drug therapy High: physical and emotional stress, trauma, inflammatory disorders
Eosinophils	1%–4%	Unchanged with aging	Low: increased adrenosteroid production High: parasitic infections, allergic reactions, autoimmune disorders
Basophils	0.5%–1%	Unchanged with aging	Low: acute allergic reactions, stress reactions High: myeloproliferative disease
Monocytes	2%–8%	Unchanged with aging	Low: drug therapy (predisposition) High: chronic inflammatory disorders, tuberculosis, chronic ulcerative colitis
Lymphocytes	20%–40%	Unchanged with aging	Low: leukemia, sepsis, systemic lupus erythematosus, chemotherapy, radiation High: chronic bacterial infection, viral infections, radiation, infectious hepatitis
Folic acid	5–25 ng/mL	Unchanged with aging	Low: malnutrition, folic acid anemia, hemolytic anemia, alcohol use disorder, liver disease, chronic kidney disease High: pernicious anemia
Vitamin B$_{12}$	160–950 pg/mL	Unchanged with aging	
Total iron binding capacity (TIBC)	250–460 mcg/dL	Unchanged with aging	Low: hypoproteinemia, cirrhosis, hemolytic capacity (TIBC) anemia, pernicious anemia High: polycythemia, iron-deficiency anemia
Iron (Fe)	M 80–180 mcg/dL F 60–160 mcg/dL	Unchanged with aging	Low: insufficient dietary iron, chronic blood loss, inadequate absorption of iron High: hemochromocytosis, hemolytic anemia, hepatitis, iron poisoning

Continued

TEST NAME	ADULT NORMALS	OLDER ADULT NORMALS	SIGNIFICANCE OF DEVIATIONS
Uric acid	M 4.0–8.5 mg/dL F 2.7–7.3 mg/dL	Values may be slightly increased	Low: lead poisoning High: gout, increased ingestion of purines, chronic kidney disease, hypothyroidism
Prothrombin time (PT)	11.0–12.5 s	Unchanged with aging	High: liver disease, vitamin K deficiency, warfarin ingestion, bile duct obstruction, salicylate intoxication
Partial thromboplastin time (PTT) Partial thromboplastin time—activated (aPTT)	PTT: 60–70 s aPTT: 30–40 s	Unchanged with aging	Low: early stages of disseminated intravascular coagulation, metastatic cancer High: coagulation factor deficiency, cirrhosis, vitamin K deficiency, heparin administration
Platelets	150,000–400,000/mm^3	Unchanged with aging	Low: hemorrhage, thrombocytopenia, systemic lupus erythematosus, pernicious anemia, chemotherapy, infection High: malignancy, polycythemia, rheumatoid arthritis, iron-deficiency anemia
Blood Chemistry			
Sodium	135–147 mEq/L	Unchanged with aging	Low: decreased intake, diarrhea, vomiting, diuretic administration, chronic kidney disease, HF, peripheral edema, ascites High: increased intake, Cushing syndrome, extensive thermal burns
Potassium	3.5–5.2 mEq/L	Unchanged with aging	Low: deficient intake, burns, diuretics, Cushing syndrome, insulin administration, ascites High: excessive dietary intake, kidney failure, infection, acidosis, dehydration
Chloride	95–106 mEq/L	Unchanged with aging	Low: overhydration, HF, vomiting, chronic gastric suction, chronic respiratory acidosis, hypokalemia, diuretic therapy High: dehydration, Cushing syndrome, kidney dysfunction, metabolic acidosis, hyperventilation
Calcium	9.0–10.5 mg/dL	Tends to decrease	Low: kidney failure, vitamin D deficiency, osteomalacia, malabsorption High: Paget disease of the bone, prolonged immobilization, lymphoma
Phosphate	3.0–4.5 mg/dL	Values may be slightly lower	Low: inadequate dietary ingestion, chronic antacid ingestion, hypercalcemia, alcohol use disorder, osteomalacia, malnutrition High: kidney failure, increased dietary intake, hypocalcemia, liver disease
Magnesium	1.3–2.1 mEq/L	Decreases 15% between third and eighth decade	Low: malnutrition, malabsorption, alcohol use disorder, disease in the renal tubules, hypoparathyroidism High: chronic kidney disease, ingestion of magnesium-containing antacids or salts, hypothyroidism
Glucose, fasting (or fasting blood sugar [FBS])	74–106 mg/dL	Age 60–90 years: 82–115 mg/dL Over age 90 years: 75–121 mg/dL	Low: hypothyroidism, liver disease, insulin overdose, starvation High: diabetes mellitus, acute stress response, diuretic therapy, corticosteroid therapy
Glucose, postprandial	Less than 140 mg/dL 2 hours after meal	Less than 160 mg/dL 2 hours after meal	Low: hypothyroidism, insulin overdose, malabsorption High: diabetes mellitus, malnutrition, Cushing syndrome, chronic kidney disease, diuretic therapy, corticosteroid therapy

TEST NAME	ADULT NORMALS	OLDER ADULT NORMALS	SIGNIFICANCE OF DEVIATIONS
Amylase	60–120 Somogyi units/dL	Values may be slightly increased	High: acute pancreatitis, perforated bowel, acute cholecystitis, diabetic ketoacidosis
Glycosylated hemoglobin (Hgb A_{1c})	4.0%–5.9%	Unchanged with aging	Low: hemolytic anemia, chronic kidney disease High: newly diagnosed diabetes, poorly controlled diabetes, nondiabetic hyperglycemia
Total protein	6.4–8.3 g/dL	Unchanged with aging	Low: liver disease, malnutrition, ascites High: hemoconcentration
Albumin	3.5–5.0 g/dL	Values may be slightly decreased	Low: malnutrition, liver disease, overhydration High: dehydration
Blood urea nitrogen (BUN)	10–20 mg/dL	Values may be slightly increased	Low: liver failure, overhydration, malnutrition High: hypovolemia, dehydration, alimentary tube feeding, kidney disease
Creatinine	M: 0.6–1.2 mg/dL F: 0.5–1.0 mg/dL	Decrease in muscle mass may cause decreased values	Low: debilitation, decreased muscle mass High: reduced renal blood flow, diabetic neuropathy, urinary tract obstruction
Creatinine clearance	M 107–139 mL/min F 87–107 mL/min	Values decrease 6.5 mL/min/ decade of life because of decline in GFR	Low: impaired kidney function, HF, cirrhosis High: high cardiac output syndromes
Cholesterol (total)	< 200 mg/dL	Increases until about middle age but decreases thereafter (or can increase abruptly in women)	Low: malabsorption, malnutrition, cholesterol-lowering medication, pernicious anemia, liver disease, hyperthyroidism High: hypercholesteremia, hyperlipidemia, hypothyroidism, uncontrolled diabetes mellitus, hypertension, stress
High-density lipoprotein (HDL)	M > 45 mg/dL F > 55 mg/dL	Unchanged with aging	Low: familial low HDL, liver disease, hypoproteinemia High: familial HDL lipoproteinemia, excessive exercise
Low-density lipoprotein (LDL)	< 130 mg/dL	Increases with aging after menopause	Low: hypolipoproteinemia High: hypothyroidism, alcohol consumption, chronic liver disease, Cushing syndrome
Alkaline phosphatase	30–120 units/L	Values may be slightly higher	Low: hypothyroidism, malnutrition, pernicious anemia High: cirrhosis, healing fracture, Paget disease
Acid phosphatase	0.13–0.63 units/L	Unchanged with aging	Low: thrombosis High: heparin administration, cirrhosis, prostate cancer
Aspartate aminotransferase (AST)	0–35 units/L	Values may be slightly higher	Low: acute kidney disease, diabetic ketoacidosis, chronic kidney dialysis High: myopathy, hepatitis, cirrhosis, multiple trauma, acute hemolytic anemia
Creatine kinase (CK)	20–200 units/L	Unchanged with aging	High: diseases or injury affecting heart muscle, skeletal muscle, and brain
Thyroid Testing			
Thyroxine (T_4)—total	M 4–12 mcg/dL F 5–12 mcg/dL	Slightly decreased	Low: hypothyroidism, malnutrition, kidney failure, cirrhosis High: hyperthyroidism, hepatitis
Triiodothyronine (T_3)	Age 20–50 years: 70–205 ng/dL Over age 50 years: 40–180 ng/dL	Values may be slightly decreased	Low: hypothyroidism, pituitary insufficiency, protein malnutrition, kidney failure, liver diseases, Cushing syndrome High: hyperthyroidism, hepatitis, hypoproteinemia
Thyroid-stimulating hormone (TSH)	2–10 mcU/mL (varies by laboratory)	Unchanged with aging	Low: pituitary dysfunction, hyperthyroidism High: primary hypothyroidism

Continued

TEST NAME	ADULT NORMALS	OLDER ADULT NORMALS	SIGNIFICANCE OF DEVIATIONS
Urine Chemistry			
Color	Yellow; amber	Unchanged with aging	Straw-colored urine indicates dilution.
Appearance	Clear	Unchanged with aging	Cloudy urine may indicate presence of pus, casts, blood, and bacteria.
Specific gravity	1.005–1.030	Values may be slightly decreased	Low: overhydration, kidney failure, diuresis, hypothermia High: dehydration, water restriction, vomiting, diarrhea
pH	4.6–8.0	Unchanged with aging	Acidic urine: diarrhea, metabolic acidosis, diabetes mellitus, respiratory acidosis, emphysema Alkaline urine: respiratory alkalosis, metabolic alkalosis, vomiting, gastric suctioning, diuretic therapy, UTI
Protein	0–8 mg/mL	Unchanged with aging	Positive: diabetes mellitus, HF, systemic lupus erythematosus, malignant hypertension
Glucose	Negative	Unchanged with aging	Positive: diabetes mellitus, Cushing syndrome, severe stress, infection, drug therapy
Ketones	Negative	Unchanged with aging	Positive: uncontrolled diabetes mellitus, starvation, excessive aspirin ingestion, high-protein diet, dehydration
Blood	Negative	Unchanged with aging	Positive: renal trauma, renal stones, cystitis, prostatitis
Leukocyte esterase	Negative	Unchanged with aging	Positive: possible UTI
Bacteria	Negative	May be seen in older adults without symptoms; evaluate for pyuria and symptoms	Positive: UTI
Arterial Blood Gases			
pH	7.35–7.45	Unchanged with aging	Low: respiratory or metabolic acidosis High: respiratory or metabolic alkalosis
Po_2	80–100 mm Hg	Decreases 25% between 30 and 80 years of age	Low: cardiac or respiratory disease
Pco_2	35–45 mm Hg	Unchanged with aging	Low: respiratory alkalosis High: respiratory acidosis
O_2 saturation	95%–100%	95%	Low: altered gas exchange
HCO_3	21–28 mEq/L	Unchanged with aging	Low: metabolic acidosis High: metabolic acidosis

HF, heart failure; *GFR*, glomerular filtration rate; *UTI*, urinary tract infection

Adapted from Pagana, K. D., Pagana, T. J., & Pagana, T. N. (2021). *Mosby's diagnostic and laboratory test reference* (15th ed.). St. Louis, MO: Elsevier.

The Geriatric Depression Scale (GDS)

GERIATRIC DEPRESSION SCALE

The Geriatric Depression Scale (GDS) was developed as a basic screening tool for depression in older adults and is used in the clinical setting. It is a short questionnaire that requires a yes or no response from the participant based on how the person feels on the day the tool is administered.

Patient _____ Examiner _____ Date _____

Directions to Patient: Please choose the best answer for how you have felt over the past week.
Directions to Examiner: Present questions VERBALLY. Circle answer given by patient. Do not show to patient.

1.	Are you basically satisfied with your life?	yes	**no (1)**
2.	Have you dropped many of your activities and interests?	**yes (1)**	no
3.	Do you feel that your life is empty?	**yes (1)**	no
4.	Do you often get bored?	**yes (1)**	no
5.	Are you hopeful about the future?	yes	**no (1)**
6.	Are you bothered by thoughts you can't get out of your head?	**yes (1)**	no
7.	Are you in good spirits most of the time?	yes	**no (1)**
8.	Are you afraid that something bad is going to happen to you?	**yes (1)**	no
9.	Do you feel happy most of the time?	yes	**no (1)**
10.	Do you often feel helpless?	**yes (1)**	no
11.	Do you often get restless and fidgety?	**yes (1)**	no
12.	Do you prefer to stay at home rather than go out and do things?	**yes (1)**	no
13.	Do you frequently worry about the future?	**yes (1)**	no
14.	Do you feel you have more problems with memory than most?	**yes (1)**	no
15.	Do you think it is wonderful to be alive now?	yes	**no (1)**
16.	Do you feel downhearted and blue?	**yes (1)**	no
17.	Do you feel pretty worthless the way you are now?	**yes (1)**	no
18.	Do you worry a lot about the past?	**yes (1)**	no
19.	Do you find life very exciting?	yes	**no (1)**
20.	Is it hard for you to get started on new projects?	**yes (1)**	no
21.	Do you feel full of energy?	yes	**no (1)**
22.	Do you feel that your situation is hopeless?	**yes (1)**	no
23.	Do you think that most people are better off than you are?	**yes (1)**	no
24.	Do you frequently get upset over little things?	**yes (1)**	no
25.	Do you frequently feel like crying?	**yes (1)**	no
26.	Do you have trouble concentrating?	**yes (1)**	no
27.	Do you enjoy getting up in the morning?	yes	**no (1)**
28.	Do you prefer to avoid social occasions?	**yes (1)**	no
29.	Is it easy for you to make decisions?	yes	**no (1)**
30.	Is your mind as clear as it used to be?	yes	**no (1)**

TOTAL: Please sum all bolded answers (worth 1 point each) for a total score. _____
Scores: 0–9 Normal, 10–19 Mild Depressive, 20–30 Severe Depressive.

From Brink, T. L., Yesavage, J. A., Lum, O., Heersema, P., Adey, M. B., & Rose, T. L. (1982). Screening tests for geriatric depression. *Clinical Gerontologist, 1*(37), 44.

Daily Nutritional Goals for Older Adults

	SOURCE OF GOAL	MEN	WOMEN
Macronutrients			
Protein (g)	RDA	56	46
Carbohydrate (g)	RDA	130	130
Dietary fiber (g)	(14 g/1000 kcal)	28	22
Added sugars	DGA	< 10% of calories	< 10% of calories
Total fat	AMDR	20%–35% of calories	20%–35% of calories
Saturated fat	DGA	< 10% of calories	< 10% of calories
Linoleic acid (g)	AI	1.6	1.1
Minerals			
Calcium (mg)	RDA	Age 51–70 years: 1000 Age 71+ years: 1200	1200
Iron (mg)	RDA	8	8
Magnesium (mg)	RDA	420	320
Phosphorus (mg)	RDA	700	700
Potassium (mg)	AI	3400	2600
Sodium (mg)	CDRR	2300	2300
Zinc (mg)	RDA	11	8
Vitamins			
Vitamin A (mg, RAE)	RDA	900	700
Vitamin E (mg, AT)	RDA	15	15
Vitamin D (IU)	RDA	Age 51–70 years: 600 Age 71+ years: 800	Age 51–70 years: 600 Age 71+ years: 800
Vitamin C (mg)	RDA	90	75
Thiamin (mg)	RDA	1.2	1.1
Riboflavin (mg)	RDA	1.3	1.1
Niacin (mg)	RDA	16	14
Vitamin B_6 (mg)	RDA	1.7	1.5
Vitamin B_{12} (mcg)	RDA	2.4	2.4
Choline (mg)	AI	550	425
Vitamin K (mcg)	AI	120	90
Folate (mcg, DFE)	RDA	400	400

AI, adequate intake; *AMDR*, acceptable macronutrient distribution range; *AT*, alpha-tocopheryl; *CDRR*, chronic disease risk reduction; *DFE*, dietary folate equivalent; *DGA*, Dietary Guidelines for Americans; *RAE*, retinol activity equivalent; *RDA*, Recommended Dietary Allowance.

Data in table are based on the following calorie consumptions per day: male, 2000 kcal/d; female, 1600 kcal/d.

Data from U.S. Department of Agriculture and U.S. Department of Health and Human Services (2020). *Dietary Guidelines for Americans* (9th ed.). December 2020. Available at DietaryGuidelines.gov

Resources for Older Adults

ORGANIZATIONS

Administration for Community Living
330 C St. SW
Washington, DC 20201
(202) 401-4634
www.acl.gov

Alzheimer's Association
225 N. Michigan Ave., Floor 17
Chicago, IL 60601
(800) 272-3900
www.alz.org

American Geriatrics Society
40 Fulton St., 18th Floor
New York, NY 10038
(212) 308-1414
www.americangeriatrics.org

American Society on Aging
605 Market St., Suite 1111
San Francisco, CA 94105
(800) 537-9728
www.asaging.org/

Center of Excellence on Elder Abuse & Neglect
University of California Irvine School of Medicine
Irvine, CA 92697
(302) 831-3525
www.centeronelderabuse.org/index.asp

Disabled American Veterans
VA Regional Office
1722 I Street NW, Room 210
Washington, DC 20024
(202) 530-9260
www.dav.org/

Justice in Aging
1444 Eye St., NW, Suite 1100
Washington, DC 20005
(202) 289-6976
www.justiceinaging.org/

National Council on Aging
251 18th Street South, Suite 500
Arlington, VA 22202
www.ncoa.org/

National Indian Council on Aging
8500 Menaul Blvd. NE, Suite B-470
Albuquerque, NM 87112
(505) 292-2001
www.nicoa.org

National Institute on Aging
Building 31, Room 5C27
31 Center Drive MSC 2292
Bethesda, MD 20892
(800) 222-2225
www.nia.nih.gov/

AGING ASSOCIATIONS AND SOCIETIES

AARP
www.aarp.org/

Alzheimer's Association
www.alz.org/

American Geriatrics Society
www.americangeriatrics.org/

American Society on Aging
www.asaging.org/

Gerontological Advanced Practice Nurses Association
www.gapna.org/

Gerontological Society of America
www.geron.org/

National Council on Aging
www.ncoa.org/

GERONTOLOGY CENTERS/EDUCATION CENTERS/INSTITUTES

Brookdale Center on Aging
www.brookdale.org/

Consortium of New York Geriatric Education Centers
www.nygec.org/

Hartford Institute for Geriatric Nursing
https://hign.org/

National Association of Geriatric Education Centers
https://n-age.org/

UAMS Donald W. Reynolds Institute on Aging
http://aging.uams.edu/

University of Iowa College of Nursing
Evidence Based Practice Guidelines (for a fee)
https://csomaycenter.uiowa.edu/practice-and-
    training#evidence-based-practices-ebp-

Wayne State University Institute of Gerontology
www.iog.wayne.edu/

STATISTICS AND GOVERNMENT SITES

Administration on Aging
https://acl.gov/about-acl/administration-aging

Department of Health and Human Services (CMS/
    AHRQ)
www.hhs.gov/

Fastats
www.cdc.gov/nchs/fastats/default.htm

National Institute on Aging
www.nia.nih.gov/

JOURNALS/PERIODICALS

Generations
www.asaging.org/

Geriatric Nursing
www.sciencedirect.com/science/journal/01974572

The Gerontologist
www.geron.org/

Journal of Gerontological Nursing
https://journals.healio.com/journal/jgn
Journals of the Gerontological Society of America
www.gerontologyjournals.org/

EDUCATIONAL RESOURCES

UCLA Geriatric Medicine
www.uclahealth.org/geriatrics/

National Institute on Aging
www.nia.nih.gov/health/exercise-physical-activity

National Institute of Diabetes and Digestive and
    Kidney Diseases
www.niddk.nih.gov/health-information/weight-
    management/healthy-eating-physical-activity-for-life

Gerontological Advanced Practice Nurses Association
www.gapna.org/

INFORMATION ON EXERCISE

American Heart Association
www.heart.org/

International Council on Active Aging
www.icaa.cc

President's Council on Fitness, Sports & Nutrition
https://health.gov/our-work/pcsfn

Robert Wood Johnson Foundation
www.rwjf.org

Glossary

A

Absorption   As in drug absorption; the process whereby a drug moves from the muscle, digestive tract, or other site of entry into the body and to the circulatory system.

Abuse   Intentional or unintentional mistreatment or harm—physical, psychological, emotional, or financial—of another person.

Adverse drug reaction   A harmful or unpleasant reaction to a medication.

Ageism   Prejudice or discrimination against a particular age group, especially older adults.

Agility   Ability to move quickly and smoothly.

Agnostic   A person who neither believes nor denies the existence of god.

Alignment   The placing or maintaining of body structures in their proper anatomic positions.

Alopecia   Partial or complete lack of hair resulting from normal aging or an endocrine disorder, drug reaction, anticancer medication, or skin disease.

Anemia   A hematologic disorder marked by a decrease in hemoglobin in the blood to abnormally low levels. It is caused by a decrease in the production of red blood cells, an increase in the destruction of red blood cells, or the loss of blood. Iron deficiency anemia results from an inadequate intake of dietary iron, and pernicious anemia results from a deficiency in intrinsic factor, which is secreted by the stomach.

Anorexia   Lack or loss of appetite resulting in the inability to eat enough.

Antioxidants   Chemicals or other agents that retard or inhibit oxidation of a substance to which they are added. Examples are vitamins, carotenoids, selenium, and phytochemicals.

Anxiety   A vague, uneasy feeling, the source of which is often nonspecific or unknown to the individual.

Aphasia   An abnormal neurologic condition in which language function is disordered or absent because of an injury to certain areas of the cerebral cortex. May be a result of stroke.

Apnea   An absence of spontaneous breathing or respiration.

Arthritis   Any inflammatory condition of the joints characterized by pain, swelling, heat, redness, or limitation of movement.

Aseptic   Free of living pathogenic organisms or infected material.

Assessment   In medicine and nursing, an evaluation or appraisal of a condition or the process of making such an evaluation, including the patient's subjective report of the symptoms and the examiner's objective findings of data obtained through laboratory tests, physical examination, and medical history.

Atheist   A person who does not believe in the existence of god.

Auscultation   A technique of assessment that uses the sense of hearing to detect sounds produced within the body, such as heart, lung, and bowel sounds.

B

Basal metabolic rate   Rate at which the body uses calories.

Biologic   Pertaining to organisms; biologic aging views aging from a genetic perspective.

Blood urea nitrogen   A measure of the amount of urea, the end product of protein metabolism, in the blood.

Body image   A person's concept of their physical appearance.

Body mass index   A measure of a person's relative size based on their height and weight.

Boredom   The state of being made weary by dullness, tedium, or repetitiveness.

C

Cachexia   General ill health and malnutrition marked by weakness and emaciation, usually associated with a severe disease such as tuberculosis or cancer.

Calorie   Unit of heat that is used to measure the available energy in consumed food.

Carbohydrates   Sugars and starches that constitute the main source of energy for all body functions, particularly brain functions, and that are necessary for the metabolism of other nutrients.

Carcinoma   Malignant epithelial neoplasm that tends to invade surrounding tissue and to metastasize to distant regions of the body.

Cardiomegaly   Enlargement of the heart, often related to heart failure.

Caries   As in dental caries, a tooth disease caused by the complex interaction of food, especially starches and sugars, with the bacteria that form dental plaque; cavities.

Cataract   Clouding of the lens of the eye, which develops over time and results in the progressive painless loss of vision.

Catastrophic reactions   Excessively emotional responses.

Catheterization   Introduction of a catheter (a hollow flexible tube) into a body cavity or organ to inject or remove a fluid.

Cheyne-Stokes respiration   An abnormal pattern of respiration characterized by alternating periods of apnea and deep, rapid breathing.

Chronologic age   The number of years a person has lived.

Circadian rhythm   A pattern based on a 24-hour cycle, especially the repetition of certain physiological phenomena, such as sleeping and eating.

Cognitive   Pertaining to the mental processes of comprehension, judgment, memory, and reasoning as contrasted with emotional processes.

Cognitive behavioral therapy   A form of psychotherapy used to replace inaccurate or negative thoughts with more positive or constructive thoughts.

Cohort   Term used by demographers to describe a group of people born within a specified time period.

Complementary protein   Two or more incomplete proteins that combine to form a complete protein.

Complete protein   A protein containing all of the essential amino acids necessary for the dietary needs of humans.

Complex grief   Grief that is complicated by adjustment disorders, such as depression, alcohol abuse, or posttraumatic stress disorder.

Confrontation   A communication technique used when there are inconsistencies in information or when verbal and nonverbal messages appear contradictory.

Confusion   A mental state characterized by disorientation regarding time, place, or person that leads to bewilderment, perplexity, lack of orderly thought, and the inability to choose or act decisively or to perform the activities of daily living.

Constipation   Difficulty in passing stools or the incomplete or infrequent passage of hard stools.

Coordination   Harmonious functioning of muscles or groups of muscles in the execution of movements.

Coping   Process by which a person deals with stress, solves problems, and makes decisions.

Creatinine A substance commonly found in blood that is formed from the metabolism of creatine. It is measured in blood and urine tests as an indicator of kidney function.

Crystallized intelligence Knowledge that comes from past learning and prior experiences.

Cultural awareness Knowledge of a people's history and ancestry and an appreciation for their artistic expressions, foods, and celebrations.

Cultural competence A set of behaviors that includes an understanding the impact of cultural values and beliefs on human experiences while maintaining awareness of one's own cultural values and their effect on the perception of self and others.

Custodial focus As in custodial care, services and care of a nonmedical nature provided on a long-term basis, usually for convalescent and chronically ill individuals.

D

Defecation The elimination of feces from the digestive tract through the rectum.

Delirium A mental disorder characterized by disturbances in cognition, attention, memory, and perception. Symptoms include confusion, disorientation, restlessness, clouding of consciousness, incoherence, fear, anxiety, and excitement. It is also often characterized by illusions; hallucinations, usually of visual origin; and sometimes delusions.

Dementia A general term for a permanent or progressive organic mental disorder characterized by personality changes, confusion, disorientation, deterioration of intellectual functioning, and impaired control of memory, judgment, and impulses.

Demographics The statistical study of human populations.

Depression A mental state of depressed mood characterized by feelings of sadness, despair, and discouragement; it may range from normal feelings of "the blues" all the way to major clinical depression. Resembling the grief and mourning that follow bereavement, the symptoms of depression include feelings of low self-esteem, guilt, and self-reproach; withdrawal from interpersonal contact; and somatic symptoms such as eating and sleeping disorders.

Dexterity Skillfulness in the use of one's hands or body; the ability to perform fine manipulative skills.

Diarrhea The frequent passage of loose, watery stools.

Dietary reference intake Developed by the U.S. National Academy of Sciences, guidelines for evaluating the diets of healthy people and estimating their optimal nutrient intake.

Distress An emotional or physical state of pain, sorrow, misery, suffering, or discomfort.

Distribution As in drug distribution, the pattern of distribution of drug molecules by various tissues after the chemical enters the circulatory system.

Diuretics Drugs that promote the formation and excretion of urine.

Diurnal Occurring daily, such as sleeping and eating.

Diversional As in diversional activity, stimulation from, interest in, or engagement in recreational or leisure activities.

Diverticulosis The presence of pouchlike herniations (diverticula) throughout the muscular layer of the colon, which develop because of weaknesses in the intestinal mucosa.

Dysarthria Difficult, poorly articulated speech due to interference in control over the muscles of speech, usually caused by neurologic damage.

Dysfunctional Unable to function normally.

Dysgeusia A distortion of the sense of taste.

Dyspareunia Discomfort during sexual intercourse.

Dysphagia Difficulty swallowing.

Dysphasia See *aphasia*.

Dyspnea A distressful sensation of uncomfortable breathing that may be caused by certain heart or respiratory conditions, strenuous exercise, or anxiety.

E

Edema The abnormal accumulation of fluid in the interstitial spaces of tissues due to increased capillary fluid pressure.

Edentulous Lacking teeth; toothless.

Electrocardiogram (ECG) A graphic record produced by an electrocardiograph, a device for recording electrical conduction through the heart.

Electrolyte An element or compound that, when melted or dissolved in water or another solvent, dissociates into ions and can conduct an electric current.

Empathy The willingness to try to understand the unique world of another person; the ability to put oneself in another person's place and to understand what he or she is feeling and thinking in various situations.

Enema The introduction of a solution into the rectum for cleansing or therapeutic purposes.

Ethical dilemmas Questions or problems related to moral values or principles.

Eustress Stress that is perceived as positive; "good stress."

Excretion As in drug excretion, the process of eliminating, shedding, or getting rid of a drug by body organs or tissues as part of natural metabolic activity.

Exudate Fluid, cell, or other substance that has been slowly discharged from cells or blood vessels through small pores or breaks in cell membranes.

F

Faith Belief in God or in a set of religious doctrines.

Fatigue A state of exhaustion or a loss of strength or endurance, such as that which may follow strenuous physical activity.

Fear A response to a perceived threat that is consciously recognized as a danger.

Fecal impaction An accumulation of hardened feces in the rectum or sigmoid colon that the individual is unable to move or pass.

Feedback Information produced by a receiver and perceived by a sender that informs the sender of the receiver's reaction to the message.

First pass effect The phase of drug absorption when oral medications take a first pass through the liver before entering the systemic circulation.

Free radical Unstable molecule produced by the body during the normal processes of respiration and metabolism or following exposure to radiation and pollution. Free radicals are suspected of causing damage to the cells, deoxyribonucleic acid, and immune system.

G

Gastroesophageal reflux disease A condition in which acidic stomach contents leak backward from the stomach into the esophagus.

Geriatrics The branch of medicine dealing with the physiological characteristics of aging and the diagnosis and treatment of diseases affecting older adults.

Gerontic nursing The nursing care and service provided to older adults.

Gerontology The study of all aspects of the aging process, including the clinical, psychological, economic, and sociologic problems of older adults and the consequences of these problems for older adults and society.

Gerontophobia The fear of aging and the refusal to accept older adults into the mainstream of society.

Geropharmacology The study of how older adults respond to medication.

Gingivitis Inflammation of the gingiva (gums), with symptoms that may include redness, swelling, and bleeding.

Glaucoma Disease characterized by increased fluid pressure (intraocular pressure) within the eye, which may result in damage to the retina.

Grief A feeling of sorrow, loss, and confusion experienced by someone who has lost a loved person or something of value.

H

Half-life The amount of time required to reduce a drug level to half of its initial value.

Halitosis   Offensive bad breath, resulting from poor oral hygiene, dental or oral infections, the ingestion of certain foods, tobacco use, or certain systemic diseases, such as diabetes, which may produce the odor of acetone on the breath.

Health maintenance   A systemic program planned to prevent illness, maintain maximal function, and promote health.

Health promotion   Lifestyle and health care practices that improve overall health and quality of life.

Heatstroke   Due to unrecognized and untreated heat exhaustion, a gradually developing condition caused by the depletion of body water or sodium.

Helplessness   A feeling of loss of control or ability, usually after repeated failures, or of being immobilized or frozen by circumstances beyond one's control, with the result that one is unable to make autonomous choices.

Hematocrit   A measure of the packed cell volume of red blood cells, expressed as a percentage of the total blood volume.

Hemianopsia   Vision loss in half of the visual field of one or both eyes.

Hemiparesis   Muscular weakness of one side of the body.

Hemiplegia   Paralysis of one side of the body.

Hemoglobin   A complex protein-iron molecule that is responsible for the transport of oxygen and carbon dioxide within the bloodstream.

Heterogeneous   Comprising many different characteristics and/or qualities.

Hiatal hernia   A condition in which part of the stomach pushes up through the diaphragm muscle.

Homogeneous   Comprising many similar characteristics and/or qualities.

Hopelessness   A state in which an individual sees only limited or no alternatives in personal choices and is unable to mobilize energy on his or her own behalf.

Hospice   A multidisciplinary system of family-centered care designed to assist the terminally ill person to be comfortable and to maintain a satisfactory lifestyle through the phases of dying.

Hyperkeratosis   Overgrowth of the epithelial layer of the skin.

Hyperthermia   A body temperature that is much higher than normal.

Hypnotics   A class of drugs often used as sedatives.

Hypothermia   A core body temperature of 95 degrees F or lower.

Hypothyroidism   Reduced function of the thyroid gland. Symptoms include cold intolerance, dry skin, dry and thin body hair, constipation, depression, and lack of energy.

Hysterectomy   Surgical removal of the uterus to treat fibroid tumors, pelvic inflammatory disease, severe recurrent endometrial hyperplasia, uterine hemorrhage, and precancerous and cancerous conditions of the uterus.

I

Imaging   Formation of a mental picture or representation of someone or something using the imagination. Medical imaging is the technique and process of imaging the interior of a body for clinical analysis and medical intervention, using techniques such as X-Ray, MRI, or others.

Immunologic   Related to the immune system. The immunologic theory of aging proposes that aging is a function of changes in the immune system, which weakens over time to make an aging person more susceptible to disease.

Incontinence   Inability to control urination or defecation.

Insomnia   Chronic inability to sleep or to remain asleep throughout the night; wakefulness; sleeplessness.

Inspection   The most commonly used method of physical assessment in which the senses of vision, smell, and hearing are used to collect data.

Intelligence   The potential ability and capacity to acquire, retain, and apply experience, understanding, knowledge, reasoning, and judgment in coping with new experiences and in solving problems.

Intercourse   Sexual intercourse between individuals; coitus.

Intermittent claudication   Cramplike pains in the calves caused by poor circulation of the blood to the leg muscles, commonly associated with atherosclerosis (whereby the tissues of the lower extremities are deprived of oxygen); manifested only at certain times, usually after walking; and relieved by rest.

Interstitial   Pertaining to the space between cells, as in interstitial fluid, or between organs.

Intracellular   Pertaining to the interior of a cell, as in intracellular fluid, a fluid within cell membranes throughout most of the body, containing dissolved solutes that are essential to electrolytic balance and healthy metabolism.

Intravascular   Pertaining to the inside of a blood vessel.

Ischemic   Related to a decreased supply of oxygenated blood, as in ischemic heart disease, a pathologic condition caused by lack of oxygen in cells of the myocardium.

Isometric   As in isometric exercise, a form of active exercise in which muscle tension is increased while pressure is applied against stable resistance.

Isotonic   As in isotonic exercise, a form of active exercise in which muscles contract and cause movement. Because there is no significant change in resistance throughout the movement, the force of contraction remains constant.

L

Laxatives   Agents that promote bowel evacuation by increasing the bulk of the feces, softening the stool, or lubricating the intestinal wall.

Leukoplakia   A precancerous, slowly developing change in a mucous membrane characterized by white, thickened, firmly attached patches that are slightly raised and sharply circumscribed.

M

Malnutrition   Any disorder of nutrition resulting from an unbalanced, insufficient, or excessive diet or from impaired absorption, assimilation, or use of foods.

Mandated reporter   A professional who is required by law to report reasonable suspicions of abuse.

Mantra   From Hinduism, a sacred verbal formula repeated in prayer, meditation, or incantation, such as the invocation of a god, a magic spell, or a syllable or portion of scripture containing mystic potentialities.

Masturbation   Sexual self-gratification; sexual activity in which the penis or clitoris is stimulated, usually to orgasm, by means other than intercourse.

Meditation   A state of consciousness in which the individual eliminates environmental stimuli from awareness so that the mind has a single focus, producing a state of relaxation and relief from stress.

Memory   The mental faculty or power that enables one to retain and to recall, through unconscious associative processes, previously experienced sensations, impressions, ideas, concepts, and all information that has been consciously learned.

Metabolism   As in drug metabolism, the transformation of a drug by the body tissues into a metabolite as the body readies the agent for elimination.

Minerals   Inorganic chemical elements required in many of the body's functions.

Morgue   A unit of a hospital or municipality with facilities for the storage and autopsy of the dead.

N

Nasogastric   Pertaining to the nose and stomach, as in nasogastric intubation, the placement of a nasogastric tube through the nose into the stomach to relieve gastric distention by removing gas, gastric secretions, or food. Such intubation serves to instill medication, food, or fluids or to obtain a specimen for laboratory analysis.

Neglect   Passive form of abuse in which caregivers fail to provide for the needs of the person under their care.

Nocturnal   Pertaining to or occurring during the night.

Nonadherence   When a patient is unwilling or unable to follow providers' recommendations about the daily timing, dosage, and frequency of medication use or other recommended health practices.

Nystagmus   Rapid, involuntary eye movement.

O

Objective data   Information obtained through the senses or measured by instruments.

Orthodox   In religion, adhering to an accepted, traditional, established faith.

Orthopnea   Dyspnea related to lying flat.

Orthostatic hypotension   Condition of low blood pressure that occurs because the circulation does not respond quickly to changes in position.

Osteoporosis   Disorder characterized by porous, brittle, fragile bones that are susceptible to breakage; it is caused by excessive loss of calcium from bone combined with insufficient replacement.

Otosclerosis   A hereditary condition of the bony labyrinth of the ear, in which spongy bone forms, resulting in hearing loss.

P

Palliative   As in palliative treatment, therapy designed to relieve or reduce the intensity of uncomfortable symptoms but not to produce a cure, such as the use of narcotics to relieve pain.

Palpation   A method of physical assessment that uses the sense of touch in the fingers and hands to obtain data.

Parasitic   Of an organism living in or on and obtaining nourishment from another organism.

Perception   The conscious recognition and interpretation of sensory stimuli that serve as a basis for understanding, learning, and knowing or for motivating a particular action or reaction.

Percussion   A technique of physical assessment in which the size, position, and density of structures under the skin are assessed by tapping the area and listening to the resonance of the sound. Depending on the amount of vibration (sound) heard, the presence of masses, fluid, or air can be determined.

Pharmacokinetics   The study of the action of drugs within the body, including the mechanisms of absorption, distribution, metabolism, and excretion; onset of action; duration of effect; biotransformation; and effects and routes of excretion of the metabolites of the drug.

Phase advance   A shifting in circadian rhythm causing a person to feel sleepy earlier in the evening and to wake up earlier in the morning.

Pigmentation   Organic color, such as melanin, produced in the body.

Polypharmacy   The prescription, administration, or use of more medications than are clinically indicated.

Powerlessness   A perceived lack of control over a current situation or problem and the person's perception that any action they might take would not affect the outcome of the particular situation.

Presbycusis   Hearing loss associated with aging, particularly of higher-pitched sounds.

Presbyopia   Found in older people, farsightedness due to the lens's loss of elasticity, thus reducing the eye's power of accommodation.

Pressure injuries   Inflammations, lesions, or ulcerations in the skin over a body prominence—occurring most commonly on the sacrum, elbows, heels, outer ankles, inner knees, hips, shoulder blades, and occipital bones—occurring mainly in high-risk patients who are most often aged, debilitated, immobilized, or cachectic.

Proactive   Creating or controlling a situation by preventing something from happening rather than by responding to it after it has happened.

Prophylactic   Preventing the spread of disease.

Prostate-specific antigen (PSA) test   A blood test used to measure the level of prostate-specific antigen, which may be present at elevated levels in patients with cancer or other diseases of the prostate, and to monitor the patient's response to therapy.

Protein   Any of a large group of naturally occurring complex organic compounds, composed of amino acids, essential for tissue repair and healing.

Proxemics   Study of the use of personal space in communication.

Pruritus   Itching; an uncomfortable sensation leading to the urge to scratch, which may result in a secondary infection.

Psychosocial   Pertaining to a combination of psychological and social factors. The psychosocial theories of aging attempt to explain why older adults have varying responses to the aging process.

Pulse deficit   The absence of palpable pulse beats in a peripheral artery for one or more heartbeats when simultaneously compared with an apical pulse measurement.

R

Rapport   Atmosphere of mutual respect and understanding.

Reactive   Acting in response to a situation rather than taking measures to prevent or control it.

Rehabilitation   The restoration of an individual or a part to normal or near normal function after a disabling disease or injury.

Rehabilitative focus   The result of high expectations and a high-level focus in planning care.

Relationships   Connections formed by the dynamic interaction of individuals who play interrelated roles.

Relaxation   As in relaxation therapy; treatment in which patients are taught to perform breathing and relaxation exercises and to concentrate on a pleasant situation.

Religious   Having belief in or reverence for God or a deity.

Reminiscence   Also called *life review*, this involves allowing the older adult to think back and reflect on past experiences.

Respite   As in respite care; allows the primary caregiver to have time away from the constant demands of caregiving, thereby decreasing caregiver stress and the risk for abuse.

Retention   The inability to urinate or defecate.

Ritual   Formal and observable ceremonies used to affirm faith and sense of belonging to a spiritual community.

Role   A socially accepted behavior pattern.

S

Scabies   Contagious disease caused by a mite, characterized by intense itching of the skin and excoriation from scratching.

Screenings   As in health screenings, which are done to identify older people in need of further, more in-depth assessment. Examples are screenings for high blood pressure, hearing problems, foot problems, and problems with activities of daily living.

Seborrheic dermatitis   An unsightly skin disorder characterized by yellow, waxy crusts that can be either dry or moist; it is caused by sebum production and occurs on the scalp, eyebrows, eyelids, ears, axillae, breasts, groin, and gluteal folds.

Seborrheic keratosis   Skin disorder in which lesions ranging in color from light tan to black appear as slightly raised, wartlike macules with distinct edges.

Sedative   An agent that decreases a person's functional activity, diminishes irritability, and allays excitement.

Self-esteem   The degree of worth and competence one attributes to oneself.

Self-hypnosis   Process of putting oneself into a trancelike state by autosuggestion, such as concentration on a single thought or object.

Senile lentigo   Skin disorder whereby clusters of melanocytes form areas of deepened pigmentation; often called *age spots* or *liver spots*.

Senile purpura   Red, purple, or brown areas commonly seen on the legs and arms, resulting from hemorrhaging as the walls of the capillaries become increasingly fragile with age.

Sexual dysfunction   A persistent impairment of a person's usual pattern of sexual functioning.

Sexuality   The sum of the physical, functional, and psychological attributes expressed by one's gender identity and sexual behavior regardless of the relationship to the sex organs or to procreation.

Shearing forces   Applied forces that causes a downward and forward pressure on the tissues beneath the skin.

Social isolation   A condition in which a feeling of aloneness is experienced, which the person acknowledges as a negative or threatening state imposed by others.

Sphincter   A circular band of muscle fibers that constricts a passage or closes a natural opening in the body, such as the external anal sphincter, which closes the anus, or the hepatic sphincter in the muscular coat of the hepatic veins near their union with the superior vena cava.

Spiritual   Of or relating to the nature of spirit; not tangible or material.

Stimuli   Things that excite or incite an organism or part to function, become active, or respond.

Stress   Any emotional, physical, social, economic, or other factor that requires a response or change.

Subjective data   Data obtained from the patient's point of view.

Sundowning   A condition in which persons with cognitive impairment (e.g., people with Alzheimer disease) and older people tend to become confused or disoriented at the end of the day, exhibiting such behaviors as wandering, combativeness, suspiciousness, hallucinations, and delusions.

Supplement   As in nutritional supplement, a nutrient added to complete, make up for a deficiency, and extend or strengthen the diet.

Symbol   An object, action, or other stimulus that represents something else by conscious association, convention, or another relationship.

T

Tachycardia   Occurs when the heart beats more rapidly than normal; can be related to factors such as decreased blood volume, increased oxygen demand by the body, pain, stress, or other factors.

Theory   An abstract statement formulated to predict, explain, or describe the relationships between concepts, constructs, or events.

Thermoregulation   The ability to maintain body temperature in a safe range, controlled by the hypothalamus.

Trace element   An element essential to nutrition or physiological processes, found in such minute quantities that analysis yields the presence of only trace amounts.

V

Vitamins   Organic compounds found naturally in foods or produced synthetically.

X

Xerosis   Dry skin caused by a decrease in the function of sebaceous and sweat gland secretion.

Xerostomia   Dryness of the mouth caused by cessation of normal salivary secretion.

Index

Note: Page numbers followed by *f* indicate figures, *t* indicate tables, and *b* indicate boxes.

A

AARP. *See* American Association of Retired Persons (AARP)
Abandonment, 24
Abdominal aortic aneurysm, 50
Absorption, drug, 141
Abuse, 22
  assessment of, 24*b*
  responses to, 24
  by unrelated caregivers, 25
Abusive behaviors, in health care settings, 26*b*
Acceptance
  in communication, 101
  of death and dying, 275*b*
Accessibility, and health promotion and maintenance, 86
Accessory muscles, with oxygenation problems, 339
Accidents. *See* Safety problems
Accommodation, 65
"Acting out" behavior, with disturbed thought processes, 203
Active listening, 101
Active range-of-motion exercises, 336*b*
Activities department for deficient diversional activities, 346
Activities of daily living (ADLs), 235–236
  with disturbed thought processes, 203, 203*f*
Activity(ies), 292*t*–293*t*, 325
  and aging, 326
  for deficient diversional activities, 345
  effects of disease processes on, 328
  negative attitudes about, 340
  normal patterns of, 325
  pacing of, 326*b*, 326
  positive attitudes about, 349
  voluntary, 326
Activity theory, 31
Activity tolerance
  nursing process/clinical judgment model for altered, 335, 336*b*
  assessment, 335
  data analysis/problem identification, 335
  planning, 336

Adaptive aids, for brushing, 306*f*
Address in communication, 101
Adenosine triphosphate (ATP), 39
Adipose tissue, 37
ADLs, 204*b*
Adrenal glands, 70
Advance directives, 18, 19*b*, 263
Adverse drug events (ADE), 140
Aerobic exercise, 39, 327
Affordable Care Act, 17
Age discrimination, 5
Ageism, 4, 216
Age-related macular degeneration, 67
Age spots, 34–35
Aggregate income, 333
Agility, 326
Aging
  activity and, 326
  alternative and complementary therapies to slow or reverse, 30*b*–31*b*
  attitudes toward, 3*b*, 3
  current knowledge about, 3*b*
  depression and, 217
  economics of, 9
  elimination and, 308
  fear of, 329
  healthy, 335*f*
  historical perspective on study of, 1
  myth *vs.* fact, 5*b*
  nutrition and, 111
  perceptions of, 64, 85, 216, 217*b*
  process of, 326
  roles, relationships, and, 231
  sexuality and, 278
  sleep and, 354
  suicide and, 218
  theories of, 29
  values about, 4*b*
"Aging eye", 65–66
Aging family members, impact of, 19*b*
"Aging in place" concept, 176
Aging population
  categorization of, 2*t*
  demographics of, 6, 8*b*
  scope of, 6
Agnostics, 255
Air exchange (respiration), 42
Air-fluidized surfaces, 297*t*–298*t*
Albumin, 117*t*

Alcohol, and sexual function, 280
Alcohol consumption, for health promotion and maintenance, 79
Alcoholism, 244
Alcohol-related problems, 303
  in older adults, 247*b*
Alcohol use disorder, 120*b*, 120
Alignment, 330
Allergic dermatitis, 37
Alopecia, 290
Altered communication ability
  nursing care plan, 208*b*
  nursing process/clinical judgment model for, 205
    assessment, 206
    data analysis/problem identification, 206
    implementation, 207
    planning, 207
Aluminum hydroxide, 149*t*
Alzheimer dementia, 61*b*
Alzheimer disease, 181
  and activity, 328
  alternative treatments for, 63
  facts about, 200*b*
  life stressors and, 62
  stages of, 200*b*
Ambulation, assistance during, 334, 334*f*
American Association of Retired Persons (AARP), 12*b*
American Indians, death in, 267*b*
American Seniors Association (ASA), 12*b*
Anemia, 52
  due to vitamin B$_{12}$ deficiency, 115
  iron-deficiency, 117
  pernicious, 118
Aneurysm, 49
Anger, related to death and dying, 275*b*
Anginal pain, with oxygenation problems, 339–340
Anorexia, during dying, 272
Antianxiety agents, 149*t*
Antibacterials, 149*t*
Antidepressants, 62–63, 149*t*
Antihypertensives, 149*t*
Antioxidant(s), 30
Antioxidant therapy, for aging, 30

Antioxidant vitamins, 115
Antipsychotics, 149t
Anxiety, 215, 360
   about dying, 268
   nursing process/clinical judgment
      model for, 223
      assessment, 224
      data analysis/problem
         identification, 224
      implementation, 224
      planning, 224
   and sleep disorders, 355
Aphasia, 102, 193, 206, 206t
Apical pulse, 173
Apnea, sleep, 355, 357b, 357
Apolipoprotein E (APOE) gene, 61
Appetite changes, assessment of, 125
Aqueous humor, 65
Areolar connective tissue, 34
Arthritis, and activity, 328
ASA. See American Seniors Association
   (ASA)
Aseptic technique for wound cleansing,
   296
Asians, roles and relationships of,
   230b
Aspiration risk, nursing process for,
   136–137
Aspirin, 149t
Assertiveness, 226f
Asset income, 11
Assisted-living centers, 338
Assistive devices, 85
   for impaired physical mobility,
      333–334, 333f
   for injury prevention, 185f
   for self-care deficits, 343
Atenolol, 149t
Atheists, 255
Atrophic vaginitis, 279
Attitudes
   about death, 263, 264b
   maintaining healthy, 83
Auditory changes, 191–192
Auricle, 67–68
Auscultation, 162, 165
Automobile accidents, 188
Autosomal dominant Alzheimer
   disease, 62
Avoidance, 245
Axillary temperature, 165

B

Baby Boomers, 8, 181, 232b, 232, 355b
Bad news, delivering, 105
Balance training, 327
Bargaining, related to death and dying,
   275b
Basal cell carcinoma, 36
Basal metabolic rate, 112
Bathing, reducing frequency of, 294
Beds to reduce pressure, 296
Behavioral signs, of stress, 243

Beliefs, 252b–253b
   about death, 263, 264b
   cultural understanding, 253b
   of older adults, 254
   in older adults, risk factors for
      alterations in values and, 257b
   spiritual, 255
   values and, 252–254
Bereavement, 275
Biocultural differences, 84
Biofeedback, for stress reduction,
   245–246
Biologic theories, of aging, 29
Bisexual, older people, 281
Bladder, 56
Bleeding, 171t–172t
Blepharitis, 66
Blood, 50
Blood chemistry, 363t–366t
Blood glucose level, 125
Blood pressure (BP), 167
   with activity intolerance, 337b
Blood tests, 80
Blood urea nitrogen, 117t, 124
Blood vessels, 46
Body fluids, 130
Body image
   nursing process/clinical judgment
      model for altered, 219
      assessment, 219
      data analysis/problem
         identification, 219
      implementation, 219
      planning, 219
Body language, 98
Body mass index (BMI), 112f, 112
Body temperature, 165–166
Bones, 37
Boredom, and sleep disorders, 360
Bowel elimination, 310
Braden scale, 292t–293t
Breast cancer, 75
Breathing, sleep disordered, 357
Broca aphasia, 206, 206t
Broca's area, 206
Bronchodilators, 149t
Brushes, long-handled, 344f
Buddhism, death in, 267b
Bulk laxatives, 312t
Bumetanide, 149t
Bureau of the Census, 6
Burn prevention, 178
Bursa, 42
Bursitis, 42
Button hook, 343f

C

Cachexia, during dying, 272
Calcitonin, 38
Calcium, 117, 117t
Call signal for injury prevention,
   186–187
Calm, 203b

Caloric intake, 111, 117
Calorie(s), 111–112
Calorie-restricted diet, for aging, 31
Cancer, 55, 302
Candidiasis, oral, 303b
Canes, 333–334, 333f
Capillary refill time, 339
Captopril, 149t
Cap, uniform, 97
Carbohydrates, 113
Cardiac arrhythmias, 48
Cardiac medication, 149t
Cardiac muscle, 38–39
Cardiac output, risk factors related to
   decreased, 338b
Cardiomegaly, 49
Cardiovascular changes, at end-of-life,
   271
Cardiovascular function, 339
Cardiovascular signs of stress, 243t
Cardiovascular system, 45
   assessment of, 162t–164t
   common disorders seen with aging
      in, 47
   expected age-related changes in, 47
Care area assessments (CAAs), 169
Care area triggers (CATs), 169
Caregiver(s)
   paid, 87
   in United States, 20b
   unpaid, 86
Caries, 301f, 301
Cartilage, 41
Cataracts, 67, 192f
Catastrophic reactions, 199
Catheterization, for urinary retention,
   316
Catheters, 322, 323f
Cellular theories, 30
Central nervous system, 58
Cephalosporins, 149t
Cerebellum, 58
Cerebrovascular accident, 63
Cerebrum, 59
Chemical restraints, 202
Chest pain, 171t–172t
Chest radiographs, 338–339
Chewing difficulties, and nutrition, 120,
   128
Cheyne-Stokes respiration, 271
Chlorpromazine, 149t
Choices and powerlessness, 226
Christianity, death in, 267b
Chronic confusion
   nursing care plan, 205b
   nursing process/clinical judgment
      model for, 197
      assessment, 200
      data analysis/problem
         identification, 201
      implementation, 201
      planning, 201
Chronic constipation, 313b

Chronic health factors and nutrition, 120
Chronic kidney disease, 58
Chronic laxative use, 310b
Chronic obstructive pulmonary disease (COPD), 43
Chronologic age, 2
Cimetidine, 149t
Circadian rhythm, 353
    sleep disorders, 358
Claudication, intermittent, with oxygenation problems, 339–340
Cleaning carts, locking of, 185
Clinical Judgment Model, 88
Clinker theory, 30
Clonidine, 149t
Clothing, for exercise, 333, 335
Clutter, as hazard, 178
Cochlea, 68
Cognition, 191, 197b
    defined, 191
    and intelligence, 192b, 192
    and language, 192
    and perception, 197b
    risk factors related to, 194b
Cognitive behavioral therapy for insomnia (CBTI), 357
Cognitive changes
    at end of life, 273
    and health promotion and maintenance, 85
Cognitive development, 192
Cognitive functioning, normal, 191
Cognitive signs of stress, 243
Cohort, 8
Collagen, 34
Combs, long-handled, 344f
Comfort measures, for pain, 210–211
Communication, 95, 206b, 206, 270b
    about death, 267
    acceptance, dignity, and respect in, 101
    address in, 101
    barriers to, 98b, 101
    clinical situation, 109b
    COVID-19 and masks, 102b
    critical thinking, 104b
    cultural considerations, 96b
    cultural differences, 103
    culture, ethnicity and, 96b
    with disturbed sensory perception, 194–195
    effective, 95
    empathy in, 101
    at end of life, 265
    formal or therapeutic, 96
    health care team, 101b
    with health care team, 106
    with impaired older adults, 102b
    improving, 96b
    informal or social, 97
    for information sharing (framing the message), 95

Communication (Continued)
    language barriers, 104b
    listening in, 101
    misunderstanding of medical jargon, 96b
    nonverbal, 97, 97f
    nurse-physician communication, 107b
    between older adult and physician, 100b
    older adult and primary care provider, 106
    with older adults, dos and don'ts in working, 96t
    pace or speed of, 99
    preventing agitation and combativeness, 103b
    preventing cultural bias in caregiving, 99b
    and self-esteem, 222
    skills and techniques of, 104
    styles of, 96b
    technology to enhance, 223b
    telephoning primary care providers, 107
    time and timing of, 99
    with visitors and families, 105
    "you" messages in, 107
Community-based residential facility (CBRF), 15
Community education programs, 317b
Community resources for disturbed thought processes, 204
Complementary health approaches, 245
    geriatric massage, 246b
    light therapy as, 201b
    music therapy as, 202b
    for postmenopausal discomforts, 279b
    prayer, 256b
    Qi gong and tai chi as, 328b
    stress reduction, 246b
    treatments for insomnia, 357b
Complementary proteins, 114–115
Complete proteins, 114–115
Complex carbohydrates, 113
Complex grief, nursing process/clinical judgment model for, 234
Compressed O_2 cylinders, 341b
Computer safety, for older adults, 180b
Concentrator, 341b
Condition change, assessment of, 169
Conduction system, 46
Cones, 65
Confrontation, 105
Confusion, 197
    acute, 197
    chronic, 197, 205b
    general approaches for, 202b
    idiopathic, 199
Conjunctiva, 64
Connective tissue theory, 30
Constipation, 171t–172t, 308–309
    assessment of, 311
    criteria for, 309

Constipation (Continued)
    defined, 309
    in dying person, 272–273
    fiber and, 309
    fluids and, 311
    new medications for, 313b
    nursing care plan for, 314b
    nursing process/critical thinking model for, 311
        assessment, 311
        data analysis/problem identification, 311
        implementation, 311
        planning, 311
    peristalsis and, 309
    positioning and, 310
    risk factors related to, 311b
    urge to defecate and, 309
    when it may be more than, 310b
Contact dermatitis, 37
Continuity, for disturbed thought processes, 202
Controlling focus, 348b, 348
Cool-down exercise, 335
Coordination, 326
Coping
    mechanisms, 243
    normal, 241
    nursing process/clinical judgment model for limited, 246, 248f
        assessment, 246
        data analysis/problem identification, 247
        implementation, 247
        planning, 247
    strategies for, 245
Coping mechanism for stress, 245b, 245
Coronary artery disease, 47
Coronary valve disease, 48
Coughing, effective, 339
COVID-19, 44
Crackles, 165
Crafts, 224f
Creams, 294
Creatinine, 117t, 124
Creative visualization, 361
Cross-cultural misunderstandings, 231
Crosslink theory, 30
Crow's feet, 35
Crushed medication, 151–152
Crystallized intelligence, 192
Cultural awareness, 253b
Cultural beliefs, for health promotion and maintenance, 84
Cultural competence, 253b
Cultural perspectives, on end-of-life, 267
Cultural values, 254
Culture, assessment and, 160b
Cushions to reduce pressure, 296
Custodial care, 15
Custodial focus, 348b, 348
Cutaneous papilloma, 34–35
Cyanosis, for oxygenation problems, 339

D

Daily physical activity, 175f
Data, health history, 161b
Deafness, 68
Death, 273
    attitudes toward, 262b, 262
    bereavement after, 275
    causes of, 261b
    communication about, 267
    funeral arrangements after, 275
    "good", 264b
    indicators of imminent, 274
    personal beliefs and attitudes about,
        264b
    recognizing imminent, 274
    stages of, Kübler-Ross, 275b
    values clarification related to, 263,
        264b
    where people die, 264
Decision-making process, 267
Decreased self-esteem
    nursing process/clinical judgment
        model for potential for, 220
        assessment, 220
        data analysis/problem
            identification, 220
        implementation, 221
        planning, 221
Defecate, urge to, and constipation, 309
Defecation
    and aging, 308
    normal patterns of, 308
Defense mechanisms for stress, 245b,
    245
Degenerative joint disease, 41
Dehydration, 130, 171t–172t
Delirium, 171t–172t, 198b
    acute, 197–198
    causes of, 197
    defined, 197
    in dying person, 273
    mnemonic assessment for, 197, 198t
    nursing interventions for, 198t
    vs. dementia, 198t
Dementia, 60, 199b
    advanced, 199
    as barrier to communication, 103
    critical thinking on, 200b
    delirium vs., 198t
    early stages of, 199
    general approaches for dealing with,
        202b
    incidence of, 199–200
    nursing interventions for, 198t
    pacing with, 201–202
    physical activity with, 201–202
    risk of injury and personal neglect
        with, 199
    and sleep disorders, 355
    types of, 199b
    wandering with, 199
Dementia with Lewy bodies (DLB),
    60–61

Demographics, 6, 8b
Denial of death and dying, 275b
Dental care, 301
Dental caries, 301
Dental examinations, 82
Dental hygiene, 305
Dental hygienist, referral to, 304
Dentures, 302
    dental examinations with, 82
    and dysphagia, 134
    learning to use, 86–87
    poor fit of, 83
Depression, 121, 171t–172t, 215, 243, 360
    about dying, 268
    and aging, 217
    goals of treatment for, 244b
    incidence of, 217–218
    related to death and dying, 275b
    and risk of suicide, 225
    signs of, 217–218
    and sleep disorders, 355
    symptoms of, 244b
Dermis, 34
Designer estrogens, 279b See
        also Estrogen receptor
        agonist-antagonists
Despair, 216
Deterministic genes, 62
Detrusor spasms, 317–318
Developmental stages, 31
Dexterity, 326
Diabetes Mellitus (DM), 72
Diabetic retinopathy, 67
Diagnosis-related group (DRG) system,
    336
Diarrhea, 171t–172t, 308, 313
    defined, 313
    in dying person, 273
    nursing process/critical thinking
        model for, 313
        assessment, 313
        data analysis/problem
            identification, 313
        implementation, 314
        planning, 314
Diazepam, 149t
Diet. See also Nutrition
    and constipation, 309
    for health promotion and
        maintenance, 79
Dietary record, for imbalanced
    nutrition, 126
Dietary Reference Intakes (DRIs), 113
Dietary restrictions, religious, 122
Dietitians, 127
Difficult conversations, 106
Digestion problems, 120
Digital rectal examination for
    constipation, 310b
Dignity in communication, 101
Digoxin, 149t
Diplopia, 67
Direct questioning, 104

Disengagement theory, 31
Disposable garment protectors, 322f
Disposable incontinence pads, 322f
Disrupted living situation
    nursing care plan for, 250b
    nursing process/clinical judgment
        model for, 248
        assessment, 249
        data analysis/problem
            identification, 249
        implementation, 249
        planning, 249
Disrupted sleep pattern
    nursing care plan, 361b
    nursing process/clinical judgment
        model for, 358
        assessment, 358
        data analysis/problem
            identification, 358
        implementation, 358
        planning, 358
Distance, in nonverbal communication,
    98
Distress, 241
Diuretics, 149t, 311b
Diurnal rhythm, 353
Diversional activity, deficient
    nursing process/clinical judgment
        model for, 345, 347f
        assessment, 345
        data analysis/problem
            identification, 345
        implementation, 345
        planning, 345
    risk factors related to, 345b
Diverticulitis, 55
Diverticulosis, 55
Documentation, 153
Donne, John, 261
"Do Not Use" list of abbreviations, 150t
"Donut hole" in prescription coverage,
    337
Doorknob turner, 343f
Doppler, 165, 167
Driving by elderly, 181b, 181
Drug absorption, 141
Drug distribution, 141
Drug excretion, 142
Drug-induced skin reactions, 288f
Drug metabolism, 142
Drug-testing methods, risks related to,
    141
Dry lips, 304–305
Dry mouth
    with aging, 302
    of dying person, 272
Dry skin, 287, 288f
Duration, of sound, 165
Dying
    amount and type of intervention, 268
    cardiovascular changes during, 271
    cognition changes during, 273
    communication during, 265

Dying (*Continued*)
 cultural perspectives on, 267
 decision making process, 267
 depression, anxiety, and fear related
  to, 268
 fatigue and sleepiness, 271
 gastrointestinal changes during,
  272
 integumentary changes during,
  273
 Maslow's hierarchy of needs, 265*f*
 pain during, 269, 269*f*
 respiratory changes during, 271
 sensory changes during, 273
 significance of pain and suffering
  during, 268
 spiritual needs during, 268*b*
 stages of, Kübler-Ross, 275*b*
 urinary changes during, 273
Dysarthria, 205
Dysgeusia, 304
Dyspareunia, 279
Dysphagia, 206
Dysphasia, 206
Dyspnea, 338
 during dying, 271

E
Ear(s), 67
 assessment of, 162*t*–164*t*
 auditory changes associated with
  aging, 68*t*
 common disorders seen with aging
  in, 68
 expected age-related changes, 68
Early retirement, 334
Eating device, 344*f*
Eccrine glands, 34
Economic risk factors for malnutrition,
  120–121
Economics of aging, 9
Economic values, 254
Economic well-being, 13
Edema, 131, 171*t*–172*t*
Edentulous, 302
Educational status, 8
Ego integrity, 216
Elder abuse, 25*b*
 in institutions, 25*b*
Elder Hostel, 347
Elderspeak, 101
Electric safety, 178
Electrolyte imbalances, 125
Elimination, 308
 and aging, 308
 normal patterns of, 308
Emesis, 171*t*–172*t*
Emollients, 294
Emotional abuse, 23
Emotional disorders, and activity, 329
Emotional signs of, stress, 243
Empathetic listening, 101
Empathy, 101

Endocrine aging, 71
 changes associated with, 71*t*
Endocrine system, 69
 common disorders seen with aging
  in, 72
 expected age-related changes in, 71
End-of-life care
 advance directives for, 263
 caregiver attitudes toward, 263
 collaborative assessment and
  interventions for, 265
 communication, 265
 costs and, 18
 cultural considerations in, 267*b*
 cultural perspectives, 267
 decision-making process, 267
 delegation and supervision of, 275*b*
 ethical dilemmas related to, 263, 264*b*
 pain, 269, 269*f*
 palliative care, 265
 patients' wishes related to, 264*b*
 physiologic changes, assessments,
  and intervention, 269
 psychosocial perspectives,
  assessments, and interventions,
  267
 religious practices regarding, 267*b*
 sedation in, 271
 values clarification related to, 263,
  264*b*
End-of-life planning, attitudes toward,
  262
Enema use in constipation, 309
Energy conservation, 337
Energy expenditure, 325
Energy-intensive activities, 337
Environmental hazards
 fire hazards as, 179
 home security as, 179
 internet safety, 179
 prevention of, 178*b*
 thermal hazards as, 182
 vehicular accidents as, 179
Environmental modification
 for activity intolerance, 337
 for disturbed sensory perception, 195
  at home, 196
 for injury prevention, 177
 for malnutrition, 127–128
 for power, 226
 for self-care deficits, 343
Epidermis, 34
Erectile dysfunction (ED), 279–280
Erikson's stages, 216*b*
Erikson's theory, 31
Error theory, 30
Erythrocytes, 50
Esophagus, 53
Estrogen receptor agonist-antagonists
  (ERAAs), 279*b*
Ethical dilemmas, 263
Ethnic disparity, 7
Eustress, 241

Evidence-based practice, 117*b*, 169*b*,
  221*b*, 357*b*
Exercise(s), 327*b*–328*b*, 333*b*
 and activity, 360
 aerobic, 327
 benefits of, 334*b*, 334
 clothing and footwear for, 333, 335
 for health promotion and
  maintenance, 79
 isometric, 330–333
 isotonic, 330–333
 normal patterns of, 325
 for older adults, 326
 programs, 335*b*
 Qi gong and tai chi as, 328*b*
 range-of-motion, 330
 schedule for, 334*b*, 334–335, 335*f*
 and sleep disorders, 360
 stretching, 327
 trapeze bar for, 333*f*
 warm-up and cool-down, 335
Expressive aphasia, 206
External physical threats, 241
External risk factors, for accidents or
  injuries, 178
External social threats, 241
External standards and self-esteem, 214
Extracellular fluid (ECF), 130
Exudate, 294
Eye contact, 99, 195*f*
Eyeglasses, verifying functionality of,
  195
Eyes, 64
 age-related macular degeneration
  and retinal detachment, 67
 assessment of, 162*t*–164*t*
 common disorders seen with aging, 66
 expected age-related changes, 65

F
Face, assessment of, 162*t*–164*t*
Facial expressions, 99
Faith, 255–256
Fall(s), 171*t*–172*t*, 175
 cultural considerations in, 178*b*
 prevention, 176, 178*b*
 risk, 317*b*
 risk, reduction, 333*b*
 risk, validated tests and tools
  available for screening and
  assessment in, 177*t*
 specific strategies to, 177
 tools to assess for, 177
Family(ies), 20*t*, 22*b*
 abuse or neglect by, 22
 caregiver choices, 4*b*
 as caregivers, 86
 communication with, 105
 cultural considerations and role of, 4*b*
 demographic changes affecting, 19*b*
 of elder with disturbed thought
  processes, 204
 impact of aging members on, 19

Family(ies) (Continued)
    separation from, 217
    teaching, 344b
Family functioning
    nursing process/clinical judgment
        model for altered, 237
        assessment, 237
        data analysis/problem
            identification, 237
        implementation, 237
        planning, 237
Family home, 335
Family support and consideration, 238b
Famotidine, 149t
FANCAPES mnemonic, for condition
    change, 171
Fasting glucose, 117t
Fat(s), 115
Fatigue, 353
    during dying, 271
    and sleep disorders, 360
Fat-soluble vitamins, 116t
Fear(s), 215
    of dying, 268
    nursing process/clinical judgment
        model for, 222
        assessment, 223
        data analysis/problem
            identification, 223
        implementation, 223
        planning, 223
Fecal impaction, 310, 313b
Fecal incontinence, 315
    nursing process/critical thinking
        model for, 315
        assessment, 315
        data analysis/problem
            identification, 315
        implementation, 316
        planning, 315
Fecal softeners, 312t
Feedback, 214
Feet, 80, 290, 293f
    tissue of, 290
Fiber, 309
Fight-or-flight response, 244–245
Finances, and health promotion and
    maintenance, 86
Financial abuse, 23
Fire hazards, 179
First pass effect, 141
Fluid, 51
Fluid balance, 111
Fluid intake, 188, 300
    and constipation, 313
    decreasing, 133
    for diarrhea, 314–315
    maintaining adequate, 130
    monitoring of, 133
    for oxygenation problems, 340
    and sleep disorders, 360–361
    and urinary retention, 316
Fluid intelligence, 192

Fluid restriction, 130
Fluid volume
    risk of deficient, 131
    risk of imbalanced, 133
    risk of overload, 131
Flurazepam, 149t
Foam overlay surfaces, 297t–298t
Folic acid, 117t
Folk medicine, 253b
Food cost, and nutrition, 120
Food intake, 187
Food likes and dislikes, for imbalanced
    nutrition, 127
Food variety, and nutrition, 121
Foot. See Feet
Foot care, 293b, 298–300
Foot problems, 293
    and activity, 328b
Footwear, for exercise, 333, 335
Formal communication, 96
Fractures, and activity, 328
Frailty syndrome, 119
Framing the message, 95
Free radical theory of aging, 30
Frequency, of sound, 165
Friction, 292t–293t
Friction rub, 162t–164t
Friends, loss of, 233f
Fulmer SPICES, for condition change,
    170
Functional foods, 118
Functional urinary incontinence, 318,
    318t
Funeral arrangements, 275
Fungal infections of nails, 291
Furosemide, 149t

G
Gait, 80
Gait belts, 334, 334f
Gas exchange problem. See
    Oxygenation problems
Gastritis, 55
Gastroesophageal reflux disease
    (GERD), 55
Gastrointestinal changes, at end-of-life,
    272
Gastrointestinal medications, 149t
Gastrointestinal signs of stress, 243t
Gastrointestinal system, 52
    assessment of, 162t–164t
Gay, older people, 281
Gel overlay, 297t–298t
Gender disparity, 7
General adaptation syndrome, 241
General inspection, 162–164
Gene theory, 29–30
Genitourinary system. See also
        Reproductive system; Urinary
        systems
    assessment of, 162t–164t
Geographic distribution of older adult
        population, 8

Geriatric, defined, 2
Geriatric Depression Scale (GDS), 367,
        367t
Geriatric massage, 246b
Geriatric nursing, introduction to, 1
Gerontic nursing, defined, 2
Gerontics, defined, 2
Gerontology, defined, 2
Gerontophobia, 4
Geropharmacology, 141
Gestures, in communication, 99
Gingivitis, 301
GI tract irritation, 118
Glaucoma, 67
Global aphasia, 206
Glucose, fasting, 117t
Glucose level, blood, 125
Good death, 263
Gout, and activity, 328
Gouty arthritis, 42
Government-subsidized housing, 336
Grandparenting, 232–233, 233f
    and grandchildren, 233f
Great imitator, 281–282
Grief, 234
Grief reactions, normal, 234b
Grieving
    nursing process/clinical judgment
        model for complicated, 234
        assessment, 234
        data analysis/problem
            identification, 235
        implementation, 235
        planning, 235
    phases of, 234t
Grip assistance, in injury prevention,
        178
Grip bars, in bathtub, 345f
Group-housing plans, 336
Growth hormone and sleep, 354
Gurgles, 162t–164t

H
Hair
    age-related changes in, 286, 287t
    amount, distribution, appearance,
        and consistency of, 290
    assessment of, 162t–164t, 286–287
    risk factors for alterations in, 294
Half-life, 142
Halitosis, 301
Haloperidol, 149t
Handrails, in injury prevention, 185f
Handwashing, 298b
Hard candy for impaired mucous
        membranes, 306
Havighurst's theory, 31
Health assessment, of older adults, 158
Health care agent, 19
Health care cost, 336
Health care dilemma, 18b
Health care directives for nonrelated
        caregivers, 282b

Health care provisions, 16
    advance directives and POLST as, 19
    costs and end-of-life care in, 336
    Medicare and Medicaid, 16
    rising costs and legislative activity
        on, 17
Health care team, communication with,
    101b
Health history, 160
Health promotion, 304
Health promotion and maintenance, 78
    factors affecting, 83
    nursing process for ineffective, 88
    recommended health practices for, 79
Health screening, 158
Hearing aids, 196f, 196
    glasses and, 196b
Hearing changes, and safety problems,
    181
Hearing examinations, 80
Hearing-impaired people, 197
    nursing interventions in home for,
        197
    special devices for, 197
Hearing impairment
    as barrier to communication, 102
    communication with, 195
Hearing loss, 193b
Heart, 46
Heart failure (HF), 48
Heat exhaustion, 183
Heatstroke, 183
Heberden nodes, 41
HECM. See Home Equity Conversion
        Mortgage (HECM)
Helplessness, 215
Hematocrit, 117t, 124
Hematology, 363t–366t
Hematopoietic system, 50
    common disorders seen with aging
        in, 52
    expected age-related changes in, 51
Hemianopsia, 195, 195f
Hemiparesis, 330
Hemiplegia, 330
Hemoglobin, 117t, 124–125
Hemorrhoids, 55
Hepatitis-B immunization, 81
Herpes zoster infection, 81
Heterogeneous society, 231
Hiatal hernia, 54
High-density lipoproteins (HDLs),
    115
Hinduism, death in, 267b
Hobbies, for deficient diversional
    activities, 346
Home Equity Conversion Mortgage
        (HECM), 11–12
Home health, 86
Home health agency, selection of, 87
Homemaker, role of, 232
Home oxygen systems, 340–341, 341b
Home remedies, 84

Home security, 179
    guidelines, 180b
Home services, types of, 87
Homogeneous society, 231
Hope
    nursing process/clinical judgment
        model for decreased, 224
        assessment, 224
        data analysis/problem
            identification, 225
        implementation, 225
        planning, 225
Hopelessness, 215
Hormone therapy, for aging, 30
Hospice care, 264–265, 265f
Hospital insurance, 336
Housing arrangements, 13
Hydralazine, 149t
Hypercalcemia, 117
Hyperkeratosis, 290
Hyperopia, 65–66
Hypertensive disease, 50
Hyperthermia, 182b, 183
    nursing process for, 187
    prevention of, 188
    symptoms of, 183
Hypnotics, for sleep disorders, 357
Hypoglycemia, 73
Hypokalemia, 118
Hypothalamus, 59
Hypothermia, 37, 182b, 182
    nursing process for, 187
    prevention of, 188
    signs of, 182b
Hypothyroidism, 62, 73
Hysterectomy, 280

Ibuprofen, 149t
Ideal, 214
Identification bracelet and medication
        administration, 148–149
Illness, 244
    atypical presentation of, 162t
Imaging for stress reduction, 247–248
Immunity, 51
Immunization, 80–81
Immunologic theory, of aging, 31
Improving communication, 96b
Incentive spirometers, 339
Income, 9
Incontinence, 308
Incontinence garments, 320–322, 322f
Incontinence pads, 320–322, 322f
Independence, loss of, 233, 336,
    340–341
Independent-living centers, 336
Infection(s), 36
    changes in integumentary system
        and, 36
    urinary tract, 316
Inflammation, changes in
    integumentary system and, 36

Influenza, 44
Influenza vaccine, 81
Informal communication, 97
Information sharing, 95
Informing, 104
Inhalation drugs, 152
Injury prevention, in home, 178b
Insomnia, 355
    medication that cause, 356t
    treatment of, 355t, 357
Inspection, 162
Intake and output (I&O)
        measurement, 132
Integumentary changes, at end-of-life,
    273
Integumentary system, 34
    common disorders seen with aging
        in, 36
    expected age-related changes, 34
Intelligence, 191–192, 192b
Intelligence quotients (IQs), 192
Intelligence tests, 192
Intensity, of sound, 165
Intentional abuse, 22
Intentional isolation, 236
Intercourse, 278
Interests for deficient diversional
        activities, 346
Intermittent claudication, 49
Internal risk factors, for accidents or
        injuries, 174
    assessment, 176
Internal threats, 241
Internal values, and self-esteem,
    214
Internet safety, 179
Interpersonal communication, 98
Interpersonal values, 254
Interpreter, 103
Interstitial fluids, 130
Intervertebral disks, 38
Interview, structuring the, 160
Intracellular fluid, 130
Intravascular fluids, 130
Introduction, Situation, Background,
        Assessment, Recommendation,
        and Readback (ISBAR-R)
        communication tool, 107b, 107,
        108b
Intruders, 180
Involuntary muscle, 38–39
Iron-deficiency anemia, 117
Iron (Fe), in diet, 117
Islam, death in, 267b
Isometric exercises, 39, 330–333
Isotonic exercises, 39, 330–333

J
Jaw pain, 302b, 339–340
Joint(s), 38, 79–80
The Joint Commission's Official
        "Do Not Use" List, 150t
Joint mobility, 330

Joint replacement surgery, and activity, 328
Judaism
  death in, 267b
  spirituality in, 256f
Jung's theory, 31–32

K

Kegel exercises, 319, 320b
Keratinized cells, 34
Kidneys, 56
Kinetic therapy, 297t–298t
Knowledge and health promotion and maintenance, 84
Kübler-Ross stages of grief, 275b
Kyphosis, 40

L

Language, 206
  cognition and, 192
Large intestine, 53
Laxatives, 309, 312t
Learning, 192
Legislation and economics of aging, 11–12
Legislative activity, 17
Lesbian, gay, bisexual, and transgendered (LGBT), older people, 281
Leukemia, 52
Leukocytes, 51
Leukoplakia, 302, 302f
Life-contract facilities, 336
Life-course theories, 31
Life expectancy, gender and ethnic disparity in, 7
Life-lease facilities, 336
Life review, and self-esteem, 221
Ligaments, 38
Light therapy, 201b
Limited coping ability, nursing process/clinical judgment model for, 246
Lipofuscin in free radical theory of aging, 30
Lipoproteins, 115
Liquid oxygen systems, 341b
Listening, 101
Liver spots, 34–35
Living will, 19
Loneliness
  nursing process/clinical judgment model for, 236
  and nutrition, 121
Loss(es), 216
Loss of power, nursing care plan, 227b
Lotions, 294, 294b–295b
Low-air loss surfaces, 297t–298t
Low-density lipoproteins (LDLs), 115
Lower respiratory tract, 42
Lung cancer, 45
Lymphatic system, 50
  common disorders seen with aging in, 52
  expected age-related changes in, 51

Lymphocytes, 51
Lymph system, 51
Lymph vessels, 51

M

Macronutrients, 368t
Magnesium hydroxide, 149t
Malabsorption, and nutrition, 120
Malnourishment, and activity, 329b
Malnutrition
  nursing process for risk for altered, 122
  and older adult, 119
  risk factors for
    economic, 120–121
    physiologic, 120
    social, 121
Mandated reporters, 345
Mantra, 247–248
Marital status, 8
Marriage and older adults, 281
Massage for stress reduction, 246b
Mastectomy, 280
Masturbation, 283
Mattresses to reduce pressure, 296
Mattress surface types, 297t–298t
Meals-on-Wheels, 121, 121f
Median income, 333
Medicaid
  and personal assets, 17b
  supplemental, 17
Medic Alert bracelet, 82
MedicAlert "panic button", 186
Medical insurance, 16
Medicare, advantage plans, 335
Medication(s), 140, 175, 184–185, 189
  absorption of, 141
  assessment and ethnicity, 148b
  Beers criteria for inappropriate use of, 144–145
  and constipation, 309
  correct, 150
  cost of, 140
  crushed, 151–152
  and diarrhea, 315
  distribution of, 141
  excretion of, 142
  half-life of, 142
  and imbalanced nutrition, 122
  independent older adults and, 154b
  list of, 82
  metabolism of, 142
  not to be chewed/crushed, 151b
  nursing assessment and, 147
  and nursing care plan, 148
  and nutrition, 120
  over-the-counter (OTC), 82, 140
  patient rights and, 153
  pharmacodynamics of, 142
  pharmacokinetics of, 141
  polypharmacy with, 147b
  to promote sleep, 360

Medication(s) (Continued)
  prophylactic, 81–82
  right documentation, 153
  right dosage form, 151
  right medication, 150
  right route, 151
  right time, 152
  safety, 311b, 313b
  safety and nonadherence issues, 155
  and sexual dysfunction, 280, 280t
  side effects, 143b
  teaching older adults, 154
  teaching sheets information, 155b
  transdermal, 152
  and urinary retention, 316
  when a patient refuses, 151b
Medication administration
  guiding rule for, 151b
  in the home, 153
  inhalation, 152
  in institutional setting, 147, 153
  nursing interventions related to, 148
  parenteral, 152
  patient rights, 153
Medication carts, locking of, 184–185
Medication error, 171t–172t
Medication risks
  factors that increase, 141b
  related to cognitive or sensory changes, 145
  related to drug-testing methods, 141
  related to financial factors, 147
  related to inadequate knowledge, 146
  related to physiologic changes of aging, 141
"Medigap", 17
Meditation, 247–248, 256b
  for stress reduction, 246b
Medulla, 58
Melanin, 34
Melanoma, 36
Melatonin, and sleep, 354
Memory, 191–192
Memory loss, 193
Men, age-related changes in, 279
Ménière disease, 69
Menopausal hormone therapy (MHT), 279
Methyldopa, 149t
MHT. See Menopausal hormone therapy (MHT)
Midbrain, 58
Middle ear, 68
Midlife crisis, 31–32
Mineral(s), 117
Minerals, 368t
Mini-Cog © instrument, 168b, 168
Minimum data set (MDS), 169
Mixed urinary incontinence, 318
Mobility, 85, 292t–293t

Mobility, altered
  nursing care plan, 336b
  nursing process/clinical judgment
    model for, 329
    assessment, 329
    data analysis/problem
      identification, 329
    implementation, 330
    planning, 329
  risk factors related to, 330b
Moisture, 292t–293t
Molecular theories, of aging, 30
Morgue, 274
Mortgages, reverse, 334
Mosque, 258, 258f
Motivation, 84
  lack of, 121
Motor vehicle accidents, 174
Mouth, suprainfections, 303b
Mucous membranes, care of aging,
  286
Muscle mass
  decrease of, 71
  loss of, 326
Muscles, 38
Muscle sense, 39
Muscle tone, decrease of, 40
Musculoskeletal signs of stress, 243t
Musculoskeletal system, 37
  assessment of, 162t–164t
  common disorders seen with aging
    in, 40, 175
Music therapy, 186b, 202b, 346b
MyPlate, 112f, 112–113

N
Nails, 290
  age-related changes in, 286, 287t
  assessment of, 162t–164t, 286–287
  care, 290
  fungal infections of, 291
  risk factors for alterations in, 294
Napping, and sleep disorders, 360
Naproxen, 149t
Nasal cannula, for oxygenation
  problems, 339, 339f
National Motorists Association, 181
Nausea, in dying person, 272
Neck, assessment of, 162t–164t
Negative attitudes, 348h, 348
Negative feedback, 214
Neglect, 22–23
  by family, 22
Nervous system, 58
  common disorders seen with aging
    in, 175
Neuroendocrine theory, 30
Neurologic condition and oral hygiene,
  303
Neurologic damage, and activity, 328
Neurologic system, assessment of,
  162t–164t
Newman's theory, 31

Niebuhr, Reinhold, 6
Night blindness, 191–192
Nighttime disruptions, 359b
Nocturia, 360–361
Nocturnal movement disorders, 355
Nodes, 51
Noise, 359
Nonadherence, nursing process for, 90
Non-English speakers, 103
Non-24-hour sleep-wake disorder, 358
Nonmelanoma, 36
Nonpowered support surface, 297t–298t
Non-rapid eye movement (NREM)
  sleep, 354
Nonrestricting sleepwear, 360f
Nonsteroidal antiinflammatory drugs
  (NSAIDs), 140, 149t
Nonverbal communication, 97, 97f
Normal activity patterns, 325
Normal elimination patterns, 308
Normal stress, 241
Normal vision, 193f
Norton risk assessment scale, 293t
Nurse
  and family interactions, 21
  teamwork and collaboration, quality
    and safety education for, 25b
Nursing care plan
  for altered communication ability,
    208b
  for altered sexual function, 283b
  for constipation, 314b
  for disrupted sleep pattern, 361b
  for impaired physical mobility, 331f
  mobility, altered, 336b
  for power loss, 227b
  for social isolation, 238b–239b
  for spiritual disconnection, 258b
Nursing home(s), insurance, 16b
Nursing Home Reform Law, 153
Nursing, implications for, 32
Nursing interventions, for health
  promotion and maintenance, 89
Nursing process/clinical judgment
  model for potential for injury,
    183
  assessment (data collection), 183
  data analysis/problem identification,
    184
  implementation, 184
  planning, 184
Nutrients
  carbohydrates as, 113
  fats as, 115
  minerals as, 117
  proteins as, 113
  vitamins as, 115
  water as, 119
Nutrition, 292t–293t, 340b
  and aging, 111
  assessment of, 121, 125
  caloric intake in, 111, 117
  coordinated care for, 121b

Nutrition (Continued)
  cultural considerations, 126b
  culture and food preferences, 127
  data analysis/problem identification,
    136
  factors affecting, 119
  implementation, 136
  nursing process for risk for altered,
    122
  in older adults, laboratory values
    used to nutritional adequacy,
    117t
  planning, 136
  social and cultural aspects of, 122,
    126
Nutritional intake, 125
  assessment of, 125
  home care/discharge planning, and
    nutrition, 126
  nursing interventions to decrease, 129
  nursing interventions to increase,
    127–129
  for oxygenation problems, 340
Nutritional supplements, for sleep
  disorders, 360
Nutritious foods, 300
Nystagmus, 69

O
Objective data, 159
Obstructive sleep apnea, 357
Occlusive peripheral vascular
  problems, 49
Occupational therapist, for dysphagia,
  134
Oils, 294
Old, defined, 2
Older adults, 250b
  active involvement of, 349b
  aspiration risk in, 136b
  attitudes toward housing for, 14b
  caregivers and sexuality of, 281
  in care planning, 249b, 249
  communication of, 342b
  computer safety for, 180b
  cruise care, 15b
  daily nutritional goals for, 368, 368t
  economic conditions of, 12b
  factors affecting drug response in,
    141t
  health assessment of
    condition change in, 169
    Internet sites for, 170b
    interviewing, 159
    minimum data set 3.0 as special
      assessments in, 169
    physical assessment, 161
    psychosocial assessment in, 168
    sensory assessment in, 168
    special assessments in, 169
    vital signs in, 165
  herbal and supplement
    considerations for, 144t

Older adults *(Continued)*
information and services, 87*b*
inadequate health maintenance, 89*b*
injury risks for, 175*b*
laboratory values for, 363, 363*t*–366*t*
marriage and, 281
plan of care for, 337*b*
potentially inappropriate medication use in, 144
privacy and personal rights of, 282
resources for, 369
aging associations and societies, 369
educational resources, 370
gerontology centers/education centers/ institutes, 369
information on exercise, 370
journals/periodicals, 370
organizations, 369
statistics and government sites, 370
rest and sleep, 360
safe driving practices for, 181*b*
screening tests for, 81*t*
self-medication and, 153
sensitivity to financial problems, 12*b*
sexual orientation of, 281
signs of experiencing abuse, 24*b*
thermoregulation risks for, 182*b*
Old person
role of, 233–234
timely assistance for, 310*b*
Oliguria, in dying person, 273
Omnibus Budget Reconciliation Act (OBRA) regulations, 185
Online psychologic assessment tools, 169*b*
Open-ended communication techniques, 104
Oral cancer, 302
risk factors for, 303*b*
symptoms of, 302*b*
Oral care, preventive, 80
Oral cavity, 52
Oral hygiene, 304
for dysphagia, 136
for fluid restriction, 132
neurologic problems and, 303
on unconscious patient, 304
Oral hygiene care plan (OHCP), 301
Oral mucous membranes
age-related changes in, 300
nursing process/clinical judgment model for altered, 303
assessment, 303
data analysis/problem identification, 303
implementation, 304
planning, 303
risk factors for problems with, 303*b*
Oral pain, 301
Oral temperature, 166
Orthopnea, 358–359
Orthostatic hypotension, 47, 167–168

Osmotic agents, 312*t*
Osteoarthritis, 41
Osteoporosis, 40
Otosclerosis, 68, 191–192
Ovaries, 70
Overflow, retention with, 316
Overflow urinary incontinence, 318
Overprotective and powerlessness, 226
Over-the-counter (OTC) medications, 82
Oxygenation problems
nursing process/clinical judgment model for, 337
assessment, 337
data analysis/problem identification, 338
implementation, 338
planning, 338
Oxygen concentrator, 340–341
Oxygen cylinder, portable, 340*f*, 341*b*
Oxygen equipment
safely precautions of, 340–341
use of, 340–341
Oxygen, supplemental, 339

P
Pace, of communication, 99
Pacific Islanders, roles and relationships of, 230*b*
Pacing with dementia, 201–202
PAD. *See* Physician assisted death (PAD) (physician assisted suicide)
Pads to reduce pressure, 296
Pain, 171*t*–172*t*, 209*b*, 269, 301
assessment of, 210, 210*t*
nursing process/clinical judgment model for, 207, 209*f*
assessment, 209
data analysis/problem identification, 210
implementation, 210
planning, 210
and nutrition, 120
with oxygenation problems, 339–340
Pain assessment in advanced dementia (PAINAD) scale, 211*t*
Pain log, 269
Pain management, end-of-life care, 270
Pain medication, 270
and exercise, 333
with oxygenation problems, 333
Pain relief, 340*b*
Palliative care, 265
Palpation, 162, 165
Pancreas, 70
Paralysis agitans, 60
Parasitic diarrhea, 315
Parathyroid glands, 70
Parenteral medications, 152
Parent, role of, 232
Parkinson disease, 60
Partner gap, 280–281
Passive range-of-motion exercises, 330

Pastoral care, 268*b*
Patient-centered care, 159*b*, 312*b*, 337
Patient education, 304–305, 335*b*
Patient Protection and Affordable Care Act (PPACA), 17
Patient rights and medication, 148
Patient teaching, 108
Penicillins, 149*t*
Pensions, 341
Perception(s), 191, 197*b*
of aging, 85, 216, 217*b*
cognition and, 197*b*
defined, 191
nursing process/clinical judgment model for altered, 194
risk factors related to, 194*b*
Perceptual functioning, normal, 191
Percussion, 162, 165
Periodontal disease, 301
Peripheral nervous system, 59
Peripheral pulse, 167
with oxygenation problems, 339
Peripheral vascular disease, 49
Peristalsis and constipation, 309
Pernicious anemia, 118
Personal rights, of older adults, 282
Personal space, in communication, 98
Personal value system, 252
Pet therapy, 347, 347*f*
Pharmacodynamics, 142
Pharmacokinetics, 141
Phase advance, 354
Phosphorus, in diet, 117
Phototherapy, 201*b*
Physical abuse, 22
Physical activity, 311
and aging, 309, 326–327
for constipation, 309
with dementia, 201–202
effects of disease processes on, 329
normal patterns of, 325
Physical assessment, body systems approach to, 162*t*–164*t*
Physical examinations, 80
Physical fitness, 327*b*
Physical mobility and health promotion and maintenance, 86
Physical restraints, 202
Physical setting, preparing the, 159
Physical signs of stress, 243, 243*t*
Physical therapy, 330*b*, 331*f*
Physician assisted death (PAD) (physician assisted suicide), 271*b*
Physician-assisted suicide, 271*b*
Physician orders for life-sustaining treatment (POLST), 18–19, 19*b*
Physiologic changes, 33
medication risks related to, 141
and safety problems, 174–175
Physiologic risk factors, for malnutrition, 120
Phytoestrogens, 279*b*
Pigmentation, 288

Pinna, 67–68
Pitch, of sound, 165
Pituitary gland, 70
Plasma, 130
Platelets, 51
Pneumonia, 44
Pneumonia vaccine, 93
Political activism, and economics of aging, 12b
Polypharmacy, 142
Pons, 58
Position changes, 295
Position, in nonverbal communication, 98
Positive attitudes, 349b, 349
Positive feedback, 214
Possessions, loss of, 233f
Postmenopausal discomfort, 279b
Postmortem care, 274
Potassium, in diet, 118
Poverty, 9
Powerlessness, 215
Power, loss of
 nursing process/clinical judgment model for, 225
  assessment, 226
  data analysis/problem identification, 226
  implementation, 226
  planning, 226
PQRST method, for pain assessment, 210, 210t
Prayer, 256b
 for stress reduction, 246b
Presbycusis, 68, 191–192
Presbyopia, 65–66, 191–192
Prescription drug coverage, 335
Prescription medications, 84
Pressure injuries, 304, 36, 171t–172t, 286, 289
 bony prominences underlying, 290f
 cultural considerations with, 287
 prevention of, 289t
 stages of, 291f, 299t
Pressure points, 295f, 295–296
Preventive overall care, 80
Primary caregivers, 86
Primary hypothyroidism, 73
Privacy, 312
 of older adults, 282
Proactive method, 245
Progeria, 33–34
Programmed theory, 29–30
Progressive relaxation, 247–248
Prophylactic medications, 81–82
 prescription and over-the-counter, 82
Propranolol, precautions related to aging, 149t
Proprioceptors, 39
Prostate cancer, 75
Prostheses, verifying functionality of, 195, 196f

Protective devices, 185, 186b
 use of, 185b–186b
Protein(s), 113
Proxemics, in communication, 98
Pruritus, 35–36, 286
Pruritus vulvae, 279
Psychological threats, 241
Psychosocial assessment, 168
Psychosocial theories, of aging, 29, 31
Psychotherapeutic medications, for disturbed thought processes, 202
Psychotropics, 149t
Public places, accessibility of, 350b
Public space, in communication, 98
Pulse, 166
 with oxygenation problems, 338
Pulse deficit, 166

Q

Qi gong, 328b
Quad cane, 333f
Quality, of sound, 165
Questioning, direct, 104

R

Radial pulse, 166
Ram's horn nails, 291
Ranitidine, 149t
Rapid eye movement (REM) sleep, 354
 sleep-behavior disorder, 358
Rapport, 95
 establishing, 159
Rashes, 288
Rate of living theory, 29–30
"Reachers", 343f
Reactive, 245
Receptive aphasia, 206
Rectal prolapse, 56
Rectal temperature, 165
Reducing fall risk, 176b
Reflection, by nursing professor, 20
Reflection for stress reduction, 246b
Reflex urinary incontinence, 318
Refraction, 65
Refusal of care, 227
Rehabilitation, 348
 after joint replacement surgery, 328
Rehabilitative focus, 342, 349b, 349
 planning care with, 350b
Relationship(s), 230
 and aging, 231
 of Asian and Pacific Islanders, 230b
 cultural considerations with, 230b
 defined, 230–231
 normal, 230
 risk factors related to changes in, 235b
 and self-image, 231
 standards for, 231
Relaxation exercises, 361
Relaxation techniques, for stress reduction, 245–246
Reliability theory, 30
Religious aspects of nutrition, 122

Religious beliefs, 268b
 for health promotion and maintenance, 84
Religious practices regarding end of life, 267b
Religious rituals, 255–256, 256f
Religious values, 255, 255f
Relocation, 248–249, 249f
Remarriage, 281
Reminiscence, and self-esteem, 221
Reproductive and genitourinary systems
 changes in men, 74
 common disorders seen with aging in, 74, 74t
 expected age-related changes in, 74
  changes in women, 74
 female reproductive organs, 73
 male reproductive organs, 73
Resident Assessment Instrument (RAI), 169
Resistance exercise, 328b
Respect in communication, 101
Respiration, 167, 338
Respiratory changes, at end-of-life, 271
Respiratory effort, with oxygenation problems, 339
Respiratory function, 339
Respiratory signs of stress, 243t
Respiratory system, 42
 assessment of, 162t–164t
 common disorders seen with aging in, 43
 expected age-related changes in, 43
Respite care, 345
Rest, 353
 clinical situation, 359b
 and incontinence, 359b
 normal, 353
 risk factors related to, 357b
Restless leg syndrome, 355
Restraints, 185
 for disturbed thought processes, 202
Restraints limit physical mobility, 330
Restricted visual field, 193f
Retention with overflow, 316
Reverse mortgages, 334
Rheumatoid arthritis, 41
Rheumatologist, 41
Right to refuse care, 227
Rising cost, 17
Rituals, 255–256, 256f
Rods, 65
Role(s), 230
 and aging, 231
 of Asian and Pacific Islanders, 230b
 cultural considerations with, 230b
 defined, 230
 of grandparents, 232–233, 233f
 of homemaker, 232
 normal, 230
 of old person, 233–234
 of parent, 232

Role(s) (Continued)
  risk factors related to changes in, 235b
  and self-image, 231
  of spouse, 233
  standards for, 231
Role conflict, internal, 231
Rome IV criteria, for constipation, 309b
Rosacea, 36–37
Rug(s), as hazards, 176
Run-out-of-program theory, 29–30

S

Safety problems
  external risk factors for, 178
  falls as, 175
  internal risk factors for, 174
  nursing process for, 183
Salivary glands, 53
Sample pain management log, 269f
Sandwich generation, 20
Scabies, 288f, 288
Sclera, 64–65
Screening tool of older person's
      prescriptions (STOPP), 145t
  criteria, 144–145
Screening tool to alert doctors to right
      treatment (START), 146t
  criteria, 144–145
Sebaceous glands, 66
Seborrheic dermatitis, 37
Seborrheic keratosis, 34–35, 35f
Secondary caregivers, 86
Secretions, clearing of, 339
Sedation, 270
Sedatives, 340, 357–358, 360
Seizures, 171t–172t
Self-care abilities
  nursing process/clinical judgment
      model for altered, 341, 342b
    assessment, 341
    data analysis/problem
        identification, 342
    implementation, 342
    planning, 342
Self-care activities, and self-esteem, 221,
      221f
Self-concept, 214
  and aging, 216, 217b
  normal, 214
  nursing process/clinical judgment
      model for altered, 218
  risk factors related to, 219b
Self-destructive behaviors, 225
Self-esteem, 214, 216f, 216
  actions to promote, 215b
  behaviors related to, 215
  communication and, 222
  external standards and, 214
  feedback and, 214
  internal values and, 214
  nursing process/clinical judgment
      model for potential for
      decreased, 220

Self-esteem (Continued)
  of older adults, 222f
  reminiscence and, 221
  self-care activities and, 221
Self health management. See also Health
      promotion and maintenance
  nursing process for inadequate, 88
Self-hypnosis, 361
  for stress reduction, 247–248
Self-identity, 214
Self-medication, 153
Self-neglect, 22
Self-perception, 214
  and aging, 216, 217b
  behaviors related to, 215
  normal, 214
  nursing process/clinical judgment
      model for altered, 218
  risk factors related to, 219b
Selye, Hans, 241
Senile lentigo, 34–35
Senile purpura, 36
Sensory changes, 188
  at end-of-life, 273
  and health promotion and
      maintenance, 85
  and nutrition, 120
  and safety problems, 188
Sensory compensation hypothesis, 192b
Sensory nerve receptors, 34
Sensory perception, 292t–293t
  nursing process/clinical judgment
      model for altered, 194
    assessment, 194
    data analysis/problem
        identification, 194
    implementation, 194
    planning, 194
Separation, from family, 217
Serenity prayer, 5–6
Sex partner, loss of, 280, 280f
Sexual dignity of confused older adults,
      283
Sexual function, altered, 278–279
  medications and, 279, 280t
  nursing care plan for, 283b–284b
  nursing process/clinical judgment
      model for altered, 282
    assessment/data collection, 282
    data analysis/problem
        identification, 283
    implementation, 283
    planning, 283
  risk factors related to, 283b
  significant impact, 278–279
Sexual health
  alcohol on, 280
  impact of illness, 280
  medications on, 280
Sexual intercourse, 278
Sexuality, 278, 279f
  caregivers and, 281
  erectile dysfunction in men, 279–280

Sexuality (Continued)
  factors that affect, 278
  loss of sex partner, 280
  marriage and, 281
  men, age-related changes in, 279
  privacy and personal rights and, 282,
      282f
  women, age-related changes in, 279
Sexually inappropriate behaviors of
      confused older adults, 283
Sexually transmitted infection (STI),
      281
Sexual orientation of older adults, 281
Shear, 292t–293t
Shearing forces, 288–289
Shingles vaccine, 81
Shoe remover, 343f
Shortness of breath (SOB), 171t–172t
Significant others, communication with,
      105
Signs indicating need for prompt
      medical attention, 82b
Silence, 100
Silver Alert programs, 204b
Simple carbohydrates, 113
Skeletal muscle, 39
Skilled care, 15
Skin
  age-related changes in, 286, 287t
  assessment of, 162t–164t, 286–287
  body diagram, 287f
  care of aging, 286
  risk factors for alterations in, 294
Skin color, 287
Skin integrity
  nursing process/clinical judgment
      model for altered, 293, 295f
    assessment, 293–294
    data analysis/problem
        identification, 294
    implementation, 294
    planning, 294
Skin irritation, 288
Skin pigmentation, 288
Skin rash, 171t–172t
Skin tags, 34–35
Skull, assessment of, 162t–164t
Sleep, 353
  and aging, 354
  bedtimes and wake-up times plan,
      359
  clinical situation, 359b
  comfort measures to promote, 360,
      360f
  hygiene practices, 356b
  and incontinence, 359b
  maintain rituals, 359
  medications used to promote, 360
  modify lighting through the day,
      359–360
  neurologic control of, 354
  normal, 353
  NREM and REM, 354

Sleep (Continued)
    nursing and medical interventions, 359
    nursing process/clinical judgment model for disrupted, 358
    and rest patterns, 360
    risk factors related to, 357b
    supervisory issues related to, 359b
Sleep apnea, 355, 357b, 357
Sleep cycle, 354b, 354f, 354
Sleep disordered breathing, 357
Sleep disorders, 355
    behaviors that contribute to, 355
    circadian rhythm in, 358
    drugs that contribute to, 360
    insomnia as, 355
    napping and, 360
    nursing care plan for, 361b
    nursing process/clinical judgment model for disrupted, 358
    REM sleep-behavior disorder as, 358
    sleep apnea as, 357
Sleep disruption, 358–359
Sleepiness, during dying, 271
Sleeping difficulties, 171t–172t
Sleep maintenance problems, 355
Sleep-rest health pattern, 353
Sleep-wake patterns, 353–354
Small intestine, 53
SMART acronym for medication assessment, 148b
Smell, 69, 174
    expected age-related changes, 69
Smoking, 79
Smooth muscle, 38–39
Snapping, 165
Soaps, 294
Social aspects, of nutrition, 122
Social communication, 97
Social interaction, 236
Social isolation, 121
    nursing care plan, 238b–239b
    nursing process/clinical judgment model for, 236, 236f
    assessment, 236
    data analysis/problem identification, 236
    implementation, 236
    planning, 236
Social risk factors, for malnutrition, 121
Social Security income, 9–10
Social Security program, 2–3
Social space, in communication, 98
Sock assist, 343f
Sodium, in diet, 118
Somatic mutation theory, 30
Space, in nonverbal communication, 98
Spasmolytics, 149t
Special assessments, 169
Special senses, 64
Specialty care facilities, 16
Specific inspection, 162–164
Speech, 206

Speech therapist, 136
    Swallowing ability, altered, 133
Speed, of communication, 99
Sphincter, 308
Spinal cord, 38
Spiritual assessment
    for nurses, 256b
    tools, 256b
Spiritual beliefs, 255, 268b
Spiritual connections, 255
Spiritual counselor, 258
Spiritual disconnection
    nursing care plan, 258b
    nursing process/clinical judgment model for, 256
    assessment, 256
    data analysis/problem identification, 257
    implementation, 257
    planning, 257
Spirituality, 253b
Spiritual objects, 257–258
Spiritual values, 255, 255f
Spirometers, 339
Spouse, role of, 233
Staffing, 349–350
Standards for roles and relationships, 231
STEADI initiative. See Stopping Elderly Accidents, Deaths, and Injuries (STEADI) initiative
Stimulant laxatives, 312, 312t
Stimuli, 191
Stokes/Gordon stress scale, 242t
Stomach, 53
Stopping Elderly Accidents, Deaths, and Injuries (STEADI) initiative, 176
Strength mobility, 330
Stress, 241
    behavioral signs of, 243
    cognitive signs of, 243
    coping or defense mechanisms, 245b
    emotional signs of, 243
    and illness, 244
    and life events, 245
    normal, 241
    physical signs of, 243, 243t
    physiologic response to, 241
    reduction, 246b
Stressors, 241
Stress-reduction strategies, 245
    for activity intolerance, 337
    geriatric massage as, 246b
    progressive relaxation, 247–248
Stress reduction techniques, 247–248, 340
Stress tolerance, risk factors related to problems with, 247b
Stress urinary incontinence, 317
Stretching exercises, 327
Stroke, 63
    and activity, 328

Subacute care facilities, 15–16
Subcutaneous tissue, 34
Subjective data, 159
Sublingual temperature, 165
Suicidal ideation, 171t–172t
Suicide, 218, 225b
    and older adults, 225b
Sulfonamides, 149t
Sundowning, 63, 199
Sundown syndrome, 199
Sun exposure, 300
Supervision, 312b
Supplemental Medicaid, 17
Supplemental oxygen, for oxygenation problems, 339, 339f
Supplemental tube feedings, 128–129
Supplement(s), to slow or reverse aging, 31
Support groups, 345
Suprainfections, 303b
Swallowing ability, altered
    nursing process for, 133
Symbols, in communication, 97
Symptoms indicating need for prompt medical attention, 82, 82b

T
Tachycardia, 337
Tai chi, 328b
Tasimelteon, 358
Taste, 69
    expected age-related changes, 69
Technology to enhance communication, 223b
Teeth, health promotion and maintenance for, 82
Temperature, 165
Tendons, 38
Terminal insomnia problems, 355
Testes, 70
Tetanus, diphtheria, pertussis vaccines, 81
Tetracyclines, 149t
Theophylline, 149t
Therapeutic communication, 96
Thermal hazards, 182
    nursing process for, 187
    risk factors for, 188
Thermoregulation, 182
Thioridazine, 149t
Thought processes, nursing process for disturbed, 204
Thrush, 303b
Thyroid gland, 70
Thyroid testing, 363t–366t
Time of communication, 99
Timing of communication, 99
Tinnitus, 68, 191–192
Tissue healing, measures to promote, 296
Tissue integrity, 288
Tissue regeneration, 296
Title, 336

Tobacco, for health promotion and maintenance, 79
Tobacco-related problems, 303
Toileting schedule
    for constipation, 316b, 316
    for fecal incontinence, 316
    for urinary elimination, 320
Tolmetin, 149t
Tone of voice, in communication, 97
Tongue, 52
Tooth decay, 301f, 301
Touch in communication, 100
Trace elements, 118
Transdermal medication, 152
    precautions when using transdermal patches, 152b
Transgender, older people, 281
Transience, 193b
Transient ischemic attacks (TIA), 63
Transportation
    for deficient diversional activities, 347
    and nutrition, 120–121
Trapeze bar, 330–333, 333f
Trends and issues, 1
    clinical situation on, 24b
Triazolam, 149t
Trust, actions that promote, 235b
Tube feeding(s), supplemental, 128–129
Tuberculosis (TB), 45
Tympanic membrane temperature, 165–166
Type 1 Diabetes Mellitus, 72
Type 2 Diabetes Mellitus, 72

U

Ulcers, 55
    medical treatment of, 55b
Uniforms, in communication, 97
Unintentional abuse, 22
Upper respiratory tract, 42
Ureters, 56
Urge urinary incontinence, 317
Urinary changes, at end-of-life, 273
Urinary function, altered, 321t
    nursing intervention for, 319
    nursing process/critical thinking model for, 319
    risk factors related to, 319b
Urinary incontinence (UI), 57, 316
    functional, 318
    mixed, 318
    overflow, 318

Urinary incontinence (UI) (Continued)
    prevention of, 317b
    reflex, 318
    risk factors associated with, 317b
    stress, 317
    urge, 317
Urinary retention, 316
Urinary signs of stress, 243t
Urinary system
    bladder, 56
    common disorders seen with aging in, 57
    expected age-related changes, 57
    kidneys, 56
    ureters, 56
Urinary tract infections (UTIs), 57, 316
Urine, characteristics of, 56
Uterine prolapse, 74

V

Vaginal infection, 75
Values, 252b–253b
    and beliefs, 252–253
    cultural, 254
    cultural understanding, 253b
    economic, 254
    interpersonal, 254
    of older adults, 254
    spiritual or religious, 255, 255f
Values clarification related to death and end-of-life care, 263, 264b
Varicose veins, 49
Vehicular accidents, 179
Vertebrae, 38
Vertebral canal, 38
Very-low-density lipoproteins (VLDLs), 115
Vision examination, 80
Visitors, communication with, 105
Visual analog scale, 209f
Visual changes, 171t–172t, 191–192
    and safety problems, 174, 184–185
Visually impaired people, 197
    nursing interventions in home for, 197
Visual pain, scales, 207, 209f
Vital signs, 165, 171t–172t
    for activity intolerance, 337
    blood pressure as, 167
    for oxygenation problems, 337
    pulse as, 166
    respiration as, 167
    temperature as, 165

Vital statistics, 329
Vitamin(s), 115, 368t
Vitamin deficiencies, 115–116, 302b
Voice, tone of, in communication, 97
Voluntary activity, 326
Voluntary muscles, 39
Volunteers, for deficient diversional activities, 346
Vomiting, in dying person, 272

W

Walker, 333–334, 333f
Wandering with dementia, 199
Warm-up exercise, 335
Water, as nutrient, 119
Water fluoridation, 301
Water overlay, 297t–298t
Water-soluble vitamins, 115, 116t
Wealth, 13
Wear-and-tear theory, 30
Weight-bearing restrictions, 330b
Weight changes, 126
Weight checks, for imbalanced nutrition, 126
Wernicke aphasia, 206, 206t
Wernicke area, 206
Western cultures, death in, 261
Wheelchair-bound patients, activity for, 334
Wheezes, 162t–164t
Whistling, 165
White blood cells (WBCs), 34
Wisdom, 192
Wold, Gloria, 338
Women, age-related changes in, 279
Wong FACES Pain Rating Scale, 209f
Wound cleansing, aseptic technique, 296
Wrinkles, 35

X

Xerosis, 35–36
Xerostomia
    with aging, 302
    in dying person, 272

Y

Yeast infection, 303b

Z

Zinc, in diet, 118
Z-track method, 118